GENETICS OF HUMAN CANCER

Progress in Cancer Research and Therapy

Volume 3

Genetics of Human Cancer

Edited by

John J. Mulvihill, M.D.
Robert W. Miller, M.D.
Joseph F. Fraumeni, Jr., M.D.

National Cancer Institute
National Institutes of Health
Bethesda, Maryland

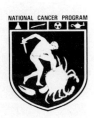

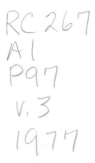

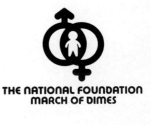

THE NATIONAL FOUNDATION
MARCH OF DIMES

Raven Press ■ New York

Raven Press, 1140 Avenue of the Americas, New York, New York 10036

Raven Press, New York 1977

Made in the United States of America

International Standard Book Number 0-89004-110-5
Library of Congress Catalog Card Number 75-44924

Foreword

The study of cancer genetics has come of age. At a time when major programs are underway to determine the environmental causes of cancer, it is important to review the genetic factors that interact with the environment to produce cancer.

Genetics is the study of inherent variability among living things. In human cancer, the science of genetics concerns differences in susceptibility and resistance to cancer, the reasons for this heterogeneity among humans, and the application of this knowledge toward cancer control.

Although an increasing number of known and potential environmental carcinogens have been identified, scientists still are unable to explain many of the differences in cancer occurrence among people: why some heavy smokers apparently are resistant to the development of lung cancer; why cancer occurs more often in some families than in others; or why some vinyl chloride workers develop angiosarcomas, but others do not.

As scientific and public interest begins to shift from a strictly environmental focus on the causes of cancer to the interactions between the individual and his surroundings, it is appropriate that the National Cancer Institute and the National Foundation–March of Dimes highlight the wide scope of information on genetics resulting from the varied interests and special perspectives of prominent experts in medical genetics, molecular biology, cellular genetics, and epidemiology.

In two cancer-related diseases, xeroderma pigmentosum and ataxia telangiectasia, specific defects in DNA repair were identified by applying laboratory tools developed in microbial systems to the study of rare patients in whom clinicians had noted an unusual sensitivity to environmental agents. The advent of new technology from molecular biology and biochemistry, combined with additional clinical and epidemiologic study of persons at high risk of cancer, may help scientists extend their knowledge of other genetic–environmental interactions and clarify fundamental mechanisms of carcinogenesis.

Frank J. Rauscher, Jr., Ph.D.
Director
National Cancer Institute
National Cancer Program

Preface

The major purpose of this volume is to summarize and evaluate the recent dramatic advances that have occurred in basic and medical genetics as they relate to oncology. The developments described in this volume should stimulate greater cooperation between geneticists and oncologists. Indeed, the recent establishment of 17 research centers for cancer and 10 for genetics in the United States provides vast resources for expanding collaboration.

The recent development of banding techniques and the visualization of sister chromatid exchanges (i.e., the interchange of identical genetic material between duplicated sections of chromosomes) opened an epoch in cytogenetics. These procedures show great potential in revealing the pathobiology of cancer development in man.

Mendelian genetics has contributed new insights into the fundamental mechanisms of carcinogenesis through investigations of patients with rare single gene traits predisposing to neoplasia. Typical are studies of cancer associated with various birth defects and immunologic deficiencies; chromosomal fragility, as in the Fanconi and Bloom syndromes; a possible excess of cancer among heterozygous carriers of genes which, in the homozygous state, predispose to malignancy; defects of DNA repair in xeroderma pigmentosum and ataxia telangiectasia; and the common embryologic origins of seemingly diverse disorders, such as neurofibromatosis, neuroblastoma, multiple endocrine adenomatosis, and perhaps small cell carcinoma of the lung. Also, the products of some genes associated with malignancies, such as *ABO, HLA,* and aryl hydrocarbon hydroxylase inducibility, may help identify persons at high risk of cancer for prevention, screening, early detection, and further research.

With regard to polygenic or multifactorial inheritance in human cancer (i.e., the interaction of many genes and environmental agents with no single factor playing a dominant role), empiric risk data have detected relatives markedly predisposed to cancer, and an interdisciplinary approach to ''cancer families'' has revealed subclinical laboratory manifestations of susceptibility.

Population genetics and epidemiology have provided etiologic clues from studies of special populations, such as inbred groups and twins, and of international and ethnic variations in cancer.

Laboratory geneticists have turned their tools to the cancer problem by hybridizing cells among species, hybridizing nucleic acid from viruses and human tumors and observing cells *in vitro* from persons prone to cancer.

These observations on patients, populations, cells, and DNA have been melded into theories and hypotheses of carcinogenesis to be tested by further investigations;

examples include the proposed mechanisms of double mutation or premutation to account for dissimilarities in familial and nonfamilial forms of cancer.

These proceedings are based on a conference cosponsored by the Epidemiology Branch of the National Cancer Institute and the National Foundation–March of Dimes.

The attendance of official delegations from collaborative efforts of the U.S.–Japan Cooperative Cancer Research Program (Analytical Epidemiology Committee) and the U.S.–U.S.S.R. Joint Working Group on Mammalian Somatic Cell Genetics Related to Neoplasia indicated the broad international appeal of this topic.

John J. Mulvihill, M.D.

Acknowledgments

We appreciate the help of many people. Early advice and encouragement concerning the conference were given by D. E. Anderson, D. Bergsma, P. S. Gerald, A. G. Knudson, Jr., V. A. McKusick, A. G. Motulsky, J. M. Opitz, and L. C. Strong, and the session chairmen were A. M. DiGeorge, J. F. Fraumeni, Jr., J. L. German, III, K. Hirschhorn, J. W. Littlefield, and R. W. Miller. T. Waller and S. Reutershan of Courtesy Associates, Inc. efficiently handled conference logistics.

In the preparation of this volume, special thanks go to the contributing authors for their high quality reports. We are grateful to our office staff: S. Trimble and D. Peterson for proofreading; J. Pearson, T. Barry, and K. Hatcher for secretarial help; and particularly W. Wade for tireless editorial assistance.

John J. Mulvihill, M.D.

Contents

Familial Cancer

Genetic Markers

Opportunities in Cancer Genetics

Postscript

Contributors

Shyam S. Agarwal
Visiting Scientist
The Institute for Cancer Research
Philadelphia, Pennsylvania 19111

David E. Anderson
Professor of Biology
The University of Texas System Cancer
  Center
M.D. Anderson Hospital and Tumor
  Institute
Houston, Texas 77030

Steven A. Atlas
Research Associate
Developmental Pharmacology Branch
National Institute of Child Health and
  Human Development
National Institutes of Health
Bethesda, Maryland 20014

William A. Blattner
Clinical Investigator
Environmental Epidemiology Branch
National Cancer Institute
Bethesda, Maryland 20014

Melvin A. Block
Chairman, Department of Surgery
Henry Ford Hospital
Detroit, Michigan 48202

Robert P. Bolande
Director, Department of Pathology
Montreal Children's Hospital
and
Professor of Pathology and Pediatrics
McGill University
Montreal, Quebec, Canada

Darrell Q. Brown
Radiobiologist
The Institute for Cancer Research
Philadelphia, Pennsylvania 19111

John T. Casagrande
Clinical Instructor of Medicine and Public
  Health
University of Southern California School of
  Medicine
Los Angeles, California 90033

James E. Cleaver
Professor of Radiology
Laboratory of Radiobiology
University of California
San Francisco, California 94143

David E. Comings
Director, Department of Medical Genetics
City of Hope National Medical Center
Duarte, California 91010

Eleanor E. Deschner
Associate Member
Memorial Sloan-Kettering Cancer Center
New York, New York 10021

Philip J. Fialkow
Chief, Medical Service
Veterans Administration Hospital
and
Professor and Vice-Chairman, Department
  of Medicine
Professor of Genetics
University of Washington
Seattle, Washington 98195

Boy Frame
Chief, Fifth Medical Division
Henry Ford Hospital
Detroit, Michigan 48202

Joseph F. Fraumeni, Jr.
Chief, Environmental Epidemiology
Branch
National Cancer Institute
Bethesda, Maryland 20014

Robert C. Gallo
Chief, Laboratory of Tumor Cell Biology
National Cancer Institute
Bethesda, Maryland 20014

Richard A. Gatti
Professor of Pediatrics
University of California School of Medicine
and
Director, Division of Pediatric Oncology
and Immunology
Cedars-Sinai Medical Center
Los Angeles, California 90048

Veeba R. Gerkins
Instructor in Pathology
University of Southern California School of
Medicine
Los Angeles, California 90033

Robert J. Gorlin
Professor and Chairman
Department of Oral Pathology
School of Dentistry
University of Minnesota
Minneapolis, Minnesota 55455

David G. Harnden
Professor, Department of Cancer Studies
University of Birmingham
Birmingham, England

Frederick Hecht
Professor of Pediatrics
Crippled Children's Division and Perinatal
Medicine
University of Oregon Health Sciences
Center
Portland, Oregon 97201

Brian E. Henderson
Professor of Pathology
University of Southern California School of
Medicine
Los Angeles, California 90033

Jürgen Herrmann
Associate Professor of Pediatrics and
Medical Genetics
Clinical Genetics Center
University of Wisconsin
Madison, Wisconsin 53706

Walter E. Heston
Head, Laboratory of Biology
National Cancer Institute
National Institutes of Health
Bethesda, Maryland 20014

Charles E. Jackson
Chief, Genetics Section
Department of Medicine
Henry Ford Hospital
Detroit, Michigan 48202

Edward J. Katz
Research Assistant
The Institute for Cancer Research
Philadelphia, Pennsylvania 19111

Mary-Claire King
Assistant Professor of Epidemiology
School of Public Health
University of California
Berkeley, California 94720

Alfred G. Knudson, Jr.
Director
The Institute for Cancer Research
Philadelphia, Pennsylvania 19111

Frederick P. Li
Head, Clinical Studies Section
Clinical Epidemiology Branch
National Cancer Institute
Sidney Farber Cancer Center
Boston, Massachusetts 02115

Martin Lipkin
Associate Member
Memorial Sloan-Kettering Cancer Center
New York, New York 10021

Lawrence A. Loeb
Associate Professor, Department of
Biochemistry
The Institute for Cancer Research
Philadelphia, Pennsylvania 19111

Anthony S. Lubiniecki
Principal Scientist
Life Sciences Division
Meloy Laboratories, Inc.
Springfield, Virginia 22151

Marvin A. Lutzner
Chief, Dermatology Branch
National Cancer Institute
National Institutes of Health
Bethesda, Maryland 20014

Henry T. Lynch
Professor and Chairman
Department of Preventive Medicine and
Public Health
Creighton University School of Medicine
Omaha, Nebraska 68178

Jane Lynch
Instructor
Department of Preventive Medicine and
Public Health
Creighton University School of Medicine
Omaha, Nebraska 68178

Patrick Lynch
Research Assistant
Department of Preventive Medicine and
Public Health
Creighton University School of Medicine
Omaha, Nebraska 68178

Barbara K. McCaw
Research Assistant Professor of Pediatrics
University of Oregon Health Sciences
Center
Portland, Oregon 97201

Max R. Mickey
Statistician
Department of Surgery
University of California School of Medicine
Los Angeles, California 90024

Robert W. Miller
Chief, Clinical Epidemiology Branch
National Cancer Institute
Bethesda, Maryland 20014

John D. Minna
Chief, National Cancer Institute-Veterans
Administration Medical Oncology
Branch
Veterans Administration Hospital
Washington, D.C. 20422

John J. Mulvihill
Head, Clinical Genetics Section
Clinical Epidemiology Branch
National Cancer Institute
Bethesda, Maryland 20014

Edmond A. Murphy
Professor of Medicine
Johns Hopkins University School of
Medicine
Baltimore, Maryland 21205

Walter E. Nance
Chairman, Department of Human Genetics
Medical College of Virginia
Richmond, Virginia 23298

Daniel W. Nebert
Chief, Developmental Pharmacology
Branch
National Institute of Child Health and
Human Development
National Institutes of Health
Bethesda, Maryland 20014

John M. Opitz
Professor of Medical Genetics and
Pediatrics
Director, Clinical Genetics Center
University of Wisconsin
Madison, Wisconsin 53706

Sondra T. Perdue
Department of Surgery
University of California School of Medicine
Los Angeles, California 90024

Nicholas L. Petrakis
Professor of Preventive Medicine
G.W. Hooper Foundation
Department of International Health
University of California School of Medicine
San Francisco, California 94143

Malcolm C. Pike
Professor, Community Medicine and
Pediatrics
University of Southern California School of
Medicine
Los Angeles, California 90033

Vincent M. Riccardi
Director, Genetics Unit
Milwaukee Children's Hospital
Medical College of Wisconsin
Milwaukee, Wisconsin 53233

Marvin M. Romsdahl
Professor of Surgery
The University of Texas System Cancer
Center
M.D. Anderson Hospital and Tumor
Institute
Houston, Texas 77030

Janet D. Rowley
Associate Professor of Medicine
Franklin McLean Memorial Research
Institute
University of Chicago
Chicago, Illinois 60637

R. Neil Schimke
Professor of Medicine and Pediatrics
University of Kansas Medical Center
College of Health Sciences and Hospital
Kansas City, Kansas 66103

William J. Schull
Professor of Population Genetics
Graduate School of Biomedical Sciences
Director, Center for Demographic and
Population Genetics
University of Texas Health Science Center
Houston, Texas 77030

Mark Skolnick
Assistant Research Professor
Department of Medical Biophysics and
Computing
University of Utah Medical Center
Salt Lake City, Utah 84132

Beatrice D. Spector
Research Specialist
Department of Laboratory Medicine and
Pathology
University of Minnesota
Minneapolis, Minnesota 55455

Louise C. Strong
Assistant Professor of Medical Genetics
Graduate School of Biomedical Sciences
University of Texas Health Science Center
and
Director, Medical Genetics Clinic
The University of Texas System
Cancer Center
M.D. Anderson Hospital and Tumor
Institute
Houston, Texas 77030

Michael Swift
Chief, Division of Medical Genetics
Department of Medicine
The Biological Sciences Research Center
University of North Carolina
Chapel Hill, North Carolina 27514

Paul I. Terasaki
Professor of Surgery
University of California School of Medicine
Los Angeles, California 90024

Josef Warkany
Professor of Research Pediatrics
Children's Hospital Research Foundation
University of Cincinnati
Cincinnati, Ohio 45229

Discussants

Arleen D. Auerbach
Carlo M. Croce
Angelo M. DiGeorge
Joseph A. DiPaolo
Roswell Eldridge
Kathryn E. Fuscaldo
Park S. Gerald
James L. German, III
Takeshi Hirayama
Kurt Hirschhorn

Noboru Kobayashi
Hilary Koprowski
John W. Littlefield
Anna T. Meadows
Arno G. Motulsky
E. E. Pogosianz
M. Nabil Rashad
Barbara H. Sanford
Joji Utsunomiya
George Yerganian

Committee on Epidemiology, U. S.–Japan Cooperative Cancer Research Program

Co-chairmen

T. Hirayama: Head, Division of Epidemiology, National Cancer Center Research Institute, Tokyo

R. W. Miller: Chief, Clinical Epidemiology Branch, National Cancer Institute, Bethesda, Maryland

A. M. DiGeorge: Professor of Pediatrics, St. Christopher's Hospital for Children, Philadelphia, Pennsylvania

K. Fukuda: Lecturer in Public Health, Sapporo Medical College, Sapporo

M. Hitosugi: Assistant Professor of Public Health, Kitasato University, Sagamihara City

N. Kobayashi: Professor of Pediatrics, Faculty of Medicine, Tokyo University, Tokyo

H. T. Lynch: Professor of Preventive Medicine and Public Health, Creighton University, Omaha, Nebraska

K. Mabuchi: Department of Epidemiology, Johns Hopkins School of Public Health, Baltimore, Maryland

J. J. Mulvihill: Head, Clinical Genetics Section, Clinical Epidemiology Branch, National Cancer Institute, Bethesda, Maryland

W. J. Schull: Director, Center for Demographic and Population Genetics, University of Texas Health Science Center, Houston, Texas

J. Utsunomiya: Assistant Professor of Surgery, Tokyo Medical–Dental University, Tokyo

T. Yoshimura: Department of Public Health, Kyushu University, Fukuoka

U.S.–U.S.S.R. Joint Working Group on Mammalian Somatic Cell Genetics Related to Neoplasia

Co-chairmen

T. King, Jr.: Director, Division of Cancer Research Resources and Centers, National Cancer Institute, Bethesda, Maryland

E. E. Pogosianz: Head, Laboratory of Cytogenetics, Cancer Research Center, Moscow

F. E. Arrighi: Section of Cell Biology, M.D. Anderson Hospital and Tumor Institute, Houston, Texas

N. P. Bochkov: Director, Institute of Medical Genetics, Moscow

J. A. DiPaolo: Biology Branch, National Cancer Institute, Bethesda, Maryland

O. J. Miller: Department of Human Genetics and Development, College of Physicians and Surgeons, Columbia University, New York, New York

B. C. Myhr: Biology Branch, National Cancer Institute, Bethesda, Maryland

W. W. Nichols: Institute for Medical Research, Camden, New Jersey

A. Sandberg: Chief of Medicine, Roswell Park Memorial Institute, Buffalo, New York

J. F. Saunders: Office of International Affairs, National Cancer Institute, Bethesda, Maryland

O. I. Sokova: Laboratory of Cytogenetics, Cancer Research Center, Moscow

A. A. Stavrovskaya: Laboratory of Cytogenetics, Cancer Research Center, Moscow

G. Yerganian: Chief, Laboratory of Cytogenetics, Sidney Farber Cancer Center, Boston, Massachusetts

V. S. Zhurkov: Institute of Medical Genetics, Moscow

Genetics of Human Cancer, edited by J. J.
Mulvihill, R. W. Miller, and J. F. Fraumeni, Jr.
Raven Press, New York, 1977.

1

Ethnic Differences in Cancer Occurrence: Genetic and Environmental Influences with Particular Reference to Neuroblastoma

Robert W. Miller

Clinical Epidemiology Branch, National Cancer Institute, Bethesda, Maryland 20014

There are marked geographic differences in cancer rates (21), even within the United States (36). Much of the variation is believed to be environmentally induced. There are, however, important differences which appear to be genetically influenced. The marked excesses or deficiencies of certain tumors in an ethnic group may fall in this category. In seeking ethnic differences in cancer occurrence it is important, as always in etiologic studies, to purify the diagnoses as fully as possible. Otherwise, key clues to etiology may be overlooked, as when registry or death certificate data are coded routinely according to anatomic site, and not by histologic type.

BLACKS

Ewing's Tumor

When all forms of bone cancer are grouped together, important ethnic differences in occurrence are obliterated. Thus, Higginson and Muir (21) found virtually no difference in the incidence of bone cancer in the U.S. population including all races as compared with U.S. blacks alone.

In 1965 we acquired death certificates for all children in the United States under 15 years of age who had died of cancer since 1960. We recoded the diagnoses according to histology, and were surprised to learn that Ewing's tumor is virtually absent in blacks (Fig. 1) (14,17,43). The finding was confirmed by data from other sources (32), including the histologically sophisticated Armed Forces Institute of Pathology (24). The rates for osteosarcoma exhibited no such difference between whites and blacks.

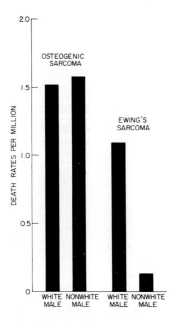

FIG. 1. Mortality rates from bone sarcoma according to histologic type in U.S. males under 15 years of age, 1960–1966, whites vs. nonwhites. The results for females were similar; 90% of nonwhites were blacks. [From Fraumeni and Glass (14).]

Data from Africa have since shown the same deficiency of Ewing's tumor in blacks (9,52) as observed in the United States. The near absence of this neoplasm in the same racial group, native in Africa and 100 or more years after "migration" to another continent, suggests genetic resistance to this form of neoplasia. The observation is of value in etiologic research and in the differential diagnosis of bone lesions in blacks.

Testicular Cancer

There is a marked deficiency of all forms of malignant tumors of the testis in U.S. blacks, as revealed by conventionally coded data from death certificates (Fig. 2). The peak in mortality at 25–29 years of age in whites is absent in blacks. The data available from Africa tend to confirm this peculiarity, which seems not to be type-specific (11,52).

Multiple Myeloma

Mortality rates for multiple myeloma among blacks are substantially higher than in whites in the United States (Fig. 3). Data from Africa are difficult to judge because the diagnosis depends so much on the availability of appropriate laboratory facilities.

It has been suggested that multiple myeloma may arise from chronic stimulation of the immune system in response to chronic infection, e.g., in patients with chronic biliary disease in whom "benign" monoclonal gammopathies first devel-

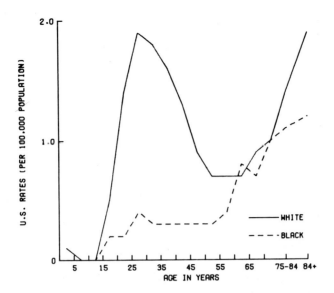

FIG. 2. Age-specific mortality from testicular cancer (ICD 178) in the United States by race, 1950–1969. Source: Special tabulation, U.S. National Vital Statistics, Epidemiology Branch, National Cancer Institute.

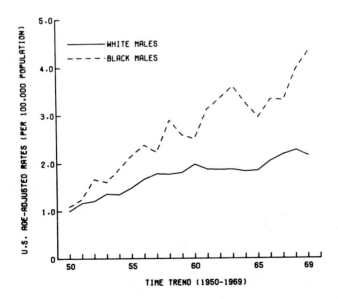

FIG. 3. Age-adjusted mortality from multiple myeloma (ICD 203) in males by race over time, 1950–1969. Findings for females were similar. Source: Special tabulation, U.S. National Vital Statistics, Epidemiology Branch, National Cancer Institute.

op and later acquire the malignant form of multiple myeloma (45).

The high rates of multiple myeloma in U.S. blacks might be explained by the higher frequency of chronic infections that blacks suffer as compared to whites, but one would then expect a social gradient in rates, greater in the poorer classes, regardless of race. Apparently, a definitive study has not yet been made in this regard. Another approach would be through retrospective study, in which one would seek more infection in patients prior to multiple myeloma than in an appropriate control group. Such an excess has been claimed (23), but was not well documented.

The high rates of multiple myeloma in U.S. blacks may be caused not by infection but by a genetic determinant. It has been found that blacks at all ages had higher levels of the three major immunoglobulins than did whites, the most prominent difference being in the IgG fraction (19). These differences may be genetic in origin because there is reportedly little influence of social class on gamma globulin levels (19).

If multiple myeloma is in part due to a genetic influence on immune status, one wonders if other type-specific cancer excesses or deficiencies in the same ethnic group can be similarly explained. For example, could an immunologic peculiarity that leads to multiple myeloma late in life suppress the development of Ewing's tumor early in life? If so, why this tumor and not others?

Acute Lymphocytic Leukemia in Childhood

Mortality rates from leukemia exhibited little variation during childhood until the 1920s, when a peak began to emerge at 4 years of age in England and Wales (6). Twenty years later, a similar peak emerged in the leukemia death rates for U.S. white children, but not for nonwhite children (6,37)—and has not as yet developed among nonwhite children (Fig. 4). The children of Japan exhibited no peak in leukemia mortality until the 1960s (Fig. 5) (38).

The cell type responsible for the peak in whites is acute lymphocytic leukemia (ALL) (6). It is this cell type in particular that occurs excessively in Down's syndrome (30,39,48), at an age 3 years younger than in the general population (30,39).

In the U.S. white population the peak declined somewhat during the 1960s (Fig. 6), perhaps because of the more conservative use of fluoroscopy and radiotherapy for benign disorders after potential hazards were described in widely publicized reports issued in 1956 by the National Academy of Sciences–National Research Council (50) and the British Medical Research Council (20).

Apparently the peak in ALL among white children is due at least in part to environmental factors. Black children are either not exposed or not susceptible. In Nigeria, the frequency of all forms of childhood leukemia was low, even after intensive search for the neoplasm (52). Only 60 cases were found among 1,325 childhood cancers, 1960–1972. The frequency of leukemia in Nigeria and in other African countries seems to be substantially less than in U.S. blacks.

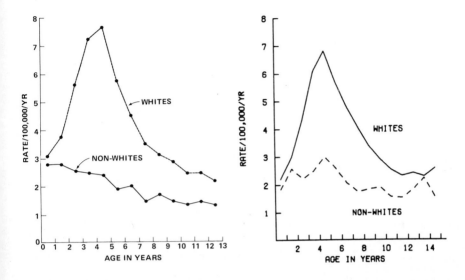

FIG. 4. Mortality from childhood leukemia by single year of age in the United States (left) 1950–1959 as compared with (right) 1960–1969, whites vs. nonwhites. Ninety percent of nonwhites were black. [Data for 1950–1959 are from Miller RW (37) and for 1960–1969 from a national registry of death certificates for childhood cancer, Epidemiology Branch, National Cancer Institute.]

Melanoma

Pigment in the skin protects against various forms of skin cancer (21), including melanoma (36). The difference in mortality from melanoma between U.S. whites and blacks is pronounced (Fig. 7). In this instance, a genetically determined racial trait, dermal pigmentation, protects against an environmental carcinogen, actinic radiation.

ARABS

Skin Cancer in Childhood

Under the auspices of the International Union Against Cancer (UICC) an international comparison was made of childhood cancer according to histologic type (41). A surprising finding came from the only contributing hospital in North Africa, the Institut Salah Aziaz, which is in Tunis. There, 14% of all childhood malignant disease was epithelioma of the skin in patients with xeroderma pigmen-

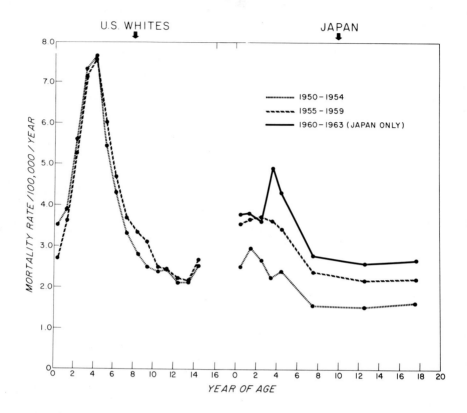

FIG. 5. Mortality from childhood leukemia according to age, U.S. whites vs. Japan, for successive intervals of time. [From Miller (38).]

tosum (XP). The relative frequency of this diagnosis is about the same as that for neuroblastoma *plus* Wilms' tumor in Europe and the United States (46,53).

The predisposition to skin cancers in patients with XP, an autosomal recessive trait, represents in a sense the opposite of the protective effect of pigmented skin. Persons with XP usually have impaired ability to repair damage to DNA produced by ultraviolet light (5). A high prevalence of XP among Arabs is well known at hospitals throughout North Africa, although references to the high frequency are difficult to find in the medical literature (35).

In this instance, a racial predisposition to cancer is caused not by a general characteristic of an ethnic group, but by a particular autosomal recessive trait, which has accumulated in a racial group.

Other such instances include (a) Bloom's syndrome among Jews who migrated from southeastern Poland and southwestern Ukraine and are at high risk of leukemia, among other cancers (15,16), and (b) ataxia-telangiectasia (AT) among Moroccan Jews in Israel (31), whose disease predisposes them to lymphoma and acute lymphocytic leukemia (25).

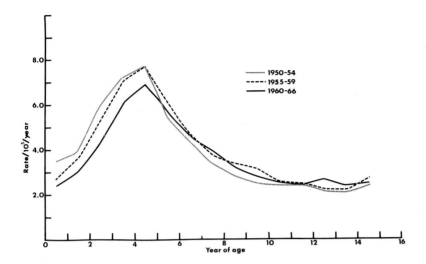

FIG. 6. Decrease in leukemia mortality among U.S. white children according to age in three successive intervals of time. [From Miller, *Lancet,* 2:1189–1190 (1969).]

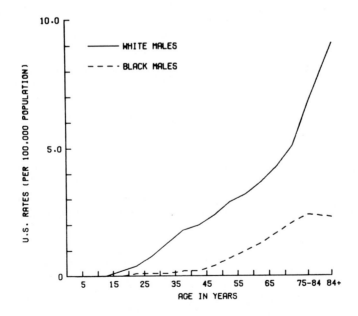

FIG. 7. Age-adjusted mortality from melanoma (ICD 190) among U.S. males, whites vs. blacks, 1950–1969. Similar differences were observed in mortality among females. Source: Special tabulation, U.S. National Vital Statistics, Epidemiology Branch, National Cancer Institute.

JAPANESE AND CHINESE

Chronic Lymphocytic Leukemia

About 25% of adult leukemia in the United States is attributable to chronic lymphocytic leukemia (CLL) (13), but this form of leukemia is rare in the Japanese (13) and Chinese (51). Adequate studies have not yet been made of migrants, either in Hawaii or on the West Coast. Thus, it is not known if the rates are increased by the occidental style of life.

CLL has not been induced by exposure to ionizing radiation in British men treated for ankylosing spondylitis (7) or in Japanese survivors of the atomic bomb (22). CLL must thus have dissimilar origins from other forms of leukemia, which *are* so induced. (In studies of cancer clusters, Nathan Mantel, formerly of National Cancer Institute, noted the value of "zero occurrences" where some cases are expected—a situation he referred to as "vacuities." Here, then, is an instance in which one might treasure his vacuities—for their etiologic importance.)

Hodgkin's Disease

Low frequency of a tumor in a racial group may be age specific. One example, already cited, is the lack of a peak in the occurrence of ALL in black children. Another is Hodgkin's disease, which has two peaks in every national group studied to date except the Japanese, among whom the first peak (at 25–29 years of age) is absent (33). Absence of the early peak in Japan led MacMahon (33) to postulate an infectious etiology for the disease in young adults and a neoplastic origin later in life. Data from other Asian peoples have not been available for comparable evaluation.

Pineal Tumors

In Japan pinealoma has been reported to be about 12 times more common than in other races (1,40). Data from the All Japan Children's Center Registration (3) also suggest a high frequency of this tumor (58 of 626 brain tumors), but interpretation is difficult because the registry is not population based, and there is referral bias. Many children with brain tumors are referred directly to neurosurgeons who do not notify the registry, whereas children with pineal tumors are usually seen first by pediatricians because the presenting signs are due to hormonal effects (N. Kobayashi, *personal communication*).

Breast Cancer

An explanation for the low rate of breast cancer in Japan has been intensively sought. An important determinant, it has been proposed (10), is the relation of three estrogen fractions to one another in young women. It is thought that estriol (E3), a noncarcinogen, impedes the carcinogenic activity of estrone (E1) and estradiol (E2). The risk of breast cancer appears to be inversely related to the "estriol ratio": E3/(E1 + E2). Among Asians (Chinese and Japanese), the ratio is high in young women, but among migrants to Hawaii it is lower, but not as low as in Caucasian Hawaiians (10). Breast cancer rates are similarly ranked. The fall in the ratio and the rise in the frequency of breast cancer with migration was taken to be "strong evidence of nongenetic determinants" (34). These observations indicate that what appeared to be a genetically determined ethnic difference in cancer occurrence is, in fact, environmentally mediated.

It would be arduous to review all tumors in all racial groups and to separate the genetic from the environmental component. From the foregoing, suffice to say, there are ethnic influences that seem to be purely genetic, and others in which the environment plays some role.

KNUDSON'S HYPOTHESIS AND INTERNATIONAL VARIATION OF CERTAIN CHILDHOOD CANCERS

In 1971, Knudson (26) proposed a two-mutation hypothesis to explain the development of retinoblastoma. He noted that the heritable form of the neoplasm was usually bilateral or otherwise multifocal, whereas sporadic cases were almost always unilateral. For heritable or multifocal retinoblastoma, there was a linear regression with respect to age at diagnosis. Data for sporadic unilateral cases formed a curvilinear regression.

These differences suggested to Knudson that two events were involved in the development of retinoblastoma: a prezygotic (germ cell) mutation plus a postzygotic (somatic cell) mutation in heritable cases, and two postzygotic mutations in sporadic cases. Subsequently, he and his co-worker presented data in support of the same mechanism in the genesis of Wilms' tumor (28), neuroblastoma, and pheochromocytoma (29). It is of interest to consider how the two-mutation hypothesis accords with geographic variations in the frequency of the three neoplasms for which some data are available.

Wilms' Tumor

It has been suggested that, of the most frequent childhood cancers, Wilms' tumor occurs with the least geographic variation in frequency, and might thus be used as a standard (reference) tumor against which the frequency of other childhood cancers can be roughly evaluated (12). The constancy of rates for Wilms' tumor is not demonstrable because of the general lack of population-based data, and relative frequencies of hospital data vary because of overwhelming real differences in frequencies (e.g., Burkitt's lymphoma comprised 60% of all childhood cancer in Nigeria [52]), or because of selective referral of patients to centers with certain specialists (e.g., retinoblastoma). Regardless of the distortion created

TABLE 1. *International comparison of Wilms' tumor, neuroblastoma, and retinoblastoma*

	Number of cases			Ratio	
	Wt	Nb	Rb	Nb/Wt	Rb/Wt
U.S. whites[a] (ref. 53)	117	146	52	1.25	0.44
Manchester, England[a] (ref. 46)	82	111	51	1.35	0.62
Israel[a]	19	27	34	1.42	1.79
Japan (ref. 3)	289	562	231	1.94	0.80
Singapore	10	16	15	1.60	1.50
Hong Kong	20	19	25	0.95	1.25
Karachi, Pakistan	19	10	34	0.53	1.79
Bombay	12	5	20	0.42	1.67
U.S. blacks[a] (ref. 53)	18	16	7	0.89	0.39
Khartoum, Sudan	17	14	41	0.82	2.41
Ibadan, Nigeria (ref. 52)	74	33	97	0.45	1.31
Uganda	98	30	110	0.31	1.12
Dakar Regional Registry[b]	60	15	69	0.25	1.15
Kenya Regional Registry[c]	45	4	35	0.09	0.78
Tanzania, 1959-1966	26	2	44	0.08	1.69
São Paulo	34	24	24	0.71	0.71
Puerto Rico[a]	75	34	63	0.45	0.84
Cali, Colombia	15	3	20	0.20	1.33

Selected data from the UICC study of childhood cancer (41). Wt, Wilms' tumor; Nb, neuroblastoma; Rb, retinoblastoma.

[a] Data from tumor registries or surveys believed to have unbiased ascertainment of cases.

[b] Includes Senegal, Cameroun, Zaire, Upper Volta, and Ivory Coast.

[c] Includes Kenya, Tanzania, Malawi, and Zambia, all for 1968-1969.

by these influences, Wilms' tumor accounted for at least 8% of all cancers in each of the many series in the UICC study (42). The variation observed from one series to another exhibited no extreme values to suggest that either the heritable or the acquired forms of Wilms' tumor were markedly excessive or deficient.

Retinoblastoma

The heritable form of retinoblastoma is transmitted as an autosomal dominant trait. Autosomal dominant mutations are thought to occur among all peoples at about the same rate. Hence, no great variation is expected geographically in the frequency of heritable retinoblastoma. At most there can be a 10% increase in the number of cases, if the effect were expressed in all persons who carry the gene. Any substantial true excess in occurrence should then be due to the form of the disease in which both mutations are postzygotic.

Table 1 shows that in the United States and Manchester, England, the numbers of cases of Wilms' tumor or neuroblastoma ran well ahead of those for retino-blastoma. In Israel, however, where ascertainment of cases was presumably comparable, the reverse occurred—there were more cases of retinoblastoma than of the other two tumors. A similar pattern was observed in Sudan, Uganda, Nigeria, Bombay, and Karachi. In Nigeria, it was noted that "most retinoblastomas were histologically undifferentiated...[whereas] the majority in the American black and English white children apparently were either moderately or well differentiated (44)." The investigators believed that children with Wilms' tumor were as likely to be referred to the hospital as were those with retinoblastoma (A. O. Williams, *personal communication*).

Therefore, it appears that retinoblastoma is more frequent in certain parts of the Indian subcontinent and Africa than elsewhere. If the excess is caused by tumors produced by two *somatic* mutations, the ratio of unilateral to bilateral tumors should prove to be substantially greater in those regions than in the United States or Europe.

Neuroblastoma

Table 1 contains the biggest surprise in the UICC study—a substantial deficiency in the occurrence of neuroblastoma in certain geographic areas, especially in the Burkitt's lymphoma belt of Africa. There was a near absence of the neoplasm in Tanzania, 1959–1966, and in the several countries covered by the Kenya Regional Registry, 1968–1969. The ratio of neuroblastoma to Wilms' tumor was 0.09, only 7% of that for U.S. whites and 10% of that for U.S. blacks. The relative frequency was less severely deficient in Uganda, Nigeria, and the countries covered by the Dakar Regional Registry. There the ratios were 25–50% of that for U.S. blacks. The ratios were also low for children in Bombay, Karachi, Cali, and Puerto Rico (where ascertainment of cases is especially good).

It is preferable, of course, to evaluate incidence rates rather than ratios of one cancer to another. From the Third National Cancer Survey in the United States, 1969–1971—the only population-based resource on children's cancer that permits racial comparisons—it was found that the annual incidence of neuroblastoma was 7.0/million blacks and 9.5/million whites (53). There was no difference between the races in the incidence of Wilms' tumor, 7.8/million.

Pathologists at the African centers where the frequency of neuroblastoma is near zero are highly skilled, so it seems unlikely that they would have difficulty in diagnosing the tumor. Referral bias might account for some underestimation of frequency, but probably not to the extent of the deficiency observed in parts of Africa.

How, then, can the strange geographic patterns for the neoplasm be explained? Knudson and Strong (29) estimated that about 22% of neuroblastoma had a heritable component. The environmental stimulus in areas with low frequencies of the neoplasm is presumably sufficient to provide the somatic mutations required for both the heritable and nonheritable forms of neuroblastoma. As suggested by Knudson and Meadows (27), something must happen to inhibit tumor development or cause fetal death of those destined to develop neuroblastoma. These authors, with data available to them only from Uganda and Nagpur, India, suggested that malaria might be such an inhibitor. It should be noted that clinical neuroblastoma sometimes undergoes spontaneous regression (4,27), and *in situ* neuroblastoma is found incidentally at autopsy under 3 months of age but not thereafter, apparently because of regression or maturation (2).

The geographic distribution of malaria does not agree well with that for low frequencies of neuroblastoma as observed in the UICC study. Thus malaria alone is not likely to account for inhibition of tumor development. Chronic infection or infestation with circulating parasites are among the characteristics of the areas where neuroblastoma is infrequent. Malaria, schistosomiasis, and trypanosomiasis are among the infestations that evoke a rapid and pronounced hypergammaglobulinemia, especially of IgG and IgM (18,47). Mention has already been made of the genetically determined higher levels of IgG in blacks as compared with whites in the United States (19). Hence, either genetic or environmental influences, or both, may affect the level of immunoglobulins transmitted by the mother to the fetus, or synthesized by the newborn—and a specific fraction may inhibit development of neuroblastoma. If so, laboratory experimentation may be revealing, e.g., the effect on human neuroblastoma cells in culture of various dilutions of hyper-gammaglobulinemic sera from patients with Burkitt's lymphoma. Cells from patients with Type IV-S neuroblastoma may be the most sensitive for such a study, because, although the tumor is widespread in the body, it regresses spontaneously (49), or responds well to therapy (8).

If a fraction of the excess of gammaglobulin produced by circulating parasites is transmitted from mother to fetus and thus inhibits development of neuroblastoma, it would represent the effect of a transplacental *anti*-carcinogen.

REFERENCES

1. Araki, C., and Matsumoto, S. (1969): Statistical reevaluation of pinealoma and related tumors in Japan. *J. Neurosurg.*, 30:146–149.
2. Beckwith, J.B., and Perrin, E.V. (1963): In situ neuroblastoma: A contribution to the natural history of neural crest tumors. *Am. J. Pathol.*, 43:1089–1104.
3. Children's Cancer Association of Japan (1975): All Japan Children's Cancer Registration, 1969–1973. Nakagawa Building, 2-4-11, Nishi-Shinbashi, Minato-ku, Tokyo.
4. Cole, W.H. (1974): Spontaneous regression of cancer: The metabolic triumph of the host? *Ann. N.Y. Acad. Sci.*, 230:111–146.
5. Combined Clinical Staff Conference (1974): Xeroderma pigmentosum. An inherited disease with sun sensitivity, multiple cutaneous neoplasms, and abnormal DNA repair. *Ann. Intern. Med.*, 80:221–248.
6. Court Brown, W.M., and Doll, R. (1961): Leukaemia in childhood and young adult life. Trends in mortality in relation to aetiology. *Br. Med. J.*, 1:981–988.
7. Court Brown, W.M., and Doll, R. (1965): Mortality from cancer and other causes after radiotherapy for ankylosing spondylitis. *Br. Med. J.*, 2:1327–1332.
8. D'Angio, G.J., Evans, A.E., and Koop, C.E. (1971): Special pattern of widespread neuroblastoma with a favorable prognosis. *Lancet*, 1:1046–1049.
9. Davies, J.N.P. (1973): Childhood tumours. In: *Tumours in a Tropical Country,* edited by A.C. Templeton, pp. 306–343. Springer-Verlag, Berlin.
10. Dickinson, L.E., MacMahon, B., Cole, P., et al. (1974): Estrogen profiles of Oriental and Caucasian women in Hawaii. *N. Engl. J. Med.*, 291:1211–1213.
11. Dodge, O.G., Owor, R., and Templeton, A.C. (1973): Tumours of the male genitalia. In: *Tumours in a Tropical Country,* edited by A.C. Templeton, p. 139. Springer-Verlag, Berlin.

12. Editorial (1973): Nephroblastoma: An index reference cancer. *Lancet,* 2:651.
13. Finch, S.C., Hoshino, T., Itoga, T., Ichimaru, M., and Ingram, R.J., Jr. (1969): Chronic lymphocytic leukemia in Hiroshima and Nagasaki, Japan. *Blood,* 33:79–86.
14. Fraumeni, J.F., Jr., and Glass, A.G. (1970): Rarity of Ewing's sarcoma among U.S. Negro children. *Lancet,* 1:366–367.
15. German, J. (1969): Bloom's syndrome. I. Genetical and clinical observations in the first twenty-seven patients. *Am. J. Hum. Genet.,* 21:196–227.
16. German, J. (1974): Bloom's syndrome. II. The prototype of genetic disorders predisposing to chromosome instability and cancer. In: *Chromosomes and Cancer,* edited by J. German, pp. 608–609. Wiley, New York.
17. Glass, A.G., and Fraumeni, J.F., Jr. (1970): Epidemiology of bone cancer in children. *J. Natl. Cancer Inst.,* 44:187–199.
18. Greenwood, B.M. (1974): Possible role of a B-cell mitogen in hypergammaglobulinaemia in malaria and trypanosomiasis. *Lancet,* 1:435–436.
19. Grundbacher, F.J. (1974): Heritability estimates and genetic and environmental correlations for the human immunoglobulins G, M, and A. *Am. J. Hum. Genet.,* 26:1–12.
20. Medical Research Council (1956): *Hazards to Man of Nuclear and Allied Radiations.* HM Stationery Office, London.
21. Higginson, J., and Muir, C.S. (1973): Epidemiology of cancer. In: *Cancer Medicine,* edited by J.F. Holland and E. Frei III, pp. 241–306. Lea & Febiger, Philadelphia.
22. Ishimaru, T., Hoshino, T., Ichimaru, M., et al. (1971): Leukemia in atomic-bomb survivors, Hiroshima and Nagasaki, 1 Oct. 1950–30 Sept. 1966. *Radiat. Res.,* 45:216–233.
23. Isobe, T., and Osserman, E.F. (1971): Pathologic conditions associated with plasma cell dyscrasias: A study of 806 cases. *Ann. NY Acad. Sci.,* 190:507–518.
24. Jensen, R.D., and Drake, R.M. (1970): Rarity of Ewing's tumor in Negroes. *Lancet,* 1:777.
25. Kersey, J., Spector, B.D., and Good, R.A. (1973): Primary immunodeficiency diseases and cancer: The Immunodeficiency Cancer Registry. *Int. J. Cancer,* 12:333–347.
26. Knudson, A.G. (1971): Mutation and cancer: Statistical study of retinoblastoma. *Proc. Natl. Acad. Sci. (USA),* 68:820–823.
27. Knudson, A.G., Jr., and Meadows, A.T. (1976): Developmental genetics of neuroblastoma. *J. Natl. Cancer Inst.,* 57:675–682.
28. Knudson, A.G., and Strong, L.C. (1972): Mutation and cancer: A model for Wilms' tumor of the kidney. *J. Natl. Cancer Inst.,* 38:313–324.
29. Knudson, A.G., and Strong, L.C. (1972): Mutation and cancer: Neuroblastoma and pheochromocytoma. *Am. J. Hum. Genet.,* 24:514–532.
30. Lashof, J.C., and Stewart, A. (1965): Oxford survey of childhood cancers. Progress report III: Leukaemia and Down's syndrome. *Mon. Bull. Ministry Health (Lond.),* 24:136–143.
31. Levin, S., and Perlov, S. (1971): Ataxia-telangiectasia in Israel with observations on its relationship to malignant disease. *Isr. J. Med. Sci.,* 12:1535–1541.
32. Linden, G., and Dunn, J.E. (1970): Ewing's sarcoma in Negroes. *Lancet,* 1:1171.
33. MacMahon, B. (1966): Epidemiology of Hodgkin's disease. *Cancer Res.* 26:1189–1200.
34. MacMahon, B., Cole, P., and Brown, J.B. (1975): Factors that influence mammary carcinogenesis. *N. Engl. J. Med.,* 292:974–975.
35. Marshall, J. (1964): *Skin Diseases in Africa,* p. 91. Maske W. Miller, Cape Town.
36. Mason, T.J., McKay, F.W., Hoover, R., Blot, W.J., and Fraumeni, J.F., Jr. (1975): *Atlas of Cancer Mortality for U.S. Counties: 1950–1969.* DHEW Publication No. (NIH) 75–780, 103 pp. Government Printing Office, Washington, D.C.
37. Miller, R.W. (1965): Environmental agents in cancer. *Yale J. Biol. Med.,* 37:487–507.
38. Miller, R.W. (1967): Childhood cancer mortality in U.S.A. and Japan. *Tohoku J. Exp. Med.,* 91:103–107.
39. Miller, R.W. (1970): Neoplasia and Down's syndrome. *Ann. NY Acad. Sci.,* 171:637–644.
40. Miller, R.W. (1971): Relation between cancer and congenital malformations. The value of small series, with a note on pineal tumors in native and migrant Japanese. *Isr. J. Med. Sci.,* 7:1461–1464.
41. Miller, R.W. (1974): Childhood cancer epidemiology: Two international activities. *Natl. Cancer Inst. Monogr.,* 40:71–74.
42. Miller, R.W. (1974): *Unpublished data.*
43. Miller, R.W., and Dalager, N.A. (1974): U.S. childhood cancer deaths by cell type, 1960–68. *J. Pediatr.,* 85:664–668.

44. Olisa, E.G., Chandra, R., Jackson, M.A., Kennedy, J., and Williams, A.O. (1975): Malignant tumors in American black and Nigerian children: A comparative study. *J. Natl. Cancer Inst.,* 55:281–284.
45. Osserman, E.F., and Takatsuki, K. (1965): Consideration regarding the pathogenesis of the plasmacytic dyscrasias. *Scand. J. Haematol.,* 4 (Suppl): 28–49.
46. Pearson, D., and Steward, J.K. (1969): Malignant disease in juveniles. *Proc. R. Soc. Med.,* 62:17–20.
47. Polednak, A.P. (1974): Connective tissue responses in Negroes in relation to disease. *Am. J. Phys. Anthropol.,* 41:49–58.
48. Rosner, F., and Lee, S.L. (1972): Down's syndrome and acute leukemia: Myeloblastic or lymphocytic? Report of forty-three cases and review of the literature. *Am. J. Med.,* 53:203–218.
49. Schwartz, A.D., Dadash-Zadeh, M., Lee, H., and Swaney, J.J. (1974): Spontaneous regression of disseminated neuroblastoma. *J. Pediatr.,* 85:760–763.
50. Summary Reports of the Committees on the Biological Effects of Atomic Radiation (1956): Washington, National Academy of Sciences–National Research Council.
51. Wells, R., and Lau, K.S. (1960): Incidence of leukaemia in Singapore, and rarity of chronic lymphocytic leukaemia in Chinese. *Br. Med. J.,* 1:759–763.
52. Williams, A.O. (1975): Tumors of childhood in Ibadan, Nigeria. *Cancer,* 36:370–378.
53. Young, J.L., Jr., and Miller, R.W. (1975): Incidence of malignant tumors in U.S. children. *J. Pediatr.,* 86:254–258.

Genetics of Human Cancer, edited by J. J.
Mulvihill, R. W. Miller, and J. F. Fraumeni, Jr.
Raven Press, New York, 1977.

2

Cancer and Inbreeding

William J. Schull

*Center for Demographic and Population Genetics, University of Texas Health Science
Center, Houston, Texas 77030*

Why, it may be asked, among all of those factors that contribute to genetic variability, should inbreeding be singled out for specific attention in this volume? A defense for its inclusion is not obvious. We generally assume inbreeding and consanguineous unions to interest geneticists largely for two reasons. First, it has long been observed that persons affected by rare, recessively inherited pathologies are frequently the products of such unions. Indeed, the rarer the phenotype, the greater is the relative proportion of consanguineous matings. This is a natural consequence of Mendelian heredity, a fact so widely accepted now that one of the criteria of inheritance associated with a single, completely recessive rare, autosomal gene is that there be an increase in the incidence of consanguinity among the parents of affected individuals. Second, it is clear that continued inbreeding must increase the frequency of homozygous classes within a population, and thereby increase the genetic variance in the absence of selection. But are either of these observations important considerations in cancerogenesis?

Knudson, et al. (6) argue that virtually all human cancers occur in a heritable as well as a nonheritable form. Most seemingly simply inherited malignancies appear, however, to be rare, autosomal dominant traits, like retinoblastoma, multiple polyposis of the colon, and the like (8). No one of the common malignant neoplasias is unequivocally identified with an increase in consanguineous marriages, although leukemia has been so reported (7). Small but possibly significant increases can, of course, go undetected, for if the coefficient of inbreeding is small relative to the frequency of the gene of interest, the increase in homozygosis that occurs with inbreeding will also be small, and a substantial sample size will be needed to demonstrate that an effect is, in fact, occurring. There are, of course, some rare recessive phenotypes with an increased risk of malignant neoplasia, (e.g., xeroderma pigmentosum), and the anticipated inbreeding effect is observed (8). Are there, however, more general effects ascribable to homozygosity per se?

We know that inbred strains of mice reared under ostensibly comparable circumstances differ significantly in cancer experiences. The same also holds true for many other laboratory animals as well, but does it hold true for human populations? Do, for example, the Amish or the Hutterites have different susceptibilities to malignancy than populations within the United States or Canada which are presumably less homozygous? If such differences do exist, can one ascribe them without qualification to increased homozygosis, or are they a reflection of differences in life styles that so frequently accompany the social or religious isolation which leads to the increased inbreeding (4)? A meaningful choice now between these alternatives is improbable for numerous reasons. Increased homozygosis is primarily a phenomenon of small populations, but efforts to estimate rates in such populations are notoriously difficult and variable. Data collected on larger populations, states, or nations are unlikely to be informative, however, since these political entities are collections of populations and the structure inherent in the true biologic units is likely to be lost. The levels of inbreeding that obtain in human populations, even those which are relatively inbred, are low (the average coefficient of inbreeding is invariably less than 0.05) when contrasted with those commonly seen in laboratory or domestic animals. Studies that may illumine these issues include (a) genealogical investigations in those populations or communities, such as the Mormons (M. Skolnick, *this volume*), Cajuns, or Iceland (3), where sufficient genealogic data exist to examine familial aggregation of neoplasia in randomly selected genealogies, and (b) scrutiny of those populations known to be more inbred than most, e.g., parts of India, Japan, or Nubia. Carcinoma of the esophagus, for example, has been observed to have a high incidence among the Saudi (1), but it is not clear whether this reflects environmental or genetic factors, or both. Many of the Saudi are or have been polygamous, and consanguineous marriages have often been favored. Liver cancer among the Bedouins presents a similar story (5). Other areas of high frequency that do not share these demographic characteristics are, however, known to exist. Does this imply that the genetic attributes of the population are of secondary importance? Clearly, even within inbred populations, it is still important to demonstrate that there is a functional relationship between the degree of inbreeding and the occurrence of disease if a hypothesis of homozygosis is to be invoked. Simple associations, although possibly titillating, are not sufficient evidence of causality. It should be noted, here, that a concomitant of an increase in homozygosis is a decline in heterozygosity. Thus, if there is validity to the argument that those individuals who are heterozygous for the rare genes that in homozygous form give rise to the simply inherited diseases such as xeroderma pigmentosum are at increased risk of other cancers, then inbred populations should exhibit lesser rates of the common cancers albeit higher ones of those malignancies associated with the rare recessive disorders.

At the codon level, most, if not all, mutations are biochemically unique, though many are functionally similar. An interesting implication of this is that so-called homozygotes that arise from nonconsanguineous unions may not really be homozygous, but in fact heterozygous for two functionally similar, but not identical, mutants. Thus, "true homozygosis" can be assumed without risk only when inbreeding occurs. This suggests that there may exist differences, say, between the individual with xeroderma pigmentosum who is the offspring of a mating of first cousins and the one who is not. One would expect the variability among cases of a given disorder that arise from consanguineous matings to be less than that among nonconsanguineous ones, since fewer genes are sampled in the former instance. These differences might manifest as differences in segregation rates secondary to differences in survivorship, severity of disease, and its biochemical manifestation. It is worth noting here that, when a rare recessive disorder occurs in an isolated inbred population, it is highly probable that all affected individuals share the same mutant, even though a clear connection between one case and another may not be establishable. Thus, inbred populations provide a means whereby numerous replications of the same mutant may be readily studied.

Finally, although the cancer burden in human populations ascribable to single gene disorders appears small (2,8), to the extent that the inducibility of aryl hydrocarbon hydroxylase can serve as a paradigm of the genotype–environment interaction which many of us hold to be so important in the etiology of cancer, it warrants noting that inbreeding that increases homozygosis could increase the frequency of neoplasia through the relative increase of individuals who respond unfavorably to a lesser level of environmental stimulation.

REFERENCES

1. Abdul Razek, M. S., and Nassar, V. H. (1974): Carcinoma of the esophagus in the Middle East. *Lab. Med. J.*, 28:149–158.
2. Anderson, D. E. (1975): Familial susceptibility. In: *Persons at High Risk of Cancer*, edited by J. F. Fraumeni, Jr., pp. 39–54. Academic Press, New York.
3. Bjarnason, O., and Magnusson, M. (1975): Linkage of the Icelandic cancer registry to an Icelandic population file. *Recent Results Cancer Res.*, 50:90–97.
4. Cross, H.E., Kennel, E.E., and Lilienfeld, A.B. (1968): Cancer of the cervix in an Amish population. *Cancer*, 21:102–108.
5. Gussarsky, J., Gross, M., and Goldberg, G. M. (1970): Liver cancer in Bedouins of the Negev. *Pathol. Microbiol. (Basel)*, 35:184–188.
6. Knudson, A. G., Strong, L. C., and Anderson, D. E. (1973): Heredity and cancer in man. *Prog. Med. Genet.*, 9:113–158.
7. Kurita, S., Kamei, Y., and Ota, K. (1974): Genetic studies on familial leukemia. *Cancer*, 34:1098–1101.
8. Mulvihill, J.J. (1975): Congenital and genetic diseases. In: *Persons at High Risk of Cancer*, edited by J.F. Fraumeni, Jr., pp. 3–38. Academic Press, New York.

Genetics of Human Cancer, edited by J. J. Mulvihill, R. W. Miller, and J. F. Fraumeni, Jr. Raven Press, New York, 1977.

3

Prospects for Population Oncogenetics

M. Skolnick

Department of Medical Biophysics and Computing, University of Utah, Salt Lake City, Utah 84132

Studies of familial predisposition to cancer have shown increased risk for cancer in relatives in some instances and the presence of single mutant genes in others. The lack of a population base in these studies precludes a rigorous analysis that could indicate a mechanism of carcinogenesis or what the underlying genetic model might be. We believe that a population-based study of the familial incidence of human cancer will elucidate some of these mechanisms. In this discussion, we review several studies that are in progress and present some preliminary results from the Utah project that demonstrate the type of insights into cancer etiology that can be derived principally from population-based studies.

Genetic factors may influence the course of malignant tumors by interacting with either the development or the elimination of malignant cell lines (7). These cell lines may start from normal cells through transformation by viruses or other carcinogens. They may also start if a transformation locus is inherited (9) and the homologous chromosome of the cell has a mutation, perhaps caused by a carcinogen, at the same locus. Sporadic cases of the same cancer can appear if two mutations occur in the same cell at the transformation locus (16). Malignant cell lines are then propagated and in some cases eliminated by the immune system. Thus, genetic predisposition to cancer may involve genes that affect the virulence of viruses, the metabolism of potential carcinogens, inheritance of a transforming gene, ability to propagate malignant cell lines, and the ability to eliminate these lines. By studying genetic predispositions for all types of cancer in a single population, we hope that the magnitude and the nature of the familial predispositions can be recognized and that this, in turn, can help us understand where in the above process genes are having their effect.

RESEARCH RESOURCES FOR POPULATION ONCOGENETICS

The study of genetic predispositions for cancer in an entire population requires special population characteristics, complete genealogical data, and accurate

19

medical information for the current generation (such as a comprehensive tumor registry). Genealogical information on large populations can be provided by several kinds of sources. The genealogy of an area can be reconstructed from parish registers of baptisms, burials, and marriages. This had been done for the Parma Valley (3,4,24-28), but in this particular area, the medical records are too diffuse to be used for the above purpose. Dr. W. J. Schull *(personal communication)* is applying these techniques to the Mexican-American community of Laredo, Texas, and they could be used wherever there is a relatively closed population with both good parish registers and medical information. A similar effort, using the vital registers and census material of Iceland (5,6), will be of particular interest because the low levels of migration make this population conform very closely to the criteria of being closed. Initial studies of ABO blood group in stomach cancer from this resource are inconclusive (6). Perhaps the most accessible source of this type of data is the Genealogical Society of the Church of Jesus Christ of Latter-day Saints (the LDS or Mormon Church) which has extensive genealogical materials for many populations.

Our initial project using their material involves creating a computerized genealogy containing approximately one million persons representing all Mormon families who migrated along the pioneer trail and settled in Utah. The Mormon population of Utah was chosen because of several unique characteristics which make it favorable for this type of study. The state was originally settled by a relatively small group of pioneers who inhabited the Salt Lake valley and started smaller settlements in other parts of the state. Until 1890 there were many polygamous marriages, and the people were extremely pronatalist, with a mean fertility per couple of seven to eight children. Thus, the original settlers are now represented by a large number of descendents. Cores of each family, typically more than a thousand descendents living today in Utah, tended to stay in the same area, and many genetic isolates exist even within larger cities. Some small towns consist of the descendents of several pioneer families where repeated marriages between families create excellent conditions for testing genetic hypotheses.

Furthermore, the population is one of the best documented in the world, having created a tremendous source of demographic material in their Genealogical Society, the largest and most active genealogical organization in the world. Founded in 1894, its primary purpose is to assist Mormons in compiling genealogical information on their ancestors. Of primary interest for this project are the more than seven million three-generation family group sheets, representing ancestors of LDS church members, and other supporting documents. To compile the family group sheets and individual records, the society has filmed and catalogued more than 75 million feet of microfilm, representing over three million printed volumes (mainly parish records and household censuses). Twenty-five million parish records have been computerized. These resources provide possibilities for extending the Utah genealogy further and for starting parallel population-based studies, particularly in Great Britain and Scandinavia.

The second major resource for this study is a tumor registry, which indicates the individuals who have developed a malignancy, the nature of the malignancy, its treatment, and the patients' response to the treatment. The Utah State Cancer Registry which we are utilizing became a statewide computerized cancer registry in 1966 and is now part of the SEER program under joint direction by Dr. C. Smart and Dr. J. L. Lyon. The registry now contains information on more than 40,000 cancer patients in Utah. Using the registry, a recent analysis of cancer incidence for Utah Mormons and non-Mormons (20) has found reduced incidence among Mormons in all smoking-related sites, plus cancer of the breast, cervix, and ovary in females, stomach in males, and colon in both sexes. Pancreatic cancer was low, and lip cancer high, for both religious categories compared with the U.S. Third National Cancer Survey, 1969 to 1971 incidence.

An additional resource is a large-scale computer system for medical research located at the LDS Hospital in conjunction with the Department of Medical Biophysics and Computing of the University of Utah. This facility, under the direction of Dr. H. Warner, has gathered extensive computerized data on more than 100,000 hospital admissions, and the system is being expanded to other hospitals. The vital statistic records are a third source for medical data, especially the death certificates which contain cause of death and are available in Utah since 1904.

PROSPECTS FOR THE UTAH RESOURCE

The first task of the Utah project is the construction of the genealogies for Utah. We are linking all Mormon families with at least one child born in Utah to form a statewide genealogy extending from 1830 to the present. This genealogy, to be created over the next two years, is being linked to the tumor registry and hospital records. Genealogies are formed by introducing three-generation family group sheets into a Data General Eclipse minicomputer, coding, verifying, and linking them on line, as well as resolving ambiguities as they appear in the linking process. There are currently 150,000 individual records in the system, with about 2,500 new entries per day. Individuals can be located in a twentieth of a second and families and pedigrees retrieved for analysis.

By linking a population-based tumor registry to a large genealogy, we can study familial clusters of cancers and evaluate the genetic components of each site or appropriate subdivision. Our initial study uses current medical records and only uses genealogy to express the degree of kinship between members in the current generation. Thus, we are trying to establish increases in kinship between people who have a type of cancer when compared with sets of controls which will be selected from the genealogy by Monte Carlo techniques [using a method under development by Dr. M. Klauber based on the Pike-Smith method (23)].

Pilot studies to test this method were carried out on 100 melanoma patients and 135 lip cancer patients. Ancestors as far back as great-great grandparents were traced where possible. Controls were drawn from the genealogy based on date and place of birth, and care was taken that the total number of ancestors found for cases and controls was about the same (22 of 30 possible ancestors on average). There were 31 pairs of lip cancer cases with at least one common ancestor and 10 melanoma pairs. The numbers of pairs in the controls were 25 and 10, indicating a small familial excess at best among lip cancer patients. However, when the degree of relationship of each pair was taken into account and accumulated, both the lip cancer and melanoma pairs showed about threefold increased kinship over controls. In other words, they represent a closer genetic relationship than control pairs. The results of this pilot study are included to demonstrate one method which will be used to evaluate increased familial incidence when the entire resource is computerized. This method will be applied both across sites and within sites by histological types.

A population-based study has the potential to answer questions about genetic predispositions which twin and kindred studies have left unanswered. Although genetic predispositions have been noted for several of the common cancers (11,18,30,33), notably premenopausal breast cancer (2,21), there has not been an attempt to identify all the familial predispositions of the various sites and to identify nonsite-specific familial predispositions. The studies of the various sites have been done on different populations, thus making comparisons difficult. We hope that extending the pilot studies to the 40,000 cases in the Utah tumor registry will give a much clearer definition of these predispositions.

In addition, most studies lack a precise reference population, and the detailed demographic knowledge of the population necessary to evaluate the results is often missing. For example, Dr. E. Gardner *(unpublished data)* recently found in a questionnaire sent to surviving breast cancer patients from the Utah Cancer Registry that 32% reported breast cancer in either a mother, a sister and/or an aunt. This figure, much higher than the usual estimate of familial breast cancer (about 8%), may be attributable to the large family size of Utah Mormons. Because there are more sisters and aunts available, the observed familial incidence would naturally be higher. This example illustrates the difficulty of dividing cases into familial and sporadic types without knowledge of the population characteristics. When the results of this questionnaire are related to the Utah genealogical project, a more accurate evaluation of the genetic predisposition to breast cancer can be made.

Studies of selected large kindreds are more valuable for identifying rare genetic syndromes than for evaluating the genetic component of common cancer. Researchers naturally gravitate toward the larger more obvious families, namely those with many cancer cases. Because of unclear ascertainment methods and population base, it is difficult to evaluate the relative frequency of families prone to cancer due to major genes and families with less well-defined genetic predispositions. In this manner, Warthin's cancer family (31,32), Lynch's breast cancer family syndrome (19), and Gardner's breast cancer family 107 (12,29) appear to be compatible with single-gene hypotheses. However, they could just as easily be due to several linked loci segregating in a particular family like a single-gene locus. By studying the pedigrees of all spouses and by integrating these cancer families into a population-based study, these models can be distinguished. In contrast, Gardner's kindred 144 (33) presented a similar familial cluster to kindred 107 initially, but on recent follow-up has not produced the same continued pattern of breast cancer. Such families will be useful in our later studies which will attempt to relate gene segregation (HLA, ABO, Gm, etc.), biochemical function, or enzyme polymorphism to cancer risk.

Twin studies have been conducted to evaluate genetic predispositions for cancer. Harvald and Hauge (13) have used the Danish twin registry, but because of the young age of some pairs, early deaths to one of the twins, a very low incidence of identified cancer in both the monozygous (MZ) and dizygous (DZ) pairs, and uncertain diagnosis, it is difficult to tell whether there is increased concordance of MZ twins or not. Site-specific comparisons and predispositions across sites would be even more difficult to detect because of the small number of cases.

Many other research goals have been outlined using the Utah population resource we are developing. We will attempt to relate cancer genetics to many other diseases (see, for example, ref. 22) using the computerized hospital records and death certificates. The Utah genealogy also gives us an excellent opportunity to study genetic and environmental interactions. Mormons are encouraged by their religion to avoid tobacco, coffee, tea, or alcohol, and therefore disease in a population which is relatively free from the effects of these substances can be studied. This is especially important for determining genetic predispositions, as the low level of some well-known carcinogens should emphasize the genetic component.

One of the best examples of genetic interaction with a carcinogen is the developing picture of aryl hydrocarbon hydroxylase (AHH) (1,14,15,17). The level of this enzyme appears to be genetically controlled, possibly by a single gene, and the risk of contracting lung cancer is reported to be directly related to the level of this enzyme (15). With the Utah genealogies and the Cancer Registry, we should be able to find large kindreds with high AHH levels and see what other sites or carcinogens are affected by this enzyme.

The resource will also be used to isolate cancer-prone and cancer-free families for biochemical and chromosome linkage studies, and risk factors will be calculated for individuals to try to develop more efficient screening programs. We are developing new methods to fit models to these data and calculate risk factors for individuals (8,10). The risk of being affected with genetic disease is quantified, given the disease status of related individuals and a postulated genetic–environmental model for the disease. This method allows us to compare theoretical models for cancer etiology *in vivo* using segments of the population from the genealogical resource. We will also have the opportunity to evaluate the recessive component globally by comparing cancer incidence among the inbred and noninbred segments of the population.

DISADVANTAGES

Clearly there are also drawbacks in undertaking a large population study. The data input is time-consuming, and the large file requires considerable attention. The confidentiality issue will vary with each population. In Utah the genealogy sheets are gathered from a public file, and both the genealogical and medical files are protected from malicious invasion by intricate coding mechanisms. The statistical analysis of the medical records will not jeopardize individual rights, but a problem arises when one desires to contact and study individual families. Our experience with these large, close-knit kindreds is that they are concerned and cooperative if there is an excess of cancer in one branch, and our problems arise from having too many branches of a kindred of several thousand individuals seeking out attention. Such large kindreds also require statistical theorems to optimize our search for answers to hypotheses, as it is often sufficient and necessary to examine only part of the family. For example, our initial design for chromosome linkage studies involves examining several branches for disease status and heterogeneity of the chromosome markers and using computer algorithms to determine which branch of the family is most informative for further study.

CONCLUSION

Thus, we hope that this and other population-based studies will be useful in evaluating the genetic component of human cancer, determining interactions between genes and the environment, fitting models to disease patterns, and linking specific biochemical markers to genetic disease.

ACKNOWLEDGMENT

This project was supported by National Institutes of Health Research Grant 16573, awarded by the National Cancer Institute, Public Health Service/DHEW. We would like to thank Dr. J. Mulvihill and K. de Nevers for helpful comments in revising this manuscript.

REFERENCES

1. Abramson, R. K., and Hutton, J. J. (1975): Effects of cigarette smoking on aryl hydrocarbon hydroxylase activity in lungs and tissues of inbred mice. *Cancer Res.*, 35:23–29.
2. Anderson, D. E. (1972): A genetic study of human breast cancer. *J. Natl. Cancer Inst.*, 48:1029–1034.
3. Barrai, I., Cavalli-Sforza, L. L., and Moroni, A. (1965): Record linkage from parish books. In: *Mathematics and Computer Science in Biology and Medicine*, pp. 51–60. John Blackburn, Ltd., London.
4. Barrai, I., Moroni, A., and Cavalli-Sforza, L. L. (1968): Further studies on record linkage from parish books. In: *Record Linkage in Medicine*, edited by E.D. Acheson, pp. 270–280. E. and S. Livingstone, Ltd., London.
5. Bjarnason, O., Fridriksson, S., and Magnusson, M. (1968): Record linkage in a self-contained community. In: *Record Linkage in Medicine*, edited by E.D. Acheson, pp. 62–68. E. and S. Livingstone, Ltd., London.
6. Bjarnason, O., and Magnusson, M. (1975): Linkage of the Icelandic Cancer Registry to an Icelandic population file. *Recent Results Cancer Res.*, 50:90–97.
7. Cairns, J. (1975): Mutation selection and the natural history of cancer. *Nature*, 255:197–200.

8. Cannings, C., Skolnick, M., de Nevers, K. and Sridharan, R. (1976): Calculation of risk factors and likelihoods for familial diseases. *Comput. Biomed. Res. (in press).*

9. Comings, D. E. (1973): A general theory of carcinogenesis. *Proc. Natl. Acad. Sci. USA,* 70:3324–3328.

10. De Nevers, K., Skolnick, M., Cannings, C., and Sridharan, R. (1975): A computer algorithm for calculation of risk factors and likelihoods. Technical report no 1. Department of Medical Biophysics and Computing, University of Utah.

11. Fraumeni, J. F., Jr. (1973): Genetic factors. In: *Cancer Medicine,* edited by J. F. Holland and E. Frei, pp. 7–15. Lea & Febiger, Philadelphia.

12. Gardner, E. J., and Stephens, F. E. (1950): Breast cancer in one family group. *Am. J. Hum. Genet.,* 2:30–40.

13. Harvald, B., and Hauge, M. (1958): Catamnestic investigation of Danish twins; survey of 3100 pairs. *Acta Genet.,* 8:287–294.

14. Kellermann, G. Luyten-Kellermann, M., and Shaw, C.R. (1973): Genetic variation of aryl hydrocarbon hydroxylase in human lymphocytes. *Am. J. Hum. Genet.,* 25:327–331.

15. Kellermann, G., Shaw, C.R., and Luyten-Kellermann, M. (1973): Aryl hydrocarbon hydroxylase inducibility and bronchogenic carcinoma. *N. Engl. J. Med.,* 289:934–937.

16. Knudson, A. G., Strong, L. C., and Anderson, D. E. (1973): Heredity and cancer in man. *Prog. Med. Genet.,* 9:113–157.

17. Kouri, R. E., Ratrie, H., and Whitmire, C. (1973): Evidence of a genetic relationship between susceptibility to 3-methylcholanthrene-induced subcutaneous tumors and inducibility of aryl hydrocarbon hydroxylase. *J. Natl. Cancer Inst.,* 51:197–200.

18. Lynch, H. T. (1967): *Hereditary Factors in Carcinoma.* Springer-Verlag, New York.

19. Lynch, H. T., Krush, A. J., and Guirgis, H. (1973): Genetic factors in families with combined gastrointestinal and breast cancer. *Am. J. Gastroenterol.,* 59:31.

20. Lyon, J. L., Klauber, M. R., Gardner, J. W., and Smart, C. R. (1976): Variation in cancer incidence by religion: Utah 1966–1970. *N. Engl. J. Med.,* 294:129–133.

21. Macklin, M. T. (1959): Comparison of the number of breast-cancer deaths observed in relatives of breast-cancer patients, and the number expected on the basis of mortality rates. *J. Natl. Cancer Inst.,* 22:927–951.

22. Miller, R. W. (1966): Relation between cancer and congenital defects in man. *N. Engl. J. Med.,* 275:87–93.

23. Pike, M. D., and Smith, P. G. (1974): A case-control approach to examine diseases for evidence of contagion, including diseases with long latent periods. *Biometrics,* 30:263–280.

24. Skolnick, M. (1971): A computer program for linking historical records. *Historical Methods Newsletter,* 4:4.

25. Skolnick, M. (1973): Resolution of ambiguities in record linking. In: *Identifying People in the Past,* edited by E. A. Wrigley, pp. 102–127. Edward Arnold, Ltd., London.

26. Skolnick, M. (1975): The construction and analysis of genealogies from parish registers with a case study of Parma Valley, Italy. Ph.D. thesis.

27. Skolnick, M., Cavalli-Sforza, L. L., Moroni, A., Siri, E., and Soliani, L. (1973): A reconstruction of historical persons from the parish registers of Parma Valley, Italy, *Genus,* 24:103–155.

28. Skolnick, M., Moroni, A., Cannings, C., and Cavalli-Sforza, L. L. (1971): The reconstruction of genealogies from parish registers. In: *Mathematics in the Archaeological and Historical Sciences,* edited by F. R. Hodson, pp. 319–334. Edinburgh University Press, Edinburgh.

29. Stephens, F. E., Gardner, E. J., and Woolf, C. M. (1958): A recheck of kindred 107 which has shown a high frequency of breast cancer. *Cancer,* 11:967–972.

30. Tokuhata, G. K. (1964): Familial factors in human lung cancer and smoking. *Am. J. Public Health,* 54:24–32.

31. Warthin, A. S. (1913): Heredity with reference to carcinoma. *Arch. Intern. Med.,* 12:546–555.

32. Warthin, A. S. (1925): The further study of a cancer family. *J. Cancer Res.,* 9:279–286.

33. Woolf, C. M., and Gardner, E. J. (1951): The familial distribution of breast cancer in a Utah kindred. *Cancer,* 4:515–520.

Genetics of Human Cancer, edited by J. J.
Mulvihill, R. W. Miller, and J. F. Fraumeni, Jr.
Raven Press, New York, 1977.

4

Relevance of Twin Studies in Cancer Research

Walter E. Nance

Department of Human Genetics, Medical College of Virginia, Richmond, Virginia 23298

The growing list of monogenic cancer syndromes provides compelling evidence for a genetic predisposition to at least some malignancies. The role of inherited genetic factors in the etiology of common forms of cancer remains controversial, however, and twin studies would seem to be one logical approach to resolving this issue. The purpose of this chapter is to review the results of previous twin studies of cancer and to describe some new approaches to the analysis of data from twins that may have relevance to cancer research.

PREVIOUS STUDIES OF CANCER IN TWINS

Classical Twin Studies

In a classical twin study of a discontinuous trait such as cancer, affected probands are ascertained, and the zygosity and health status of the co-twins are determined retrospectively. If a greater concordance rate is observed in monozygotic (MZ) than in dizygotic (DZ) twins, a genetic influence is inferred. The unreliability of concordance rates derived from case reports in the medical literature is widely recognized. However, even in studies based on preexisting twin or cancer registries, there may be serious problems in defining the method of ascertainment accurately, and, as a consequence, there is no general agreement as to the appropriate method of estimating concordance rates (1,8,27). The interpretation of data from previous twin studies is further complicated by the overlap of cases reported by several investigators.

Table 1 summarizes the results of three studies of cancer in twins. The earlier studies of Busk et al. (2), and of Nielsen and Clemmesen (24) are not included in the table because they were drawn from the same population of Danish twins as those included in the later studies of Harvald and Hauge (5). Twins in the former studies were ascertained from the Danish cancer registry in 1947 and 1955, whereas those in the latter study were obtained through a systematic survey of

27

TABLE 1. *Cancer in twins: Summary of three studies*

| Study (ref. no., yr) | No. of pairs | | Concordance rate (%) | | | |
| | | | Pairwise | | Proband | |
	MZ	DZ	MZ	DZ	MZ	DZ
Jarvik and Falek (10,1962)	26	25	11.5	4.0	20.7	7.7
Harvald and Hauge (5,1963)	153	620	6.5	6.9	12.8	13.1
Cederlöf et al. (3,1970)	227	418	4.8	4.5	9.2	8.7

6,893 of 37,914 twin pairs born in Denmark between 1870 and 1910. Whether the concordance rates are calculated by the pairwise or the casewise method (27), the two large Scandinavian surveys (Table 1) agree in showing rather low concordance rates in twins of both types, with no suggestion of a significant difference between the two zygosity classes. Jarvik and Falek (10) found more evidence for a genetic effect in their small series of twins with cancer. Most of the subjects included in this study were ascertained from a panel of older twins, selected for survivalship beyond the age of 60. Conceivably, the age distribution of the sample may account for the difference in the results. Alternatively, there may be relevant genetic differences between the populations of Scandinavia and New York, or environmental differences may exist that elicit the expression of an underlying genetic variation.

Studies of Specific Neoplasms

Although the overall evidence for a genetic influence on cancer from the studies is not impressive, some authors have suggested that concordance for site may indicate a genetic predisposition to certain types of cancer (3). Data on large numbers of twins with specific neoplasms or combinations of neoplasms that have been ascertained in an unbiased manner would obviously be of great interest, particularly if the cancers were classified by histologic subtypes. Table 2 gives concordance rates for tumors at three different sites. Except for the concordance rate reported by von Verschuer (30) for a small series of gastrointestinal cancers in MZ twins, which is so high as to suggest ascertainment bias, the reported concordance rates for breast cancer and gastrointestinal cancer are relatively low, despite other evidence that genetic factors are of etiologic importance in some patients with tumors at these sites. The data on childhood leukemia were taken from two series in which affected twins were ascertained by matching birth and death certificates for two large samples of twins born in the northeastern United States (18) and California (9), respectively. Because the twins were not studied individually, the overall distribution of MZ and DZ pairs had to be estimated by the Weinberg method. An additional group of patients included in the study of MacMahon and Levy (18) who were not ascertained through the vital statistics survey has been omitted from the tabulation because the group included a concordant pair who were probands in the later study of Jackson et al. (9). In the total

TABLE 2. *Cancer in twins: Specific sites*

Study (ref. no., yr)	No. of pairs		Concordance rate (%)			
			Pairwise		Proband	
	MZ	DZ	MZ	DZ	MZ	DZ
Gastrointestinal cancer						
Harvald and Hauge (5,1963)	52	152	3.8	2.0	7.4	3.9
Verschuer (30,1956)	5	17	60.0	5.9	75.0	11.1
Breast cancer						
Harvald and Hauge (5,1963)	19	41	10.5	7.3	19.0	13.6
Verschuer (30,1956)	18	37	5.5	2.7	10.5	5.3
Childhood leukemia						
MacMahon and Levy (18,1964)	18[a]	34[a]	16.7	0	28.6	0
Jackson et al. (9,1969)	8[a]	40[a]	25.0	0	46.0	0

[a] Estimated by Weinberg's method.

sample of 100 twin pairs, all five concordant pairs were like-sexed, and whenever additional observations were available, they suggested monozygosity. The estimated number of MZ pairs in the pooled sample was 26. Although the data are consistent with a prenatal origin of some cases of childhood leukemia, as noted by Zuelzer and Cox (31), this does not necessarily imply an inherited genetic predisposition to leukemia. Since MZ twins often share a common placental blood supply, the observed concordance could reflect a single postzygotic prenatal oncogenic event. To support this view, Zuelzer and Cox compiled the reported age of onset for 21 pairs of twins with concordant leukemia described in the medical literature. In more than half the pairs, leukemia was diagnosed during the first year of life, in contrast to the usual peak between 3 and 5 years for childhood leukemia. However, even if concordance merely indicates that the leukemogenic event occurred before birth, these cases do provide an interesting insight into the pathogenesis of acute leukemia of childhood. The fact that in at least one concordant pair reported by McMahon and Levy (18) the diagnosis was not made until the twins were 7 years old suggests that acute leukemia of childhood may sometimes have a protracted latent period (4).

The two population-based studies also illustrate the unreliability of concordance rates taken from individual case reports. In a recent survey of the world literature Keith and Brown (12) found that among 29 MZ twin pairs with leukemia, both twins were affected in 17 pairs. Among 11 MZ pairs in which leukemia was diagnosed in the neonatal period, 10 were reported to be concordant. Finally, among all the reported cases in their review only seven of the 62 pairs were unlike-sexed twins whereas unlike-sexed twins accounted for 37 of the 100 pairs in the population-based studies.

If placental vascular anastomoses account for high concordance for perinatal leukemia in MZ twins, the true pairwise concordance rate probably does not exceed 70% because at least 30% of MZ twins have dichorionic membranes in which vascular anastomoses are very uncommon even between monozygotic twins. When the parents of an affected newborn MZ twin with leukemia are counseled, a knowledge of the disposition of the fetal membranes is obviously of importance in assigning an accurate risk figure for the co-twin. In the absence of vascular anastomosis, the concordance rate for MZ twins may not be substantially greater than that for DZ twins.

Incidence of Cancer in Twins

The question of whether cancer occurs more or less frequently in twins than in singletons is difficult to answer because of the increased infant mortality of twins, the changing incidence of both DZ twinning and cancer, and the increased exposure of twin-born infants to X-radiation during fetal life. Most authors have found a modest deficiency of twins among cancer patients (10). In a careful analysis of twin data from the Oxford survey of childhood cancers, Hewitt et al. (7) found a 9% deficiency of unlike-sexed twins and a 28% deficiency of like-sexed twins. Among twins without a history of irradiation *in utero,* the relative deficiency of like-sexed twins was even greater; indeed in this group, there were more affected unlike-sexed, 21, than like-sexed pairs, 17. The authors postulated a prenatal loss of MZ twins with cancer-prone genotypes and cited five examples of twin probands with childhood cancer whose co-twins had been stillborn to support their view. However, since like- and unlike-sexed DZ twins are expected to occur in approximately equal numbers, this hypothesis cannot explain the absolute excess of unlike-sexed pairs that was observed. An alternative possibility which should at least be considered is that there may be prenatal hormonal interactions between unlike-sexed twins that predispose to the later development of some forms of cancer.

Cancer of the Ovary in Unlike-Sexed DZ Twins

Table 3 compares the prevalence of cancer involving the sex organs for like-sexed and unlike-sexed DZ twins using data taken from the study of Harvald and Hauge (5). The prevalence of cancer of the ovary in female DZ twins from unlike-sexed pairs appears to be almost three times greater than the rate observed in DZ females from like-sexed pairs. Among 2,525 female twins from unlike-sexed pairs 17 (0.67%) had cancer of the ovary, whereas only 6 (0.23%) of the 2,608 female DZ twins from like-sexed pairs were similarly affected. As the frequency of twin-born individuals among those surviving infancy is 1.8%, of whom about 60% are DZ twins, these findings suggest that at least 1.5% of all ovarian cancers occur in women who shared their intrauterine environment with a male co-twin. Exposure of the developing female fetus to exogenous hormones is known to have oncogenic potential in the case of diethylstilbestrol, where treatment of the pregnant mother results in a vastly increased risk of cancer of the vagina in the daughter (6). Analogously, it seems possible that fetal androgens

TABLE 3. *Comparison of cancer rates for selected organs in like-sexed and unlike-sexed DZ twins*

Number of twins (individuals)		Prevalence of cancer ($\times 10^{-3}$)				
		Female breast	Ovary	Uterus	Prostate	Testis
Unlike-sexed twins						
Males	2,525	—	—	—	2.38	1.19
Females	2,525	21.78	0.73	9.11	—	—
Like-sexed twins						
Males	2,610	—	—	—	3.49	1.91
Females	2,608	16.87	2.30	12.27	—	—
Like- vs. unlike-sexed twins						
p		> 0.10	0.017	> 0.25	> 0.50	> 0.75

From Harvald and Hauge (5).

may have an oncogenic effect on the ovaries of females of unlike-sexed twins. The bovine freemartin provides ample evidence for the dysmorphogenic effects that fetal androgens can have on a female fetus (17). Although the ''freemartin'' condition does not occur in man, even in those rare cases in which vascular anastomoses exist between the placentae of unlike-sexed twins (23), this finding obviously does not exclude a delayed oncogenic effect. Other examples of prenatal interactions between heterosexual twins have been reported for birthweight (26) and enzyme levels (19) that presumably have an endocrinologic basis.

Summary

In the aggregate, studies of cancer in twins have provided surprisingly little evidence to support the view that inherited differences among individuals play a major role in the etiology of cancer. The results do not imply that genetic mechanisms or changes in the genetic material are irrelevant to cancer; nor do they exclude the possibility that certain cancers may be initiated by an interaction of the environment with multiple mutant genes, some of which may be transmitted in the germ line. It is possible that, at a genetic or molecular level, apparently uniform types of cancer may be extremely heterogeneous. Under these circumstances, individuals of a particular genotype could have a markedly increased risk, say from 10^{-4} to 10^{-2}, for a specific rare form of cancer without its ever being detected in a twin study. The recognition of genetic predispositions of this type could, nevertheless, be of great value in the design of cost effective screening programs.

NEW USES FOR TWINS IN CANCER RESEARCH

Concordance Analysis of Identical Twins

Morton has pointed out that, whereas the concordance rate of MZ twins should provide the best possible estimate of the penetrance of inherited genetic traits, sporadic and nonpenetrant cases are confounded in conditions that are etiologically heterogeneous since two parameters cannot be estimated with a single statistic (20). Nevertheless, the elegant study of Tattersall and Pyke on diabetes (29) shows how concordance in MZ twins can be used to define etiologic heterogeneity in diseases with complex causes. These authors found that among 96 MZ twins with diabetes the concordance rate was much higher in late onset than in early onset diabetes (Table 4) with nearly two-thirds of the early onset cases being discordant. Furthermore, in 75% of the concordant pairs, the interval between diagnosis had been less than 3 years whereas half the discordant pairs had remained so for more than 10 years. The authors concluded that diabetes is etiologically heterogeneous with the concordant pairs representing largely genetic cases and the discordant pairs largely environmentally determined cases. In keeping with this interpretation, a family history of diabetes was found to be more common among the concordant pairs.

Application of this approach to the study of cancer in twins can be regarded as an extension of Knudson's two-hit model (13,14), which permits the analysis of cancers involving unpaired organs. In the twin model, concordance in MZ twins replaces bilateral or multicentric disease as an indication of the presence of a germ-line mutation, which would be expected to be associated with early onset as well as an increased incidence of a positive family history of cancer. For tumors that are clearly inherited, the concordance rate in MZ twins is a measure of the penetrance. For example, if twin data were available for medullary carcinoma of the thyroid, the concordance rate in familial cases would yield an estimate of the penetrance of the gene. When combined with similar observations from nonfamilial cases, the data would permit estimation of the relative incidence of cases attributable to germinal and somatic mutation. An example of this approach is the case of familial Wilms' tumor in discordant MZ twins and one affected sib reported by Juberg et al. (11). Whereas the authors favored an environmental interpretation, Knudson and Strong (16) point out that the family history is also consistent with a genetic etiology. In families such as this, the concordance rate in MZ twins would provide the best possible estimate of penetrance.

For the special case in which penetrance depends on a second random somatic mutation, the cumulative age of onset should follow a single negative exponential

TABLE 4. *Concordance for diabetes in identical twins*

Age of onset (yr)	Concordant pairs		Discordant pairs	
	Number	Affected parent	Number	Affected parent
<40	31	6	28	1
>40	34	15	3	0
Total	65	21	31	1

From Tattersall and Pyke (29).

TABLE 5. *Age of onset in first affected twin and interval between diagnosis in 21 concordant MZ pairs with leukemia*

Age of onset in first affected twin	Interval between diagnosis	Rank order		
		Onset	Interval	Interval > 3 mo.
4 mo	0	1	1	—
5 mo	0	2	1	—
5 mo	1 wk	2	7	—
5½ mo	0	4	1	—
6 mo	1 mo	5	8	—
6 mo	12 mo	5	16	4
7 mo	1 mo	7	8	—
9 mo	1 mo	8	8	—
10 mo	0	9	1	—
11 mo	4 mo	10	13	1
2 yr 6 mo	18 mo	11	18	6
3 yr 3 mo	3 mo	12	11	—
3 yr 6 mo	5 mo	13	14	2
3 yr 10 mo	12 mo	14	16	4
4 yr 2 mo	0	15	1	—
4 yr 6 mo	9 mo	16	15	3
7 yr 9 mo	21 mo	17	19	7
45 yr	5 yr	18	20	8
56 yr	0	19	1	—
56 yr	15 yr	19	21	9
64 yr	3 mo	21	11	—

From Keith and Brown (12).

curve, as is true of bilateral familial tumors (13). However, in the twin model, an additional test of the somatic mutation hypothesis is provided by the expectation that there should be a correlation between the age of onset and the interval between onset in concordant twin pairs. A correlation is expected because the age of onset will be dominated by the intrinsic overall rate of complementary onco-genic mutations, although it may also be influenced by other factors, such as the number of target cells and the efficiency of repair, which could show considerable variation among twin pairs. On the other hand, the within-pair interval will more nearly reflect the effects of the intrinsic mutation rate. These relationships are illustrated by the data shown in Table 5, which gives the age of onset of the first affected twin and interval between diagnosis for 21 pairs of twins who were concordant for leukemia. The mean ages of onset ranged between 4 months and 64 years and the intervals between diagnosis from less than 1 week to 15 years. A nonparametric rank correlation test for the entire data set showed $r = 0.398$, 19 DF, which falls short of significance at the 5% level. However, inspection of the data shows that throughout the whole range of ages of onset, there are twin pairs in which the interval between diagnosis is very short. If all cases in which the interval between diagnosis was less than 4 months are omitted, the rank correlation in the remaining nine pairs is substantially increased to $r = 0.725$ (7 DF

$p < 0.05$). The omissions include four older pairs as well as eight pairs in which the initial age of onset was less than 1 year, which, as noted previously, may arise from a single prenatal oncogenic process. These findings raise the possibility that leukemia in concordant twins may be etiologically heterogeneous. In one group, there is a correlation between age of onset and interval between diagnosis as predicted by the two-hit model, whereas in another group, the interval between onset is very short regardless of the age of onset. In this group, single gene mutations, environmental factors, or some other mechanism may govern the penetrance and age of onset. No consistent histologic pattern was apparent in the four older pairs with short intervals between diagnosis. They included pairs who were concordant for chronic lymphocytic, chronic myelocytic, acute lymphocytic, and acute myelocytic leukemia, respectively.

Analysis of the Families of Identical Twins

The significance of host factors in cancer susceptibility is an important question from both a practical and theoretic point of view. If all individuals who are exposed to oncogenic agents are not equally liable to develop cancer, identification of specific genetic risk factors could provide the basis for an effective program of screening and disease prevention. Host factors that could contribute to cancer liability include variation in the efficiency of genetic repair mechanisms, variation in relevant immune mechanisms, or variation in the metabolism of potentially oncogenic compounds. A new model has recently been described for the genetic analysis of continuously distributed metric traits of this type (21,22). The method involves a systematic study of the families of identical twins. These families include individuals who share one-quarter of their genes (the offspring of the twins who are related to each other in the same way as half-sibs), half their genes (the full-sib relationship), all the genes (the MZ twins), and none of their genes (the spouses of the twins). Exploitation of these and other unique relationships that exist with these families permits the resolution of genetic and environmental influences and a partitioning of the genetic variance into its additive, dominant, epistatic, and maternal effects. Table 6 shows the genetic interpretation of several variance components that can be derived from the genetic relationships that exist within these families. The mean squares associated with each of these variance components provides an equation of estimation from which the genetic and environmental parameters of interest may be estimated by the least square technique. In Table 7 the results of analyses of total dermal ridge count and of birthweight are given. In keeping with previous evidence, the analyses demonstrate that total ridge count is determined largely by additive genetic factors, whereas maternal effects make a major contribution to the observed variation in birthweight. Application of this model could permit an accurate estimation of the relative contributions of genetic and environmental factors to any quantitative trait that is thought to influence cancer risk.

TABLE 6. *Genetic interpretation of variance components derived from relationships in families of MZ twins*

Variance component		Constituent genetic and environmental variance components						
		V_A	V_D	V_{AA}	V_M	V_{EH}	V_{ES}	V_{EW}
Offspring data								
1. $\sigma^2_A\sigma$:	Among ♂ half-sibships	1/4	0	1/16	0	1	0	0
2. $\sigma^2_B\sigma$:	Between sibships— Within ♂ half-sibships	1/4	1/4	3/16	1	0	1	0
3. σ^2_W :	Within sibships	1/2	3/4	3/4	0	0	0	1
4. σ^2_B♀:	Between sibships— Within ♀ half-sibships	1/4	1/4	3/16	0	0	1	0
5. σ^2_A♀:	Among ♀ half-sibships	1/4	0	1/16	1	1	0	0
Parental data								
6. σ^2_{AT}:	Among twin pairs	1	1	1	1	1	0	0
7. σ^2_{WT}:	Within twin pairs	0	0	0	0	0	1	1
8. σ^2_{HW}:	Husband–wife covariance	0	0	0	0	1	1	0
9. σ^2_{SS}:	Spouse-spouse covariance	0	0	0	0	1	0	0

V_A, V_D, V_{AA}, V_M = additive, dominant, epistatic, and maternal components of the genetic variance; V_{EH}, V_{ES}, V_{EW} = environmental variance components.

Studies of Discordant MZ Twins

Twins who are discordant for cancer provide a unique opportunity to study simultaneously a single human genotype before and after the onset of cancer. If cancer is assumed to arise from an acquired change in the genetic material or from an environmental cause, comparison of an affected individual with a twin who is identical in every way except for that change should facilitate the recognition of very subtle differences. In contrast, if the cancer is caused by a genetic predis-

TABLE 7. *Genetic analysis of data on total ridge count and birthweight from families of identical twins*

Variable	No. of half-sibships	No. of offspring	Genetic and environmental variance components		
			V_A	V_M	V_{EW}
Birthweight	57	308			
Component estimate			44,230	74,283	168,862
Standard error			±46,200	±31,582	±26,290
Total variance (%)			15.4	25.8	58.8
Ridge count	64	302			
Component estimate			1,777	68	431
Standard error			±258	±219	±75
Total variance (%)			78.1	3.0	18.9

position, careful study of the unaffected co-twin may reveal preexisting or early diagnostic signs or symptoms. Osborne and DeGeorge's analysis of infectious disease in twins with cancer is an example of this type of study (25). A medical history of previous viral and nonviral infections was elicited from 46 pairs of MZ twins who were discordant for benign or for malignant neoplasms. As shown in Table 8 the twin pairs with benign tumor showed no difference in prior illness with either viral or nonviral infections. However, among 16 pairs of twins who were discordant for malignant disease as well as discordant for their history of viral illnesses, the twin affected with cancer had the positive history of viral illness in 14 cases, while the reverse was true in two pairs. No similar effects were observed for nonviral infections. Although not shown in the table, it was of interest that in none of eight pairs who were concordant for neoplastic disease was there a history of discordance for viral illnesses. Although there are obviously many potential biases in anamnestic studies of this type, conceivably careful immunologic testing could provide objective evidence for the apparent differences in prior exposure to viral illness.

In some cases, the careful study of individual twin pairs has provided important information about the pathogenesis of cancer. Several pairs of identical twins have now been described who were discordant both for chronic myelogenous leukemia and for the Philadelphia chromosome, strongly suggesting that this chromosome rearrangement is postzygotic in origin (15). In a similar manner, the demonstration by Spiegelman et al. of viral specific DNA in the leukocytes of the affected member of two discordant MZ twin pairs with leukemia provides compelling evidence for the etiologic significance of the finding (28). If we knew what to look for, similar insights could doubtless be derived from other twins who are discordant for cancer, and the systematic study of twin pairs of this type would seem to be a very promising area of clinical research.

TABLE 8. *Distribution of disease in twins discordant for neoplastic and infectious disease*

Type of disease	Twin I Twin II	Neoplasia/ infection + + − −	Neoplasia/ infection + − − +	χ^2	p
Malignant neoplasia					
Viral infections		14	2	7.56	<0.01
Other infections		6	5	0.09	>0.5
Benign neoplasia					
Viral infections		6	6	0.00	>0.5
Other infections		3	4	0.14	>0.5

From Osborne and DeGeorge (25).

CONCLUSION

In conclusion, although the existence of numerous monogenic syndromes has firmly established the importance of genetic factors in the etiology of certain rare forms of cancer, twin studies have provided surprisingly little evidence that inherited genetic differences are of major importance as an immediate cause of most common cancers. In contrast, twin and twin family studies hold great promise for the genetic analysis of quantitative risk factors, and the systematic investigation of identical twins who are discordant for cancer provides a unique opportunity to identify genetic and environmental factors that are of etiologic importance in specific forms of cancer.

ACKNOWLEDGMENTS

This is paper No. 12 from the Department of Human Genetics of the Medical College of Virginia, Richmond, Virginia 23298, and was supported in part by Grant No. HD-10291 from the National Foundation–March of Dimes and the MCV–VCU Cancer Center. I gratefully acknowledge the advice of Dr. Roger Flora and Dr. John Mulvihill and the assistance of Phyllis Winter.

REFERENCES

1. Allen, G. (1965): Twin research: Problems and prospects. *Prog. Med. Genet.,* 4:242–269.
2. Busk, T., Clemmesen, J., and Nielsen, A. (1948): Twin studies and other genetical investigations in the Danish cancer registry. *Br. J. Cancer,* 2:156–163.
3. Cederlöf, R., Floderus, B., and Friberg, L. (1970): Cancer in MZ and DZ twins. *Acta Genet. Med. Gemellol. (Roma),* 19:69–74.
4. Clarkson, B. D., and Boyse, E. A. (1971): Possible explanation of the high concordance for acute leukemia in monozygous twins. *Lancet,* 1:699–701.
5. Harvald, B., and Hauge, M. (1963): Heredity of cancer elucidated by a study of unselected twins. *JAMA,* 186:749–753.
6. Herbst, A. L., Ulfelder, H., and Poskanzer, D. C. (1971): Adenocarcinoma of the vagina: Association of maternal stilbestrol therapy with tumor appearance in young women. *N. Engl. J. Med.,* 284:878–881.
7. Hewett, D., Lashof, J. C., and Stewart, A. M. (1966): Childhood cancer in twins. *Cancer,* 19:157–161.
8. Hrubec, Z., and Allen, G. (1975): Methods and interpretation of twin concordance data. *Am. J. Hum. Genet.,* 27:808–809.
9. Jackson, E. W., Norris, F. D., and Klauber, M. R. (1969): Childhood leukemia in California-born twins. *Cancer,* 23:913–919.
10. Jarvik, L. F., and Falek, A. (1962): Comparative data on cancer in aging twins. *Cancer,* 15:1009–1018.
11. Juberg, R. C., St. Martin, E. C., and Hundley, J. R. (1975): Familial occurrence of Wilms' tumor: Nephroblastoma in one of monozygous twins and in another sibling. *Am. J. Hum. Genet.,* 27:155–164.
12. Keith, L., and Brown, E. (1971): Epidemiologic study of leukemia in twins (1929-1969). *Acta Genet. Med. Gemellol. (Roma),* 20:9–20.
13. Knudson, A. G. (1971): Mutation and cancer: Statistical study of retinoblastoma. *Proc. Natl. Acad. Sci. USA,* 68:820–823.
14. Knudson, A. G. (1975): Genetics of human cancer. *Genetics,* 79 (Suppl.): 305–316.
15. Knudson, A. G., Strong, L. C., and Anderson, D. E. (1973): Heredity and cancer in man. *Prog. Med. Genet.,* 9:113–158.

16. Knudson, A. G., and Strong, L.C. (1975): Familial Wilms' tumor. *Am. J. Hum. Genet.,* 27:809–810.
17. Lillie, F. R. (1917): The freemartin: A study of the action of sex hormones in the fetal life of cattle. *J. Exp. Zool.,* 23:371–452.
18. MacMahon, B., and Levy, M. A. (1964): Prenatal origin of childhood leukemia. *N. Engl. J. Med.,* 270:1082–1085.
19. McCune, S. A. (1974): T-RNA synthetase from erythrocytes and placentae of normal twins. PhD thesis, Indiana University, pp. 1–152.
20. Morton, N. E. (1962): Segregation and linkage. In: *Methodology in Human Genetics,* edited by W. J. Burdette, pp. 17–52. Holden-Day, San Francisco.
21. Nance, W. E. (1976): Genetic studies of the offspring of identical twins. *Acta Genet. Med. Gemellol. (Roma). (in press).*
22. Nance, W. E., Nakata, M., Paul, T. D., and Yu, P. (1974): The use of twin studies in the analysis of phenotypic traits in man. In: *Congenital Defects: New Directions in Research,* edited by D. T. Janerich, R. G. Skalko, and J. H. Porter, pp. 23–49. Academic Press, New York.
23. Nichols, J. W., Jenkins, W. J., and Marsh, W. L. (1957): Human blood chimeras: A study of surviving twins. *Br. Med. J.,* 1:1458.
24. Nielsen, A., and Clemmesen, J. (1957): Twin studies in the Danish cancer registry, 1942-55. *Br. J. Cancer,* 11:327–336.
25. Osborne, R. H., and DeGeorge, F. V. (1967): Cancer and contagious disease in twins, *Cancer,* 20:263–270.
26. Ounsted, M. (1972): Gender and intrauterine growth. In: *Gender Differences: Their Ontogeny and Significance,* edited by C. Ounsted and D. C. Taylor, pp. 177–201. Churchill Livingstone, Edinburgh.
27. Smith, C. (1974): Concordance in twins: Methods and interpretation. *Am. J. Hum. Genet.,* 26:454–466.
28. Spiegelman, S., Axel, R., Baxt, W., Kufe, D., and Schlom, J. (1975): The molecular genetics of human cancer and its etiologic implications. *Genetics,* 79 (Suppl.):317–338.
29. Tattersall, R. B., and Pyke, D. A. (1972): Diabetes in identical twins. *Lancet,* 2:1120–1125.
30. Von Verschuer, O. F. (1956): Cancer in twins. *Ger. Med. Mon.,* 1:302–304.
31. Zuelzer, W. W., and Cox, D. E. (1969): Genetic aspects of leukemia. *Semin. Hematol.,* 6:228–249.

Discussion

Hecht: Dr. Miller suggested that the increased IgG levels in blacks protect against one kind of tumor but predispose to another later in life. Is there any evidence that persons with heritable tumors of one type are protected against tumors of another type?

Miller: I know of none. My suggestion was based on traditional medical school training: try to account for all of the patient's signs and symptoms by one diagnosis. I was attempting to follow the same convention for findings within an ethnic group.

I should like to ask Dr. Schull a question. What about determining the frequency of consanguineous parentage of persons with a cancer that occurs excessively in a country where cousin marriages are unrestricted? I am thinking specifically of pinealoma in Japan. Dr. Kobayashi has 58 cases in his series. Should he determine if the parents were more often cousins than is usual?

Schull: I am sure he could. Presumably there are appropriate statistics for consanguinity rates by administrative district in Japan from the 1970 census that include questions about cousin marriages. A major difficulty may be in finding appropriate controls for comparison with the case series.

Murphy: Dr. Miller, you reported that the peak in leukemia mortality among children with Down's syndrome is 3 or 4 years earlier than it is among children in the general population. It occurs to me, looking at these graphs, that there is much more positive skewness in the population with Down's syndrome. In accord with the target theory for the induction of neoplasia, a multiple-hit process may be involved, and the more hits required, the greater will be the symmetry of the distribution. Have you, in fact, tried fitting multiple-hit curves to the data that you reported for Down's syndrome as compared with the general population?

Miller: I have not, but I think it is an interesting idea, and I will ask our statisticians about it. [Subsequently, Dr. A. Lubiniecki examined the data, Chapter 7.]

Herrmann: Along the same lines, it may be that heterogeneity is a greater factor in sporadic cases than in familial cases. It would be of interest to know if the proportion of sporadic and familial cases is similar from one country to another for each of the tumors you mentioned [Wilms' tumor, neuroblastoma, and retinoblastoma].

Miller: From the data available, we cannot classify the cases as sporadic versus familial or unifocal versus multifocal. If excesses of the nonheritable form of retinoblastoma did occur in certain areas of the world, one would expect that the ratio of unilateral to bilateral tumors would be greater than it is in the United States or in other countries where there is no such excess.

Heston: Dr. Miller reported several groups that had reduced frequencies of neuroblastoma and speculated that it might be due to heavy infestation with parasites. The observation reminds me that we have an animal model for studying this. Sabine from Australia obtained mice from us, C3H-A^{vy} and C3H-A^{vy} fB strains, that have a very high incidence of hepatoma and mammary tumors. In Australia, no such neoplasms developed—not because the experiment was done across the equator but because in Australia the mice were put only on pine shavings, whereas we had kept them on pine and cedar shavings. When Sabine put them on pine and cedar shavings, he too observed tumors and concluded that cedar shavings were carcinogenic—that message has gone all over the world. Well, cedar

39

shavings are not carcinogenic. His mice failed to get tumors on the pine shavings alone because the animals became infested with ectoparasites. We used cedar shavings to keep them from getting ectoparasites, and when we put our mice on pine alone and used other methods to prevent ectoparasites, tumors developed just as they had when we used cedar shavings as protection against the parasites. It is evident that his mice failed to get tumors because they were infested [*J. Natl. Cancer Inst.,* 54:1011–1014 (1975)].

In looking at Dr. Miller's data, I thought that in some areas other tumors were reduced in frequency also, not just neuroblastoma. Is that correct?

Miller: Wilms' tumor seemed to be reduced relative to retinoblastoma, but one is then faced with the question: is the frequency of Wilms' tumor reduced, or is that for retinoblastoma elevated? We really do not know the answer because we do not have population-based data, only very rough ratios. Generally speaking, where the circumstances of life are less favorable, the frequency of neuroblastoma is low, whereas the frequencies of retinoblastoma and lymphoma tend to be high. There appears to be a reciprocal relationship between the occurrence of neuroblastoma and the occurrence of retinoblastoma or lymphoma.

Bolande: In Kenya, a high proportion of childhood deaths are due to measles, usually complicated by bacterial infection. Generally this effect is thought to be due to diminished T and B cell function related to marginal malnutrition. How does that accord with your concept of a protective factor?

Miller: If you are asking about a competing risk such as infection that might claim the life of a child destined to develop neuroblastoma before such a diagnosis can be made, the answer is yes, that is a possibility. The high frequency of bacterial complications of measles later in childhood might still accord with my speculation that the *newborn* is protected by passive immunity through maternal hypergammaglobulinemia induced by parasites that might inhibit neuroblastoma development.

Knudson: At a meeting on neuroblastoma in Philadelphia in May 1975, Dr. Voûte from the Netherlands said that two of the first three urinalyses he performed on children with Burkitt's lymphoma had very high levels of catecholamines [suggesting that neuroblastoma might be misdiagnosed as Burkitt's lymphoma].

Miller: Yes, [but such confusion could not have occurred in other places where the frequency of neuroblastoma was low, for example, India, Pakistan, or Puerto Rico].

Nance: Are there quantitative risk factors that could be measured through our model for twins? Are there, for example, simple tests that could be performed on a population basis, or at least on the basis of family studies, to quantitate the ability of normal individuals to repair DNA? Are there measures of immunologic responses that are relevant to cancer? Is there a battery of immunologic tests that can be applied in family studies to dissect the genetic and environmental components of these risk factors? [See chapter by Blattner.]

Another possibility concerns determination of the levels of mutagenic compounds in the urine. It is generally assumed that these compounds are a reflection of environmental exposure, but one could ask the question: is there a genetic component to the levels of mutagenic compounds excreted in the urine? This is the kind of problem for which twin studies would be most useful.

Miller: As I understand it, you are suggesting that a patient with environmentally induced cancer might be evaluated to determine if he is excreting a mutagen in his urine, as measured by the *Salmonella* system of Ames for example. With what patients would you start?

Nance: We would start with normal twins and their families and ask the question: is there genetic or environmental variation in the levels of compounds observed in the urine?

Miller: How about starting with patients whose cancers are known to be environmentally induced?

Nance: Well, I think that might be of considerable interest from another point of view, but I think the value of studying offspring of identical twins is that it allows you to separate the genetic and environmental influences in a way that is superior to methods previously available.

Hecht: For clinicians who are not mathematically inclined, will the panel tell us in simple terms what the risk of acute leukemia is in a monozygotic twin after his co-twin develops the neoplasm?

Fraumeni: Dr. Miller reported one of the major studies on this subject [*J. Natl. Cancer Inst.,* 46:203–209 (1971)]. I should like to ask if he has comments on the possible mechanisms involved in the excess concordance for childhood leukemia in identical twins.

Miller: A possible explanation has been offered by B. D. Clarkson and E. A. Boyse [*Lancet,* 1:699–701 (1971)], based on the diminishing concordance rates for leukemia in identical twins from 100%, when the first twin is affected under 1 year of age, to no increase above that for siblings in general when the first twin is affected after age 6. The suggestion advanced by Clarkson and Boyse was that the high concordance of leukemia among infants reflects the prenatal origins of leukemia in one twin and cross-transfusion of leukemic cells through their shared circulation. In older twins, such prenatal origins and *in utero* transplantation are less likely, and the concordance rate falls.

Nance: It should be noted that if the twins have separate placentas as is true for about 20% of monozygotic twins, the risk of concordance for leukemia is drastically reduced if the transfusion hypothesis is correct. For this reason, knowledge of the placentation would be of great importance in counseling the parents of an affected identical twin.

Rashad: In Hawaii where I work, we can make some interesting observations on cancer incidence according to racial groups. During the 1850s, many workers migrated from China, Japan, Korea, Puerto Rico, Portugal, the Philippine Islands, and the mainland United States and bred with the native inbred Polynesian Hawaiians. In 1942, a complete record was made of the population for civil defense purposes; the cohort being followed has five well represented racial groups—Caucasians, Japanese, Chinese, Filipinos, and part-Hawaiians. Data now include height and weight by age and race as well as blood type. Information was supplemented by vital statistics documents linked to the Hawaii Tumor Registry established in 1960. Results to date show that Filipinos have the lowest rates for most sites, and the highest rates vary by site. For cancer of the uterine cervix, part-Hawaiians had the highest rate of invasive carcinoma, whereas Caucasians had the highest rate of *in situ* disease. Japanese were highest for stomach cancer, Chinese for colon and rectal carcinoma, part-Hawaiians for lung and corpus uteri, and Caucasians for breast, urinary bladder, and prostate cancer.

Genetics of Human Cancer, edited by J. J.
Mulvihill, R. W. Miller, and J. F. Fraumeni, Jr.
Raven Press, New York, 1977.

5

Childhood Tumors and Their Relationship to Birth Defects

Robert Paul Bolande

*Department of Pathology, Montreal Children's Hospital, and Departments of Pathology
and Pediatrics, McGill University, Montreal, Quebec, Canada*

In recent years, varied and interesting relationships have been shown between congenital malformations and neoplasms. The extent and complexity of these relationships are beginning now to gain appreciation, as more and more associations are documented. Indeed, the kinship of teratogenesis and oncogenesis appears of fundamental importance in developmental pathobiology. Its appreciation may add significantly to the understanding of the neoplastic process. It is my purpose to examine the existing body of data concerning these relationships and to consider how in certain instances they may account for the pathogenesis of neoplastic disorders.

I shall be concerned primarily with structurally demonstrable anomalies of organs and tissues, rather than with those teratologic disorders whose primary or sole manifestations are congenital derangements or insufficiency of cell function.

TUMORS OF EARLY LIFE

General Features

In order to deal effectively with this area, we must consider the peculiarities and unique features of neoplasms of early life, distinguishing them from those occurring in adulthood. The common adult cancers arise within mature tissue; yet this phenomenon appears to occur most often in cells retaining an ability to multiply and regenerate in adulthood. Other adult cancers may arise in developmentally anomalous tissue, or their appearance is predetermined by inborn or acquired defects. The most common solid tumors of infancy and childhood are characterized by cellular features indicating an origin in abnormal embryogenesis. When malignant, they are rapidly progressive and highly lethal. The susceptibility of the

43

young host to the malignant process has been repeatedly demonstrated by an enhanced growth of transplanted tumors in young animals. Moreover, oncogenic viruses and chemical carcinogens more readily induce tumors in a young host than in a mature one (39). Paradoxically, regression and cytodifferentiation occur most often in human tumors of early life (13,15,38,129).

Human tumors characteristic of early life may be manifested by an overgrowth of well-differentiated cells and tissues, in either orderly or chaotic arrangements. The cells may be indigenous or alien to the site of involvement. Other tumors are composed of persistent embryonal or fetal tissues, indicating a failure of proper maturation or cytodifferentiation in intrauterine or postnatal life. The most important tumors of this sort are the hamartomas, hamartoses, choristomas, teratomas, and embryomas (13,129). Some tumors that are initially nonmalignant may become the seat of malignant transformation in later life. In other instances, tumors may persist in a latent or cryptic form for long periods after birth, becoming manifest later in childhood or even in adult life.

Characteristics of Major Tumors

Wilms' Tumor

General features.

Wilms' tumor is a malignant embryoma of the kidney derived from metanephric blastema. As such, it is composed of an admixture of mesoblastic stroma and primitive nephronoblastic epithelium arranged in sheets and nests containing prominent foci of poorly formed or dysplastic tubules and glomeruli. It occurs in about one out of 10,000 live births; or six or seven per year per million in children under age 15 (130). Wilms' tumor is discovered most often between 3 and 4 years of age, at which time it is extremely malignant. At this age, it accounts for about 20% of malignant tumors (51). Cure rates in tumors treated during the 1950s by nephrectomy and irradiation were on the order of 30% (115). The addition of chemotherapy to the regimen resulted in cure rates well in excess of 50% (84,115). Cure rates for cases presenting under 1 year of age have always been much better, generally over 80% (2,69).

Wilms' tumors are bilateral in 5 to 10% of cases. Bond (21) has shown that the average age of patients with bilateral Wilms' tumor is 15 months, which is much younger than the peak age of incidence of unilateral Wilms' tumor. Bilateral Wilms' tumors may develop simultaneously or sequentially. Sequential bilateral tumors, where involvement of the contralateral kidney becomes apparent some time after the treatment of an ostensibly unilateral tumor, are much less common than simultaneous bilateral tumors.

Congenital and infantile congeners of Wilms' tumor.

Primary renal tumors of infants and children are generally diagnosed as Wilms' tumor. They are thus presumed to be possessed of an implacably malignant potentiality, and are vigorously treated. In reality, this group of tumors is not monolithic, showing considerable variability in clinical behavior and morphologic characteristics, particularly when detected at birth or within the first few months of life. At this point of development, renal neoplasia is expressed in several clinical and pathologic forms, all of which are significantly less aggressive than conventional Wilms' tumor, if not completely benign. Indeed the cryptic presence of these entities in most series of Wilms' tumors has, in the past, largely accounted for the enhanced survival statistics generally recorded in cases under 1 year of age. Furthermore, careful review of the literature based on an appreciation of these lesions fails to demonstrate evidence of a truly life-threatening, metastasizing Wilms' tumor of conventional morphology occurring within the first few months of life (14,19,128). It would be foolhardy to assert that such a lesion does not exist, only that it must be exceedingly rare and not well described. A few recent reports seem to have confirmed its existence (128).

Three more-or-less distinct clinicopathologic entities are distinguishable from conventional Wilms' tumor in the first months of life (19; Table 1). The foremost of these is the *congenital mesoblastic nephroma of infancy* (14,19) or mesoblastic nephroma, sometimes referred to as fetal renal mesenchymal hamartoma (128) or leiomyomatous hamartoma (12,67). The tumor is typically detected at birth or shortly thereafter by virtue of its huge size (Fig. 1). It is predominantly composed of a fibrous or mesenchymal stroma in which bizarre and dysplastic tubules are focally and irregularly scattered (Fig. 2). The tumor is essentially benign and is curable by nephrectomy alone, although a few cases showing locally invasive and recurrent behavior have been encountered (9,19,20,40). This tumor is the most common form of congenital renal neoplasia. It was often misdiagnosed as "congenital Wilms' tumor" in the past.

Less appreciated is a group of well-differentiated epithelial nephroblastomata. These tumors are essentially monomorphic and are composed of well-differentiated, nephroblastic epithelium forming discrete, closely apposed tubules, microcysts, or papillary forms without intervening mesoblastic stroma (Figs. 3 and 4). These are also relatively benign (28).

These tumors may be viewed as cytodifferentiated kindred of conventional Wilms' tumor evolving from metanephric blastema during fetal life. As such, the neoplastic process may be initiated earlier in development than conventional Wilms' tumors.

TABLE 1. *Congenital and infantile congeners of Wilms' tumor*

Congenital mesoblastic nephroma of infancy
Well differentiated epithelial nephroblastoma
Monomorphic epithelial Wilms' tumor
Polycystic nephroblastoma or cystic Wilms' tumor
Nephroblastomatosis and nodular renal blastema

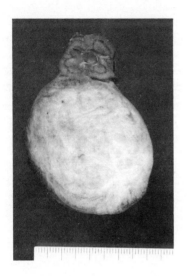

FIG. 1. Mesoblastic nephroma of infancy. This tumor was present in the kidney of a neonate. Hemisection indicates that most of the kidney is replaced by a poorly encapsulated tumor mass. The tumor is homogenously pale yellowish-gray and rubbery-firm in consistency.

In recent years, still another important type of congenital renal disease has been recognized that is referred to as *nephroblastomatosis* or *nodular renal blastema* (23,62,99). It is generally viewed as intermediate between malformation and true neoplasia. This disease is characterized by the presence of discrete subcapsular clusters of primitive metanephric epithelium (Fig. 5). Although the lesion may affect one kidney, it is more often bilateral. The nodules are often microscopic, so they are identified only as incidental findings at autopsy. These are referred to as nodular renal blastema. They are found in 1 out of 200 to 1 out of 400 pediatric autopsies under 4 months of age. After this time, they generally disappear from the general pediatric autopsy population, suggesting that many of the lesions regress.

Sometimes the lesion may be massive and confluent, replacing, in the extreme situation, the entire outer portion of the renal cortex; this is called *massive nephroblastomatosis* (Fig. 6). External examination shows bilateral renal enlargement and an exaggerated, bizarre pattern of fetal lobulation. A number of cases fitting this description have been reported as bilateral Wilms' tumor, and prolonged survival has been observed following treatment (19).

The ultimate fate and progression of nephroblastomatosis is unclear and controversial, in particular its relationship to the development of frank Wilms' tumor. A number of investigators regard these lesions as nephroblastoma *"in situ,"* emphasizing that a certain proportion of these congenital lesions may give rise to Wilms' tumor later in life (99,108).

Bove et al. (23) found foci of nodular renal blastema in about 17% of kidneys removed for unilateral Wilms' tumor. In five of these eight cases, the Wilms' tumor was bilateral. In their Wilms' tumor population, the incidence of nodular renal blastema is about 50 times greater than the general autopsy population. In a

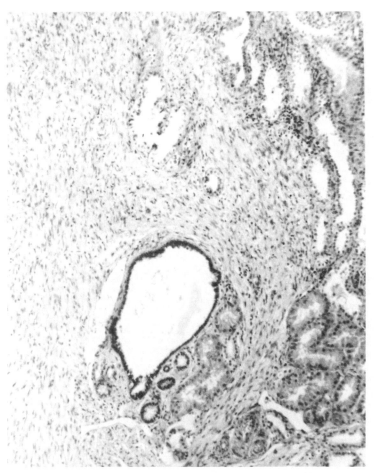

FIG. 2. Mesoblastic nephroma of infancy. The tumor is composed of a fibroblastic mesenchyme in which are embedded entrapped normal nephrons and cystic, dysplastic tubules. Note how the tumor infiltrates the surrounding kidney. There is no encapsulation. H & E stain. × 155.

recent review and expanded description of this complex of lesions, Bove and McAdams emphasized their pathogenetic relationship to Wilms' tumor by showing that multifocal metanephric abnormalities of the nodular blastemal type were detectable in all their cases of bilateral Wilms' tumor (24).

Kidneys with nephroblastomatosis often show closely associated cortical cystic and dysplastic areas. This strongly indicates that many of the primitive metanephric nodules may regress by cytodifferentiation into innocuous renal lesions (19,24).

Familial Wilms' tumor.

Familial Wilms' tumor occurring in siblings has been reported by a number of authors. Brown et al. (26) even reported cases of Wilms' tumor affecting four

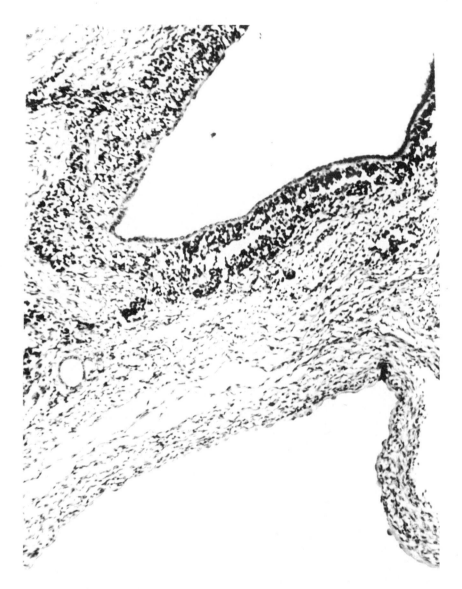

FIG. 3. Polycystic nephroblastoma (cystic Wilms' tumor). The tumor is composed of numerous large cysts often lined by flattened cuboidal epithelium. The cysts are separated by broad fibrous septae. Focally rests of primitive metanephric blastema may be present. H & E stain. × 200.

individuals in three successive generations of one family.

Knudson and Strong (71) reviewed and analyzed these familial occurrences of Wilms' tumor. They estimated that about 62% of Wilms' tumors are nonhereditary, whereas in the remainder, genetic factors are involved. In familial Wilms' tumor, the incidence of bilaterality is much greater, and the median age at

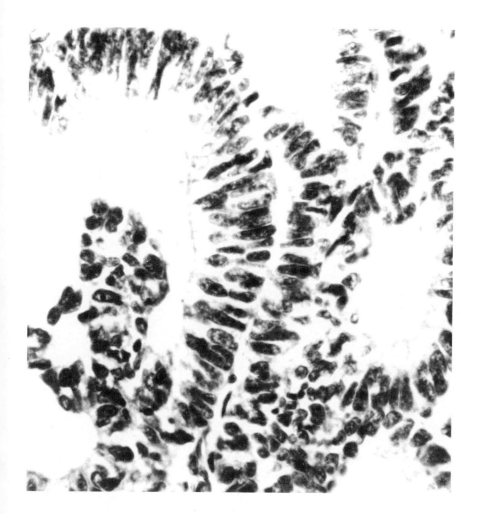

FIG. 4. Well differentiated epithelial nephroblastoma. This tumor is composed of well differentiated epithelial tubules, with no intervening stroma. The epithelial cells are well differentiated with brush borders and discrete basement membranes. H & E stain. × 1,000.

diagnosis of the tumor(s) is significantly younger. The authors hypothesized that the development of familial Wilms' tumor is partly determined by an autosomal dominant gene. It is likely that some familial cases of bilateral Wilms' tumor are in reality either diffuse nephroblastomatosis or frank Wilms' tumor arising in relation to nephroblastomatosis.

Neuroblastoma

General features.

Neuroblastoma is a clinically important and common malignant embryoma of early life estimated to occur in approximately 1 in 10,000 live births (6). Recent

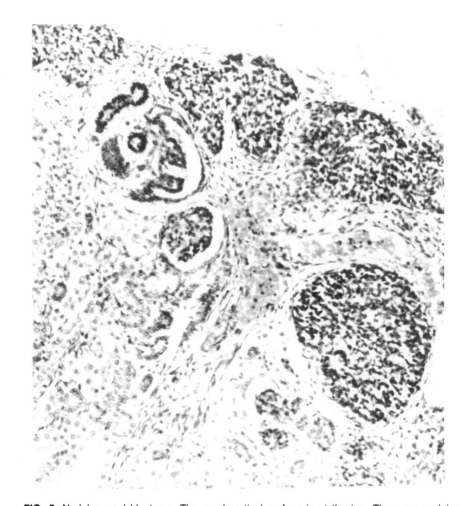

FIG. 5. Nodular renal blastema. The renal cortical surface is at the top. There are nodular aggregates of immature metanephric epithelium scattered throughout the renal cortex, mostly in the immediate subcapsular zone. Note the subjacent cystic and dysplastic nephron units. H & E stain. × 250.

studies show that it occurs at a rate of 9 per year per million children under age 15 (130).

It is formed of primitive neuroblasts derived from the neural crest. The tumor arises in the adrenal medulla or from some part of the abdominal, thoracic, pelvic, or cervical chains of autonomic ganglia. The organ of Zuckerkandl is an important extraadrenal site of origin. Although neuroblastoma may be an extremely lethal malignant tumor, particularly when it appears after 1 year of age, it is characterized by higher cure rates under 1 year of age (Table 2) and a remarkable incidence of spontaneous regression when clinically manifested at birth or within the first

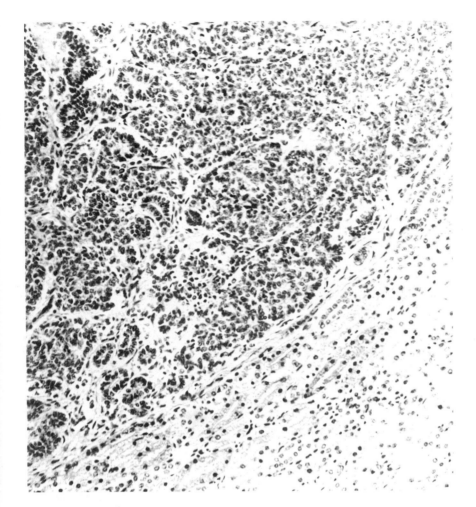

FIG. 6. Nephroblastomatosis. This is representative of the massive confluent form of the disease. In both kidneys, the blastematous foci become markedly hyperplastic and confluent, growing inward from the cortex and compressing the normal kidney tissue. This shows the deep junction of the nephroblastomatosis and normal kidney. The cells show evidence of tubular differentiation. The demarcation from the kidney is sharp. There is not as yet evidence of malignant transformation to Wilms' tumor. H & E stain. × 154.

few months of life (1,5,105,114). Spontaneous regression may heavily influence the excellent cure rates documented in this period of development.

Regression and cytodifferentiation.

Regression occurs in three fashions: disappearance by cytolysis, hemorrhagic necrosis leading to fibrocalcific residua, and cytodifferentiation to ganglioneuroma and ganglioneurofibroma. Nowhere is such regressive behavior displayed as

TABLE 2. *Survival and age in neuroblastoma*

Age of onset	2-Year (%) survival
Neonatal or congenital	62–70
Before 1 year of age	35
Second year	19
After second year	5

Data pooled from Bachmann and Kroll (1); Becker et al. (5); Schneider et al. (105,114).

dramatically and regularly as in *congenital neuroblastoma*. This phenomenon is all the more outstanding in the presence of the widespread cutaneous and visceral metastases that characterize this disease (5,100,105). Regressive behavior occurs in congenital neuroblastoma even in the presence of osseous metastases; skeletal involvement is an ominous prognostic sign in the more common forms of neuroblastoma occurring in later life (100).

Maturation to ganglioneuroma through cytodifferentiation is the best documented form of regression. Cytodifferentiation is characterized by a transformation of primitive neuroblasts into mature ganglion cells. These cells become embedded in a dense, proliferating stroma of neuroid connective tissue having the appearance of a neurofibroma or schwannoma (Fig. 7). With progressive degeneration and loss of these ganglion cells in later life, the lesion becomes virtually indistinguishable from neurofibroma. In cases where cytodifferentiation of this sort occurs in multiple foci, particularly in the skin, the condition produced closely resembles von Recklinghausen's disease (16,53).

Familial neuroblastoma.

There is little epidemiologic evidence to suggest that neuroblastoma has a heredofamilial basis, although familial recurrence has been described in some 29 cases (27,53,72). Despite the rarity of familial neuroblastoma, it remains possible that genetic factors exist in its pathogenesis, which are obscured in several ways. Knudson and Amromin (70) have hypothesized that neuroblastoma is the result of a dominant mutant gene, and that the early lethality of the disease in the past may have obscured this possibility. Today, with improved therapy, offspring of survivors may more clearly display evidence of genetic transmission of the tumor. In addition to lethality, spontaneous regression or transformation to forms no longer recognizable as neuroblastomatous in origin (ganglioneuroma, neurofibroma, pheochromocytoma) may obscure genetic factors at work (16,53).

Neuroblastoma "in situ."

The condition entitled neuroblastoma *"in situ"* merits special consideration in any discussion of neuroblastoma. Neuroblastoma *"in situ"* refers to prominent nodular aggregates of primitive neuroblasts in the central portion of the adrenal

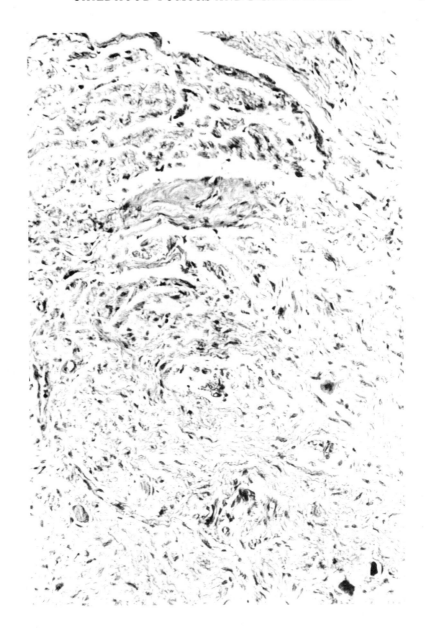

FIG. 7. Cytodifferentiation of congenital neuroblastoma. This is a skin nodule removed from a 10-year-old girl who was born with disseminated neuroblastoma. There were numerous nodules of the skin and viscera, which spontaneously regressed leaving a number of subcutaneous nodules. These are composed of schwannian or neurofibromatoid stroma. Only rare degenerating ganglion cells can be identified that are indicative of the neuroblastomatous origin of the lesion. There is now a striking pathologic resemblance to von Recklinghausen's disease. H & E stain. × 250.

glands incidentally found in perinatal autopsies (6). Depending on the intensity of search and the minimum size of the lesion acceptable to the investigator, neuroblastoma *"in situ"* has been estimated to occur at anywhere from one in 10 to one in 500 pediatric autopsies (6,54,108,119).

It is generally agreed that the nodules are no longer identifiable after 3 months of age, having either regressed or cytodifferentiated into patterns indistinguishable from the normal constituents of the adrenal medulla. A recent study suggests that such lesions are almost universally present in fetuses of 10 to 30 weeks' gestation, but generally regress following 20 weeks' gestation (119).

Neuroblastoma *"in situ"* particularly over 2000 μm in size probably represents a precursor or latent form of overt neuroblastoma (Fig. 8). If this is true, its prevalence at birth as compared to the much lower incidence of clinically overt neuroblastoma, suggests a sizable frequency of incipient neuroblastoma regression. The possibility of this pathogenetic relationship should be appreciated when attempting to delineate heredofamilial patterns and teratogenic relationships in neuroblastoma.

Neuroblastoma and the concept of neurocristopathy.

The neural crest origin of neuroblastoma, the similarity of its regressed and differentiated forms to von Recklinghausen's disease, and its occasional concurrence with that disease as well as pheochromocytoma, nonchromaffin paragangliomas, and Hirschsprung's disease place it prominently among the so-called *neurocristopathies* (18). This term has been used to designate a group of dysgenetic, hamartomatous, and neoplastic conditions, occurring as individual lesions or as constellations of multiple, variegated lesions forming distinct syndromes or complexes. These are all pathogenetically united by a shared origin in the maldevelopment of the neural crest and its derivatives.

Retinoblastoma

Retinoblastoma is an embryoma formed of the precursors of rod and cone cells of the retina. These tumors arise in the posterior portions of the inner and outer nuclear layers of the retina; may be multifocal and bilateral, and occur in about 1 in 18,000 live-born children in the United States (30). Mortality is associated with direct extension into the cranial cavity to involve the brain and leptomeninges. Hematogenous metastases to bone, lymph nodes, liver, spleen, and kidney may occur. The mortality of this tumor has been so sharply reduced by prompt enucleation of the affected globe, coupled with irradiation and chemotherapy, that many affected individuals have lived to procreate.

The tumor, being of neuroectodermal origin, shares many similarities with neuroblastoma both in histologic appearance and behavior. Spontaneous regression occurs in retinoblastoma as in neuroblastoma, and appears to be heralded by hemorrhagic necrosis of the tumor leading to fibrotic and calcified residua (13).

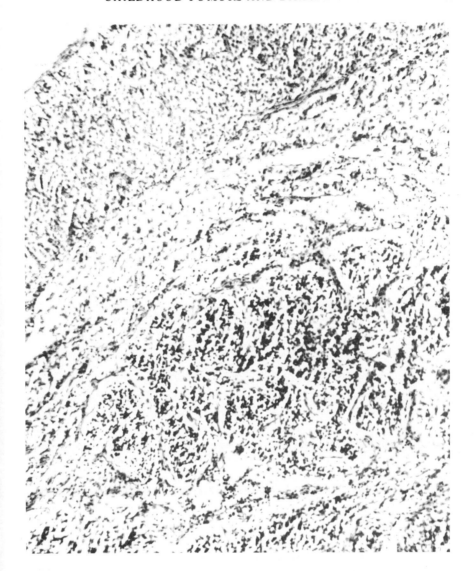

FIG. 8. Neuroblastoma *in situ*. Large mass of neuroblasts incidentally discovered in the adrenal gland of a newborn infant dying of perinatal anoxia. Note how the mass compresses the fetal adrenal cortex *(upper left)*. H & E stain. × 200.

Retinoblastoma is most notable among the embryomas of early life for its striking hereditary pattern, best shown in offspring of parents cured of the disease, particularly where the parent had bilateral tumors. In such bilateral retinoblastomas, the offspring are affected in a manner consistent with the inheritance of a dominant gene. Yet offspring of unilateral cases may also develop bilateral tumors and vice versa. Analysis of data indicates that 60% of all retinoblastomas are unilateral and nonhereditary, 15% are unilateral and hereditary, and 25% are bilateral and hereditary. In hereditary cases, the tumors tend to appear a year earlier than the nonhereditary cases (72). It must be emphasized that the majority of retinoblastomas are sporadic and without risk to the offspring of tumor, although such cases may be associated with a spectrum of malformations, especially the 13q- syndrome (66). Retinoblastoma kinships have been described, where children cured of their ocular lesions subsequently developed osteogenic sarcoma of the long bones (52,104).

Sacrococcygeal Teratoma

Sacrococcygeal teratoma is the most important teratoma clinically manifested in the newborn infant. It occurs in 1 out of 20,000 to 40,000 live births and is four times more frequent in females. Under 4 months of age, less than 10% are malignant, whereas after this time over 70% are malignant (15,48,120). Malignant growth is most often manifested as embryonal carcinoma or yolk-sac carcinoma. The development of malignancy shows no sex predilection.

Other Tumors

In addition to the examples cited above, hepatoblastoma occurring in infancy may have a better prognosis than in later childhood (64). Similarly, yolk-sac carcinoma of the infantile testis has an excellent survival following orchiectomy (97). This favorable prognosis is surprising considering this tumor's bizarre and embryonal histologic features. If the same tumor appears after 2 years of age it is very malignant. Congenital leukemia as in Down's syndrome is characterized by spontaneous remissions. The extent of spontaneous regressions in retinoblastoma has not been established.

The Benignity of Neonatal and Infantile Tumors

It would thus appear that many tumors manifest at birth or shortly thereafter display surprisingly benign behavior, sometimes despite extremely malignant cellular features; whereas a tumor of identical morphologic features in later life is highly lethal (Table 3). The realization of these facts about tumors in early life has led us to postulate that an *oncogenic period of grace* exists, beginning *in utero* and extending through the first months of postnatal life. During this time the host is resistant to the full expression or progression of malignant disease (15). Neoplasms seem repressed during this period, tending toward benignity through arrested growth, regression, or cytodifferentiation. The mechanisms responsible for this are unknown.

TABLE 3. *Tumors of infancy showing benign or regressive tendencies*

Congenital and infantile congeners of Wilms' tumor

Neuroblastoma

    Congenital and infantile neuroblastomas

    Neuroblastoma *in situ*

Sacrococcygeal teratoma before 4 months of age

Yolk-sac carcinoma of infantile testis before 2 years of age

Hepatoblastoma before 1 year of age

Congenital leukemia

Adrenocortical carcinoma with hemihypertrophy under 1 year of age

Retinoblastoma?

THE ASSOCIATION OF NEOPLASMS WITH MALFORMATIONS

General Features

It is now well established that a variety of congenital malformations are antecedents of neoplasms in man (17,124). The elucidation of many of these important relationships is largely due to the pioneering epidemiologic studies of R. W. Miller and co-workers at the National Cancer Institute (88,90).

In an analysis of 371 carefully studied cases of childhood malignant disease at the University of Tokyo (73), 41% of the children showed evidence of congenital malformation, in contrast to a 13% incidence in children without malignant neoplasms. Wilms' tumor showed the highest incidence (58%), followed by lymphoreticular malignancies (48%), hepatoblastoma (45%), leukemia (44%), neuroblastoma and retinoblastoma (35% each), brain tumors (28%), and testicular-ovarian tumors (17%). Berry et al. (10) could find no significant increase in anomalies in neuroblastoma, Wilms' tumor, and hepatoblastoma, but the search for malformation was not as detailed as in the Japanese study.

The Origin of Neoplasms in Congenitally Anomalous Tissue

An important factor predisposing to cancer in later life is the presence of developmentally anomalous tissue. Thus cancer may develop in heterotopias (fetal rests and choristomas), developmental vestiges, hamartomas, and dysgenetic gonads (13,17,129).

Tumors Arising in Developmental Vestiges and Heterotopias

Developmental vestiges are the residua of transient structures of normal embryogenesis (129). Examples of tumors arising in developmental vestiges are well established histogenetically (13,17,124,129). The craniopharyngioma develops from parapituitary vestiges of Rathke's pouch. Chordoma is derived from notochordal remnants persisting within the nucleus pulposus. Residua of the mesonephric or Wolffian ducts (vaginal adenosis) in the female give rise to a peculiar papillary adenocarcinoma of the vagina, cervix, uterus, ovary, and broad ligament in young girls. A number of very rare carcinomas have been described developing in various and sundry vestiges such as branchial cleft cysts, thyroglossal duct cysts, gut duplications, and urachal remnants.

Tumors Arising in Undescended Testes and Dysgenetic Gonads (Table 4)

Cryptorchidism affects 0.28% of the male population. The incidence of tumor is 15 to 40 times more common in undescended testes than it is in intrascrotal testes. Between 3 and 11% of all testicular neoplasms develop in cryptorchid testes (68). The most common tumor that develops is seminoma. It has been suggested that the extrascrotal testis is a minimal manifestation of disordered sexual differentiation, as undescended testes are the rule in male pseudohermaphroditism. It has been further suggested that foci of testicular dysgenesis are present in undescended testes, and it is from these foci that tumors arise in later life, typically after puberty (109).

Aberrant sexual development favors the development of gonadal neoplasms in later life. The undescended testes of male pseudohermaphrodites share the susceptibility to seminoma seen in cryptorchid normal males. Sixty percent of tumors occurring in undescended testes of male pseudohermaphrodites are seminomas (49). By contrast, Sertoli cell tumors or hyperplasias are more common in the feminizing estrogenic testes of the testicular feminization syndrome (91), although a variety of tumors of the testes may occur in this condition.

A unique form of neoplasm occurring in dysgenetic gonads is the gonadoblastoma or gonocytoma (107,117). The gonadoblastoma is defined by Scully (107) as a neoplasm containing an intimate admixture of germ cells and elements resembling immature granulosa or Sertoli cells. The cell nests and masses resemble huge Call–Exner bodies; they are subject to marked calcification. The tumor may progress into or be associated with a dysgerminoma–seminoma type of pattern. This neoplastic process is often bilateral. Less frequently, embryonal teratoma, embryonal carcinoma, endodermal sinus tumor, or choriocarcinoma may supervene. It has been estimated that gonadoblastomas and/or dysgerminomas develop in 30 to 40% of dysgenetic gonads (57,116). Most of the tumors arise in a gonad of indeterminate nature, but 22% develop in a primitive atretic ovary and 18% in a cryptorchid, dysgenetic testis (107). Eighty percent of gonadoblastomas develop in phenotypic females, often showing some evidence of virilization or primary amenorrhea. The remainder develop in phenotypic males with cryptorchidism, hypospadias, and female internal secondary sex characteristics. Buccal smears are chromatin negative in most gonadoblastoma patients, the majority exhibiting a normal male karyotype. A lesser number show an XO/XY form of mosaicism. Although some of the individuals may have one or more features of Turner's syndrome, gonadoblastomas have not been shown to occur in XO individuals. The presence of a Y chromosome in the karyotype seems to be necessary to increase the expectation of gonadoblastoma.

Bilateral benign testicular teratomas have been reported in infant brothers with 47 XXY Klinefelter's syndrome (55). The occurrence of teratomas in Klinefelter's syndrome has been reported in other individuals suggesting that this concurrence may not be fortuitous (98).

Malignant Transformation in Hamartomas

Hamartomas are often the seat of malignant transformation. This usually occurs later in life. It is difficult to determine the actual increase in susceptibility to cancer over nonhamartomatous tissue. In some hamartomas the development of cancer is striking. Thirty percent of von Recklinghausen's neurofibroma cases may develop sarcomatous transformation after age 50 (25). Virtually all patients with multiple familial polyposis of the intestine eventually develop carcinoma of the colon. Malignancy seems to be documented more frequently in genetically determined hamartoses, rather than in sporadic, isolated lesions.

The Increased Expectancy of Neoplasms in Specific Teratologic Disorders (Table 5)

Aniridia — Wilms' Tumor

Aniridia is a dominantly inherited condition affecting no more than 1 out of 50,000 of the general population (43,88,90). About 30% of cases are sporadic and are presumed to represent new germinal mutations. The presence of this congenital anomaly somehow renders the affected child prone to the development of Wilms' tumor. Aniridia is present in 1 out of 80 Wilms' tumor cases. The sporadic aniridias seem more at risk, as about a third of these develop Wilms' tumor.

Additional but less common features of the aniridia–Wilms' tumor syndrome are microcephaly, physical and mental retardation, anomalies of the genitourinary tract, recurved aural pinnae, and a variety of hamartomas including hemangiomas, exostoses, and lipomas. The risk of developing Wilms' tumor seems highest when sporadic aniridia is accompanied by genitourinary tract malformations and mental retardation.

Hemihypertrophy

Congenital hemihypertrophy is a condition characterized by gross asymmetry of the body. Although detectable at birth, it usually becomes more apparent with increasing age. It seems to occur more often on the right side. Children who are afflicted with it are at an unusually high risk for the development of one of three types of malignancy: Wilms' tumor (41,43), hepatoblastoma (44), and adrenocortical neoplasia (42,56,103). Whereas the majority of tumors develop on the hypertrophied side of the body, 30% develop contralaterally. It has also been shown that an excessive concurrence of pigmented nevi and vascular hamartomas exists with hemihypertrophy.

Some 16 cases of adrenocortical neoplasia occurring in hemihypertrophy have been described. These cases often present as an endocrinopathy—Cushing's syndrome or precocious puberty. Those patients who have their tumors diagnosed and removed under 1 year of age have a better prognosis than those diagnosed and treated later in life (56). One of the surviving patients subsequently developed a fatal Wilms' tumor (103). These observations underline the necessity of early diagnosis of hemihypertrophy and of close surveillance of affected individuals.

Meadows et al. (85) recently reported a mother with hemihypertrophy who gave birth to three children developing Wilms' tumor. The fourth child had shown no evidence of Wilms' tumor but had a double collecting system of one kidney. None of the offspring showed hemihypertrophy. These workers also documented another family with hemihypertrophy in which one child developed Wilms' tumor.

Omphalocele-Macroglossia Syndrome (Beckwith–Wiedemann Syndrome)

Beckwith et al. (7) and Wiedemann (127) independently described a complex constellation of anomalies including omphalocele, macroglossia, bilateral cytomegaly of the fetal adrenal cortex, hyperplasia of gonadal interstitial cells, renal medullary dysplasia, and hyperplastic visceromegaly in several other organs, including the kidneys and pancreas. The pancreas exhibits islet hyperplasia. In some cases, neonatal hypoglycemia is present which may prove fatal. Postnatal development may also be associated with the development of hemihypertrophy. As in isolated hemihypertrophy, Beckwith's syndrome has been found to be excessively associated with adrenocortical carcinoma and Wilms' tumor (8). Cutaneous vascular nevi may also occur.

Nevoid Basal Cell Carcinoma Syndrome

The nevoid basal cell carcinoma syndrome is another clear example of a teratologic-neoplastic syndrome. The principal features of the syndrome consist of multiple basal cell carcinomas of the skin, multiple epithelial-lined jaw cysts, and multiple skeletal anomalies including scoliosis, spina bifida, bifid ribs, fused and hemivertebrae, and dolichocephaly with prominent supraorbital ridges and frontal eminences, a broad nasal root, and bridging of the sella turcica. There may be agenesis of the corpus callosum and low intelligence. Ocular abnormalities may include congenital cataracts, coloboma, and glaucoma. In addition, there may be dyskeratosis of the palms and soles (63,106,123).

Most important is the neoplastic predisposition. Frank basal cell carcinomas may appear before 15 years of age, whereas ordinary basal cell carcinoma typically does not appear until after 50 years. In addition 20% of children with the nevoid basal cell carcinoma syndrome develop medulloblastoma at an early age (72,93). Lipomas and fibromas may also be present.

The nevoid basal cell carcinoma syndrome is inherited as an autosomal dominant with a high degree of penetrance. The syndrome has been estimated to occur in from 1 to 2% of patients with multiple basal cell carcinomas, cystic epitheliomas, and/or odontogenic cysts (72).

Genitourinary Tract Malformations with Wilms' Tumor

There is an excessive concurrence of Wilms' tumor and genitourinary tract malformations. Approximately 6% of patients with Wilms' tumor exhibit upper urinary tract anomalies including horseshoe kidneys, ectopic or solitary kidneys, hypoplastic kidney, and duplication of the upper urinary tract (65,89). These teratologic associations appear to be most common with simultaneously developing, bilateral Wilms' tumor (69).

In addition, Wilms' tumor has been described in association with male pseudohermaphroditism manifested by cryptorchidism and hypospadias (31,78,113). Baraket et al (3) have suggested that in addition to Wilms' tumor, an unusual concurrence of congenital "nephron disorders" may occur in this teratologic-neoplastic complex. Nephron disorders refer to nephropathies manifested as the congenital nephrotic syndrome and infantile glomerulonephritis. The various combinations of pseudohermaphroditism, congenital nephron disorders, and Wilms' tumor appear linked by common teratogenic factors, all affecting renal embryogenesis.

Poland Syndrome and Leukemia

An unusual concurrence of Poland syndrome and leukemia has recently been appreciated (77). The Poland syndrome consists of unilateral aplasia of the sternal portion of the pectoralis major muscle and ipsilateral symbrachydactyly (syndactyly and short digits of the hand). Thus far, at least six instances of acute leukemia have been described with this teratologic disorder.

Nephroblastomatosis, Nodular Renal Blastema, and Related Anomalies

There is a distinct association of these lesions with teratologic disorders. Bove et al. (23) showed that five of eight infants with nodular renal blastema had trisomy 18 and its characteristic constellation of anomalies including horseshoe or cystic kidneys. Bilateral nephroblastomatosis has also been described in association with splenic agenesis and malformation of the liver (122). Sotelo-Avila and Gooch have recently documented that nephroblastomatosis occurs in Beckwith's syndrome (110). Liban and Kozenitzky (79) and Perlman et al. (96) have described familial nephroblastomatosis occurring in an Israeli sibship which displayed a unique teratologic syndrome characterized by fetal gigantism, visceromegaly, hypoglycemia, hyperplasia of the islets of Langerhans, and bizarre facies. In addition to the nephroblastomatosis, some have also shown metanephric hamartomas and isolated nodular renal blastemata deep in the kidney substance. This syndrome bears a superficial resemblance to Beckwith's syndrome. Recently Mankad et al. (83) reported a case of diffuse bilateral nephroblastomatosis occurring in the Klippel–Trenaunay syndrome, i.e., cutaneous hemangiomas with bony and soft tissue hypertrophy of extremities.

As has been suggested earlier the nephroblastomatosis complex must be sharply distinguished from Wilms' tumor, and in particular bilateral Wilms' tumor. It is my impression that bilateral nephroblastomatosis or Wilms' tumor arising in it shows the most striking teratologic associations and heredofamilial tendencies.

Congenital Heart Disease and Neoplasia

Isolated case reports have appeared in the literature suggesting an association between neuroblastoma *"in situ"* with a variety of anomalies, including congenital heart disease (10), adrenal cyst (118), and trisomy D (94). Chatten and Voorhess (27) in their review of the rare instances of familial neuroblastoma, reported a kinship in which three sisters died of neuroblastoma. One of these girls had a concurrent patent ductus arteriosus and hypertrophic pyloric stenosis. An unaffected brother died in infancy of long segment aganglionosis of the colon and ileum and showed a neuroblastoma *"in situ"* in one adrenal at autopsy. In the original study of Beckwith and Perrin (6) defining neuroblastoma *"in situ,"* nine of the 13 infants they described had severe malformations; seven of these had congenital heart disease. Their observations have suggested an association of neuroblastoma and/or neuroblastoma *"in situ"* with congenital heart disease, but the concurrence has not been substantiated.

Although about six cases of Wilms' tumor associated with congenital heart malformations have been reported (47,81), excessive concurrence cannot be documented. Long-term follow-up of 779 patients who had undergone corrective surgery for tetralogy of Fallot did not demonstrate evidence of excess cancer development (92).

The case reported by Lynch and Green (81) merits some special consideration. A 6-year-old child with corrected transposition of the great vessels and Ebstein's anomaly developed fatal bilateral Wilms' tumor. The mother had Sipple's syndrome (pheochromocytoma and medullary thyroid carcinoma), one of the complex neurocristopathies (18). This seems to be a unique event.

Sacrococcygeal Teratoma and Anomalies

Hickey and Layton (61) reviewed the English literature on sacrococcygeal teratoma from 1938 to 1954, and in an analysis of 112 patients found 11% associated with congenital anomalies. The anomalies were largely along the longitudinal axis of the body (anencephaly, spina bifida, patent urachus, cleft palate, rectovaginal fistulas, meningoceles, spinal anomalies, and undescended testicles). A strong familial history of twinning was present in 14% of the cases. Berry et al. (10), reviewing the concurrence of anomalies in a series of 350 pediatric tumors, found the most significant increase in incidence in sacrococcygeal teratoma as compared to the Wilms' tumor, neuroblastoma, and hepatoblastoma groups. The associated defects included imperforate anus, rectovaginal fistula, ectopia vesicae with epispadias, tracheoesophageal fistulae, talipes equinovarus, and hydrocephalus. These anomalies, present in six out of 63 sacrococcygeal teratomas, were mainly defects of the hindgut and cloacal regions, and as such could be attributed to local growth disturbances secondary to the presence of the teratoma during intrauterine development. If these "local" anomalies are excluded, the incidence of anomalies does not significantly differ from that of the general tumor population.

More recently, Fraumeni et al. (45) also found that infants with sacrococcygeal teratoma were prone to pelvic malformations, involving the lower vertebrae, lower genitourinary system, and anorectum. In addition to meningoceles, spina bifida, sacral defects, hypospadias, and imperforate anus, recorded in other series, there were also instances of genitourinary tract and hindgut duplications or "twinnings." These workers suggested that the pelvic anomalies might be due not to local effects of tumor growth, but to some embryopathic process resulting in the teratoma.

Cytogenetic Abnormalities

Specific chromosomal abnormalities are directly related to teratologic syndromes and in selected instances are associated with an increased incidence of neoplasms (elsewhere in this volume). In addition, chromosome instability, fragility, and breakage without specific karyotype abnormality occurs in another group of teratologic and growth disorders. These recessively inherited syndromes are associated with a high incidence of neoplasms (elsewhere in this volume).

The Teratogenicity of Carcinogens

General Observations

A striking observation has emerged from the enormous body of data on experimental carcinogenesis: many agents known to be carcinogenic postnatally are teratogenic to the fetus or embryo. DiPaolo and Kotin (33) listed 26 chemical agents that had been tested for both carcinogenic and teratogenic activity in animals. Of 20 listed as carcinogenic, 19 had been shown to be teratogenic. Direct evidence for the carcinogenicity of teratogenic agents given or experienced during intrauterine life is nonetheless very limited. Stewart et al. (112) in the Oxford survey of childhood malignancies showed that the frequency of three prenatal events—direct fetal radiation, maternal virus infection, and threatened

TABLE 4. *Tumors in dysgenetic gonads*

Condition	Clinical features	Karyotype	Gonad	Tumor
Male, normal	Normal	XY	Undescended testis	Seminoma
Male, pseudohermaphrodite	Undescended testes Hypospadias Variable internal genitalia	XY or mosaics with Y chromosome	Undescended testes	Seminoma, gonadoblastoma
Testicular feminization syndrome	Normal female habitus, vagina No uterus or tubes Undescended testes	XY	Dysgenetic testes	Sertoli cell or tubular adenoma
Pure gonadal dysgenesis	Eunuchoid female habitus Uterus and fallopian tubes	XY or mosaics	Dysgenetic testes	Gonadoblastoma, dysgerminoma, seminoma
Female pseudohermaphrodite, nonadrenal	Female habitus with variable masculinization	XY or XO/XY and other mosaics with Y chromosome	Streak ovaries or indeterminate gonads	Gonadoblastoma, dysgerminoma
Mixed gonadal dysgenesis	Asymmetric gonads and internal genitalia Ambiguous external genitalia	XO/XY and other mosaics with Y chromosome	Streak or indeterminate gonad on one side Contralateral testis	Gonadoblastoma Seminoma, sertoli cell adenoma
True hermaphrodite	Variable external and internal genitalia and secondary characteristics Usually male habitus	XX or mosaicism	Bilateral ovotestes asymmetrical testis and ovary Ovotestis and contralateral ovary or testis	Dysgerminoma

TABLE 5. *Specific teratologic disorders associated with neoplasm*

Anomaly	Tumor
Aniridia	Wilms' tumor
Hemihypertrophy	Wilms' tumor Hepatoblastoma Adrenocortical carcinoma
Beckwith's syndrome	Adrenocortical carcinoma Wilms' tumor + nephroblastomatosis
Genitourinary tract malformations	Wilms' tumor Nephroblastomatosis
Nevoid basal cell carcinoma syndrome	Basal cell carcinoma Medulloblastoma Rhabdomyosarcoma
Poland syndrome	Leukemia
Mongolism (21 trisomy)	Leukemia Retinoblastoma
13 q- syndrome	Retinoblastoma
Fanconi's anemia	Leukemia Squamous cell carcinoma Hepatoma (androgen-induced)
Bloom's syndrome	Leukemia Gastrointestinal carcinoma
Ataxia-telangiectasia	Lymphoma Leukemia Others

abortion—was slightly but significantly higher for children dying of cancer than for a group of healthy children of comparable age.

Irradiation

A sizable body of information has accumulated on the postnatal oncogenicity and prenatal teratogenicity of irradiation. The data concerning the true oncogenicity of prenatal radiation are equivocal. A late increase in tumor incidence has been observed in animals and man. MacMahon (82) and Stewart and Kneale (111) have shown that a slight excess of childhood cancer appears in the offspring of mothers receiving prenatal diagnostic obstetric X-rays. An improved reanalysis of the data from the 1958 Oxford survey showed again that the relative risk for all types of pediatric malignancy was increased about 1.5 times. The risk declined as the number and dose of X-rays diminished (11).

Studies of survivors of the atomic bomb explosion at Hiroshima and Nagasaki showed that those heavily exposed to radioactive fallout during intrauterine life have not experienced an excess incidence of tumors thus far. Individuals exposed during childhood or as adults showed an excess of leukemia and other cancers (87).

Chemical Agents

The animal experiments aimed at showing carcinogenicity in the fetus, in addition to or separate from teratogenicity, are hampered by a high incidence of fetal death, abortion, and resorption, particularly when the agent is administered to the mother early in gestation or injected intraamniotically. Often in this type of experiment, the surviving offspring are not observed long enough for evidence of tumor development. The administration of dibenzathracene, urethan, benzpyrene, and alkylnitrosoamines has been followed by an increased incidence of tumors in offspring (102).

Urethan.

Urethan readily traverses the placenta and persists briefly in the fetus. Experiments in which a single dose is administered to gestating mice on sequential days of gestation make it possible to study the varying spectrum of teratogenic and oncogenic effects. Administration of urethan between 7 and 11 days tends to produce offspring with profound brain, tail, and lung anomalies. The critical period for carcinogenesis comes later, between days 13 to 17 of gestation, during which an increasing number of offspring are produced who develop multiple hepatomas and papillary adenomas of the lung; these tumors appear histologically benign and are of limited growth potentiality. The number and incidence of these tumors of the lung increase with advancing gestation until days 15 to 17 after which the susceptibility to the oncogenic effects of urethan diminishes until birth (32,95,121).

Alkylnitrosoureas.

Of great importance are the investigations carried out by Druckrey and co-workers (35,36) with alkylnitrosoureas, especially ethylnitrosourea. These alkylating agents are highly effective fetal carcinogens when given even as a single injection to gestating rats and hamsters. In 90 to 100% of offspring, multiple neurogenic tumors develop, which are evidenced by the death of the animal at 150 to 600 days after birth. The tumors involve the peripheral and central nervous systems and consist of multiple neurinomas, gliomas, and ependymomas of varying degrees of differentiation (29,35,74,125). There is a certain resemblance to von Recklinghausen's disease in the human.

The fetus appears to be 50 times more sensitive to the effect of these carcinogens than does the adult animal. In order to test the susceptibility to oncogenesis at different stages of development, a series of pregnant rats was given a single dose of ethylnitrosourea on each day of pregnancy. It was found that tumors could be induced only after the 12th day of gestation. After this time, there was an abrupt increase in tumors, the greatest number being induced between 18 and 22 days of gestation. Beginning shortly before and accelerating after birth, there was a rapid decrease in susceptibility to the carcinogenic action of the agent (74). With high intravenous doses given on the 15th day of gestation, a high incidence of malformations of the paws (oligodactyly and syndactyly) occurred in the newborns (35). The characteristic neurogenic tumors did not become apparent until 5 to 6 months after birth. On the other hand, when ethylnitrosourea was given to pregnant hamsters on the eighth day of gestation, severe malformations of the entire cephalic region, eye, and thorax developed, along with a high incidence of fetal death and resorption (50); carcinogenesis was not apparent. More recent experiments have shown that malformations of the brain (microcephaly, exencephaly, and encephalocele) can be produced by alkylnitrosoureas in rats prior to 11½ days gestation after which time no teratogenic effects could be noted (75). Diwan and Meier (34) showed that transplacental treatment of mice with alkylnitrosoureas induces tumors in several strains of mice. The most commonly produced tumors were pulmonary adenomas and leukemia. The most sensitive period for the inducibility of neoplasm was between 16 and 18 days of gestation. As the injections were begun on the 12th day of gestation, teratogenicity was not observed.

The experiments cited, which are only representative of the investigations going on with these agents, are of importance in delineating the temporal relationships between oncogenic and teratogenic reactions to intrauterine injury. It seems clear that carcinogenesis tends to be maximal in the latter stages of gestation, occurring only after organogenesis is complete. Prior to this time, teratogenesis is the prevalent response (102).

Estrogens.
The first clear example of transplacental carcinogenesis in man was elucidated by Herbst et al. (58,59). They showed that a rare and peculiar clear cell cervicovaginal adenocarcinoma developed in adolescent girls whose mothers had been given stilbestrol during their gestation for the prevention of threatened abortion. Since their original report, numerous articles have appeared confirming this association. The tumor is a papillary adenocarcinoma with clear cells (Fig. 9). It is thought to arise by malignant transformation of Müllerian or Wolffian duct vestiges known as vaginal adenosis (4,58). Vaginal adenosis is characterized by the presence of foci of endocervical and endometrial-like glands immediately beneath the vaginal squamous mucosa usually along the anterior wall of the vagina. The conclusion that these developmental vestiges are precursors of the clear cell carcinoma is based on their frequent presence in the vagina adjacent to clear cell carcinoma and on histologic evidence of dysplastic changes in adenosis leading to carcinoma (4).

Herbst et al. (60) conducted a prospective study on the effects of prenatal exposure to stilbestrol on young females. In these individuals, a marked increase in benign vaginal lesions was detected: transverse fibrous ridges of the vagina (22%), abnormal vaginal mucosa (56%), and biopsy-proved vaginal adenosis (35%). The incidence of vaginal adenosis was highest when stilbestrol was given in early pregnancy; it did not develop if therapy was begun after 18 weeks gestation. These lesions were virtually nonexistent in an untreated, age-matched control population.

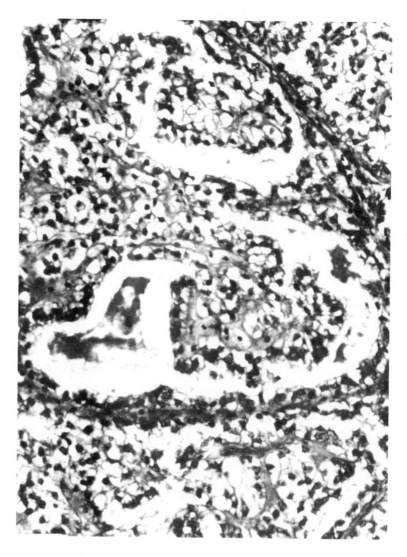

FIG. 9. Adolescent clear cell adenocarcinoma of the vagina (induced by diethylstilbestrol). The tumor is papillary and composed of clear or "hobnail" cells lining the neoplastic acini. H & E stain. × 400.

The actual risk of exposed girls developing adenocarcinoma is not certain. It has been estimated at lower than 0.1%. Lanier et al. (76) suggest that it is no greater than 4 per 1,000 for all girls whose mothers received estrogens, but in the first trimester, the incidence may reach 9 per 1,000.

The oncogenicity of estrogens has been previously shown in mice, rats, guinea pigs, and hamsters (33). Gardner (46) reported epidermoid carcinomas of the cervix and vagina in mice after intravaginal installation of estrogen. Meissner et al. (86) reported endometrial hyperplasia and carcinoma in young rabbits given diethystilbestrol intramuscularly. Dunn and Greene (37) showed that the injections of estrogens into newborn mice produced carcinomas of the cervix and vagina.

The teratogenicity of estrogens is also appreciated. They typically produce abnormalities in somatosexual differentiation. Paradoxical masculinization of female offspring has been described in humans and rodents (22). This may include retention of Wolffian duct remnants. It thus seems likely that stilbestrol given to pregnant women significantly elicits anomalies in primitive sex duct development and involution, and thus accounts for the presence of vaginal adenosis.

Pathogenetic Theories Relating Oncogenesis and Teratogenesis

It is clear that linkages between oncogenesis and teratogenesis are numerous and varied. An adequate explanation for all these relationships is not clear, yet certain speculations seem indicated.

Timing of Teratogenic-Oncogenic Insult

It seems clear from the experimental studies cited that the timing of the initiating events may be critical in determining the outcome. The degree of cytodifferentiation and the metabolic or immunologic state of the organism may determine whether the effect is teratogenic, oncogenic, or both. Additional variables might be the changing placental permeability of an agent and its persistence in both the mother and fetus.

I thus tend to view teratogenesis and oncogenesis as different developmental stages in the intrauterine reaction to a special type of injury, with teratogenesis being the more primitive reaction. The effect of an inciting agent or influence in early gestation is teratogenic, with a gradual shifting toward combined oncogenic-teratogenic forms in later gestation and, ultimately, pure oncogenic expression following late gestational or postnatal exposure. In man, the excessive coexistence of tumors and anomalies could be explained on this basis, depending on the initiation and persistence of the agent's effect on the host.

Dysgenetic Tissues as Cancer Precursors

A primary teratologic event in the fetus may in some fashion predispose the organism to a secondary oncogenic induction in later life. This might explain the neoplastic transformation occurring in some hamartomas, developmental vestiges, heterotopias, and dysgenetic tissues. It is also possible that these structures harbor a latent oncogenic agent, which may have even been originally responsible for the anomaly in intrauterine life. Environmental insults in later life (e.g., trauma, infection, hormonal or metabolic change) might cause a derepression or activation of this cryptic genome and result in the production of cancer. The heightened hormonal stimulation accompanying puberty might be partly responsible for the development of tumors in dysgenetic gonads. These anomalous tissues are probably unable to respond appropriately to increasing levels or cyclical fluctuations in sex hormones; this might result in a predisposition for malignant transformation. A similar mechanism may be involved in the development of the adolescent carcinoma of the vagina induced by stilbestrol therapy during gestation. Here vestiges of anomalous sex duct differentiation (vaginal adenosis) may also respond to the hormonal stimulation of puberty by tumor formation.

The "Two-Hit" Theory

The "two-hit" theory of carcinogenesis as proposed by Knudson et al. (71,72) is not difficult to integrate into the relationships between teratogenesis and oncogenesis if the first hit were expressed as an heritable anomaly or a constellation of anomalies and the second hit expressed as the appearance of tumor. The increased risk of tumor in certain teratologic conditions would depend on a heightened susceptibility of the defective genome to the oncogenic transformation of the second hit. The theory may be further applicable in nonhereditary combinations of anomaly and tumor as well. Here one must assume a postzygotic initiation of the sequence of events.

CONCLUSION

The peculiarities of neonatal and infantile tumors of man suggest that an oncogenic stimulus exerted on the embryo and fetus is often expressed as a relatively benign tumor tending toward arrested growth, regression, and cytodifferentiation. Indeed, some of these tumors approach hamartomas in their appearance and behavior. This pattern is anticipated in the early months of postnatal life, suggesting that up to then malignant growth is repressed or diverted into relatively innocuous forms. How this modification of the full development and progression of neoplasms is effected is unknown; maybe antimitotic, cytolytic, or cytodifferentiative influences are exerted maximally on tumor cells in the fetus and newborn. It is also possible that total derepression of an inborn cancer does not occur until later in life for unknown environmental or genetic reasons.

From a slightly different perspective, this phenomenon may reflect the shifting pattern of fetal reaction to intrauterine oncogenic-teratogenic insult. If early intrauterine stimulation results in teratogenesis, and late gestational or postnatal injury results in tumor, intermediate phases might well result in combinations of anomalies, hamartomas, or a benign congenital tumor. Sequential or persistent stimuli the timing of which would influence the pathologic results are also possible. It seems likely that certain dysgenetic and hamartoid tissues are more susceptible to malignant transformation than are normal tissues.

These various phenomena in pediatric oncology suggest new lines of research aimed at delineating the precise cellular or subcellular mechanism that may have general applicability to the problem of cancer at any age.

REFERENCES

1. Bachmann, K. D., and Kroll, W. (1962): Über das pränatal enstandene. Neuroblastoma sympathicum. *Z. Kinderheilkd.*, 103:61–72.
2. Bachmann, K. D., and Kroll, W. (1969). Der Wilms-Tumor in Ersten Lebensjahr insbesondere über 62 Nephroblastome des Neugeborenen. *Dtsch. Med. Wochenschr.*, 94:2598–2601.
3. Barakat, A. Y., Papadopoulou, Z. L., Chandra, R. S., Hollerman, C. E., and Calcagno, P. (1974): Pseudohermaphroditism, nephron disorder and Wilms' tumor: A unifying concept. *Pediatrics*, 54:366–369.
4. Barber, H. R. K., and Sommers, S. C. (1974): Vaginal adenosis, dysplasia and clear cell adenocarcinoma after diethylstilbestrol treatment in pregnancy. *Obstet. Gynecol.*, 43:645–652.
5. Becker, J. M., Schneider, K. M., and Krasna, I. H. (1970): Neonatal neuroblastoma. *Prog. Clin. Cancer*, 4:382–386.
6. Beckwith, J. B., and Perrin, E. V. (1963): In situ neuroblastomas: A contribution to the natural history of neural crest tumors. *Am. J. Pathol.*, 43:1089–1104.
7. Beckwith, J. B., Wang, C. I., Donnell, G. N. et al. (1964): Hyperplastic fetal visceromegaly with macroglossia, omphalocele, cytomegaly of fetal adrenal cortex and other abnormalities. *J. Pediatr.*, 65:1053a.
8. Beckwith, J. B. (1969): Macroglossia, omphalocele, adrenal cytomegaly, gigantism and hyperplastic visceromegaly. *Birth Defects*, 5(2):188–196.
9. Beckwith, J. B. (1974): Mesenchymal renal neoplasms revisited. *J. Pediatr. Surg.*, 9:803–805.
10. Berry, C. L., Keeling, J., and Hilton, C. (1970): Coincidence of congenital malformation and embryonic tumors of childhood. *Arch. Dis. Child.*, 45:229–231.
11. Bithell, J. F., and Stewart, A. M. (1975): Pre-natal irradiation and childhood malignancy: A review of British data from the Oxford survey. *Br. J. Cancer*, 31:271–287.
12. Bogdan, R., Taylor, D. E. M., and Mostofi, F. K. (1973): Leiomyomatous hamartoma of the kidney. *Cancer*, 31:462–467.
13. Bolande, R. P. (1967): *Cellular Aspects of Developmental Pathology.* Lea and Febiger, Philadelphia.
14. Bolande, R. P., Brough, A. J., and Izant, R. J. Jr. (1967): Congenital mesoblastic nephroma of infancy. *Pediatrics*, 40:272–278.
15. Bolande, R. P. (1971): Benignity of neonatal tumors and the concept of cancer repression in early life. *Am. J. Dis. Child.*, 122:12–14.
16. Bolande, R. P., and Towler, W. F. (1970): A possible relationship of neuroblastoma to von Recklinghausen's disease. *Cancer*, 26:162–175.
17. Bolande, R. P. (1973): Relationships between teratogenesis and oncogenesis. In: *Pathobiology of Development*, edited by E. V. Perrin and M. Finegold, pp. 114–134. Williams & Wilkins, Baltimore.
18. Bolande, R. P. (1974): The neurocristopathies. A unifying concept of disease arising in neural crest maldevelopment. *Hum. Pathol.*, 5:409–429.
19. Bolande, R. P. (1974): Congenital and infantile neoplasia of the kidney. *Lancet*, 2:1497–1498.
20. Bolande, R. P. (1974): Letter to the editor: Congenital mesoblastic nephroma. *Arch. Pathol.*, 98:357.
21. Bond, J. (1975): Bilateral Wilms' tumor. *Lancet*, 2:482–484.
22. Bongiovanni, A. M., DiGeorge, A. M., and Grumbach, M. M. (1959): Masculinization of the female infant associated with estrogenic therapy alone during gestation: Four cases. *J. Clin. Endocrinol. Metab.*, 19:1004–1011.
23. Bove, K. E., Koffler, H., and McAdams, J. (1969): Nodular renal blastema. Definition and possible significance. *Cancer*, 24:323–332.
24. Bove, K. E., and McAdams, J. (1976): The nephroblastomatosis complex and its relationship to Wilms' tumor. *Perspect. Pediatr. Pathol.*, 3:185–223.
25. Brasfield, R. D. and Das Gupta, T. K. (1972): Von Recklinghausen's disease: A clinico-pathological entity. *Am. Surg.*, 175:86–104.

26. Brown, W. T., Puranik, S. R., Altman, D. H., and Hardin, H. C., Jr. (1972): Wilms' tumor in three successive generations. *Surgery*, 72:756–761.

27. Chatten, J., and Voorhess, M. L. (1967): Familial neuroblastoma: Report of a kindred with multiple disorders. *N. Engl. J Med.*, 277:1230–1236.

28. Chatten, J. (1976): Well differentiated epithelial nephroblastomata. *Perspect. Pediatr. Pathol.*, 3:225–254.

29. Cravioto, J. F., Weiss, J. F., Weiss, K de C., Goebel, H. H., and Rensehoss, J. (1973): Biological characteristics of peripheral nerve tumors induced with ethylnitrosourea. *Acta Neuropathol. (Berl.)*, 23:265–280.

30. Devesa, S. S. (1975): The incidence of retinoblastoma. *Am. J. Ophthalmol.*, 80:263–265.

31. DiGeorge, A. M., and Harley, R. D. (1966): The association of aniridia, Wilms' tumor and genital abnormalities. *Arch. Ophthalmol.*, 75:796–798.

32. DiPaolo, J. A. (1962): Effects of oxygen concentration on carcinogenesis induced by transplacental urethan. *Cancer Res.*, 22:299–304.

33. DiPaolo, J. A., and Kotin, P. (1966): Teratogenesis-oncogenesis. A study of possible relationships. *Arch. Pathol.*, 81:3–23.

34. Diwan, B. A., and Meier, H. (1974): Strain and age dependent transplacental carcinogenesis by 1-ethyl-1-nitrosourea in inbred strains of mice. *Cancer Res.*, 34:764–767.

35. Druckrey, H., Ivankovic, S., and Preussmann, R. (1966): Teratogenic and carcinogenic effects in the offspring after a single injection of ethylnitrosourea to pregnant rats. *Nature*, 210:1378–1379.

36. Druckrey, H. (1973): Specific carcinogenic and teratogenic effects of indirect alkylating methyl and ethyl components, and their dependency on stages of oncogenic development. *Xenobiotica* 3:271–303.

37. Dunn, T. B., and Greene, A. W. (1963): Cysts of epididymis, cancer of the cervix, granular cell myoblastoma, and other lesions after estrogen injections in newborn mice. *J. Natl. Cancer Inst.*, 31:425–455.

38. Everson, T. C., and Cole, W. H. (1966): *Spontaneous Regression of Cancer*. Saunders, Philadelphia.

39. Foulds, L. (1969): *Neoplastic Development. Vol. 1.* Academic Press, New York.

40. Fu, Y.-S., and Kay, S. (1973): Congenital mesoblastic nephroma and its recurrence. *Arch. Pathol.*, 96:66–70.

41. Fraumeni, J. F., Jr., and Glass, A. G. (1968): Wilms' tumor and congenital aniridia. *JAMA*, 206:825–828.

42. Fraumeni, J. F., Jr., Li, F. P., and Dalager, N. (1973): Teratomas in children: Epidemiologic features. *J. Natl. Cancer Inst.*, 15:1425–1430.

43. Fraumeni, J. F., Jr., and Miller, R. W. (1967): Adrenocortical neoplasms with hemihypertrophy, brain tumors and others. *J. Pediatr.*, 70:129–138.

44. Fraumeni, J. F., Jr., Miller, R. W., and Hill, J. A. (1968): Primary carcinoma of the liver in childhood: An epidemiological study. *J. Natl. Cancer Inst.*, 40:1087–1099.

45. Fraumeni, J. F., Jr., Geiser, C. F., and Manning, M. D. (1967): Wilm's tumor and congenital hemihypertrophy: A report of five new cases and review of literature. *Pediatrics*, 40:886–899.

46. Gardner, W. U. (1959): Carcinoma of the uterine cervix and upper vagina: Induction under experimental conditions. *Ann. N.Y. Acad. Sci.*, 75:543–564.

47. Gaulin, E. (1951): Simultaneous Wilms' tumor in identical twins. *J. Urol.*, 66:547–550.

48. Ghazali, S. (1973): Presacral teratomas in children. *J. Pediatr. Surg.*, 8:915–918.

49. Gilbert, J. B. (1942): Studies in malignant testis tumors. VIII. Tumors in pseudo-hermaphrodites: A review of sixty cases and a case report. *J. Urol.*, 48:665–672.

50. Givelber, H., and DiPaolo, J. A. (1969): Teratogenic effects of N-ethyl-N-nitrosourea in the Syrian hamster. *Cancer Res.*, 29:1151–1155.

51. Glenn, J. F., and Rhame, R. C. (1961): Wilms' tumor: Epidemiological experience. *J. Urol.*, 85:911–918.

52. Gordon, H. (1974): Family studies in retinoblastoma. *Birth Defects*, 10(10):185–190.

53. Griffin, M. E., and Bolande, R. P. (1969): Familial neuroblastoma with regression and maturation to ganglioneurofibroma. *Pediatrics*, 43:377–382.

54. Guin, G. H., Gilbert, E. E., and Jones, B. (1969): Incidental neuroblastoma in infants. *Am. J. Clin. Pathol.*, 51:126–135.

55. Gustavson, K.-H., Gamstorp, I., and Mearling, S. (1975): Bilateral teratoma of testis in two brothers with 47,XXY Klinefelter's syndrome. *Clin. Genet.*, 8:5–10.

56. Haicken, B. N., Schulman, N. H., and Schneider, K. M. (1973): Adrenocortical carcinoma and congenital hemihypertrophy. *J. Pediatr.*, 83:284–285.

57. Hamerton, J. L. (1971): Abnormal sex chromosome complements in the female. *In: Human Cytogenetics, Vol. II*, p. 65. Academic Press, New York.

58. Herbst, A. L., and Scully, R. E. (1970): Adenocarcinoma of the vagina in adolescence. A report of 7 cases including 6 clear-cell carcinomas (so-called mesonephromas). *Cancer*, 25:745–757.

59. Herbst, A. L., Ulfelder, H., and Poskanzer, D. C. (1971): Adenocarcinoma of the vagina: Association of maternal stilbestrol therapy with tumor appearance in young women. *N. Engl. J. Med.*, 284:878–881.

60. Herbst, A. L., Poskanzer, D. C., Robboy, S. J., Friedlander, L., and Scully, R. E. (1975): Prenatal exposure to stilbestrol. *N. Engl. J. Med.*, 292:334–339.

61. Hickey, R. C., and Layton, J. M. (1954): Sacrococcygeal teratoma. *Cancer*, 7:1031–1043.

62. Hou, L. T., and Holman, R. L. (1961): Bilateral nephroblastomatosis in a premature infant. *J. Pathol. Bacteriol.*, 82:249–255.

63. Howell, J. B., and Anderson, D. E. (1972): The nevoid basal cell carcinoma syndrome. *In: Cancer of the Skin*, edited by A. Andrade, S. L. Gumport, G. L. Popkin, and T. D. Rees. Saunders, Philadelphia.

64. Ishak, I. G., and Glunz, P. R. (1967): Hepatoblastoma and hepatocarcinoma in infancy and childhood. *Cancer*, 20:396–422.

65. Jagasia, K. H., and Thurman, W. G. (1965): Congenital anomalies of the kidney in association with Wilms' tumor. *Pediatrics*, 35:338–340.

66. Jensen, R. D., and Miller, R. W. (1971): Retinoblastoma: Epidemiological characteristics. *N. Engl. J. Med.*, 285:307–311.

67. Kay, S., Pratt, C. B., and Salzberg, A. M. (1965): Hamartoma (leiomyomatous type) of the kidney. *Cancer*, 19:1825–1832.

68. Kissane, J., and Smith, M. (1967): *Pathology of Infancy and Childhood.* Mosby, St. Louis.

69. Klapproth, H. J. (1959): Wilms' tumor: A report of 45 cases and an analysis of 1351 cases reported in the world literature from 1940 to 1958. *J. Urol.*, 81:633–648.

70. Knudson, A. G., and Amromin, G. D. (1966): Neuroblastomas and ganglioneuroma in a child with neurofibromatosis. Implications for the mutational origin of neuroblastomas. *Cancer*, 19:1032–1037.

71. Knudson, A. G., and Strong, L. C. (1972): Mutation and cancer: A model for Wilms' tumor of the kidney. *J. Natl. Cancer Inst.*, 48:313–324.

72. Knudson, A. G., Strong, L. C., and Anderson, D. E. (1973): Heredity and cancer in man. *Prog. Med. Genet.* 9:113–158.

73. Kobayashi, N., Furukawa, T., and Takatsu, T. (1968): Congenital anomalies in children with malignancy. *Paediatr. Univ. Tokyo*, 16:31–37.

74. Koestner, A., Swanberg, J. A., and Wechsler, W. (1971): Transplacental production with ethylnitrosourea of neoplasms of the nervous system in Sprague-Dawley rats. *Am. J. Pathol.*, 63:37–56.

75. Koyama, T. J., Hanada, H., and Matsumoto, S. (1970): Methylnitrosourea-induced malformations of brain in SD-JCL rat. *Arch. Neurol.*, 22:342–347.

76. Lanier, A. P., Noller, K. L., Decker, D. G., Elveback, L. K., and Kurland, L. T. (1973): Cancer and stilbestrol: A follow-up of 1719 persons exposed to estrogens in utero and born 1943-1959. *Mayo Clin. Proc.*, 48:793–798.

77. Lanzkowsky, P. (1975): Absence of pectoralis major muscle in association with acute leukemia. *J. Pediatr.*, 86:817–818.

78. Le Marec, B., Lautridou, A., Urvoy, M., Renault, A., Fonlupp, Jr., Dary, J., Ardouin, M., and Coutel, Y. (1971): Un cas d'association de nephroblastome avec aniridie et malformations genitales. *Arch. Fr. Pediatr.*, 28:457.

79. Liban, E., and Kozenitzky, I. L. (1970): Metanephric hamartomas and nephroblastomatosis in siblings. *Cancer*, 25:885–888.

80. Lowry, W. S. (1974): Passive immunity against cancer. *Lancet*, 1:602–603.

81. Lynch, H. T., and Green, G. S. (1968): Wilms' tumor and congenital heart disease. *Am. J. Dis. Child.*, 115:723–727.

82. MacMahon, B. (1962): Prenatal exposure and childhood cancer. *J. Natl. Cancer Inst.*, 28:1173–1191.

83. Mankad, V. N., Gray, G. F. and Miller, D. R. (1974): Bilateral nephroblastomatosis and

      Klippel-Trenaunay syndrome. *Cancer,* 33:1462–1467.
 84. Martin, J., and Rickham, P. P. (1974): Wilms' tumor—an improved prognosis. *Arch. Dis. Child.,* 49:459–462.
 85. Meadows, A. T., Leichtenfeld, J. L., and Koop, C. E. (1974): Wilms' tumor in three children of a woman with congenital hemihypertrophy. *N. Engl. J. Med.,* 291:23–24.
 86. Meissner, W. A., Sommers, S. C., and Sherman, G. (1957): Endometrial hyperplasia, endometrial carcinoma and endometriosis produced experimentally by estrogen. *Cancer,* 10:500–509.
 87. Miller, R. W. (1956): Delayed effects occurring within the first decade after exposure of young individuals to the Hiroshima atomic bomb. *Pediatrics,* 18:1–18.
 88. Miller, R. W. (1969): Childhood cancer and congenital defects. A study of U.S. death certificates during 1960-1966. *Pediatr. Res.,* 3:389–397.
 89. Miller, R. W., Fraumeni, J. F., Jr., and Manning, M. D. (1964): Association of Wilms' tumor with aniridia, hemihypertrophy and other congenital malformations. *N. Engl. J. Med.,* 270:922–927.
 90. Miller, R. W. (1966): Relation between cancer and congenital defects in man. *N. Engl. J. Med.,* 275:87–93.
 91. Morris, J. M. (1953): The syndrome of testicular feminization in male pseudohermaphrodites. *Am. J. Obstet. Gynecol.,* 65:1192–1211.
 92. Mulvihill, J. J., Miller, R. W., and Taussig, H. B. (1973): Long-time observations on the Blalock-Taussig operation. V. Neoplasms in tetralogy of Fallot. *Johns Hopkins Med. J.* 133:16–18.
 93. Neblett, C. R., Waltz, T. A., and Anderson, D. E. (1971): Neurological involvement in the nevoid basal cell carcinoma syndrome. *J. Neurosurg.,* 35:577–584.
 94. Nevin, N. C., Dodge, J. A., and Allen, I. V. (1972): Two cases of trisomy D associated with adrenal tumors. *J. Med. Genet.,* 9:119–122.
 95. Nomura T., and Ikamoto, E. (1972): Transplacental carcinogenesis by urethan in mice: Teratogenesis and carcinogenesis in relation to organogenesis. *Gann,* 63:731–742.
 96. Perlman, M., Levin, M., and Wittels, B. (1975): Syndrome of fetal gigantism, renal hamartomas and nephroblastomatosis with Wilms' tumor. *Cancer,* 35:1212–1217.
 97. Pierce, G. B., Bullock, W. K., and Huntington, R. W., Jr. (1970): Yolk-sac tumors of the testis. *Cancer,* 25:644–658.
 98. Pierson, M., Gilgenkantz, O., Saborio, M., and Worms, A. M. (1975): Syndrome de Klinefelter, trilogie de Fallot, tératome du médiastin, puberté précoce. *Arch. Fr. Pediatr.,* 32:297.
 99. Potter, E. L. (1972): *Normal and Abnormal Development of the Kidney.* Year Book Medical Publ., Chicago.
100. Reilly, D., Nesbitt, M. D., and Krivit, W. (1968): Care of three patients who had skeletal mestastases in disseminated neuroblastoma. *Pediatrics,* 41:47–51.
101. Reisman, M., Goldenberg, E. D., and Gordon, J. (1966): Congenital heart disease and neuroblastoma. *Am. J. Dis. Child.,* 11:308–310.
102. Rice, J. M. (1973): An overview of transplacental carcinogenesis. *Teratology,* 8:113–125.
103. Riedel, H. A. (1952): Adrenogenital syndrome in a child due to adrenocortical tumor. *Pediatrics,* 10:19–27.
104. Schimke, R. N. (1974): Retinoblastoma and osteogenic sarcoma in siblings. *Cancer,* 34:2077–2079.
105. Schneider, K. M., Becker, J. M., and Krasna, I. H. (1965): Neonatal neuroblastoma. *Pediatrics,* 36:359–366.
106. Schwartz, S. H., Blankenship, B. J., and Stout, R. A. (1970): Multiple basal cell nevus syndrome. *J. Oral Surg.,* 28:523–527.
107. Scully, R. E. (1970): Gonadoblastoma: A review of 74 cases. *Cancer,* 25:1340–1356.
108. Shanklin, D. P., and Sotelo-Avila, C. (1969): In situ tumors in fetuses, newborns and young infants. *Biol. Neonate,* 14:286–316.
109. Sohval, A. R. (1956): Testicular dysgenesis in relation to neoplasm of the testicle. *J. Urol.,* 75:285–291.
110. Sotelo-Avila, C., and Gooch, M. (1976): Neoplasia in Beckwith's syndrome. *Perspect. Pediatr. Pathol.,* 3:255–272.
111. Stewart. A. M., and Kneale, G. W. (1970): Age distribution of cancers caused by obstetrical x-rays and their relevance to cancer latent periods. *Lancet,* 2:4–8.

112. Stewart, A. M., Webb, J., and Hewitt, D. (1958): A survey of childhood malignancies. *Br. Med. J.*, 1:1495–1508.
113. Stump, T. A., and Garrett, R. H. (1954): Bilateral Wilms' tumor in a male pseudohermaphrodite. *J. Urol.*, 72:1146–1152.
114. Survey on neuroblastoma among the surgical Fellows of the American Academy of Pediatrics (1968): *J. Pediatr. Surg.*, 3:191–193.
115. Sutow, W., Gehan, E. A., Heyn, R. M., Kung, F. H., Miller, R. W., Murphy, M. L., and Traggis, D. G. (1970): Comparison of survival curves, 1956 versus 1962, in children with Wilms' tumor and neuroblastoma. *Pediatrics*, 32:800–811.
116. Talerman, A. (1971): Gonadoblastoma and dysgerminoma in two siblings with dysgenetic gonads. *Obstet. Gynecol.*, 38:416–426.
117. Teter, J., and Boczkowski, K. (1967): Occurrence of tumors in dysgenetic gonads. *Cancer*, 20:1301–1310.
118. Tubergen, D. G., and Heyn, R. M. (1970): In situ neuroblastoma associated with an adrenal cyst. *J. Pediatr.*, 76:451–453.
119. Turkel, S. B., and Itabashi, H. H. (1974): The natural history of neuroblastic cells in the fetal adrenal gland. *Am. J. Pathol.*, 76:225–244.
120. Vaez-Zadeh, K., Sieber, W. K., Sherman, F. E., and Kieswetter, W. B. (1972): Sacrococcygeal teratomas in children. *J. Pediatr. Surg.*, 7:152–156.
121. Vessilinovitch, S. D., Mihailovich, M., and Pietra, G. (1967): The prenatal exposure of mice to urethan and the consequent development of tumors in various tissues. *Cancer Res.*, 27:2333–2337.
122. Vlachos, J., and Tsakraklides, V. (1968): A case of renal dysplasia and its relation to bilateral nephroblastomatosis. *J. Pathol. Bacteriol.*, 95:550–562.
123. Walike, J. W., and Karas, R. P. (1961): Nevoid basal cell carcinoma syndrome. *Laryngoscope*, 79:478–487.
124. Warkany, J. (1971): *Congenital Malformations: Notes and Comments.* Year Book Medical Publ., Chicago.
125. Wechsler, W., Kleinhues, P., Matsumoto, S., Zülch, K. J., Ivankovic, S., Preussman, R., and Druckrey, H. (1969): Pathology of experimental neurogenic tumors induced during prenatal and postnatal life. *Ann. N.Y. Acad. Sci.*, 159:360–408.
126. Wexler, H. A., Poole, C. A., and Fujacco, R. M. (1975): Metastatic neonatal Wilm's tumor: A case report with review of the literature. *Pediatr. Radiol.*, 3:179–181.
127. Wiedemann, H. R. (1964): Complexe malformatif familial avec hernie ombilicale et macroglossie un "syndrome nouveau." *J. Genet. Hum.*, 13:223–232.
128. Wigger, H. J. (1969): Fetal hamartoma of the kidney. *Am. J. Clin. Pathol.*, 51:323–337.
129. Willis, R. A. (1962): *The Borderland of Pathology and Embryology,* 2nd ed. Butterworths, Washington.
130. Young, J. L., and Miller, R. W. (1975): Incidence of malignant tumors in U.S. children. *J. Pediatr.*, 86:254–258.

Genetics of Human Cancer, edited by J. J.
Mulvihill, R. W. Miller, and J. F. Fraumeni, Jr.
Raven Press, New York, 1977.

6

Cancer and Congenital Malformations:
Another View

Robert W. Miller

Clinical Epidemiology Branch, National Cancer Institute, Bethesda, Maryland 20014

Traditionally, there have been two main approaches in epidemiology:

1. Retrospective: looking backward into the patients' histories to learn the cause of disease [e.g., stilbestrol as a transplacental carcinogen (6), and most chemical inducers of cancer or malformations in man (14)].

2. Prospective: looking forward, that is, following persons over time after exposure to an agent known or suspected to have a delayed effect on health (e.g., the Japanese atomic bomb survivors).

It seems to me that an equally important approach might be termed "laterospective," looking sideways for collateral disease in the patient or his family. Identification of such disease may lead to new understanding of etiology. The laterospective approach led to the discovery that Down's syndrome predisposed to leukemia, and the realization that, since Down's syndrome is prezygotically determined, so, to some extent, must be the leukemia with which it is associated.

With that in mind, in 1964 we examined the hospital records of 440 children with Wilms' tumor to see with what malformations it was associated (15). Cases with congenital hemihypertrophy had already been reported in the European literature. We found three such cases in our series, and a previously undescribed association of Wilms' tumor with congenital absence of the iris of the eyes (aniridia)—six cases—found simply by reviewing medical charts at half a dozen hospitals. The frequency of the eye defect, about 1 in 75, contrasted with the usual incidence of aniridia at birth, 1 in 75,000. These findings have both clinical and research implications. Clinicians look for the tumor early in patients with the anomalies, and etiologists look for the cause of the tumor from what is known about the causes of the malformations with which it occurs excessively.

The list of disorders associated with Wilms' tumor has continued to grow (Table 1). One constellation consists of four manifestations of excess growth seen together or in various combinations: malignant growths, benign developmental

TABLE 1. *Disorders that occur excessively with Wilms' tumor, and in various combinations with one another*

1. Congenital hemihypertrophy
2. Hamartomas
3. Congenital visceral cytomegaly syndrome of Beckwith and Wiedemann
4. Adrenal cortical neoplasia
5. Primary liver cancer
6. Urinary tract malformations
7. Aniridia syndrome
8. Male pseudohermaphroditism
9. Nephron disorder (congenital nephrosis and nephritis)

From Barakat et al. (1); Filippi and McKusick (2); Fraumeni et al. (3,4); Irving (8); and Miller et al. (15).

tumors (hamartomas), visceral cytomegaly (Wiedemann–Beckwith's syndrome), and hyperplasia (congenital hemihypertrophy) (13). Separate from this group is another constellation in which Wilms' tumor is associated with aniridia (15), or with male pseudohermaphroditism and a nephron disorder (congenital nephrosis) (1). The Wilms' tumor constellations overlap only in relation to urinary tract malformations, e.g., hypospadias, duplication of the ureters, or horseshoe kidney. These anomalies in turn are, or may be, linked with renal dysplasia, which in theory gives rise to the cancer.

By contrast, groups with inborn or acquired high risk of leukemia have cytogenetic abnormalities as a feature in common (5,12), whereas high risk of lymphoma is associated with preexistent cell-mediated immunodeficiency (Fig. 1) (7,9). Groups at high risk of leukemia are not at high risk of lymphoma, but among

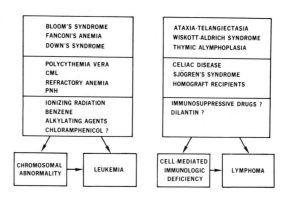

FIG. 1. Etiologic separation of leukemia from lymphoma according to the feature in common (inborn or acquired) of groups at high risk. The constellations have essentially no overlap except for ataxia-telangiectasia, which predisposes primarily to lymphoma and far less so to acute lymphocytic leukemia.

those at high risk of lymphoma, there is a relatively small increase in the frequency of leukemia, particularly among patients with ataxia-telangiectasia (9).

Each of the three childhood neoplasms mentioned (Wilms' tumor, leukemia, and lymphoma) is part of a constellation, essentially separate from the others. By contrast, neuroblastoma has no strong link with any preexistent disorder, but case reports indicate some connection with multiple neurofibromatosis and possibly with disorders of the sympathetic nervous system, such as aganglionic megacolon (10,11). These distinctions should be useful in studies of oncogenic mechanisms, the definition of which may lead to new concepts of prevention.

REFERENCES

1. Barakat, A. Y., Papadopoulou, Z. L., Chandra, R. S., Hollerman, C. E., and Calcagno, P. L. (1974): Pseudohermaphroditism, nephron disorder and Wilms' tumor: A unifying concept. *Pediatrics,* 54:366–369.
2. Filippi, G., and McKusick, V. A. (1970): The Beckwith-Wiedemann syndrome (the exomphalos-macroglossia-gigantism syndrome). Report of two cases and review of the literature. *Medicine,* 49:279–298.
3. Fraumeni, J. F., Jr., and Miller, R. W. (1967): Adrenocortical neoplasms with hemihypertrophy, brain tumors, and other disorders. *J. Pediatr.,* 70:129–138.
4. Fraumeni, J. F., Jr., Miller, R. W., and Hill, J. A. (1968): Primary carcinoma of the liver in childhood: An epidemiologic study. *J. Natl. Cancer Inst.,* 40:1087–1099.
5. German, J. (1972): Genes which increase chromosomal instability in somatic cells and predispose to cancer. *Prog. Med. Genet.,* 8:61–101.
6. Herbst, A. L., Ulfelder, H., and Poskanzer, D. C. (1971): Adenocarcinoma of the vagina: Association of maternal stilbestrol therapy with tumor appearance in young women. *N. Engl. J. Med.,* 284:878–881.
7. Hoover, R., and Fraumeni, J. F., Jr. (1973): Risk of cancer in renal-transplant recipients. *Lancet,* 2:55–57.
8. Irving, I. (1970): The "EMG" syndrome (exomphalos, macroglossia, gigantism). *Prog. Pediatr. Surg.,* 1:1–61.
9. Kersey, J., Spector, B. D., and Good, R. A. (1973): Primary immunodeficiency diseases and cancer: The Immunodeficiency Cancer Registry. *Int. J. Cancer,* 12:333–347.
10. Knudson, A. G., and Meadows, A. T. (1976): Developmental genetics of neuroblastoma, *J. Natl. Cancer Inst.,* 57:675–682.
11. Meadows, A. T., and Knudson, A. G., Jr. (1976): Heterochromia and neuroblastoma. *J. Pediatr.,* 88:168.
12. Miller, R. W. (1967): Persons at exceptionally high risk of leukemia. *Cancer Res.,* 27 (Part 1):2420–2423.
13. Miller, R. W. (1973): Etiology of childhood cancer. In: *Clinical Pediatric Oncology,* edited by W. W. Sutow, T. J. Vietti, and D. J. Fernbach, pp. 7–18. St. Louis, Mo.
14. Miller, R. W. (1974): How environmental effects on child health are recognized. *Pediatrics,* 53:792–796.
15. Miller, R. W., Fraumeni, J. F., Jr., and Manning, M. D. (1964): Association of Wilms' tumor with aniridia, hemihypertrophy and other congenital malformations. *N. Engl. J. Med.,* 270:922–927.

Discussion

German: Dr. Kobayashi, will you tell us about your registration of childhood cancer in Japan?

Kobayashi: We have seven registration centers for malignancies in children to cover the entire nation. We are looking for significant differences in occurrences in various respects, but especially in relation to major and minor malformations. We divided congenital malformations with several cancers into four groups: no malformations, minor malformations, major malformations, and major with minor malformations. We found significant differences in the frequencies of malformations when leukemia was compared with Wilms' tumor or with malignant teratoma, and when lymphoma was compared with Wilms' tumor.

Rashad: In Hawaii, the information on a birth certificate includes sex, father's and mother's age and race, birthweight, presence or absence of pregnancy or labor complications, congenital malformations obvious at birth, birth injury, and previous reproductive history. Linking death and birth records provided such information on 318 cases of cancer. Compared with the total birth cohort, the cancer cases had a significant excess of congenital malformations and previous pregnancy wastage. In addition, their birthweight was significantly higher than the average of the total population.

Hecht: Dr. Miller, you emphasized the association of preexistent cytogenetic defects with leukemia and cell-mediated immunologic deficiency with lymphoma. At first I thought this made no sense, but on second thought you may be right. Is there, for example, an increase of lymphoma in Down's syndrome?

Miller: There is no such increase. There is no substantial excess of lymphoma to match the marked increase in leukemia in atomic bomb survivors, to cite another example. There is one exception to the dichotomy between persons at high risk of lymphoma versus those at high risk of leukemia, and you pointed it out [*Lancet,* 2:1193 (1966)]: acute lymphocytic leukemia occurs in patients with ataxia-telangiectasia, but not nearly to the extent that lymphoma occurs excessively in this syndrome.

Hecht: What you are saying is that there is a little overlap but very little.

Miller: Exactly.

Gatti: Dr. Bolande, we know that the incidence of neuroblastoma *in situ* is very high in autopsies of infants under 3 months of age, but not thereafter. Has anyone measured the occurrence of such neuroblastoma in premature infants?

Bolande: Neuroblastic rests in the fetal adrenal usually disappear after 30 weeks of gestation. One may occasionally see, after this time, neuroblastic aggregates less than 2,000 μm in diameter, but most observers have set this size as the minimum required before designating it a bona fide mass that may be precursive of neuroblastoma, rather than some sort of developmental vestige.

German: You spoke of hamartomas becoming neoplastic. Do you think that the cells throughout the benign lesion change their character, or do you think the neoplasm begins just in one area? In other words, is the malignant change unifocal or multifocal within a benign tumor?

Bolande: With regard to cytodifferentiation of neuroblastoma, I think the original neuroblast is bipotential, so it can produce mature neurons or it may produce Schwann cells. As time goes on, one sees a progressive interstitial deposition of Schwann cells that gradually can press out the neuroblastic constituents. The remaining neuronal elements undergo eosinophilic degeneration, cytolysis, and eventually disappear. I think this process occurs uniformly throughout congenital tumors. I cannot say that this happens uniformly in every regressing neuroblastoma; perhaps it does. Usually we do not have the chance to sample every lesion sequentially.

German: I am trying to relate your observations to our thinking about the unicellular origin for most malignant tumors and for apparently some benign tumors, such as meningioma. I am having some difficulty in thinking about the biological process. Is there a sudden change in the patient that causes a change in the character of the cells wherever they are located in the body?

Bolande: I believe so, but I do not know what the change is. I think one of the best examples concerns hamartomas in the intestines, where these lesions may appear quite dysplastic. The cytologic character of the lesion permits objective separation of the type that occurs in familial polyposis from that of Peutz-Jeghers' syndrome—the latter having a much lower frequency of malignant transformation. Its lesion is a very quiescent looking benign, well differentiated hamartoma, in contrast to the hamartomas of multiple polyposis, which are indeed dysplastic, with a piling up of cells, hyperchromatism, and many atypical cellular features very early in life. I think the same would hold true for many genodermatoses.

Knudson: Dr. Bove of Cincinnati has made some new observations of renal abnormalities that accompany Wilms' tumor [*Perspect. Pediatr. Pathol.*, 3:185–223 *(1976)*]. About 33% of patients with Wilms' tumor have multifocal developmental lesions in their kidneys. Some of these are called metanephric hamartomas. There are also advanced lesions that indicate healing and degeneration of glomeruli, among other changes. These lesions were found in all nine cases with bilateral Wilms' tumor. In the total series of 69 cases, 23 showed these lesions, a figure which is in agreement with an estimate by Dr. Strong and me that 38% of Wilms' tumors are due to a dominant gene. The observation raises the possibility that prezygotically determined cases of Wilms' tumor have renal lesions due to the action of a single gene that is inherited and that a second mutation postzygotically gives rise to the tumor.

Bolande: It is important to emphasize this group of tumors because familial or bilateral Wilms' tumors exhibit a greater association with teratologic disorders than unifocal Wilms' tumors.

Yerganian: Dr. Bolande, how do you view the primitive mesenchymal derivative?

Bolande: I do not think it is a fibrosarcoma, although it has been called that in the past. I view it as the earliest initiation of the true oncogenic process *in utero,* when the kidney is entirely mesodermal. It starts as a mesenchymal structure that then differentiates into metanephric epithelium. I believe it to be a highly cytodifferentiated sibling of Wilms' tumor originating rather early *in utero*—earlier than the other lesions we have discussed. I call this "mesoblastic nephroma" to distinguish it clearly from congenital Wilms' tumor in particular. It is the cryptic presence of the three congeners that, before the era of chemotherapy, accounted almost entirely for the enhanced survival of children with Wilms' tumor under 1 year of age. Mesoblastic nephroma is the commonest true neoplasm of the newborn kidney.

Hirayama: Dr. Miller, in your attractive hypothesis concerning a transplacental anticarcinogen, is there a relationship to the regression of neuroblastoma (e.g., Everson, T. C., and Cole, W. H.: *Spontaneous Regression of Cancer.* Philadelphia: W. B. Saunders, 1966)?

Miller: Such regression may possibly be a consequence of a transplacental anticarcinogen.

Littlefield: Can someone bring us up to date on the immunologic basis for the regression of neuroblastoma—work that was of such interest a few years ago?

Meadows: At the Children's Hospital in Philadelphia, pretreatment sera from 16 children with neuroblastoma were assayed for α_1-antitrypsin, haptoglobin, C3 component of complement, and orosomucoid. The mean values of these acute phase reactants were elevated in patients who died or relapsed and normal in survivors free of disease [*Proc. Am. Assoc. Cancer Res.* 16:189 (1975)].

Gatti: With regard to neuroblastoma, one must remember that the newborn animal in general is very prone to become tolerant. Thus, not only are these systems complicated, but so too is the antigen–antibody complex formation and its role in oncogenesis. I think we must stop extrapolating to the newborn infant and begin to make the necessary studies that pertain specifically to these very young subjects.

Riccardi: We recently studied the chromosomes of two children with Wilms' tumor, aniridia, and urinary tract malformations (one of them was a male pseudohermaphrodite). Both had 11p-, with the breakpoint in the same place. One had been studied in 1965, before banding techniques were available, and was said to have normal chromosomes. It is important to study all patients with the Wilms' tumor-aniridia syndrome to determine if they, or a portion of the group, have this abnormality.

Genetics of Human Cancer, edited by J. J. Mulvihill, R. W. Miller, and J. F. Fraumeni, Jr. Raven Press, New York, 1977.

7

Target Theory Applied to Acute Leukemia in Down's Syndrome and the General Population

A. S. Lubiniecki

Life Sciences Division, Meloy Laboratories, Inc., Springfield, Virginia 22151

Down's syndrome (DS) is well known to be associated with increased risk of leukemia (2–5,7). Several studies based on death certificates have also suggested that the modal age of leukemia mortality is lower in DS patients than in the general population (4,5). As suggested by Murphy *(this volume),* these epidemiological findings were subjected to target theory analysis using data in the literature. Although inconclusive, the results suggest imperfections of current data.

Data on childhood leukemia mortality in 97 DS patients in England and Wales and in the general U.S. population came from death certificate studies by Lashof and Stewart (4) and Miller (5). Information on morbidity and survival time in the general population and in 31 cases of acute lymphatic leukemia (ALL) among DS patients was obtained, respectively, from Fraumeni et al. (1) and from the Acute Leukemia Group B by Rosner and Lee (6). Both sets of data were examined through the first 15 years of life.

Figure 1 shows that the cumulative frequency distribution of leukemia mortality with time in DS is greater than that in the general population. The exact mathematical description of these data is complicated since in the general population the curve does not extrapolate to 100% and both populations are curvilinear. To a first approximation, however, the logarithmic complement of mortality appears to be a linear function of time in both populations. The slopes of the two regression lines are significantly different ($p < 0.0005$).

The greater leukemia mortality in DS patients in Fig. 1 would seem to result from an increased morbidity of leukemia. An alternative explanation—decreased survival following diagnosis—is not supported by available data: survival time with leukemia is virtually identical in DS compared with the general population (Fig. 2). In leukemia associated with DS (6), survival time seems independent of age at diagnosis. Confounding factors may certainly be operating; for example, death from congenital heart disease or the leukemoid reaction of neonatal DS may influence

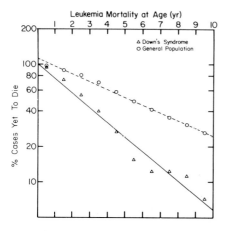

FIG. 1 Mortality from leukemia through age 15 years in DS compared to the general population. [From Lashof and Stewart (4); and Miller (5).]

morbidity and mortality figures. However, these factors are generally considered significant only in the DS population under 1 year of age.

Nonetheless, mortality data suggest that DS patients are at high risk of leukemia. Indeed, this is common knowledge, yet data on the morbidity of ALL do not support this suggestion (Fig. 3). Both sets of data possess initial shoulders and are clearly not consistent with single-hit models. The general population data become approximately linear with advancing age; the erratic nature of the Down's syndrome curve in the later childhood years probably reflects the small sample size (31 cases) on which data are available. Virtually identical curves are generated when all leukemia is considered for both populations instead of just ALL.

In general, assuming some survivors, one expects data from comparable populations to have a steeper (more negative) slope for morbidity than for mortality, as shown for leukemia in the general population (Figs. 1 and 3). The anomalous finding is the virtually identical curves for incidence and mortality in DS, despite the contrary evidence presented earlier. The DS data shown in Figs. 1 and 3 are from limited studies of two different parameters and from two different countries and times; however, leukemia mortality in DS is reportedly similar in England and Wales, 1943–1964 (4), and in the United States, 1960–1966 (5). Also, both sets of data show a peculiar inflection point at about 5 to 6 years of age. This is of unknown origin or significance.

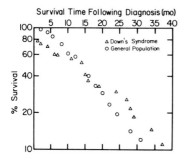

FIG. 2 Survival following diagnosis of acute lymphoblastic leukemia through age 15 years in DS compared to the general population. [From Fraumeni et al. (1); and Rosner and Lee (6).]

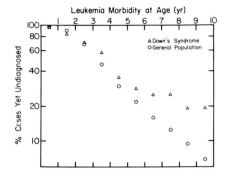

FIG. 3. Morbidity of acute lymphoblastic leukemia through age 15 years in DS compared to the normal population. [From Fraumeni et al. (1); and Rosner and Lee (6).]

One obvious discrepancy is the lower frequency of very young leukemic cases (2 to 3 years) with DS in the morbidity study (6) in comparison with data from death certificates. These differences are seen in the median age at diagnosis of ALL: 4.3 years in DS patients referred to Acute Leukemia Group B (6) versus 3.8 years in the general cohort seen at the Boston Children's Cancer Research Foundation (1). This may reflect a possible referral bias in the report of cases of ALL to Acute Leukemia Group B. Alternatively, the generally accepted notion of an excess of "leukemia" in DS under 3 years of age could be an artifact from deaths certified as due to leukemia, whereas the true diagnosis is a leukemoid reaction either overtreated or accompanying death from concomitant disease at a later point in time. Further studies might approach this question, thereby furnishing data suitable for the target theory analysis requested by Murphy.

ACKNOWLEDGMENTS

The author wishes to thank Drs. R. W. Miller, J. J. Mulvihill, W. J. Blot, and B. J. Stone of the Epidemiology Branches, National Cancer Institute, for helpful discussions of many epidemiologic and statistical facets of this report.

REFERENCES

1. Fraumeni, J. F., Jr., Manning, M. D., and Mitus, W. J. (1971): Acute childhood leukemia: Epidemiologic study by cell type of 1,263 cases at the Children's Cancer Research Foundation in Boston, 1947–1965. *J. Natl. Cancer Inst.*, 46:461–470.
2. Holland, W. W., Doll, R., and Carter, C. O. (1962): The mortality from leukemia and other cancers among patients with Down's syndrome (mongols) and among their parents. *Br. J. Cancer*, 16:178–186.
3. Jackson, E. W., Turner, J. H., Klauber, M. R., and Norris, F. D. (1968): Down's syndrome: Variation of leukemia occurrence in institutionalized populations. *J. Chronic Dis.*, 21:247–253.
4. Lashof, J. C., and Stewart, A. (1965): Oxford survey of childhood cancers. Progress report III: Leukemia and Down's syndrome. *Monthly Bull. Ministry Health (Lond.)*, 24:136–143.
5. Miller, R. W. (1970): Neoplasia and Down's syndrome. *Ann. N.Y. Acad. Sci.*, 171:637–644.
6. Rosner, F., and Lee, S. L. (1972): Down's syndrome and acute leukemia: Myeloblastic or lymphoblastic? *Am. J. Med.*, 53:203–218.
7. Wald, N. W., Barges, W. H., Li, C. C., Turner, J. H., and Harnois, M. C. (1961): Leukemia associated with mongolism. *Lancet*, 1:1228.

Genetics of Human Cancer, edited by J. J.
Mulvihill, R. W. Miller, and J. F. Fraumeni, Jr.
Raven Press, New York, 1977.

8

Cytogenetics of Human Neoplasia

D. G. Harnden

Department of Cancer Studies, University of Birmingham, Birmingham, England

The longstanding interest in the cytogenetics of human neoplasia stems from two basic observations. First, the chromosomes of tumor cells are often, but not always, abnormal and second, the occurrence of chromosomal abnormalities—whether induced or spontaneous—is frequently associated with subsequent neoplasia. This paper is not concerned with documenting in detail the chromosome changes that are present in tumor cells or the association between chromosome aberrations and the induction of cancer, since this field has recently been reviewed (33).

Rather, I shall try to summarize the situation, drawing particular attention to recent results from my own laboratory and to recent work by others—a sort of biased review. There are two fundamental questions: (1) What part do chromosome changes play in the genesis of the neoplastic process? and (2) What part do chromosome changes play in the developing neoplasm? The question often asked is, "Are chromosome changes themselves visible manifestations of the primary initiation event in neoplasia?" I would prefer to consider the role of chromosome changes in the dynamic process that leads from normal tissue to overt cancer, considering events both before and after the recognition of malignant cells. Furthermore, one should not necessarily expect all cancers to be the same; the group of neoplastic diseases is as varied as the group of infectious diseases, and by comparison one should expect a wide range of biological processes underlying these diseases.

THE ROLE OF CHROMOSOME CHANGE IN PREDISPOSITION TO MALIGNANCY

Does the occurrence or presence of chromosomal abnormalities in nonneoplastic tissue make it more likely that neoplastic change will follow? The association between the occurrence of chromosome aberrations and neoplastic disease is so strong that it is easy to assume some sort of causal relationship. Let us examine this assumption. It is clear that the presence of chromosome abnormalities in an otherwise normal tissue does not necessarily mean that neoplastic disease is already present. The lymphocyte clones in patients with ataxia telangiectasia (AT) are a good example; virtually all the lymphocytes may be grossly abnormal even at a time when there is no clinical or pathological evidence of hematologic disease (52,90). Similarly patients with polycythemia vera frequently have a large number of cells with a specific chromosome abnormality (98). On the other hand, both these conditions have an increased risk of neoplasia and one must ask whether there is something about the progress of the disease that makes it more likely that neoplasia will occur. In this section I therefore deal with both induced and spontaneous chromosome changes associated with malignant change.

Induced Chromosome Abnormalities

Radiation

Agents that cause chromosome abnormalities are commonly carcinogenic but the correlation is far from universal. The induction of cancer by ionizing radiation is well documented (60). Ionizing radiation also causes a wide range of chromosome aberrations; the incidence is proportional to dose (22,23) and the type of aberration is normally related to the stage of the cell cycle at which the radiation is administered. Chromatid-type aberrations follow irradiation in the G2 phase while, normally, irradiation in the G1 phase causes chromosome-type aberrations. Patients with AT show clinical evidence of sensitivity to radiation (18) and we have recently shown that AT cells are radiosensitive and that there is a high frequency of chromatid-type aberrations following G1 irradiation of lymphocytes from these patients (115,116). This suggests that, unlike the chromosomes of normal subjects which behave as a single linear structure in G1, the chromosomes of these cancer-prone patients behave as if there are two parallel threads in the chromatid (Fig. 1). By estimating relative DNA content using a scanning microdensitometer, we have ruled out the possibility that there are post-S-phase cells present in AT peripheral blood. The most probable explanation is, therefore, that single strand lesions are created in the DNA by G1 X-irradiation and that, unlike those in normal cells, the lesions remain available for exchange so long that an exchange is probable. Using gradient centrifugation techniques we have found no evidence of an excess of single-strand breaks in irradiated AT DNA.

The majority of cells damaged by irradiation will probably not survive, but there is now strong evidence for clones of chromosomally marked cells in patients who have been irradiated. In the case of lymphocytes in thorotrast-treated patients (14) or bone marrow cells from ^{32}P irradiated patients (69), these clones clearly exist *in vivo*. Fibroblasts cultured from irradiated skin contain clones of cytogenetically abnormal cells (7,20,120) but the significance of these clones is unclear. We have confirmed that such clones exist in cells from irradiated skin (113) and are also present in skin cells from patients treated with chemicals

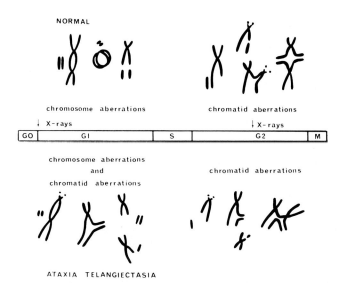

FIG. 1. Schematic representation of chromosome aberrations that are found in lymphocytes from patients with AT and from normal controls at the first mitosis following X-irradiation in either the G1 or the G2 phase of the cell cycle.

(P. Benn, *personal communication*) and in cells from control skin (47,70). Whether or not these clones are present *in vivo* will be difficult to determine. It is certain, therefore, that ionizing radiation leads to chromosome damage, including clone formation, and that tumors induced by radiation show chromosome changes (including the Ph[1] in radiation-induced chronic myeloid leukemia (CML) (117) but so far no one has succeeded in linking the chromosome damage induced by radiation and that seen in radiation-induced tumors.

Viruses

It is now well documented that viruses induce chromosome damage [see (46) for review]. As a broad generalization, one can say that only those viruses which cause chromosome rearrangements are associated with the production of neoplasms. Most of the damage associated with viruses such as measles will almost certainly lead to cell death. Much more interesting are those situations that lead to chromosome rearrangements, but even there it is curious that some viruses regularly lead to stem line proliferation (e.g., adenovirus type 2 in rat cells), whereas others produce continuing instability (e.g., SV-40 in human cells). Surprisingly little work has been done with human cells, though the progress of changes, some specific, in SV-40-infected human cells was well documented many years ago (85). Of particular interest at present is the possible localization of the genome of SV-40 virus at one specific chromosomal site in human transformed cells (15,17). In the lines studied so far, the virus appears to be located on chromosome 7. Although this does seem an intriguing possibility, the evidence presented to date does not altogether rule out the possibility that the SV-40 virus genome may be present on several chromosomes and that chromosome 7 is preferentially retained for reasons unconnected with cellular transformation. There is already some evidence for the preferential retention of chromosome 7 (16). If specific chromosomal localization sites can be recognized for oncogenic viruses, then this could make the study of the cytogenetics of human tumors much more meaningful. For example, is there any connection between the preferential retention of chromosome 7 in SV-40-transformed cells and the apparent preferential loss of 7 in myeloproliferative disorders?

Also of considerable interest at present is the recognition that adenovirus type 12 produces a lesion on chromosome 17 at the locus of the gene for thymidine kinase, which the virus requires for its own synthesis (73). This phenomenon may help in elucidating the specificity of chromosome abnormalities, e.g., there is evidence for the preferential involvement of chromosome 17 in CML (39), and it is possible to speculate that such specificity may be due to the requirement for particular genes at some point in the genesis of the neoplasm.

Chemical Substances

It has been known for many years that a whole range of substances, some of which are carcinogenic, will cause damage to human chromosomes *in vitro.* Evidence that accidental exposure of people to chemical substances in their environment will cause damage is much less convincing; but, many drugs are known to cause chromosome damage *in vivo* (13). A recent development in this field is the use of the production of sister chromatid exchanges as a means of assessing the activity of particular chemical compounds. This system has proved in some cases to be several orders of magnitude more sensitive than chromosome damage as a measure of assessing the damaging effect of a chemical on cellular DNA (94). However, activity in this system does not necessarily correlate with carcinogenic activity, e.g., mitomycin C is highly active while its carcinogenic activity is quite insignificant. The need to develop such a system is quite clear since, in too many cases, the recognition of a chromosome damaging potential comes after epidemiological evidence that the substance is a carcinogen, e.g., vinyl chloride (29,97). However, when the demonstration of chromosome damage comes prior to any evidence of carcinogenicity in man, e.g., nitrophenylene diamines (108), the problems that arise in attempting to show that the chromosome damage is of significance are great because at present we simply do not understand the relationship between chemically induced chromosome damage and cancer. It would seem wise, by analogy with ionizing radiation, to assume that increasing damage at higher dose levels indicates higher risk. Cytogenetic studies may therefore play an important part in screening for environmental carcinogens and may be useful in recognizing specially susceptible individuals. However, it may be difficult to distinguish between a hereditary susceptibility to neoplasia and a common exposure to an environmental agent as in the family (122) where three out of five siblings had a neoplasm, but two of these, and one unaffected sib, all worked in a polluted atmosphere in a shoe factory. The relationship between the observed chromosome damage and the familial incidence of neoplasia is not clear.

Chromosome Breakage Syndromes

In these syndromes—Fanconi's anemia (107), Bloom's syndrome (35), and AT (45,51)—spontaneous breakage of the chromosomes occurs in peripheral blood lymphocytes and in cultured fibroblasts. Chromosome breakage has also been reported in fibroblasts from patients with xeroderma pigmentosum (36,59), porokeratosis of Mibelli (114), and nevoid basal cell carcinoma syndrome (43), and in lymphocytes of patients with scleroderma (21) and incontinentia pigmenti (40). The lesions in Fanconi's anemia are apparently random. In AT they are clearly nonrandom (90), and specifically involve the region 14q12; the distal portion of 14 is translocated most often to the other 14, but sometimes to the X or 7. The parallel with the specific translocations involving chromosome 22 in CML is striking; yet the tandem type of translocation (14/14), common in AT, seems rare in CML despite one report of a tandem 22/22 translocation, which was likely constitutional (27). It is possible that particular aberrations are selected but the regular occurrence of these aberrations could suggest some sort of preferential translocation.

Similarly in Bloom's syndrome, the chromosome abnormalities are nonrandom, preferentially involving chromatid exchange between homologous chromosomes (34). This could be due to some sort of somatic pairing; the increased frequency of sister chromatid exchanges in bromodeoxyuridine-treated cells may also be an important indication of how these specific rearrangements arise (11).

Constitutional Chromosome Aberrations

While *induced* aberrations are associated with neoplasia, so also are some chromosomal abnormalities which are present in *all* cells of the body. The association between Down's syndrome and leukemia is well established (55,79), but the association with solid neoplasms is less certain, although isolated case reports occur with regularity (66). Patients with Klinefelter's syndrome have an increased incidence of breast carcinoma (48,106) but the suggested association with leukemia may be no more than chance (109). The link between dysgerminoma and females with XY sex chromosomes or at least an XY cell line now seems well established (86,95).

An additional example is probably the chromosome 13 long arm deletion observed in all cells of some patients with retinoblastoma. The deletion has been defined by Orye et al. (89) as an interstitial deletion of the region q21 on chromosome 13. The regularity of the occurrence suggests that the association is meaningful. However, it is curious that the chromosome deletion is not seen constitutionally in most patients [although it may be seen in most tumors (49)]. Ladda et al. (67) report normally banded chromosomes in seven bilateral (five familial) and five unilateral cases. In some families, individuals inherit the disease as a simple Mendelian dominant gene, whereas in others it appears to be sporadic.

It is interesting to note that the original lesion, whether it is a single gene or a chromosomal deletion, depends on the differentiated state of the cell and also on the occurrence of a second, probably mutational, event before its effects can be manifest (65).

Another area of interest is the reported occurrence of cancer in patients with translocations. For example, Langlands and Maclean (68) report a patient with a 14/21 translocation who had two primary lymphoreticular neoplasms many years apart. Garson and Milligan (32) describe a 4/14 translocation in a patient with acute lymphoblastic leukemia but also in his relatives. Other similar instances have been reported [e.g., a ring-1 chromosome and acute myelogenous leukemia (AML) (8), a B/C translocation and bilateral Wilms' tumor (37)], but whether the frequency of such associations is greater than chance is not clear. O'Riordan et al. (88) found eight patients with translocations among 3,086 patients with cancer but did not consider this to be greater than chance expectation. Likewise, it was originally thought that the deleted G chromosome, called the Christchurch (Ch^1) chromosome (26,41), was similar to the Ph^1 chromosome, but now it seems more likely to be an example of a constitutional abnormality that predisposes to chronic lymphatic leukemia, if it has any significance at all.

Clone Formation Prior to Neoplasia

It is certain that clones of cells may form prior to the onset of neoplasia. When clones arise *in vivo,* this could indicate the establishment of a population of cells with a proliferative advantage in which a neoplastic population could arise. The significance of clones recognized *in vitro* is more tenuous. Nevertheless our finding clones in a high proportion of early passage fibroblasts cultured from the skin of normal persons, together with the absence of clones from embryo skin fibroblasts, suggests that aneuploid clones may be present *in vivo* even in normal individuals (47). For this reason, it is suggested that previous reports of clones among patients with chromosomal instability syndromes must be examined closely. These could have arisen *in vitro* but they are also consistent with the ideas of Burnet (9), who has postulated that exposure to environmental agents is not an adequate explanation for somatic mutation and that a process of intrinsic mutagenesis may be responsible for the generation of mutant clones in all individuals. The critical questions are whether or not the *frequency* of clones is increased in cancer-susceptible individuals and whether or not the clones occur *in vivo.* It seems possible that, as they grow older, individuals may accumulate populations of cells (some clonal) with abnormal chromosomes and these populations of cells may be the regions prone to neoplasia.

The Significance of DNA Repair in the Origin of Chromosome Abnormalities

Dramatic chromosome changes have been described by Huang et al. (59) and German et al. (36) in cultured cells from patients with xeroderma pigmentosum. It

is interesting to speculate that the defect of DNA repair, now so well documented (12) might lead to these aberrations. Further, a slow rate of DNA synthesis has
been reported by Hand and German in Bloom's syndrome (42) and by Taylor et
al. in AT (115), using cytogenetic evidence. It has recently been reported that AT
cells are inefficient in the excision of γ- and X-ray-induced single strand
damage in DNA (M. Paterson, *personal communication*). The interesting possibility is emerging that defects in the process of DNA repair may be an important
means of generating chromosomal diversity in a cell population. A positive
correlation between nonrepairable DNA damage in xeroderma pigmentosum cells
and the subsequent appearance of chromosome aberrations has been reported by
Sasaki (105).

THE SIGNIFICANCE OF CHROMOSOME ABNORMALITIES IN CANCER CELLS

Do All Tumor Cells Have Abnormal Chromosomes?

It is generally agreed that where human neoplasms have been examined directly
and where it is reasonably certain that the tumor cells themselves are being
examined the chromosomes are usually found to be abnormal. Exceptions are
common enough to be no longer surprising and one cannot therefore say that the
presence of abnormal chromosomes is an *invariable* feature of tumor cells. In the
acute leukemias, for example, it has always been clear from a study of conventionally stained preparations that a proportion of cases had an apparently normal
chromosome complement; but those who believe chromosome changes to be of
fundamental significance in neoplasia have argued that the chromosome changes
are there but just not recognizable by current techniques. Banding techniques now
give us better resolution but the same arguments can still be applied; for example,
Mitelman and Brandt (80) have shown that five out of their six patients with
chromosomes which were apparently normal by conventional staining methods
also appeared normal following G-banding. The sixth patient was found to have
an additional chromosome 8 and to be lacking an X chromosome. One can
nevertheless argue that those cases with normal banding patterns have chromosome changes below the level of resolution by this method of staining. We are
not, however, discussing changes in the DNA, and it is only reasonable to accept
that some human neoplasms have normal chromosomes even using the most
refined techniques available.

The Pattern of Chromosome Abnormalities in Tumor Cells

After accepting that chromosome changes are present in only some tumors, the
next question to ask is whether or not there is any discernible pattern. The general
impression gained using conventional staining techniques has been that for most

tumors there is no overall pattern. Some tumors are polyploid or at least hyper-diploid, whereas others are near diploid or pseudodiploid. A few are hypodiploid. Some histological types of tumor may more often be of one type than another, e.g., it is unusual for a meningioma to be hyperdiploid (75). Simple aneuploidy seems to be one of the commonest changes observed with just the addition or elimination of one or more chromosomes (38), but chromosome rearrangements (e.g., translocations) do commonly occur in tumors, and these may be very complex. A preparation which, by normal staining procedures, may appear to have a small number of "marker" chromosomes may, in fact, have many aberrations the origin of which may be quite obscure. As a general rule, tumors of the same histological type do not have similar chromosome changes. However, within a single tumor many of the cells may have similar or even identical abnormal chromosome patterns suggesting a common origin for these cells. It has been postulated that we should look for patterns in a different way. Rowley (101) has hypothesized that the chromosomal change is determined by the particular etiologic agent.

Nonrandom Change in the Chromosomes of Cancer Cells

Those cases wherein chromosome changes are not random are, therefore, all the more interesting. The classic example has always been the Ph[1] chromosome in chronic myeloid leukemia; but, even before the advent of banding, it was apparent that other specific changes did occur (44). More recent studies have confirmed these specificities which, in some cases, have become more precise.

Leukemias and Preleukemic Conditions

The specificity of the Ph[1] chromosome has been confirmed with time and I shall consider here only the more recent developments. Most striking of these is the recognition that the Ph[1] chromosome results from a translocation (100). Normally, material from the long arm of chromosome 22 is translocated to the long arm of chromosome 9 (Fig. 2) but translocations to other sites have been reported, e.g., 2, 13, 17, 19, and 22 (50). The concept of a translocation requiring two specific lesions regularly in close spatial proximity raises numerous questions about the nature of the loci at these two points and their physiological role within these cells. We are, however, as far from understanding this as we are from answering questions about the relationship between this translocation event and the origin of the neoplastic process. The source of the abnormal cells is a matter of some interest. Recent findings again suggest that the spleen may be the site of generation of many of the abnormal cells (4,82). The current trials of splenectomy following splenic irradiation will be watched with interest and should be followed carefully cytogenetically.

Whatever the precise role of the Ph[1] chromosome, the clone with the abnormal chromosome does not respond, during the active phase of the disease, to normal

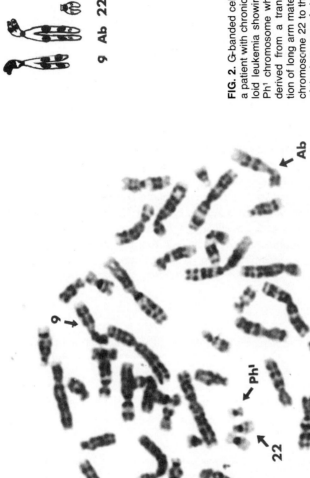

9   Ab   22   Phⁱ

FIG. 2. G-banded cell from a patient with chronic myeloid leukemia showing the Phⁱ chromosome which is derived from a translocation of long arm material of chromosome 22 to the end of the long arm of chromosome 9. (Courtesy of Peter Benn.)

regulatory mechanisms. Remission in CML is not due to elimination of the clone (110) but to restoration of regulatory control over the abnormal clone. However, in general, conditions within the clone favor the generation of further abnormalities. Pedersen (91) has shown that in early CML the loss and gain of chromosomes is random. These new abnormalities may pre- or postdate the blastic crisis, but most often they occur at about the same time (39,92,93). It is a reasonable assumption that progression by subclonal evolution is occurring and that in many cases this may be visualized as chromosomal evolution. The recent demonstration that these further changes also show specificity adds considerable interest. Specific changes such as the loss of the Y (57,70) and the formation of an isochromosome of the long arms of chromosome 17 (6,81) have, of course, been recognized for some time; however, attention has recently focused on the C group of chromosomes not only in CML but also in AML, polycythemia vera and other conditions. The additional C group chromosome, previously recognized in many cells, has been identified as an 8 with surprising regularity in all of these conditions (28,31,58,103). Although chromosomes 9, 10, 11, 12 and X may occasionally be added, this does not occur as frequently as an additional 8. Likewise when a C chromosome is lost, it is almost always a number 7, and equally surprising, it seems that 6 is seldom either lost or duplicated. Evidence is also emerging that not only is the loss or gain of chromosomes specific but also the rearrangement. For example, Rowley (102) draws attention to a specific breakpoint at 8q22 in three of her cases.

Testicular Tumors

In 1967, Martineau (78) reported the occurrence of a long submetacentric marker in eight out of nine patients with testicular tumors (seminomas), but so far no banding studies have been reported on these tumors.

Burkitt's Tumor and Other Lymphomas

A long D-like acrocentric marker has been described in Burkitt's tumor and cell lines derived from it (61). It now seems clear that a chromosome 14 with an additional terminal band (62,74) is present in many such cases. The origin is not yet clear but Zech (123) has suggested that the extra band arises as a translocation of the terminal band from a chromosome 8. This specific abnormality has not so far been recognized in lymphoid cell lines derived from patients with infectious mononucleosis or other lymphoproliferative diseases. Steel (112) concluded that the long acrocentric chromosomes seen in these cases were all of different origin. Although this specific aberration is not found regularly in other lymphomas, it does now appear that there is some specificity. Reeves (98) reports that, among ten cases, five had a deletion of chromosome 3 and three had a chromosome 9 with an apparent deletion distal to the band q22.

Meningiomas

Meningiomas have been carefully studied and the majority have a hypodiploid stem line; the G group chromosome missing in many cases is a 22 (75,77). Even in the rare hyperdiploid cases, there is a relative deficiency of chromosome 22 (76). The significance of this specific aberration is unknown but the chromosome involved is the one involved in the production of the Ph[1] chromosome. Weiss et al. (121) have recognized S V-40 T antigen in meningioma cells which have specifically lost chromosomes 22, although they have never had S V-40 in their laboratory. This curious observation requires confirmation but recalls the earlier recognition of the deletion of a G group chromosome in S V-40-transformed cells (85).

Precancerous Lesions

A number of conditions, though they do not display the criteria of malignancy, are so frequently followed by malignancy that they must be considered premalignant. Chromosomal abnormalities have been recognized in carcinoma *in situ* of the uterine cervix (111), sporadic and familial colonic polyps (83), benign tumors of the nervous system (77), and preleukemic hematological disorders (87,96,104), including polycythemia vera (99), thrombocythemia (53), and multiple myeloma (1). Trisomy 2 has been reported in a hydatidiform mole, but this is not necessarily associated with the neoplastic potential of the mole (56). Such observations strengthen the concept that the chromosomal abnormalities seen in malignant neoplasms may be the consequence of cellular selection from within an inherently unstable cellular population.

Clone Formation in Tumors

This would be an appropriate point at which to consider the chromosomal evidence of clone formation in human neoplasms in general and the part played by chromosome changes in determining the pattern of clonal evolution. The finding of the same unusual chromosome abnormality in all the cells of a tumor has been put forward for a long time as evidence that cancers are clonally derived. It is not necessary to go over the evidence here, but it is generally accepted that cells with an unusual chromosome abnormality represent the progeny of a single cell, that there may be one or more clones within a tumor (2) and that, ultimately, one clone may come to predominate (39). This concept is supported by two other pieces of evidence. Gahrton et al. (30) have shown that in cells from patients with CML the pattern of occurrence of chromosomes with fluorescent markers (i.e., chromosomes with polymorphisms) strongly suggests that it is always the same member of a chromosome pair that is involved in a rearrangement or other abnormality. It is therefore more probable that all the abnormal cells were the progeny of a single cell rather than the result of multiple aberrations of the same type. Gartler, Fialkow and their colleagues, using X-linked markers, have demonstrated the clonal origin of abnormal cells in CML and a number of other neoplasms (24). The argument that the apparent clonal nature of the cells in CML results from selection of cells of one particular glucose-6-phosphate dehydrogenase phenotype (A) was removed by the demonstration by Barr and Fialkow (5) that the other variant (B) of glucose-6-phosphate dehydrogenase was present in the cells of at least one CML patient. Some neoplasms have been shown to be multicellular in origin, e.g., hereditary neurofibromas (25). Even in CML, where evidence in favor of clonal origin of the leukemic cells comes from a study of chromosome mosaics (84), at least one case could support a multiclonal origin (118).

In CML the clone must either have a considerable proliferative advantage over normal elements or arise at a very early stage in embryogenesis. Both possibilities have intriguing implications. If the former is true, then there is a clone with a proliferative advantage which obeys (in the case of erythroid and thrombocyte precursors) normal regulatory controls. If the latter, then the myeloid cells must remain under normal control for prolonged periods in spite of having the Ph^1 chromosome. Evidence favors the idea that the development of the Ph^1 chromosome neither initiates the neoplasia nor results from it. Rather it is a marker of a preexisting abnormal clone within which neoplasia is more likely to arise [cf. the 14q12 clones in ataxia telangiectasia (72)]. Evidence that it preexists comes from cases of polycythemia (119) and thrombocythemia with the Ph^1 (64) and also from rare normal individuals with the Ph^1 (3,10,54). It seems possible that many normal people have the Ph^1 chromosome in their bone marrow, but to substantiate this hypothesis would require many thousand chromosome studies on the bone marrow of normal individuals.

Given the clonal nature of the cell population in many tumors, what is its significance? Fialkow points out that, while clonal proliferation may indicate that the neoplasm has had its origin in a single cell, it is equally compatible with the idea that one particular clone may be selected out from within a population of variable chromosomal structure. Evidence to support this latter idea comes from various sources. Older evidence of sequential emergence of different clones in acute leukemia may support this concept but it is open to the criticism that the clones often emerge following treatment and may therefore be a special case. However, in some cases it can be shown that the clone was not induced by therapy. For example, Jonasson et al. (63) describe a case of AML with a trisomy 8 clone which was clearly present prior to treatment and which reappeared (complicated by two translocations) at the time of relapse. Thus, generally there seems little doubt that cell selection and clone formation play an important part in tumor progression. This general area seems to be a fruitful one for further investigation. It is particularly important to determine whether or not clones, even without cytogenetic markers, are formed in normal tissues *in vivo* and to explore the reasons for the emergence of only certain clones with particular abnormal karyotypes in AT and in the leukemias.

CONCLUSION

The association of some constitutional chromosome aberrations with neoplasia, e.g., Down's and Klinefelter's syndromes, may be indirect and due to hormonal imbalance or other physiologic factors. In other cases, the aberrations may themselves be a manifestation of instability of the genome. The chromosome breakage syndromes and those with defects of DNA repair may exert their effect by generating a population of enormous cellular diversity. Environmental agents could similarly lead to the production of a population of variable unstable cells. It may be from within this population of cells that clones of cells with malignant potential are selected by an interplay between the cells and the response of the host. Clonal evolution may precede the recognition of neoplasia but certainly plays an important role in the progression of the neoplasm following malignant transformation. This progression will be influenced by a variety of factors including host responses and treatment, but in many cases seems to lead to a more highly malignant line of cells.

ACKNOWLEDGMENTS

I am grateful to the British Cancer Research Campaign for their support for this work, to Jennifer Oxford for reading the manuscript, to Malcolm Taylor and Peter Benn for allowing me to quote unpublished results, and to Peter Benn for Fig. 2.

REFERENCES

1. Anday, G. J., Fishkin, B., and Gabor, E. P. (1974): Cytogenetic studies in multiple myeloma. *J. Natl. Cancer Inst.*, 52:1069–1079.
2. Atkin, N. B., Baker, M. C., Robinson, R., and Gaze, S. E. (1974): Chromosome studies on 14 near-diploid carcinomas of the ovary. *Eur. J. Cancer*, 10:143–146.
3. Baccarani, M., Zaccaria, A., and Tura, S. (1973): Letter. Philadelphia-chromosome-positive preleukaemic state. *Lancet*, 2:1094.
4. Baccarani, M., Zaccaria, A., and Tura, S. (1974): Letter. Splenic lymphocytes in chronic myeloid leukaemia. *Lancet*, 2:401.
5. Barr, R. D., and Fialkow, P. J. (1973): Clonal origin of chronic myelocytic leukemia. *N. Engl. J. Med.*, 289:307–309.
6. Bauke, J. (1973): Klonal Evolution in Spätstadium der chronischen myeloischen leukämie. *Dtsch. Med. Wochenschr.*, 98:1956–1959.
7. Bigger, T. R. L., Savage, J. R. K., and Watson, G. E. (1972): A scheme for characterising ASG banding and an illustration of its use in identifying complex chromosomal rearrangements in irradiated human skin. *Chromosoma*, 39:297–310.
8. Bobrow, M., Emerson, P. M., Spriggs, A. I., and Ellis, H. L. (1973): Ring-1 chromosome, microcephalic dwarfism, and acute myeloid leukemia. *Am. J. Dis. Child.*, 126:257–260.
9. Burnet, M. (1974): *Intrinsic Mutagenesis. A Genetic Approach in Ageing.* Medical and Technical Publishing Co. Ltd., Lancaster.
10. Canellos, G. P., and Whang-Peng, J. (1972): Philadelphia chromosome positive preleukaemic state. *Lancet*, 2:1227–1228.
11. Chaganti, R. S. K., Schonberg, S., and German, J. (1974): A manifold increase in sister chromatid exchanges in Bloom's syndrome lymphocytes. *Proc. Natl. Acad. Sci. USA*, 71:4508–4512.

12.   Cleaver, J. E. (1973): DNA repair with purines and pyrimidines in radiation and carcinogen-damaged normal and xeroderma pigmentosum human cells. *Cancer Res., 33*:362–369.

13.   Cohen, M. M., and Shaw, M. W. (1965): Specific effects of viruses and antimetabolites on mammalian chromosomes. In: *The Chromosome: Structural and Functional Aspects,* edited by C. J. Dawe, pp. 50–66. Waverley Press, Baltimore.

14.   Court Brown, W. M., Buckton, K. E., Langlands, A. O., and Woodcock, G. E. (1967): The identification of lymphocyte clones, with chromosome structural aberrations in irradiated men and women. *Int. J. Radiat. Biol.,* 13:155–168.

15.   Croce, C. M., and Koprowski, H. (1974): Somatic cell hybrids between mouse peritoneal macrophages and SV40-transformed human cells. I. Positive control of the transformed phentotype by the human chromosome 7 carrying the SV40 genome. *J. Exp. Med.,* 140:1221–1229.

16.   Croce, C. M., Knowles, B. B., and Koprowski, H. (1973): Preferential retention of the human chromosome C-7 in human—(thymidine kinase deficient) mouse hybrid cells. *Exp. Cell. Res.,* 82:457–461.

17.   Croce, C. M., Huebner, K., Girardi, A. J., and Koprowski, H. (1974): Genetics of cell transformation by simian virus 40. *Cold Spring Harbor Symp. Quant. Biol.,* 34:335–343.

18.   Cunliffe, P. N., Mann, J. R., Cameron, A. H., Roberts, K. D., and Ward, H. W. C. (1974): Radiosensitivity in ataxia telangiectasia. *Br. J. Radiol.,* 48:374–376.

19.   Deaton, J. G. (1973): The mortality rate and causes of death among institutionalised mongols in Texas. *J. Ment. Defic. Res.,* 17:117–122.

20.   Engel, E., Flexner, J. M., Engel-de-Montmollin, M. L., and Frank, H. E. (1964): Blood and skin chromosomal alterations of a clonal type in a leukemic man previously irradiated for a lung carcinoma. *Cytogenetics,* 3:228–251.

21.   Emerit, I., Housset, E., de Grouchy, J., and Camus, J. P. (1971): Chromosomal breakage in diffuse scleroderma. *Eur. J. Clin. Biol. Res.,* 16:684–694.

22.   Evans, H. J. (1974): Effects of ionizing radiation on mammalian chromosomes. In: *Chromosomes and Cancer,* edited by J. German, pp. 191–237. Wiley, New York.

23.   Evans H. J., and Adams, A. (1973): X-ray induced chromosome aberrations in human lymphocytes irradiated *in vitro*: The influence of exposure conditions, genotype and age on aberration yields. In: *Advances in Radiation Research,* edited by J. F. Duplan and A. Chapiro, pp. 335–348. Gordon and Breach, New York.

24.   Fialkow, P. J. (1974): The origin and development of human tumors studied with cell markers. *N. Engl. J. Med.,* 291:26–35.

25.   Fialkow, P. J., Sagebiel, R. W., Gartler, S. M., and Rimoin, D. L. (1971): Multiple cell origin of hereditary neurofibromas. *N. Engl. J. Med.,* 284:298–300.

26.   Fitzgerald, P. H., and Homer, J. W. (1969): Third case of chronic lymphocytic leukemia in a carrier of the inherited Ch[1] chromosome. *Br. Med. J.,* 3:752–754.

27.   Foerster, W., Medau, H. J., and Löffler, H. (1974): Chronische Myeloische Leukämie mit Philadelphia-chromosom und tandem-translokation AM 2. Chromosom NR 22; 46, XX, tan (22q+:22q-). *Klin Wochenschr.,* 52:123–126.

28.   Ford, J. H., Pittman, S. M., and Gunz, F. W. (1974): Letter. Consistent chromosome abnormalities in acute leukaemia. *Br. Med. J.,* 4:227–228.

29.   Funes-Cravioto, F., Lambert, B., Lindsten, J., Ehrenberg, L., Natarajan, A. T., and Osterman-Golkar, S. (1975): Chromosome aberrations in workers exposed to vinyl chloride. *Lancet,* 1:459.

30.   Gahrton, G., Lindsten, J., and Zech, L. (1974): Clonal origin of the Philadelphia chromosome from either the paternal or the maternal chromosome number 22. *Blood,* 43:837–840.

31.   Gahrton, G., Lindsten, J., and Zech, L. (1974): Involvement of chromosome 8, 9, 19 and 22 in Ph[1] positive and Ph[1] negative chronic myelocytic leukemia in the chronic or blastic stage. *Acta Med. Scand.,* 196:355–360.

32.   Garson, O. M., and Milligan, W. J. (1974): Acute leukemia associated with an abnormal genotype. *Scand. J. Haematol.,* 12:256–262.

33.   German, J. (ed) (1974): *Chromosomes and Cancer.* Wiley, New York.

34.   German, J. (1974): Bloom's syndrome. The prototype of human genetic disorders predisposing to chromosome instability and cancer. In: *Chromosomes and Cancer,* edited by J. German, pp. 601–617. Wiley, New York.

35.   German, J., Archibald, R., and Bloom, D. (1965): Chromosomal breakage in a rare and probably genetically determined syndrome of man. *Science,* 148:506–507.

36. German, J., Gilleran, T. G., Setlow, R. B., and Regan, J. D. (1973): Mutant karyotypes in a culture of cells from a man with xeroderma pigmentosum. *Ann. Genet.,* 16:23–27.
37. Giangiacomo, J., Penchansky, L., Monteleone, P. L., and Thompson, J. (1975): Bilateral neonatal Wilms' tumor with B-C chromosomal translocation. *J. Pediatr.,* 86:98–102.
38. Granberg, I., Gupta, S., and Zech, L. (1973): Chromosome analyses of a metastatic gastric carcinoma including quinacrine fluorescence. *Hereditas,* 75:189–194.
39. de Grouchy, J., and Turleau, C. (1974): Clonal evolution in the myeloid leukemias. In: *Chromosomes and Cancer,* edited by J. German, pp. 287–311. Wiley, New York.
40. de Grouchy, J., Bonnette, J., Brussieu, J., Roidot, M., and Begin, P. (1972): Cassures chromosomiques dans l'incontinentia pigmenti. Étude d'une famille. *Ann. Génét.,* 15:61–65.
41. Gunz, F. W., Fitzgerald, P. H., and Adams, A. (1962): An abnormal chromosome in chronic lymphatic leukaemia. *Br. Med. J.,* 2:1097–1099.
42. Hand, R., and German, J. (1974): A retarded rate of DNA chain growth in Bloom's syndrome. *Proc. Natl. Acad. Sci. USA,* 72:758–762.
43. Happle, R., and Hoehn, H. (1973): Cytogenetic studies on cultured fibroblast-like cells derived from basal cell carcinoma tissue. *Clin. Genet.,* 4:17–24.
44. Harnden, D. G. (1972): Specificity of acquired chromosome damage in man. In: *Proc. 4th Int. Cong. Hum. Genet.,* edited by J. de Grouchy, F. J. G. Ebling, and I. W. Henderson, pp. 177–187. Excerpta Medica, Amsterdam.
45. Harnden, D. G. (1974): Ataxia telangiectasia: Cytogenetic and cancer aspects. In: *Chromosomes and Cancer,* edited by J. German, pp. 616–636. Wiley, New York.
46. Harnden, D. G. (1974): Viruses, chromosomes, and tumours: The interaction between viruses and chromosomes. In: *Chromosomes and Cancer,* edited by J. German, pp. 151–190. Wiley, New York.
47. Harnden, D. G., Benn, P. A., Oxford, J. M., Taylor, A. M. R., and Webb, T. P. (1976): Cytogenetically marked clones in human fibroblasts cultured from normal subjects. *Somatic Cell Genetics,* 2:55–62.
48. Harnden, D. G., Maclean, N., and Langlands, A. O. (1971): Carcinoma of the breast and Klinefelter's syndrome. *J. Med. Genet.,* 8:460–461.
49. Hashem, N., and Khalifa, S. H. (1975): Retinoblastoma. A model of hereditary fragile chromosomal regions. *Hum. Hered.,* 25:33–49.
50. Hayata, I., Kakati, S., and Sandberg, A. A. (1975): Letter. Another translocation related to the Ph^1 chromosome. *Lancet,* 1:1300.
51. Hecht, F., Koler, R. D., Rigas, D. A., Dahnke, G. S., Case, M. P., Tisdale, V., and Miller, R. W. (1966): Leukaemia and lymphocytes in ataxia telangiectasia. *Lancet,* 2:1193.
52. Hecht, F., McCaw, B. K., and Koler, R. D. (1973): Ataxia telangiectasia—clonal growth of translocation lymphocytes. *N. Engl. J. Med.,* 289:286–291.
53. Herrmann, R. P., Gallon, W., Jackson, J. M., and Woodliff, H. J. (1973): Idiopathic thrombocythaemia; a review of seven cases in Western Australia. *Aust. N.Z. J. Med.,* 3:489–494.
54. Hirschhorn, K. (1968): Cytogenetic alterations in leukemia. In: *Perspectives in Leukemia,* edited by W. Demashek and R. M. Dutcher, pp. 113–122. Grune & Stratton, New York.
55. Holland, W. W., Doll, R., and Carter, C. O. (1962): The mortality from leukaemia and other cancers among patients with Down's syndrome (mongols) and among their parents. *Br. J. Cancer,* 16:177–186.
56. Honoré, L. H., Dill, F. J., and Poland, B. J. (1974): The association of hydatidiform mole and trisomy 2. *Obstet. Gynecol.,* 43:232–237.
57. Hossfeld, D. K., and Wendehorst, E. (1974): Ph^1-negative chronic myelocytic leukaemia with a missing Y chromosome. *Acta Haematol. (Basel),* 52:232–237.
58. Hsu, L. Y., Alter, A. V., and Hirschhorn, K. (1974): Trisomy 8 in bone marrow cells of patients with polycythemia vera and myelogenous leukemia. *Clin. Genet.,* 6:258–264.
59. Huang, C. C., Banerjee, A., and Hou, Y. (1975): Chromosomal instability in cell lines derived from patients with xeroderma pigmentosum. *Proc. Soc. Exp. Biol. Med.,* 148:1244–1248.
60. Jablon, S., and Kato, H. (1972): Studies of the mortality of A-bomb survivors: 5. Radiation dose and mortality 1950-1970. *Radiat. Res.,* 50:649–698.
61. Jacobs, P. A., Tough, I. M., and Wright, D. A. (1963): Cytogenetic studies in Burkitt's lymphoma. *Lancet,* 2:1144–1146.
62. Jarvis, J. E. (1974): Herpesviruses and oncogenesis. *Nature,* 252:348.

63. Jonasson, J., Gahrton, G., Lindsten, J., Simonsson-Lindemalm, C., and Zech, L. (1974): Trisomy 8 in acute myeloblastic leukemia and sideroachrestic anemia. *Blood,* 43:557–563.
64. Kemp, N. H., Stafford, J. L., and Tanner, R. (1964): Chromosomal studies during early and terminal chronic myeloid leukaemia. *Br. Med. J.,* 1:1010–1014.
65. Knudson, A. G. (1971): Mutation and cancer. Statistical study of retinoblastoma. *Proc. Natl. Acad. Sci. USA,* 68:820–823.
66. Kuni, C. C. (1973): Extra-adrenal pheochromocytoma with metastasis in Down's syndrome. *J. Pediatr.,* 83:835–836.
67. Ladda, R., Atkins, L., Littlefield, J., and Pruett, R. (1973): Retinoblastoma: Chromosome banding in patients with heritable tumour. *Lancet,* 2:506.
68. Langlands, A. O., and Maclean, N. (1976): Lymphoma of the thyroid. An unusual clinical course in a patient possessing a 14/21 translocation. *Cancer,* 38:259–267.
69. Lawler, S. D., Millard, R. E., and Kay, H. E. M. (1970): Further cytogenetical investigation in polycythaemia vera. *Eur. J. Cancer,* 6:223–233.
70. Lawler, S. D., Lobb, D. S., and Wiltshaw, E. (1974): Philadelphia-chromosome-positive bone marrow cells showing loss of the Y in males with chronic myeloid leukaemia. *Br. J. Haematol.,* 27:247–252.
71. Littlefield, L. G., and Mailhes, J. B. (1975): Observations of *de novo* clones of cytogenetically aberrant cells in primary fibroblast cell strains from phenotypically normal women. *Am. J. Hum. Genet.,* 27:190–197.
72. McCaw, B. K., Hecht, F., Harnden, D. G., and Teplitz, R. (1975): Somatic rearrangement of chromosome 14 in human lymphocytes. *Proc. Natl. Acad. Sci. USA,* 72:2071–2075.
73. McDougall, J. K., Dunn, A. R., and Gallimore, P. H. (1974): Recent studies on the characteristics of adenovirus-infected and transformed cells. *Cold Spring Harbor Symp. Quant. Biol.,* 34:591–600.
74. Manolov, G., and Manolova, Y. (1972): Marker band in one chromosome 14 from Burkitt lymphomas. *Nature,* 237:33–34.
75. Mark, J. (1973): Karyotype patterns in human meningiomas. A comparison between studies with G- and Q-banding techniques. *Hereditas,* 75:213–219.
76. Mark, J. (1973): The fluorescence karyotypes of three human meningiomas with hyperdiploid-hypotriploid stemlines. *Acta Neuropathol. (Berl),* 25:46–53.
77. Mark, J. (1974): The human meningioma: A benign tumor with specific chromosome characteristics. In: *Chromosomes and Cancer,* edited by J. German, pp. 497–517. Wiley, New York.
78. Martineau, M. (1967): Chromosomes in testicular tumours. *Lancet,* 1:386.
79. Miller, R. W. (1970): Neoplasia and Down's syndrome. *Ann. N. Y. Acad. Sci.,* 171:637–644.
80. Mitelman, F., and Brandt, L. (1974): Chromosome banding pattern in acute myeloid leukaemia. *Scand. J. Haematol.,* 13:321–330.
81. Mitelman, F., Brandt, L., and Levan, G. (1973): Letter. Identification of isochromosome 17 in acute myeloid leukaemia. *Lancet,* 2:972.
82. Mitelman, F., Brandt, L., and Nilsson, P. G. (1974): Cytogenetic evidence for splenic origin of blastic transformation in chronic myeloid leukaemia. *Scand. J. Haematol.,* 13:87–92.
83. Mitelman, F., Mark, J., Nilsson, P. G., Dencker, H., Norryd, C., and Tranberg, K. G. (1974): Chromosome banding pattern in human colonic polyps. *Hereditas,* 78:63–68.
84. Moore, M. A., Ekert, E., Fitzgerald, M. G., and Carmichael, A. (1974): Evidence for the clonal origin of chronic myeloid leukemia from a sex chromosome mosaic: Clinical, cytogenetic and marrow culture studies. *Blood,* 43:15–22.
85. Moorhead, P. S., and Saksela, E. (1963): Non-random chromosome aberrations in SV40-transformed human cells. *J. Cell. Comp. Physiol.,* 62:57–83.
86. Mulvihill, J. J., Wade, W. M., and Miller, R. W. (1975): Gonadoblastoma in dysgenetic gonads with a Y chromosome. *Lancet,* 1:863.
87. Nowell, P. C. (1971): Marrow chromosome studies in "preleukemia," further correlation with clinical course. *Cancer,* 28:513–518.
88. O'Riordan, M. L., Langlands, A. O., and Harnden, D. G. (1972): Further studies on the frequency of constitutional chromosome aberrations in patients with malignant disease. *Eur. J. Cancer,* 8:373–379.
89. Orye, E., Delbeke, M. J., and Vandenabeele, B. (1974): Retinoblastoma and long arm deletion of chromosome 13. Attempts to define the deleted segment. *Clin. Genet.,* 5:457–464.
90. Oxford, J. M., Harnden, D. G., Parrington, J. M., and Delhanty, J. D. A. (1975): Specific

chromosome aberrations in ataxia telangiectasia. *J. Med. Genet.*, 12:251–262.
91. Pedersen, B. (1973): The karyotype evolution in chronic granulocytic leukaemia. I. The chromosomes gained and lost during initiation of the evolution. *Eur. J. Cancer*, 9:503–507.
92. Pedersen, B. (1973): The karyotype evolution in chronic granulocytic leukaemia—II. The chromosome and karyotype pattern of advanced evolution. *Eur. J. Cancer*, 9:509–513.
93. Pedersen, B. (1973): The blastic crisis of chronic myeloid leukaemia: Acute transformation of a preleukaemic condition? *Br. J. Haematol.*, 25:141–145.
94. Perry, P., and Evans, H. J. (1975): Cytological detection of mutagen-carcinogen exposure by sister chromatid exchange. *Nature*, 258:121–125.
95. Philip, J. (1975): Letter. Gonadoblastoma in dysgenetic gonads with a Y chromosome. *Lancet*, 1.1244.
96. Pierre, R. V. (1974): Preleukemic states. *Semin. Hematol.*, 11:73–92.
97. Purchase, I. F. H., Richardson, C. R., and Anderson, D. (1975): Chromosomal and dominant lethal effects of vinyl chloride. *Lancet*, 2:410–411.
98. Reeves, B. R. (1973): Cytogenetics of malignant lymphomas. Studies utilising a Giemsa-banding technique. *Humangenetik*, 20:231–250.
99. Reeves, B. R., Lobb, D. S., and Lawler, S. D. (1972): Identity of the abnormal F-group chromosome associated with polycythaemia vera. *Humangenetik*, 14:159–161.
100. Rowley, J. D. (1973): Letter. A new consistent chromosomal abnormality in chronic myelogenous leukaemia identified by quinacrine fluorescence and Giemsa staining. *Nature*, 243:290–293.
101. Rowley, J. D. (1974): Editorial. Do human tumors show a chromosome pattern specific for each etiologic agent? *J. Natl. Cancer Inst.*, 52:315–320.
102. Rowley, J. D. (1974): Letter. Missing sex chromosomes and translocations in acute leukaemia. *Lancet*, 2:835–836.
103. Rowley, J. D. (1975): Non-random chromosomal abnormalities in hematologic disorders of man. *Proc. Natl. Acad. Sci. USA*, 72:152–156.
104. Rowley, J. D., Blaisdell, R. K., and Jacobson, L. O. (1966): Chromosome studies in preleukemia. I. Aneuploidy in group C-chromosomes in 3 patients. *Blood*, 27:782–799.
105. Sasaki, M. S. (1973): DNA repair capacity and susceptibility to chromosome breakage in xeroderma pigmentosum cells. *Mutat. Res.*, 20:291–293.
106. Scheike, O. (1975): Male breast cancer. *Acta Pathol. Microbiol. Scand. (A) (Suppl.)*, 251:3–35.
107. Schroeder, T. M., Anschütz, F., and Knopp, A. (1964): Spontane Chromosomenaberrationen bei der familiärer Panmyelopathie (Typus Fanconi). *Humangenetik*, 1:194–196.
108. Searle, C. E., Harnden, D. G., Venitt, S., and Gyde, O. H. B. (1975): Carcinogenicity and mutagenicity tests of some hair colourants and constituents. *Nature*, 255:506–507.
109. Sohn, K. Y., and Boggs, D. R. (1974): Klinefelter's syndrome, LSD usage and acute lymphoblastic leukemia. *Clin. Genet.*, 6:20–22.
110. Spiers, A. S., Galton, D. A., Kaur, J., and Goldman, J. M. (1975): Thioguanine as primary treatment for chronic granulocytic leukaemia. *Lancet*, 1:829–832.
111. Spriggs, A. I. (1974): Cytogenetics of cancer and precancerous states of cervix uteri. In: *Chromosomes and Cancer*, edited by J. German, pp. 423–450. Wiley, New York.
112. Steel, C. M. (1971): Non-identity of apparently similar chromosome aberration in human lymphoblastic cell lines. *Nature*, 233:555–556.
113. Taylor, A. M. R. (1973): Inherited and induced variation in the chromosomes of human cells in primary culture. PhD thesis. University of Birmingham.
114. Taylor, A. M. R., Harnden, D. G., and Fairburn, E. A. (1973): Chromosomal instability associated with susceptibility to malignant disease in patients with porokeratosis of Mibelli. *J. Natl. Cancer Inst.*, 51:371–378.
115. Taylor, A. M. R., Metcalfe, J., Oxford, J. M., and Arlett, C. (1976): Cell survival and chromosome damage in ataxia telangiectasia following X-irradiation. *Heredity*, 36:283.
116. Taylor, A. M. R., Harnden, D. G., Arlett, C. F., Harcourt, S. A., Lehmann, A. R., Stevens, S., and Bridges, B. A. (1975): Ataxia telangiectasia: A human mutation with abnormal radiation sensitivity. *Nature*, 258:427–429.
117. Tough, I. M. (1965): Cytogenetic studies in cases of chronic myeloid leukaemia with previous history of radiation. In: *Current Research in Leukaemia*, edited by F. G. J. Hayhoe, Cambridge University Press, London.
118. Tough, I. M., Court Brown, W. M., Baikie, A. G., Buckton, K. E., Harnden, D. G., Jacobs,

P. A., King, M. J., and McBride, J. A. (1961): Cytogenetic studies in chronic myeloid leukaemia and acute leukaemia associated with mongolism. *Lancet,* 1:411–417.

119. Verhest, A., and van Schoubroek, F. (1973): Letter. Philadelphia-chromosome-positive preleukaemic state. *Lancet,* 2:1386.

120. Visfeldt, J. (1966): Clone formation in tissue culture. *Acta Path. Microbiol. Scand.,* 68:305–312.

121. Weiss, A.F., Portmann, R., Fischer, H., Simon, J., and Zang, K. D. (1975): Simian virus 40-related antigens in three human meningiomas with defined chromosome loss. *Proc. Natl. Acad. Sci. USA,* 72:609–613.

122. Wurster-Hill, D. H., Cornwell, G. G., and McIntyre O. R. (1974): Chromosomal aberrations and neoplasm—a family study. *Cancer,* 33:72–81.

123. Zech, L. (1974): Non-random distribution of chromosome abnormalities in tissues of neoplastic origin. *11th Int. Cancer Cong. Abstr.* 644.

Discussion

Gerald: Concerning the malignancy in XY females, who are in general XO/XY mosaics, I wonder if any of these tumors have been karyotyped? Are they XO, XY, or mosaic?

Harnden: First, I think it is wrong to say that these tumors occur in mosaics only; they occur also in testicular feminization and gonadal dysgenesis where the entire karyotype is XY. But, I don't know of even one tumor from such a patient that has been karyotyped.

Hirschhorn: In one patient with XYY/XY/XO mosaicism, the tumor was XY.

Herrmann: I know of eight reported Down's syndrome (DS) patients with retinoblastoma. Does that exceed expectation by chance? I think so.

Harnden: I agree. On the other hand, the association of testicular cancer in a few DS patients seems by chance. (Ed.: In the United States retinoblastoma occurs in one of 18,000 births and 5,000 cases of DS are born annually; so, one DS patient with retinoblastoma would be expected every 3 years, and the eight published cases does not seem excessive.)

Croce: The preferential retention of chromosome 7 in somatic cell hybrids has nothing to do with the presence of integrated SV-40 on chromosome 7. If a mouse cell deficient in thymidine kinase is crossed with a normal tumor cell, about 80% of the clones retain chromosome 7. That is *not* 100%, which means that chromosomes *can* be lost from the hybrid cell. If the same mouse cell line is crossed with the same human cell, this time transformed by SV-40, again 80% of the hybrid clones retain human chromosome 7, and those that retain it express SV-40-induced antigen. Even if a normal parental mouse cell line is used for hybridization, all the hybrid cells that retain chromosome 7 transform *in vitro* (i.e., clonal formation in soft agar) and behave *in vivo* as tumorigenic cells (i.e., produce tumors when injected in nude mice). Clones or subclones from the same cross that lack chromosome 7 behave normally *in vitro* and do not cause tumors in nude mice.

Koprowski: Dr. Harnden mentioned the presence of SV-40 in meningiomas. The evidence, in fact, comes from only one laboratory and is based on supposedly specific immunofluorescent staining for SV-40 T antigen in human meningioma cells [*Proc. Natl. Acad. Sci. USA,* 72:609–613 (1975)]. These results have not been confirmed in other laboratories, and two meningiomas studied by us showed no evidence for presence of SV-40 T antigen. I think there is some evidence for the role of SV-40 in human pathology based on two isolations of the virus from cases of progressive multifocal leukoencephalopathy (PML); on the other hand, no more isolations of SV-40 from PML were reported but another papovavirus, the JC virus, was being incriminated in the etiology of PML in many more cases than SV-40 [*N. Engl. J. Med.,* 289:1278–1282 (1973).]

Genetics of Human Cancer, edited by J. J.
Mulvihill, R. W. Miller, and J. F. Fraumeni, Jr.
Raven Press, New York, 1977.

9

Chromosome Instability Syndromes

Frederick Hecht and *Barbara Kaiser McCaw

*Crippled Children's Division and Perinatal Medicine, *Department of Pediatrics, and Division of Medical Genetics, University of Oregon Health Sciences Center, Portland, Oregon 97201*

At least three terms have been employed to designate a group of disorders —chromosome *instability* syndromes, chromosome *fragility* syndromes, and chromosome *breakage* syndromes. "Breakage" means an increase of chromosome breaks; this is not the case in all of these syndromes. "Fragility" implies an increase in spontaneous or induced chromosome damage; this is also not true of each of these conditions. "Instability," a more encompassing word, suggests impaired chromosome stability. We prefer the term chromosome instability syndromes.

Another key feature of the chromosome instability syndromes is that they all predispose to cancer. These two features of rare diseases—chromosome instability and cancer predisposition—continue to spark studies to clarify the genetics and genesis of cancer.

Various criteria can be used to classify the chromosome instability syndromes—their genetic mode of transmission, their chromosome characteristics, and the type of cancer to which they predispose. We find history, especially the year 1970, useful in separating the syndromes into two groups: (a) the *classic* chromosome instability syndromes, described before 1970, and (b) the *new* chromosome instability syndromes, described since 1970 (Table 1).

CLASSIC CHROMOSOME INSTABILITY SYNDROMES (1–3)

The classic chromosome instability syndromes are Bloom's syndrome, Fanconi's syndrome, ataxia-telangiectasia, and xeroderma pigmentosum.

Bloom's Syndrome (4–16)

This is a rare genetic disorder characterized by growth retardation and a telangiectatic, erythematous rash on the face.

TABLE 1. *Chromosome instability syndromes*

Syndrome	Genetics
Classic	
Bloom's syndrome	Autosomal recessive
Fanconi's syndrome	Autosomal recessive
Ataxia-telangiectasia	Autosomal recessive
Xeroderma pigmentosum	Autosomal recessive
New	
Porokeratosis of Mibelli	Autosomal dominant
Nevoid basal cell carcinoma syndrome	Autosomal dominant
Incontinentia pigmenti	Dominant ?
Scleroderma	Multifactorial

Clinical Picture

Patients with Bloom's syndrome are born at term and appear normal but small. They are short throughout life, even though the growth rate is normal; adult height is usually less than 5 ft. The body has normal proportions. The face is narrow with a relatively prominent nose and hypoplastic malar areas and chin. As children, they have scanty subcutaneous fat and a delicate, rather adult appearance.

The skin looks normal at birth. A sun-sensitive reddish rash appears over the face and other exposed areas during infancy. The rash contains telangiectases —dilated blood vessels. The skin reddens and blisters form, break, and crust, leaving scars.

Intelligence and sexual development are normal. Males may be infertile (no females have mated).

Immunologic Picture

Many patients have serious respiratory and intestinal infections. The immune system is impaired with regard to both delayed hypersensitivity and immunoglobulin production; however, detailed immunologic data are not yet available.

Risk of Cancer

The risk of cancer is increased in Bloom's syndrome. Primary cancer develops in approximately one in every six patients. About half the cancers are acute leukemias, nonlymphocytic in type. It is not known whether relatives of patients have an increased risk of malignancy.

Genetics

Bloom's syndrome is an autosomal recessive condition. Roughly half of all cases have been Ashkenazi Jews. Founder effect is evident—the affected Ashkenazi Jews have been traced to a small area at the present Polish-Ukrainian border. The heterozygote cannot be detected.

Cytogenetics

The cytogenetic hallmark of Bloom's syndrome is the quadriradial figure, which is rarely seen in other chromosomal instability syndromes. Lymphocytes and fibroblasts show an increase in quadriradials. The quadriradials are usually symmetric and involve homologous chromosomes. They arise from equal exchange of chromatid segments, usually at the centromere. The chromosomes contributing to quadriradials are apparently specific, e.g., number 1 is more frequently involved than number 2.

The tendency to homologous interchanges may be correlated with the increased tendency for sister chromatid exchange, also seen in Bloom's syndrome.

During life the proportion of quadriradial and other chromatid exchange figures remains constant, whereas there is a gradual rise in the frequency of monocentric and dicentric chromosomes. This leads to an increasing proportion of micronuclei and hence to increased premature chromosome condensation with pulverization.

Comment

Bloom's syndrome is the prototype of a whole class of disorders that show chromosome instability and predispose to cancer. Although the precise mode of action of the Bloom's allele is unknown, the Bloom's locus may prove to be one gene site in a polygenic system governing the etiology of human cancer.

Fanconi's Anemia (17–34)

Fanconi described several syndromes. His syndrome of osteomalacia with renal overflow of glucose phosphate and amino acids is *not* associated with chromosome instability. Fanconi's syndrome of anemia (also termed Fanconi's pancytopenia or Fanconi's constitutional infantile panmyelopathy) is a chromosome instability syndrome—the only one associated with progressive marrow failure.

Clinical Picture

All marrow elements are usually affected. There is progressive underproduction of red cells, white cells, and platelets leading to anemia, leukopenia, and thrombocytopenia. This in turn leads to increasing lassitude, risk of infection, and bleeding.

Congenital malformations are a distinctive feature of Fanconi's syndrome. Hypoplasia or aplasia of the radius and thumb are most characteristic. Other skeletal malformations and anomalies of the heart and kidney also occur. Length at birth is normal. Growth may become retarded, but not as severely as in Bloom's syndrome.

Immunologic Picture

Immunologic deficiency related to leukopenia occurs. Beyond this, little is known immunologically about Fanconi's anemia patients.

Risk of Cancer

For almost 20 years it has been recognized that Fanconi's syndrome is accompanied by an increased risk of acute leukemia, especially myelomonocytic. Pancytopenia may allow mutant clones to establish themselves with greater ease than usual. Affected patients are also at high risk for squamous cell carcinoma of mucocutaneous junctions, such as around the mouth and anus, and for hepatic adenoma especially following prolonged androgen therapy of their pancytopenia.

Genetics

Fanconi's syndrome is an autosomal recessive condition like the other classic chromosome instability syndromes. The Fanconi gene may be more common than the Bloom gene. It certainly appears to be more ecumenical; it shows no clear concentration in European Jews or other ethnic groups. Carriers of the Fanconi gene cannot be unequivocally identified by any laboratory test.

Cytogenetics

Patients show increased chromosome breakage and rearrangement. This is most evident in fresh bone marrow preparations and in lymphocytes cultured for short periods of time such as 2 to 3 days, but it is also seen in fibroblasts cultured for longer periods. Symmetric quadriradials are *not* a notable feature of Fanconi's syndrome; if quadriradials are found, they tend to be asymmetric. Breaks are usually chromatid in type and are generally *not* located at the centromere. Loss of chromosome material is often evident. There is *no* increase in sister chromatid exchange.

Comment

Why are Fanconi's patients predisposed to chromosome instability *and* cancer? The tendency to chromosome breakage may itself promote cancer. Or the chromosome breaks may make the cells more susceptible to viral or chemical oncogens, or both. Viral transformation induced by SV-40 and perhaps adenovirus 12 is easier in fibroblasts from Fanconi's syndrome patients than normal.

Close relatives of Fanconi's patients show an increased incidence of cancer. Obligate male heterozygotes, for example, have a risk of malignancy more than three times that of the general population. This finding provides support for the hypothesis that the chromosome instability loci may be among the gene sites controlling susceptibility to cancer. The precise enzymatic basis for Fanconi's syndrome is not yet clear.

Ataxia-Telangiectasia (35–74)

Features of this dramatic disorder, recognized for over 30 years, are so varied that workers focus first on one manifestation and then on another, but rarely keep the whole picture in view. At least 300 patients with ataxia-telangiectasia (AT) are known.

Clinical Picture

The cardinal findings associated with AT are progressive cerebellar ataxia, oculocutaneous telangiectases, and recurrent sinopulmonary infections. Most clinicians consider ataxia and oculocutaneous telangiectases as prerequisite to the diagnosis. Only half of our 20 to 25 patients have had sinopulmonary disease.

At birth and during the first year of life patients with AT appear normal. Wobbliness is first evident when the child begins to walk and progresses to severe, incapacitating ataxia. The eyes show nystagmoid movement. The face loses expression and becomes sad, drooping, and drooling. Speech is progressively impaired. Movements of the hands and arms become choreoathetoid; deep tendon reflexes diminish. Intelligence is usually not grossly impaired, since cortical damage is slight compared to that in the cerebellum.

Oculocutaneous telangiectases typically become apparent between 3 and 6 years of age. The bulbar conjunctivae appear reddened, as if the child had been crying. The prominent facial telangiectases have the same butterfly pattern as in Bloom's syndrome. They are most evident over the malar prominences and nose. They may also involve the eyelids, ears, nape of the neck, upper back, antecubital and popliteal fossae, and the dorsum of the hands and feet. Exposure to sunlight increases the tendency for telangiectases to develop, as in Bloom's syndrome. The telangiectases rupture, leaving progressive subtle scarring, pits, and freckles.

Pathology

Telangiectases in the central nervous system are *not* characteristic of AT. At autopsy in AT there is uniform cerebellar cortical atrophy involving both the Purkinje layer and the internal granular layer. There is often demyelinization of the dorsal spinal cerebellar tracks and the posterior columns.

Immunologic Picture

The lymphoid system is generally hypoplastic; the thymus and lymph nodes are small or absent. T lymphocytes are diminished in number resulting in impaired cellular immunity and absent or prolonged delayed hypersensitivity. B lymphocytes are usually impaired with most patients having low or absent IgA and IgE. Levels of IgG and IgM vary, but may be above normal.

Although immunologists see AT as a genetic immunopathy, immunologic defects fail to explain the ataxia and telangiectases.

Risk of Cancer

AT is associated with an increased risk of malignancy. The types of malignancies reported in this condition are listed in Table 2.

Most of the cancers reported in AT involve the lymphoreticular system. Lymphocytic leukemia and lymphomas are most common. The lymphomas may be of the Hodgkin's or non-Hodgkin's type, such as lymphosarcoma and reticulum cell sarcoma. Undifferentiated small cell lymphomas of the Burkitt's type have not been reported in AT.

An AT patient had a 14/14 translocation clone of lymphocytes that constituted about 20% of all lymphocytes sampled. The patient developed chronic lymphocytic leukemia. During relapse, 100% of the cells sampled from peripheral blood were leukemic and showed only one of the two number 14 chromosomes, namely, one with extra material on its long arm (14q+). The evolution of the leukemic clone from the preexisting translocation clone was, we believe, in no way fortuitous. We believe that the leukemic transformation was intimately connected to the loss of a chromosome 14, i.e., to the loss of the 14q- chromosome.

The solid tumors reported in AT range from dysgerminomas to gliomas (Table 2). The number of such cases reported to date is small; it is not clear whether they are coincidental or meaningful.

The absolute risk of malignancy in AT is not known. Of course, AT patients with cancer are more likely to be reported. Many patients with AT die of

TABLE 2. *Malignancies in ataxia-telangiectasia*

Common	Also reported
Acute lymphatic leukemia	Frontal cystic mixed glioma
Chronic lymphatic leukemia	Cerebellar medulloblastoma
Hodgkin's disease	Carcinoma of the pyloris
Reticulum cell sarcoma	Adenocarcinoma of the stomach
Lymphosarcoma	Dysgerminoma, bilateral
Other lymphomas	

From Harnden (46).

infections, and it is not known whether they would have developed a malignancy. There is, however, no doubt that the risk of malignancy, at least of the reticuloendothelial system, is greatly increased in AT.

Genetics

AT is inherited as an autosomal recessive condition, as are the other classic chromosome instability syndromes.

We suspect very strongly that AT is *genetically heterogeneous*. Tendency to infection is one criterion by which we can split AT into two or more genetically separate disorders (Table 3).

The best known form is accompanied by recurrent sinopulmonary infections. We designate this type I. In families with multiple patients, we have observed that if the first affected child has serious respiratory infections, so will all subsequent affected sibs. Approximately half of the patients with AT whom we have seen in Washington, Oregon, and California are *not* prone to infection. We term this type II. Here too we have consistently noted that if the firstborn with AT is spared sinopulmonary infection, subsequent affected sibs will likewise have no such difficulty.

There thus appears to be 100% concordance for progressive pulmonary disease. There is incidentally no apparent correlation between the IgA level in AT patients and their tendency to infection.

Type III is represented by a pair of sibs we have seen with mild ataxia of a nonprogressive nature, oculocutaneous telangiectases, mental retardation sufficient to result in institutionalization, and no undue tendency to infection.

There are at least two other disorders that may be confounded with AT. For the sake of completeness, we class them tentatively as types IV and V. Type IV comprises ataxia of the diplegic type and defective cellular immunity (45). Two sibs—a brother and sister—were affected. The boy died of a brain abscess at age 5. The sister was vaccinated for smallpox, acquired vaccinia gangrenosa at 15 months of age, was treated, and recovered only to die of generalized chickenpox at 4 years of age. It should be noted that these particular infectious problems are not reported in the classic type I AT.

TABLE 3. *Heterogeneity of ataxia-telangiectasia*

Type I.	Ataxia-telangiectasia *with* recurrent sinopulmonary infections
Type II.	Ataxia-telangiectasia *without* recurrent sinopulmonary infections
Type III.	Ataxia-telangiectasia *without* recurrent sinopulmonary infections, but *with* mental retardation (ataxia is nonprogressive)
Type IV.	Ataxic diplegia *with* defective cellular immunity
Type V.	Ataxia, intermittent, with pyruvate decarboxylase deficiency (dehydrogenase)

Type V AT is clinically separable from the other types in that the cerebellar ataxia, choreoathetosis, and anomalous eye movements occur intermittently (36,55,74). Fever may precipitate neurologic attacks, during which serum levels of pyruvic acid, alanine, and phenylalanine are increased. Enzyme assays demonstrate a deficiency of pyruvate decarboxylase. Thiamine may be beneficial in preventing attacks or in lessening their severity.

Another possible criterion by which females with AT may be separable into two genetic disorders is the presence or absence of ovarian failure.

Just as all that glitters is not necessarily gold, so we need to be cautious in grouping patients with either ataxia or telangiectasia, or both, into the same narrow genetic niche. At present, we do *not* know whether types I to V represent different alleles at the same locus, genetic compounds (like some of the storage disease patients), or rare alleles at separate loci.

Cytogenetics

The modal karyotype in AT is normal, which is the case in all of the chromosome instability syndromes. In many patients, increased chromosome breakage is evident in lymphocytes and, less strikingly, in fibroblasts. Breakage is of the chromosomal type, involving both chromatids at homologous sites. We have found but not reported previously that the breaks are apparently random in location. This is in contrast to Bloom's syndrome where the breaks are predominantly located near the centromere and are nonrandom with regard to chromosomes involved.

The level of chromosome breakage often fluctuates. At birth and in early infancy there may be no detectable increase in breakage. It may rise perceptibly and then decline to normal levels in later years. The reasons for these fluctuations in chromosome breakage are not well understood. Clones that are known to arise in AT patients may play a role, as may viruses or other clastogenic agents.

Pseudodiploid clones are usually common in AT. For example, we followed clinically and cytogenetically a young man with AT for almost 5 years until his death of progressive pulmonary insufficiency. When first studied (at age 18 years) a small percentage (1 to 2%) of his lymphocytes had a D/D translocation of the t(14q−;14q+) type. Over the 5 years, the translocation clone of lymphocytes increased to become the predominant type of peripheral lymphocyte, eventually constituting over 70% of sampled lymphocytes. There was a gradual decline in chromosome breakage and a concomitant rise in mitotic activity. Dicentric chromosomes, as observed in Bloom's and Fanconi's syndromes, also become more frequent. Significantly, our patient never developed leukemia or other malignancy, although two of his affected sibs had died of acute lymphocytic leukemia.

A number of other AT patients have subsequently been found to harbor pseudodiploid clones. Most patients have clones marked by a translocation involving chromosome 14. The break in chromosome 14 is always in the long arm at the q11-q12 region. In the translocation, the other involved chromosomes have been 7, 8, 14, and X. There is no apparent loss or gain of genetic material. The only

AT patient reported with a nontranslocation clone has a ring 14 chromosome marker (56).

The common denominator among AT pseudodiploid clones appears therefore to be either loss of material from the long arm (q) of chromosome 14 or more likely position effect (i.e., a change in the genetic activity of the distal portion of 14q due to repositioning of that segment in the genome).

Cytogenetic studies are difficult because AT lymphocytes grow sluggishly and are relatively unresponsive to phytohemagglutinin and other mitogens.

AT fibroblasts have a prolonged doubling time and dally unduly in the S phase of the cell cycle (67), providing further evidence that the AT gene is expressed in fibroblasts. We believe that fibroblasts may provide a useful tool for exploring the obscure biochemistry of the AT cell in search of the basic genetic lesion.

Comment

AT has many interesting aspects. The convergence of progressive neurologic, vascular, and infectious diseases is unusual. So are the profound immune deficiency and the tendency to lymphoid cancer.

Careful clinical observations in AT have stimulated equally careful pathology studies. The resultant clinical and pathologic observations have stimulated incisive thinking in cell biology. The converse is equally true. For example, in 1967 a child with AT and a lymphoma was reported because of an unexpectedly severe reaction to radiotherapy (43). A year later a similar case was described (61), and in 1975 a third case (40). We know of other unreported cases of AT patients with hypersensitivity to radiation treatment (and to corticosteroid therapy) given for malignancy. These clinical observations prompted investigation of AT cells (71). On exposure to X-irradiation, fibroblasts *in vitro* had a marked reduction in cell survival as compared to normal cells. An endonuclease for repair of X-ray-induced DNA damage may, as Harnden has suggested (47), be missing in AT fibroblasts, similar to the deficient enzyme for ultraviolet (UV) damage in xeroderma pigmentosum. Thus, may AT and the other chromosome instability syndromes provide opportunities to correlate clinical, cellular, and subcellular observations.

Xeroderma Pigmentosum (75–95)

The combined clinical and laboratory approach has been fruitful in xeroderma pigmentosum (XP), and is discussed in greater detail elsewhere (J. E. Cleaver, *this volume*).

Clinical Picture

Patients are hypersensitive to sunlight in early childhood. They freckle easily. More serious is their tendency to reddening, blistering, and scarring of exposed skin areas. Most serious is their predisposition to develop myriad basal and squamous cell carcinomata. Families with such children would do well to move *en masse* to western Oregon to avoid the sun and to enjoy the endless gray mist and drizzle of our area! Other preventative measures include attention to protective clothing, a broad-brimmed hat, special sun screens, and frequent whole body examinations by an alert dermatologist.

Genetics

XP is inherited, like the other three classic chromosome instability syndromes, in autosomal recessive fashion. Parental consanguinity is common, suggesting that the gene or genes are infrequent.

So far, at least four complementation groups have been postulated, mainly through experimental fusion of various XP cells. According to the observed percentage of normal DNA repair rates, the groups are designated A ($< 2\%$), B (3 to 7%), C (10 to 25%), and D (25 to 55%). Group E might be temporarily reserved for the syndrome of xeroderma pigmentosum associated with normal rates of UV-induced DNA repair. Several such patients are known. This may, however, represent a mutation at a separate locus.

The syndrome of XP and mental retardation called the De Sanctis–Cacchione syndrome may be a genocopy due to homozygosity for rare alleles at another locus (90–95). In somatic cell hybridization studies, cells from a patient with this condition complemented classic XP cells completely with regard to DNA repair. This type of complementation, as in groups *A* to *D,* could be interlocus or interallelic. Thus, to date, there is no incontrovertible evidence for more than one XP locus.

The De Sanctis–Cacchione syndrome could also represent coincidence of XP and a genetically separate (nonallelic) form of mental retardation. (All three patients with XP plus mental retardation whom we have seen were offspring of first cousin matings.) Alternatively, one can postulate that the basic biochemical lesion in De Sanctis–Cacchione syndrome affects both skin and brain cells.

Cytogenetics

There is no spontaneous increase in chromosome or chromatid fragility. Nor can one induce a significant increase in breakage *in vitro,* to our knowledge, in XP cells.

XP cells do, however, have a defect in DNA repair after UV-irradiation.

NEW CHROMOSOME INSTABILITY SYNDROMES

Chromosome instability has been recently found in other genetic syndromes, but is less well documented. In the cases of porokeratosis of Mibelli and nevoid basal cell carcinoma syndrome, there have only been one or two chromosome studies.

Porokeratosis of Mibelli (96–100)

Clinical Picture

This is a rare genodermatosis with crater-like lesions surrounded by horny ridges, which tend to become malignant.

Genetics

An autosomal dominant trait, this condition and the following one are clearly inherited in a different fashion from the four classic chromosome instability syndromes (Table 1).

Cytogenetics

Chromosome breaks and rearrangements have been observed *only* in cells cultured from the skin lesions, not in fibroblasts cultured from normal areas of skin, or in lymphocytes.

Nevoid Basal Cell Carcinoma Syndrome (101–109)

This disorder is characterized by multiple basal cell nevi, odontogenic keratocysts, and skeletal anomalies.

Clinical Picture

The basal cell nevi are myriad, some resembling seborrheic keratoses. The face may be distinctive with frontal and biparietal bossing, lateral displacement of the inner canthi, jaw cysts, and mildly protruding jaw. The palms and soles may show pits. The skeletal malformations may include vertebral anomalies, fused ribs, and short fourth and fifth metacarpals.

Radiographically, there are lamellar calcifications of the falx cerebri and the jaw cysts. Ovarian fibromata tend to calcify.

The patients are supposedly unresponsive to parathormone.

Genetics

The syndrome is an autosomal dominant trait; there may also be a much rarer autosomal recessive form.

Cytogenetics

There are increased chromosome breaks; several laboratories have reported this finding.

Risk of Cancer

The most frequent malignancies reported in this syndrome are basal cell carcinomas. Brain tumors (particularly medulloblastomas) and ovarian carcinoma have also been reported.

Incontinentia Pigmenti (110–120)

This is a mysterious disease with a constellation of diverse findings.

Clinical Picture

It is characterized by skin pigmentation anomalies in combination with a variety of malformations, suggesting features of Fanconi's syndrome and AT. The pigmentary anomaly is, however, distinctive. At first, it resembles tattooing with inflammation. It is usually evident at birth or shortly thereafter. In its full form, the pigmentary disturbance has the swirling appearance of multicolored marble. Histologically, it was suggested that the basal layer of the epidermis is "incontinent" of melanin. A variety of malformations may involve the eyes, dentitia, heart, and skeleton. Mental retardation is still a debatable feature.

Genetics

It is clear that incontinentia pigmenti behaves as a Mendelian dominant. Despite many reported families with the condition, no affected males have been definitively identified. Several putative cases in males have been claimed.

The salient possibilities are, in order of probability, an X-linked dominant gene lethal in the male, an autosomal dominant gene lethal in the male, and cytoplasmic (or other nonchromosomal) inheritance.

Cytogenetics

Chromosome breaks have been reported in several families segregating for incontinentia pigmenti.

Risk of Cancer

We are aware of only two affected patients with cancer—a 4-month-old girl with acute myelogenous leukemia (120), and a 14-year-old girl with pheochromocytoma (114).

Scleroderma (121–123)

Scleroderma is a generalized disorder of connective tissue and perhaps an autoimmune disease.

Genetics

Scleroderma is clearly not a simple Mendelian trait. It is presumably multifactorial; it does show some familial clustering and so may have in part a genetic basis.

Cytogenetics

Lymphocytes from scleroderma patients have been found to manifest increased chromosome breakage. This tendency is also present in marrow cells on direct preparation, suggesting that it is present *in vivo*. Experiments mixing control and test cells and serum suggest that a breakage factor may exist in the serum of patients with scleroderma.

Risk of Cancer

There is a clearly increased risk of cancer. By 1975, over 25 patients with scleroderma (progressive systemic sclerosis) were reported with alveolar cell adenocarcinoma of the lung. Striking features of the association are the 7 to 1 female:male ratio (compared to 2 or 3 to 1 for scleroderma in general) and positive correlation with the intensity of sclerodermic interstitial pulmonary fibrosis.

CONCLUSION

We have presented a general overview of knowledge pertinent to the chromosome instability syndromes.

The *classic* syndromes—Bloom's syndrome, Fanconi's syndrome, ataxia-telangiectasia, and xeroderma pigmentosum—have been and continue to be heuristic models.

The *new* chromosome instability syndromes are inherited differently and so are presumably caused by different types of genetic lesions, such as defects in receptor site or structural protein. The chromosome breakage in scleroderma may be simply the result of a serum factor.

The old and new chromosome instability syndromes continue to offer opportunities for gaining insight into the mechanisms of human chromosome stability and into the pathogenesis of human cancer.

ACKNOWLEDGMENT

This work has been supported by grants CA 16747 and HD 05082 from the National Institutes of Health.

REFERENCES

General
1.   German, J. (1969): Chromosomal breakage syndromes. *Birth Defects,* 5(5):117–131.

2.   German, J. (1972): Genes which increase chromosomal instability in somatic cells and predispose to cancer. *Prog. Med. Genet.,* 8:61–101.
3.   German, J. (1973): Oncogenic implications of chromosomal instability. *Hosp. Prac.,* 8:93–104.

Bloom's Syndrome

4.   Bloom, D. (1966): The syndrome of congenital telangiectatic erythema and stunted growth. *J. Pediatr.,* 68:103–113.
5.   Chaganti, R. S. K., Schonberg, S., and German, J. (1974): A manyfold increase in sister chromatid exchanges in Bloom's syndrome lymphocytes. *Proc. Natl. Acad. Sci. USA,* 71:4508–4512.
6.   Ferrera, A. (1972): Goltz's syndrome. *Am. J. Dis. Child.,* 123:262.
7.   Ferrera, A., Fontana, V. J., and Numsen, G. (1967): Bloom's syndrome in Oriental male. *NY State J. Med.,* 67:3258–3262.
8.   German, J. (1969): Bloom's syndrome. I. Genetical and clinical observations in the first twenty-seven patients. *Am. J. Hum. Genet.,* 21:196–226.
9.   German, J., Archibald, R., and Bloom, D. (1965): Chromosomal breakage in a rare and probably genetically determined syndrome of man. *Science,* 148:506–507.
10. German, J., and Crippa, L. P. (1966): Chromosomal breakage in diploid cell lines from Bloom's syndrome and Fanconi's anaemia. *Ann. Genet. (Paris),* 9:143–154.
11. Landau, J. W., Sasaki, M. S., Newcomer, V. D., and Norman, A. (1966): Bloom's syndrome. The syndrome of telangiectatic erythema and growth retardation. *Arch. Dermatol.,* 94:687–694.
12. Rauh, J. L., and Soukup, S. W. (1968): Bloom's syndrome. *Am. J. Dis. Child.,* 116:409–413.
13. Sawitsky, A., Bloom, D., and German, J. (1966): Chromosomal breakage and acute leukemia in congenital telangiectatic erythema and stunted growth. *Ann. Intern. Med.,* 65:487–495.
14. Schroeder, T. M. (1975): Sister chromatid exchanges and chromatid interchanges in Bloom's syndrome. *Humangenetik,* 30:317–323.
15. Sperling, K., Goll, U., Kunze, J., Lüdtke, E. K., Tolksdorf, M., and Obe, G. (1976): Cytogenetic investigations in a new case of Bloom's syndrome. *Hum. Genet.,* 31:47–52.
16. Szalay, G. C. (1963): Dwarfism with skin manifestations. *J. Pediatr.,* 62:686–695.

Fanconi's Anemia

17. Bernstein, M. S., Hunter, R. L., and Yachnin, S. (1971): Hepatoma and peliosis hepatis developing in a patient with Fanconi's anemia. *N. Engl. J. Med.,* 284:1135–1136.
18. Bloom, G. E., Warner, S., Gerald, P. S., and Diamond, L. K. (1966): Chromosome abnormalities in constitutional aplastic anemia. *N. Engl. J. Med.,* 274:8–14.
19. Brunetti, P., Neuci, G. G., Vaccaro, R., Puxeddu, A., and Migliorini, E. (1966): Fanconi's anemia. *Lancet,* 2:1194–1195.
20. de Grouchy, J., de Nava, C., Marchand, J. C., Feingold, J., and Turleau, C. (1972): Cytogenetic and biochemical studies of eight cases of Fanconi's anemia. *Ann. Genet. (Paris),* 15:29–40.
21. Fanconi, G. (1966): Familial constitutional panmyelocytopathy, Fanconi's anemia (F.A.). I. Clinical aspects. *Semin. Hematol.,* 4:233–240.
22. Garriga, S., and Crosby, W. H. (1959): The incidence of leukemia in families of patients with hypoplasia of the marrow. *Blood,* 14:1008–1014.
23. German, J., and Crippa, L. P. (1966): Chromosomal breakage in diploid cell lines from Bloom's syndrome and Fanconi's anaemia. *Ann. Genet. (Paris),* 9:143–154.
24. Lohr, G. W., Waller, H. D., Anschütz, F., and Knopp, A. (1965): Biochemische Defekte in den Blutzellen bei familiärer Panmyelopathie (Typ Fanconi). *Humangenetik,* 1:383–387.
25. McDonald, R., and Goldschmidt, B. (1960): Pancytopenia with congenital defects (Fanconi's anemia). *Arch. Dis. Child.,* 35:367–372.

26. Sasaki, M. S. (1975): Is Fanconi's anaemia defective in a process essential to the repair of DNA cross links? *Nature,* 257:501–503.
27. Schmid, W. (1967): Familial constitutional panmyelocytopathy, Fanconi's anemia (F.A.). II. A discussion of the cytogenetic findings in Fanconi's anemia. *Semin. Hematol.,* 4:241–249.
28. Swift, M. (1971): Fanconi's anaemia in the genetics of neoplasia. *Nature,* 230:370–373.
29. Swift, M. R., and Hirschhorn, K. (1966): Fanconi's anemia: Inherited susceptibility to chromosome breakage in various tissues. *Ann. Intern. Med.,* 65:496–503.
30. Swift, M. R., Sholman, L., and Gilmour, D. (1972): Diabetes mellitus and the gene for Fanconi's anemia. *Science,* 178:308–310.
31. Swift, M., Cohen, J., and Pinlchham, R. (1974): Maximum-likelihood method for estimating the disease predisposition of heterozygotes. *Am. J. Hum. Genet.,* 26:304–317
32. von Koskull, H., and Aula, P. (1973): Nonrandom distribution of chromosome breaks in Fanconi's anemia. *Cytogenet. Cell Genet.,* 12:423–434.
33. Zachmann, M., Illig, R., and Prader, A. (1972): Fanconi's anemia with isolated growth hormone deficiency. *J. Pediatr.,* 80:159.
34. Zaizov, R., Matoth, Y., and Mamon, Z. (1969): Familial aplastic anemia without congenital malformations. *Acta Paediatr. Scand.,* 58:151–156.

Ataxia-Telangiectasia

35. Ammann, A. J., Cain, W. A., Ishizaka, K., Hong, R., and Good, R. A. (1969): Immunoglobulin E deficiency in ataxia-telangiectasia. *N. Engl. J. Med.,* 281:469–472.
36. Blass, J. P., Avigan, J., and Uhlendorf, B. W. (1970): A defect in pyruvate decarboxylase in a child with an intermittent movement disorder. *J. Clin. Invest.,* 49:423–432.
37. Blass, J. P., Kark, R. A. P., and Engel, W. K. (1971): Clinical studies of a patient with pyruvate dehydroxylase deficiency. *Arch. Neurol.,* 25:449–460.
38. Boder, E., and Sedgwick, R. P. (1958): Ataxia-telangiectasia: A familial syndrome of progressive cerebellar ataxia, oculocutaneous telangiectasia and frequent pulmonary infection. *Pediatrics,* 21:526–554.
39. Cohen, M. M., Dagan, J., and Shaham, M. (1975): Chromosome studies in families with ataxia telangiectasia. *Am. J. Hum. Genet.,* 27:27A.
40. Cunliffe, P. N., Mann, J. R., Cameron, A. H., and Roberts, K. D. (1975): Radiosensitivity in A-T. *Br. J. Radiol.,* 48:374–376.
41. Eisen, A. H., Karpati, G., Laszlo, T., Andermann, F., Robb, J. P., and Bacal, H. L. (1965): Immunologic deficiency in ataxia telangiectasia. *N. Engl. J. Med.,* 272:18–22.
42. Feigin, R. D., Vietti, T. J., Wyatt, R. G., Kaufman, D. G., and Smith, C. H. (1970): Ataxia telangiectasia with granulocytopenia. *J. Pediatr.,* 77:431–438.
43. Gotoff, S. P., Amirmokro, E., and Liebner, E. J. (1967): Ataxia telangiectasia. Neoplasia, untoward response to X-irradiation, and tuberous sclerosis. *Am. J. Dis. Child.,* 114:617–625.
44. Haerer, A. F., Jackson, J. F., and Evers, C. G. (1969): Ataxia-telangiectasia with gastric adenocarcinoma. *JAMA,* 210:1884–1887.
45. Hagberg, A., Hansson, O., Liden, S., and Nilsson, K. (1970): Familial ataxic diplegia with deficient cellular immunity. A new clinical entity. *Acta Paediatr. Scand.,* 59:545–550.
46. Harnden, D. G. (1974): Ataxia telangiectasia syndrome: Cytogenetic and cancer aspects. In: *Chromosomes and Cancer,* edited by J. German, pp. 619–636. Wiley, New York.
47. Harnden, D. G.: Cytogenetics of human neoplasia. *This volume.*
48. Hecht, F., Koler, R. D., Rigas, D. A., Dahnke, G. S., Case, M. P., Tisdale, V., and Miller, R. W. (1966): Leukaemia and lymphocytes in ataxia-telangiectasia. *Lancet,* 2:1193.
49. Hecht, F., McCaw, B. K., and Koler, R. D. (1973): Ataxia-telangiectasia clonal growth of translocation lymphocytes. *N. Engl. J. Med.,* 289:286–291.
50. Hecht, F., McCaw, B. K., Peakman, D., and Robinson, A. (1975): Non-random occurrence of 7-14 translocations in human lymphocyte cultures. *Nature,* 225:243–244.
51. Hoar, D. I., and Sargent, P. (1975): Chemical mutagen hypersensitivity in ataxia telangiectasia. *Am. J. Hum. Genet.,* 27:44A.
52. Korein, J., Steinman, P. A., and Senz, E. H. (1961): Ataxia-telangiectasia: Report of a case and review of the literature. *Arch. Neurol.,* 4:272–280.
53. Levin, S., and Perlov, S. (1971): Ataxia-telangiectasia in Israel, with observations on its relationship to malignant disease. *Isr. J. Med. Sci.,* 7:1535–1541.

54. Lisker, R., and Cobo, A. (1970): Chromosome breakage in ataxia-telangiectasia. *Lancet*, 1:618.

55. Lonsdale, D., Faulkner, W. R., Price, J. M., and Smeby, R. R. (1969): Intermittent cerebellar ataxia associated with hyperpyruvic acidemia, hyperphenylalaninemia and hyperalaninuria. *Pediatrics*, 43:1025–1034.

56. McCaw, B. K., Hecht, F., Harnden, D. G., and Teplitz, R. L. (1975): Somatic rearrangement of chromosome 14 in human lymphocytes. *Proc. Natl. Acad. Sci. USA*, 72:2071–2075.

57. McFarlin, D. E., Strober, W., and Waldmann, T. A. (1972): Ataxia-telangiectasia. *Medicine (Baltimore)*, 51:281–314.

58. McKusick, V. A., and Cross, H. E. (1966): Ataxia-telangiectasia and Swiss-type agammaglobulinemia. Two genetic disorders of the immune mechanism in related Amish sibships. *JAMA*, 195:739–745.

59. Miller, M. E., and Chatten, J. (1967): Ovarian changes in ataxia telangiectasia. *Acta Paediatr. Scand.*, 56:559–561.

60. Miller, R. W. (1963): Down's syndrome (mongolism), other congenital malformations and cancers among the sibs of leukemic children. *N. Engl. J. Med.*, 268:393–401.

61. Morgan, J. L., Holcomb, T. M., and Morrissey, R. W. (1968): Radiation reaction in ataxia telangiectasia. *Am. J. Dis. Child.*, 116:557–558.

62. Peterson, R. D. A., Kelly, W. D., and Good, R. A. (1964): Ataxia-telangiectasia: Its association with a defective thymus, immunological-deficiency disease and malignancy. *Lancet*, 1:1189–1193.

63. Rary, J. M., Bender, M. A., and Kelly, T. E. (1974): Cytogenetic studies of ataxia-telangiectasia. *Am. J. Hum Genet.*, 26:70A.

64. Reye, C., and Mosman, N. S. W. (1960): Ataxia-telangiectasia. *Am. J. Dis. Child.*, 99:238–247.

65. Schalch, D. S., McFarlin, D.E., and Barlow, M.H. (1970): An unusual form of diabetes mellitus in ataxia telangiectasia. *N. Engl. J. Med.*, 282:1396–1402.

66. Shuster, J., Hart, Z., Stimson, C. W., Brough, A. J., and Poulik, M. D. (1966): Ataxia-telangiectasia with cerebellar tumor. *Pediatrics*, 37:776–786.

67. Siegel, E. B., Elmore, E., and Swift, M. (1975): Growth and cell cycle abnormalities of cultured fibroblasts of ataxia-telangiectasia patients. *Am. J. Hum. Genet.*, 27:81A.

68. Sourander, P., Bonnevier, J. O., and Olsson, Y. (1966): A case of ataxia telangiectasia with lesions in the spinal cord. *Acta Neurol. Scand.*, 42:354–366.

69. Swift, M., Cohen, J., and Pinlchham, R. (1974): Maximum-likelihood method for estimating the disease predisposition of heterozygotes. *Am. J. Hum. Genet.*, 26:304–317.

70. Tadjoedin, M. K., and Fraser, F. C. (1965): Heredity of ataxia telangiectasia (Louis-Bar syndrome). *Am. J. Dis. Child.*, 110:64–68.

71. Taylor, A. M. R., Harnden, D. G., Arlett, C. F., Harcourt, S. A., Lehmann, A.R., Stevens, S., and Bridges, B. A. (1975): Ataxia telangiectasia: A human mutation with abnormal radiation sensitivity. *Nature*, 258:427–429.

72. Taylor, A. M. R., Metcalfe, J. A., Oxford, J. M., and Harnden, D. G. (1976): Is chromatid-type damage in ataxia telangiectasia after irradiation at G_0 a consequence of defective repair? *Nature*, 260:441–443.

73. Waldmann, T. A., and McIntire, K. R. (1972): Serum-alpha-fetoprotein levels in patients with ataxia-telangiectasia. *Lancet*, 2:1112–1115.

74. Willems, J. L., Monnens, L. A. H., Trijbels, J. M. G., Sengers, R. C. A., and Veerkamp, J. H. (1974): Pyruvate decarboxylase deficiency in liver. *N. Engl. J. Med.*, 290:406–407.

Xeroderma Pigmentosum

75. Burnet, F. M. (1974): Intrinsic mutagenesis, an interpretation of the pathogenesis of xeroderma pigmentosum. *Lancet*, 2:495–498.

76. Cleaver, J. E. (1977): *This volume*.

77. Cleaver, J. E. (1968): Defective repair replication of DNA in xeroderma pigmentosum. *Nature*, 218:652–656.

78. Cleaver, J. E. (1973): Xeroderma pigmentosum. Progress and regress. *J. Invest. Dermatol.*, 60:374–380.

79. Cleaver, J. E. (1972): Xeroderma pigmentosum: Variants with normal DNA repair and normal sensitivity to ultraviolet light. *J. Invest. Dermatol.*, 58:124–128.

80. Cleaver, J. E., and Bootsma, D. (1975): Xeroderma pigmentosum: Biochemical and genetic characteristics. *Annu. Rev. Genet.*, 9:19–38.

81. Cockayne, E. A. (1933): *Inherited Abnormalities of the Skin and its Appendages.* Oxford Univ. Press, London.

82. de Grouchy, J., de Nava, C., Feingold, J., Frezal, J., and Lamy, M. (1967): Asynchronie chromosomique dans un cas de xeroderma pigmentosum. *Ann. Genet. (Paris)*, 10:224–225.

83. German, J., Gilleran, T. G., La Rock, J., and Regan, J. D. (1970): Mutant clones amidst normal cells in cultures of xeroderma pigmentosum skin. *Am. J. Hum. Genet.*, 22:10a.

84. Goldstein, S., and Lin, C. C. (1972): Survival and DNA repair of somatic cell hybrids after ultraviolet irradiation. *Nature [New Biol.]*, 239:142–145.

85. Kraemer, K. H., Coon, H. G., Petinga, R. A., Barrett, S. F., Rahe, A. E., and Robbins, J. H. (1975): Genetic heterogeneity in xeroderma pigmentosum: Complementation groups and their relationship to DNA repair rates. *Proc. Natl. Acad. Sci. USA*, 72:59–63.

86. Macklin, M. T. (1944): Xeroderma pigmentosum: Report of a case and consideration of incomplete sex linkage in inheritance of the disease. *Arch. Dermatol. Syph.*, 49:157–171.

87. Regan, J. D., Setlow, R. B., Kaback, M. M., Howell, R. R., Klein, E., and Burgess, G. (1971): Xeroderma pigmentosum: A rapid sensitive method for prenatal diagnosis. *Science*, 174:147–150.

88. Robbins, J. H., Kraemer, K. H., Lutzner, M. A., Festoff, B. W., and Coon, H. G. (1974): Xeroderma pigmentosum: An inherited disease with sun sensitivity, multiple cutaneous neoplasms, and abnormal DNA repair. *Ann. Intern. Med.*, 80:221–248.

89. Wolff, S., Bodycote, J., Thomas, G. H., and Cleaver, J. E. (1975): Sister chromatid exchange in xeroderma pigmentosum. *Genetics*, 81:349–355.

Xeroderma Pigmentosum with Mental Deficiency (De Sanctis–Cacchione Syndrome)

90. Deweerdt-Kastelein, E. A., Keijzer, W., and Bootsma, D. (1972): Genetic heterogeneity of xeroderma pigmentosum demonstrated by somatic cell hybridization. *Nature [New Biol.]*, 238:80–83.

91. Elsasser, G., Greusberg, O., and Theml, F. (1950): Das Xeroderms pigmentosum und die 'xerodermische Idiotie.' *Arch. Dermatol.*, 188:651–655.

92. Reed, W. B., Landing, B. H., Sugarman, G. I., Cleaver, J. E., and Malnyk, J. (1969): Xeroderma pigmentosum. Clinical and laboratory investigation of its basic defect. *JAMA*, 207:2073–2079.

93. Reed, W. B., May, S. B., and Nickel, W. R. (1965): Xeroderma pigmentosum with neurological complications. *Arch. Dermatol.*, 91:224–226.

94. Robbins, J. H., Kraemer, K. H., Lutzner, M. A., Festoff, B. W., and Coon, H. G. (1974): Xeroderma pigmentosum: An inherited disease with sun sensitivity, multiple cutaneous neoplasms and abnormal DNA repair. *Ann. Intern. Med.*, 80:221–248.

95. Yano, K. (1950): Xeroderma pigmentosum mit Storungen des Zentralnervensystems: Eine histopathologische Untersuchung. *Folia Psychiatr. Neurol. Jpn.*, 4:143–151.

Porokeratosis of Mibelli

96. Bloom, D., and Abramowitz, E. W. (1943): Porokeratosis mibelli: Report of three cases in one family: Histologic studies. *Arch. Dermatol. Syph.*, 47:1–15.

97. Cort, D. F., and Abdul-Aziz, A. H. (1972): Epithelioma arising in porokeratosis of Mibelli. *Br. J. Plast. Surg.*, 25:318–328.

98. Harnden, D. G., Taylor, A. M. R., and Oxford, J. M. (1973): Chromosomal instability in cells cultured from patients susceptible to cancer. *Genetics*, 74:S109.

99. Reed, R. J., and Leone, P. (1970): Porokeratosis—a mutant clonal keratosis of the epidermis. Histogenesis. *Arch. Dermatol.*, 101:340–347.

100. Saunders, T. S. (1961): Porokeratosis. A disease of epidermal eccrine-sweat-duct units. *Arch. Dermatol.*, 84:980–988.

Nevoid Basal Cell Carcinoma Syndrome

101. Anderson, D. E., and Cook, W. A. (1966): Jaw cysts and basal cell nevus syndrome. *J. Oral Surg.*, 24:15–26.
102. Anderson, D. E., Taylor, W. B., Falls, H. F., and Davidson, R. T. (1967): The nevoid basal cell carcinoma syndrome. *Am. J. Hum. Genet.*, 19:12–22.
103. Berlin, N. I., Van Scott, E. J., Clendenning, W. E., Archard, H. O., Block, J. B., Witkop, C. J., and Haynes, H. A. (1966): Basal cell nevus syndrome. *Ann. Intern. Med.*, 64:403–421.
104. Cawson, R. A., and Kerr, G. A. (1964): The syndrome of jaw cysts, basal cell tumours and skeletal anomalies. *Proc. R. Soc. Med.*, 57:799–801.
105. Gorlin, R. J., and Goltz, R. W. (1960): Multiple nevoid basal-cell epithelioma, jaw cysts and bifid rib: A syndrome. *N. Engl. J. Med.*, 262:908–912.
106. Gorlin, R. J., and Pindborg, J. J. (1964): Multiple basal nevi, odontogenic keratocysts and skeletal anomalies. In: *Syndromes of the Head and Neck*, pp 400–409. Blakiston Division, McGraw-Hill, New York.
107. Horland, A. A., Wolman, S. R., and Cox, R. P. (1975): Cytogenetic studies in patients with the basal cell nevus syndrome and their relatives. *Am. J. Hum. Genet.*, 27:47A.
108. Lile, H. A., Rogers, J. F., and Gerald, B. (1968): The basal cell nevus syndrome. *Am. J. Roentgenol.*, 103:214–217.
109. Rater, C. J., Selke, A. C., and Van Epps, E. F. (1968): Basal cell nevus syndrome. *Am. J. Roentgenol.*, 103:589–594.

Incontinentia Pigmenti

110. Cantu, J. M., del Castillo, V., Jiminez, M., and Ruiz-Barquin, E. (1973): Chromosomal instability in incontinentia pigmenti. *Ann. Genet. (Paris)*, 16:117–119.
111. Carney, R. G., and Carney, R. G., Jr. (1970): Incontinentia pigmenti. *Arch. Dermatol.*, 102:157–162.
112. Carney, R. G. (1976): Incontinentia pigmenti: A world statistical analysis. *Arch. Dermatol.*, 112:535–542.
113. de Grouchy, J., Bonnette, J., Brussieux, J., Roidot, M., and Begin, P. (1972): Cassures chromosomiques dans l'incontinentia pigmenti. Etude d'une famille. *Ann. Genet. (Paris)*, 15:61–65.
114. Fischbein, F. I., Schub, M., and Lesko, W. S. (1972): Incontinentia pigmenti: Pheochromocytoma and ocular abnormalities. *Am. J. Ophthalmol.*, 93:961–964.
115. Garrod, A. E. (1906): Peculiar pigmentation of the skin in an infant. *Trans. Clin. Soc. Lond.*, 39:216.
116. Haber, H. (1952): The Bloch-Sulzberger syndrome (incontinentia pigmenti). *Br. J. Dermatol.*, 64:129–140.
117. Iancu, T., Komlos, L., Shabtay, F., Elian, E., Halbrecht, I., and Book, J. A. (1975): Incontinentia pigmenti. *Clin. Genet.*, 7:103–110.
118. Lenz, W. (1961): *Medizinische Genetik. Eine Eiführung in ihre Grundlagen und Probleme*, p. 89. Georg Thieme Verlag, Stuttgart.
119. Reed, W. B., Carter, C., and Cohen, T. M. (1967): Incontinentia pigmenti. *Dermatologica*, 134:243–250.
120. Rivera, R., Cangir, A., and Strong, L. (1975): Incontinentia pigmenti (Bloch-Sulzberger syndrome) associated with acute granulocytic leukemia. *South. Med. J.*, 68:1391–1394.

Scleroderma

121. Emerit, I., and Housset, E. (1973): Chromosome studies on bone marrow from patients with systemic sclerosis. Evidence for chromosomal breakage *in vivo*. *Biomedicine*, 19:550–554.

122. Emerit, I., Levy, A., and Housset, E. (1973): Chromosomal breakage in scleroderma. Possible presence of a breakage factor in the serum of patients. *Ann. Genet. (Paris),* 16:135–138.
123. Godeau, P., deSaint-Maur, P., Herreman, G., Rault, P., Cenac, A., and Rosenthal, P. (1974): Carcinome bronchiolo-alvéolaire et sclérodermie. *Sem. Hop. Paris,* 50:1161–1168.

Discussion

Cleaver: It is worth emphasizing a couple of points about the karyology of xeroderma pigmentosum (XP). Namely, it has a normal karyotype and a normal frequency of sister chromatid exchanges, and it does *not* fit into the same category as other chromosomal instability syndromes. Likewise, when low frequencies of chromosomal aberrations are seen in cultured fibroblasts, very careful quality control is required to rule out a nonspecific effect from mycoplasma infection or some such technical problem.

German: But, the question is whether or not certain environmental conditions can increase the frequency of chromosomal arrangements in XP cells? For example, Dr. Stich in Canada has shown dramatic breakage and rearrangement after treatment with *N*-acetoxy-2-acetylaminofluorene [*Nature [New Biol.]*, 238:9–10 (1972)].

Cleaver: That is a different situation. In XP, the frequency of spontaneous abnormalities in the untreated cell is quite different from that in ataxia-telangiectasia (AT) or Bloom's syndrome. After exposure to a known agent, both chromatid exchanges and aberrations are undoubtedly increased, but, that is a different question.

German: However that is the important fact, that, for example, under ultraviolet radiation (which is what the skin does receive), there is more chromosome mutation than in normal cells.

Cleaver: Yes, but I want to emphasize that spontaneous phenomena and those induced by chemicals or radiation may not necessarily be the same.

Harnden: To further emphasize Dr. Cleaver's point, chromosomal abnormalities occur in cultured fibroblasts even from normal individuals. Thus, it is not enough to look at cells from XP or any other syndrome, to see breaks, and say chromosomal breakage is associated with the syndrome. You must look at the phenomena quantitatively. At the same time, I should add that embryo cells do not show clone formation such as we have observed in normal fibroblasts under identical conditions.

Hecht: What you are saying is the point I was making: with our present ignorance, we have to be cautious about accepting unconfirmed reports. I think we all agree that these syndromes are good models of single-gene disorders that predispose to malignancy.

Comings: Dr. Hecht, how specific is this 14p12 band? In how many cases of AT has it been found? Has Dr. Cohen in Israel found it in his patients? Is the same region involved in Burkitt's lymphoma?

Hecht: When a pseudodiploid clone is found in a patient with AT it seems to involve chromosome 14. So far, every reported case involves a translocation of chromosome 14, except one that has a ring 14, presumably arising from breaks in the long and short arms. Thus, in every case, the same region is involved in a translocation in which the distal portion of 14 is moved off to a small number of sites.

Concerning Burkitt's lymphoma, the original work from Sweden on African Burkitt's has held up elsewhere and has been confirmed in nonAfrican Burkitt's as well, both in Sweden and the United States. In Burkitt's (in contrast to AT), the change in 14q is the *addition* of material from chromosome 8. So, an interesting paradox arises to challenge someone like you. In AT, chromosome 14 is broken near the centromere, and material is moved away, i.e., chromosome 14 is shortened in AT. In Burkitt's and some lymphomas, material is tacked on at the end of chromosome 14, i.e., chromosome 14 is lengthened in Burkitt's. What does this mean at the molecular level? The common denominator is that the same chromosome is involved every time a lymphoid disorder is found with a marker clone.

Genetics of Human Cancer, edited by J. J.
Mulvihill, R. W. Miller, and J. F. Fraumeni, Jr.
Raven Press, New York, 1977.

10

Are Nonrandom Karyotypic Changes Related to Etiologic Agents?

Janet D. Rowley

*Department of Medicine, The University of Chicago, Chicago, Illinois 60637; and The
Franklin McLean Memorial Research Institute, Chicago, Illinois 60637*

At the present time, there is not one shred of evidence to support the hypothesis that, in human tumors, specific chromosomal abnormalities might be related to particular etiologic agents. Nevertheless, I believe that this hypothesis merits consideration for two reasons. First, there is evidence from animal tumors that supports this notion, and second, the concept can be tested with techniques that are currently available.

The hypothesis was proposed (34) as a possible explanation for nonrandom chromosomal changes that have been observed in a variety of human neoplasms, some malignant, others benign. Some of the evidence was obtained prior to the application of the new banding techniques; with these techniques, however, more precise information has been obtained. This chapter covers three areas: first, the evidence for nonrandom changes; second, the evidence in animals relating nonrandom changes to specific etiologic agents; and finally, the human neoplasms that, in my view, offer the most promising opportunities for the investigation of this question in humans.

NONRANDOM CHROMOSOMAL ABNORMALITIES IN HEMATOLOGIC DISORDERS

This subject has been reviewed briefly by Harnden (12). Additional data regarding nonrandom chromosomal changes in both chronic myelogenous leukemia and acute leukemia are available and should be presented.

Chronic Myelogenous Leukemia (CML)

Chronic Phase

It is now accepted that the Ph^1 chromosome, which is found in patients with CML, represents a translocation rather than a deletion (33). The karyotypes of 187 Ph^1-positive patients have been examined with banding techniques (see ref. 36 for review). The original report on the translocation and a number of reports confirming the observation noted that in 173 of these patients the translocation occurred only between chromosomes 9 and 22. Measurement of the DNA content of the Ph^1 and the 9 with the additional material (9q+) demonstrates no detectable loss of chromosomal material when these chromosomes are compared to their normal homologs (23). Recently, 14 cases with either unusual or complex translocations, accounting for 7.5% of all Ph^1-positive patients, were detected. In eight of these, the translocation involved No. 22 and some other chromosome, namely, Nos. 2, 13, 16, 17, 19, 21, or an unidentified chromosome (7,10,13,15,26,36). In one patient, the translocation occurred between an abnormal 9 and a 22 (13). Five cases have also been reported in which the rearrangement involved three chromosomes; in all these cases, two of the chromosomes were 9 and 22 with breaks in the usual band (13,18,30). Thus, among the 187 Ph^1-positive patients whose cells have been examined with banding, there appear to be 14 who showed an unusual chromosomal rearrangement; No. 9, with a break in band q34, was involved in six of these 14; therefore, only eight of 187 Ph^1-positive patients had a normal No. 9. The explanation for the great specificity of the translocation involving 9 and 22 remains an enigma.

Acute Phase

The complex karyotypic changes that occur in the acute phase of CML can now be determined with the use of banding. Bone marrow chromosomes from 63 patients with Ph^1-positive CML, who were in the acute phase, have been analyzed with banding techniques (13,36). Twelve showed no change in their karyotype, whereas 51 patients showed additional chromosomal abnormalities. The gains or, more rarely, losses of particular chromosomes observed in 46 patients who had relatively complete analyses are summarized in Table 1.

The table shows that the single most common change is the addition of a second Ph^1 (22q—) chromosome, an event that occurred in more than 50% of the patients. Prior to banding, the most commonly observed abnormality was an additional C group chromosome. The use of banding reveals that, although different additional C group chromosomes are present, one pair, No. 8, is involved much more frequently than the remainder. Of 25 patients whose cells contained additional C's, 19 had an additional No. 8 (Table 1). In 12 patients, this was the only abnormality involving a C, whereas in seven others a second additional C was contributed by some other pair. The i(17q) appears to be the second most common structural rearrangement, after the 9;22 translocation, as it was observed in 12 patients.

TABLE 1. *Chromosome changes in 46 patients in acute phase of CML* [a]

	Chromosome no.																						
	3	4	5	6	7	8	9	10	11	12	X	C	13	14	16	17	i(17q)	18	19	21	22	22q-[b]	Mar
No. of patients with gain	1	?	1	3	2	19	3	5	4	4	2	6	2	4	2	2		12	3	10	4	1	27 8
No. of patients with loss					1		1		1	1	1				1	2			1				

[a]Updated from ref. 36.
[b]Includes two dicentric Ph[1] chromosomes.

Except in four cases, it was found to be associated with an additional No. 8 (four times) or an additional unidentified C (four times). Without exception, the additional F noted in 10 patients was a No. 19.

Acute Leukemia

Prior to banding, the chromosomal pattern in acute leukemia, both myelogenous and lymphocytic, appeared to be so variable that chromosomal changes were assumed to be an epiphenomenon. Furthermore, abnormal karyotypes were observed in only 30 to 50% of patients (review, ref. 36).

I have recently completed a study of the karyotype (with banding) of 50 patients with acute nonlymphocytic leukemia (37). Twenty-five patients showed an abnormal karyotype in the initial examination; although there was considerable variability, some patterns tended to recur. The presence of nonrandom patterns becomes much more apparent if published data on chromosomal abnormalities determined with banding techniques are added to my own.

The data from the 23 patients in my series whose cells could be analyzed completely, together with the published data from 37 patients (36), provide information on the banding patterns in 60 patients. There is a surprisingly narrow range of modal chromosome numbers in this group, with 22 individuals having 45 chromosomes, 15 having 46, and 14 having 47; five patients had 42 to 44 and four patients had 48 to 50 chromosomes. The chromosomal abnormalities can be grouped into three major types: gain of one autosome, loss of one autosome, and balanced translocations.

Prior to banding, the frequent involvement of C and G group chromosomes and the absence of F group involvement had been noted. The use of banding confirms these observations and demonstrates that there is a nonrandom pattern within both the C and G groups as to the particular chromosomes involved (Fig. 1). Thirteen patients had one extra autosome, identified as No. 8 in 10 cases. Nine patients showed loss of one autosome, which was identified as No. 7 in six. The other

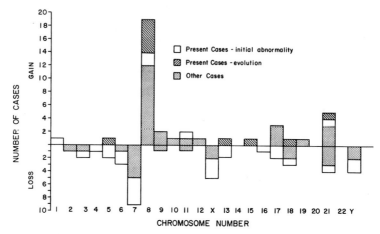

FIG. 1. Summary of gains and losses of whole chromosomes observed in patients with acute leukemia. (From ref. 37, with permission.)

chromosomal changes that occurred in more than a few patients were the loss of an X chromosome in five, the gain or loss of a No. 21 in five and four patients, respectively, and the loss of the Y chromosome in four patients. Balanced translocations involving No. 8 (with or without loss of sex chromosomes) were seen in six patients, and balanced translocations of other chromosomes were noted in nine others, giving a total of 15.

The evidence for nonrandom involvement of particular chromosomes in other tumors has been summarized by Harnden (12) and others (21,34,35). It appears that only certain chromosomes are abnormal in a particular tumor, and that these same chromosomes may be aneuploid in a variety of tumors (21,35).

EXPERIMENTAL EVIDENCE RELATING NONRANDOM CHANGES TO ETIOLOGIC AGENTS

In my view, the evidence for nonrandom changes is very convincing, and we must now search for mechanisms producing these changes. We must also look for some plausible explanation for the malignancy of these chromosomally abnormal cells. One possible mechanism, namely, that specific karyotypic changes are related to specific agents, is explored more fully in this chapter. An alternative hypothesis, which states that malignancy represents an imbalance between genes concerned with the expression or suppression of malignancy (2,17,45), has received much attention; it is outside the scope of this presentation and therefore is not discussed.

Chromosomal Patterns in Specific Tumors

Nonrandom chromosomal abnormalities occur in some animals exposed to chemical and viral mutagenic agents. For example (Fig. 2), when leukemia (32,43,44), sarcomas (27), and epithelial tumors (1) were induced by 7,12-dimethylbenz[a]anthracene (DMBA) and 6,8,12- and 7,8,12-trimethylbenz[a]anthracene in rats, trisomy for the largest telocentric chromosome (A2) was observed; trisomy for a metacentric chromosome was less frequent (32,43). An analysis of the banding pattern of DMBA-induced sarcomas has shown that additional material of chromosome A2 was present in 12 of 13 tumors (19). A different, but very consistent karyotypic pattern was seen in sarcomas induced in the rat by Rous sarcoma virus (RSV) (29). Some Rous sarcomas in the rat may show a normal karyotype initially. On independent serial propagation of these tumors, however, the same nonrandom karyotypic changes are noted in the different passages (25). The pattern of karyotypic evolution involved additions of one medium-sized telocentric chromosome, followed by one medium and one small subtelocentric chromosome. Chromosomes most frequently abnormal in DMBA-induced tumors were rarely abnormal in RSV-induced tumors, and vice versa. *The sarcomas produced by DMBA and RSV were histologically indistinguishable.*

A similar phenomenon was observed in the Chinese hamster. One or more additional chromosomes belonging to three pairs (Nos. 5, 6, or 10) were found in most sarcomas induced by RSV (16), whereas No. 11 was the most frequent addition in cells from DMBA-induced sarcomas (28) in the same inbred Chinese hamster strain.

These observations led Mitelman et al. (29) to propose that the specific chromosomal abnormalities are associated with particular etiologic agents, and that the chromosomal change is independent of the type of tumor produced. Further research has shown that this is a somewhat oversimplified view, because the karyotypic changes in sarcomas produced by other polycyclic hydrocarbons,

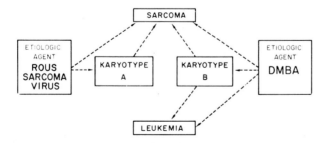

FIG. 2. Although histologically identical, sarcomas induced in rats by *different* agents have *different* chromosomal abnormalities; whereas, two different malignancies induced by the *same* agent have *identical* karyotypes. [From Rowley, J. D. (1975): Nonrandom chromosomal abnormalities in hematologic disorders of man. *Proc. Natl. Acad. Sci. USA,* 72:152–156, *with permission*].

such as methylcholanthrene (MC) or benzo(a)pyrene (BP), although still nonrandom and frequently involving chromosome A2, are more complex and show greater variability (20).

Even in experimental animals, some chromosomal variability is present in tumors induced with a single, known oncogenic agent. It may be significant, however, that chromosomal variability is lower in inbred (20 to 30%) than in random-bred (approximately 50%) animals.

It should be acknowledged that not all investigators have observed nonrandom changes. Some of the data are presented in a recent review by DiPaolo (4).

Mechanisms for Agent-Chromosome Specificity

One mechanism that could account for the specificity of the chromosomal abnormalities observed with different oncogenic agents is suggested by Sugiyama (42). He noted that two regions on the long telocentric chromosome (A2), which is frequently present in a trisomic state in DMBA-induced rat leukemia, were specifically vulnerable to the chromosome-damaging action of DMBA. These same regions were late-replicating and heterochromatic. It has been known for some time that such regions show preferential susceptibility to mutagenic agents (40). In addition, Levan and Levan (20) remarked on the very interesting relationship between chromosomal changes and carcinogenicity. In the rat, the order of carcinogenic potency is DMBA > MC > BP (31); the frequency of nonrandom changes shows the same order, with DMBA producing the most consistent and BP the least consistent karyotypic changes. Although the significance of this relationship is unknown, Levan and Levan have suggested that, if a given mutagen is more potent as a carcinogen, it may attack certain genes more selectively in the induction of malignancy (20).

HUMAN TUMORS WITH A KNOWN ETIOLOGY

Whereas there is no evidence in man at the present time that links any specific chromosomal abnormality with a particular carcinogen, we needn't remain so ignorant. There are a number of patients in whom this hypothesis could be tested.

Human Tumors with a Known Environmental Cause

Present Knowledge

A number of human tumors are associated with known environmental carcinogens. Some of these associations have been recognized for many years; they include skin cancer and exposure to soots, tars, and oils; lung cancer and exposure to asbestos or benzo(a)pyrene and other polycyclic aromatic hydrocarbons in industry, in cigarette smoke, and polluted city air; and urinary bladder cancer from benzidine and β-naphthylamine (see ref. 24 for review). More recently, it has been recognized that girls whose mothers received diethylstilbestrol (DES) in early pregnancy have vaginal adenosis and a high risk of developing adenocarcinoma of the vagina and cervix (14); individuals who received X-ray therapy for enlarged tonsils, adenoids, or thymus, or for acne are prone to carcinoma of the thyroid (6). Workers exposed to vinyl chloride show an increased incidence of hepatic angiosarcomas (3), and those exposed to chloromethyl methyl ether (CMME) have an increased incidence of lung cancer, usually the oat cell type (8).

Many of these tumors are otherwise rare, and, to my knowledge, none has been studied with cytogenetic techniques. The nearest approach to such a study was a report on the DNA content of cells from DES-induced vaginal adenosis (three patients) and adenocarcinoma (three patients), which showed that the DNA content of the former was in the diploid–tetraploid range, whereas cells from the latter showed an aneuploid amount of DNA (22). The authors concluded that the ''diploid'' (and therefore ''normal'') state of the adenosis cells indicated that these cells were unlikely to be the source for the adenocarcinoma. However, Granberg et al. (11) studied a uterine adenocarcinoma and found a consistent chromosomal abnormality $(46,XX,+3,-D)$ in cells with a diploid amount of nuclear DNA. Thus, measurements of DNA cannot reveal consistent chromosomal changes that are the result of reciprocal translocations, nor do they detect gains and losses of chromosomes of relatively similar size.

Areas for Future Research

For an answer to the question whether there are nonrandom chromosomal changes in environmentally induced human tumors, the following four criteria should be met with regard to the tumors selected.

1. There should be a relatively specific association between the tumor and the carcinogenic agent.

2. Relatively few tumors should occur in the same site without a known exposure to the agent; alternatively, exposed and nonexposed groups should be clearly distinguishable on the basis of clinical history or the specific histologic appearance of the tumor.

3. The tumors should be relatively frequent (preferably at least 10 to 20 cases per year) in the United States.

4. Surgical specimens should be available for cytogenetic analysis.

The tumors that appear to be among the most promising candidates for investigation at the present time are included in Table 2.

Workers exposed to asbestos dust provide a particularly important population for study because they show an increased incidence of several types of tumors and therefore may provide evidence in man that could be compared with that obtained for DMBA-induced tumors in rats. The tumors observed in asbestos workers include not only lung cancer, but mesotheliomas of the pleura and peritoneum,

TABLE 2.

Tumors[a]	Population at risk
1. Thyroid carcinoma (6)	Patients who received X-rays for enlarged tonsils, adenoids, thymus, or for acne
2. Lung cancer, mesotheliomas of pleura and peritoneum, and gastric cancer (24,38,39)	Workers exposed to asbestos
3 Oat cell cancers of lung (8)	Workers exposed to halo ethers
4. Hepatic angiosarcoma (3)	Workers exposed to vinyl chloride
5. Clear cell adenocarcinoma of the vagina (14)	Daughters of mothers who received diethylstilbestrol early in pregnancy
6. Urinary bladder carcinoma (24)	Workers exposed to polycyclic aromatic compounds

[a]References appear in parentheses.

and gastric and colon cancer as well. These individuals also show pulmonary fibrosis and pleural thickening (asbestosis), so that abnormal, possibly premalignant, tissue is also available for chromosomal analysis. Present evidence indicates that the increased risk of bronchogenic carcinoma in workers exposed to asbestos dust is confined to smokers (39). One could thus compare the karyotypes of lung cancers from these two populations to determine whether the chromosomal changes are similar or different.

Although there is no information on the karyotype of any of these environmentally induced tumors, there is evidence that some of the agents discussed previously cause chromosomal damage. An increased incidence of chromosomal aberrations has been detected in cultured lymphocytes obtained from workers exposed to vinyl chloride (9). It has also been reported recently that Chinese hamster cells cultured with asbestos fibers show an increased frequency of polyploids, fragments, and other structural rearrangements (41). These changes were not observed in control cells exposed to fiber glass or glass powder. It has also been reported that carcinogenic substances produce banding of mammalian chromosomes, whereas noncarcinogenic substances do not (5).

As we are unwittingly exposed to an increasing variety of environmental pollutants, some of which are carcinogenic, information regarding the relationship of etiologic agent and tumor formation becomes critically important.

ACKNOWLEDGMENTS

This work was supported in part by the Leukemia Research Foundation of Chicago, and the Otho S. A. Sprague Memorial Institute.

REFERENCES

1. Ahlstrom, U. (1974): Chromosomes of primary carcinomas induced by 7,12-dimethylbenz(a)-anthracene in the rat. *Hereditas,* 78:235–244.
2. Codish, S. D., and Paul, B. (1974): Reversible appearance of a specific chromosome which suppresses malignancy. *Nature,* 252:610–612.
3. Creech, J. L., Jr., and Johnson, M. M. (1974): Angiosarcoma of liver in the manufacture of polyvinyl chloride. *J. Occup. Med.,* 16:150–151.
4. DiPaolo, J. A. (1975): Karyological instability of neoplastic somatic cells. *In Vitro,* 11:89–96.
5. DiPaolo, J. A., and Popescu, N. C. (1974): Chromosome bands induced in human and Syrian hamster cells by chemical carcinogens. *Br. J. Cancer,* 30:103–108.
6. Duffy, B. J., and Fitzgerald, P. J. (1950): Thyroid cancer in childhood and adolescence: Report on 28 cases. *J. Clin. Endocrinol.,* 10:1296–1308.
7. Engel, E., McGee, B. J., Flexner, J. M., and Krantz, S. B. (1975): Chromosome band analysis in 19 cases of chronic myeloid leukemia: 9 chronic, 10 blastic, two with Ph[1] (22q–) translocation on 17 short arm. *Ann. Genet.,* 18:239–240.
8. Figueroa, W. G., Raszkowski, R., and Weiss, W. (1973): Lung cancer in chloromethyl ether workers. *N. Eng. J. Med.,* 288:1096–1097.
9. Funes Cravioto, F., Lambert, B., Lindsten, J., Ehrenberg, L., Natorajan, A. T., and Osterman-Golkan, S. (1975): Chromosome aberrations in workers exposed to vinyl chloride. *Lancet,* 1:459.
10. Gahrton, G., Zech, L. and Lindsten, J. (1974): A new variant translocation (19q+,22q–) in chronic myelocytic leukemia. *Exp. Cell. Res.,* 86:214–216.
11. Granberg, I., Gupta, S., Joelsson, I., and Sprenger, E. (1974): Chromosome and nuclear DNA study of a uterine adenocarcinoma and its metastases. *Acta Pathol. Microbiol. Scand.* [A], 82:1–6.
12. Harnden, D. G. (1976): Cytogenetics of human neoplasm. *This volume.*
13. Hayata, I., Sakurai, M., Kakati, S., and Sandberg, A. A. (1975): Chromosomes and causation of human cancer and leukemia. XVI. Banding studies of chronic myelocytic leukemia, including five unusual Ph[1] translocations. *Cancer,* 36:1177–1191.
14. Herbst, A. L., Uhfelder, H., and Poskanzer, D. C. (1971): Adenocarcinoma of the vagina. *N. Engl. J. Med.,* 284:878–881.
15. Ishihara, T., Kohno, S. I., and Kumatori, T. (1974): Ph[1] translocation involving chromosomes 21 and 22. *Br. J. Cancer,* 29:340–342.
16. Kato, R. (1968): The chromosomes of forty-two primary Rous sarcomas of the Chinese hamster. *Hereditas,* 59:63–119.
17. Klein, G., Bregula, U., Weiner, F., and Harris, H. (1971): The analysis of malignancy by cell fusion. I. Hybrids between tumor cells and L cell derivatives. *J. Cell Sci.,* 8:659–672.
18. Lawler, S. D., Lobb, D. S., and Wiltshaw, E. (1974): Philadelphia chromosome positive bone-marrow cells showing loss of the Y in males with chronic myeloid leukaemia. *Br. J. Haemat.,* 27:247–252.
19. Levan, G., Ahlstrom, U., and Mitelman, F. (1974): The specificity of chromosome A2 involvement in DMBA-induced rat sarcomas. *Hereditas,* 77:262–280.
20. Levan, G., and Levan, A. (1975): Specific chromosome changes in malignancy: Studies in rat sarcomas induced by two polycyclic hydrocarbons. *Hereditas,* 79:161–198.
21. Levan, G., and Mitelman, F. (1975): Clustering of aberrations of specific chromosomes in human neoplasms. *Hereditas,* 79:156–160.
22. Lewis, J. L., Nordquist, S. R. B., and Richard, R. M. (1973): Studies of nuclear DNA in vaginal adenosis and clear-cell adenocarcinoma. *Am. J. Obstet. Gynecol.,* 115:737–750.
23. Mayall, B. H., Carrano, A. V., and Rowley, J. D. (1974): DNA cytophotometry of chromosomes in a case of chronic myelogenous leukemia. *Clin. Chem.,* 20:1080–1085.
24. Miller, J. A. (1970): Carcinogenesis by chemicals: An overview. *Cancer Res.,* 30:559–576.
25. Mitelman, F. (1972): Predetermined sequential chromosome changes in serial transplantation of Rous rat sarcomas. *Acta Pathol. Microbiol. Scand.* [A], 80:313–328.
26. Mitelman, F. (1974): Heterogeneity of Ph[1] in chronic myeloid leukaemia. *Hereditas,* 76:315–316.
27. Mitelman, F., and Levan, G. (1972): The chromosomes of primary 7,12-dimethylbenz(a)anthra-cene-induced rat sarcomas. *Hereditas,* 71:325–334.
28. Mitelman, F., Mark, J., and Levan, G. (1972): Chromosomes of six primary sarcomas induced

in the Chinese hamster by 7,12-dimethylbenz(a)anthracene. *Hereditas,* 72:311–318.

29. Mitelman, F., Mark, J., Levan, G., and Levan, A. (1972): Tumor etiology and chromosome pattern. *Science,* 176:1340–1341.

30. Nowell, P. C., Jensen, J., and Gardner, F. (1975): Two complex translocations in chronic granulocytic leukemia involving chromosomes 22,9, and a third chromosome. *Humangenetik,* 30:13–21.

31. Rees, E. D. (1969): Chromosomal aberrations in rat marrow cells following intravenous poly-cyclic hydrocarbons: Possible basis for a carcinogen bioassy. *Univ. Kentucky Tobacco Health Res. Inst. Proc. Tobacco Health Workshop,* pp.18–23.

32. Rees, E. D., Majumdar, S. K., and Shuck, A. (1970): Changes in chromosomes of bone marrow after intravenous injections of 7,12-dimethylbenz(a)anthracene and related compounds. *Proc. Natl. Acad. Sci. USA,* 66:1228–1235.

33. Rowley, J. D. (1973): A new consistent chromosomal abnormality in chronic myelogenous leukemia. *Nature,* 243:290–293.

34. Rowley, J. D. (1974): Do human tumors show a chromosome pattern specific for each etiologic agent? *J. Natl. Cancer Inst.,* 52:315–320.

35. Rowley, J. D. (1975): Abnormalities of chromosome 1 in myeloproliferative disorders. *Cancer,* 36:1748–1757.

36. Rowley, J. D. (1976): Population cytogenetics of leukemia. In: *Population Cytogenetics,* edited by I. H. Porter and E. B. Hook, Academic Press, New York *(In press.)*

37. Rowley, J. D., and Potter, D. (1976): Chromosomal banding patterns in acute non-lymphocytic leukemia. *Blood,* 47:705–721.

38. Selikoff, I. J., and Hammond, E. C. (1975): Multiple risk factors in environmental cancer. In: *Persons at High Risk of Cancer,* edited by J. F. Fraumeni, Jr. pp. 467–483. Academic Press, New York.

39. Selikoff, I. J., Churg, J., and Hammond, E. C. (1964): Relation between exposure to asbestos and mesothelioma. *N. Engl. J. Med.,* 272:560–565.

40. Shaw, M. W., and Cohen, M. M. (1965): Chromosome exchanges in human leukocytes inducted by mitomycin C. *Genetics,* 51:181–190.

41. Sincock, A., and Seabright, M. (1975): Induction of chromosome changes in Chinese hamster cells by exposure to asbestos fibers. *Nature,* 257:56–58.

42. Sugiyama, T., (1971): Specific vulnerability of the largest telocentric chromosome of rat bone marrow cells to 7,12-dimethylbenz(a)anthracene. *J. Natl. Cancer Inst.,* 47:1267–1273.

43. Sugiyama, T., Kurita, Y., and Nishizuka, Y. (1967): Chromosome abnormality in rat leukemia induced by 7,12-dimethylbenz(a)anthracene. *Science,* 158:1058–1059.

44. Sugiyama, T., Kurita, Y., and Nishizuka, Y. (1969): Biological studies on 7,12-dimethyl-benz(a)anthracene-induced rat leukemia with special reference to the specific chromosomal abnor-malities. *Cancer Res.,* 29:1117–1124.

45. Yamamoto, T., Rabinowitz, Z., and Sachs, L. (1973): Identification of the chromosomes that control malignancy. *Nature* [*New Biol.*], 243:247–250.

Discussion

Nance: In acute leukemia, do the karyotypes correlate in any way with the clinical features, such as survival, response to treatment, etc.?

Rowley: As Dr. Sandberg found [*Cancer,* 33:1548–1557 (1974)] and we confirmed, patients with an abnormal karyotype respond more poorly to chemotherapy and have a shorter median survival than do patients with normal karyotypes. This is particularly true in acute myeloblastic leukemias as compared with acute myelomonoblastic. We and others are looking into the significance of the possible presence of the gene for glutathione reductase on chromosome 8.

Pogosianz: Maybe it would interest this audience to know our Russian data on some of the human hematologic neoplasias. I should say, for those who are not cytogeneticists, that all sorts of geneticists were very excited with the data that came from the Levans' laboratory and Dr. Rowley's work involving nonrandom distribution of chromosomal changes in malignancy. So, it is interesting to have data from different laboratories in different countries.

In our laboratory, Drs. E. E. Prigogina and E. V. Fleishman carried out chromosome studies in 54 cases of human hemoblastoses [*Humangenetik,* 30:109–119 (1975)]. Out of 19 cases of acute leukemia studied with G-banding technique, 11 had normal karyotypes, and 8 were aneuploid. Among the aneuploid were two cases each with chromosomes 7, 8, and 21 involved.

All 21 patients with chronic myelogenous leukemia had 9;22 translocation. This was the only abnormality in six cases; whereas eight also had involvement of chromosome 17 (iso 17q). Trisomy 8 and 19 were added to the i(17q) marker in a progressive fashion, especially during blast crisis. Half of the cases had these patterns and half had a different pattern. So, we agree with Dr. Rowley that not all chronic myelogenous leukemias are alike. Whether the differences reflect different etiologic agents, no one knows.

Finally, we have six cases of chronic lymphatic leukemias (two with chromosomal abnormalities, one involving chromosome 14, one a 14q+), and eight cases of lymphosarcoma (four with abnormalities, three involving chromosome 14, one with chromosome 14q+). Altogether, aneuploidy was seen in six of these 14 cases of lymphoreticular malignancy, and four had an abnormality of chromosome 14.

Hirschhorn: Dr. Pogosianz, did you test for Epstein–Barr virus in your patients, in particular in the two cases with 14q+ in the lymphoma group?

Pogosianz: We do not have data on Epstein–Barr viral antibodies. If you are implying that the two cases have Burkitt's lymphoma, I can say there are no known cases of typical Burkitt's lymphoma in our country. It could be that 14q+ is found in lymphomas other than Burkitt's or that our patients had atypical Burkitt's lymphoma.

Rowley: It is nice to get confirmation from another country, the Soviet Union. I say this because Ford and Gunz from Australia have recently reported that the most consistent abnormality they see in acute leukemia is an additional chromosome 9 and a missing chromosome 8 [*J. Natl. Cancer Inst.,* 55:761–765, (1975)]. This contrasts with our findings and raises the question of a different climate or etiologic agent. Alternatively, I might suggest that it is difficult to distinguish chromosome 8 from 9 in leukemic cells using Giesma banding alone as Ford and Gunz did. A further reason for uncertainty is their observation that the chromosomal abnormality persisted even in remission. Most other laboratories have reported that patients in good clinical remission lose their chromosomally abnormal cell line, so perhaps the Australian patients were not in remission.

Hecht: Dr. Hirschhorn's question concerning the Soviet experience with 14q+, lymphoid tumors and the Epstein–Barr virus is another way of getting back to Dr. Rowley's hypothesis relating the pattern of chromosomal abnormalities to the etiologic agent. I am afraid that such simple thinking is not going to get us far in man because there is overwhelming evidence, I think, that the type of chromosomal aberration pertains to the *cell type* of the malignancy and not to its *etiology.* Rowley and others have clearly shown the nonrandom association of erythromyeloid malignancy with abnormalities of chromosomes 8, 22, and 9; whereas lymphoid tumors seem to involve preferentially chromosome 14 as reported from the Soviet Union, Great Britain, Sweden, Japan, and the United States. The chromosomal pattern looks quite cell-specific, although it does not rule out the idea that it is also agent-specific. For example, not all 14q+ tumors are positive for Epstein–Barr virus; we have some that are negative.

German: In the Levans' report cited by Dr. Rowley to support her hypothesis, I was impressed that the karyotypes of tumors induced by certain chemicals were far less specific than, for example, the 14q12 band in Burkitt's lymphoma in humans. Rather, certain morphologically similar chromosomes had the tendency to become trisomic or monosomic following treatment with certain agents.

Rowley: To the contrary, the Levans did careful Giesma banding on the tumors induced by polycyclic hydrocarbons. They felt they sometimes observed reliably consistent patterns even to the point of identifying trisomy of particular regions of the rat chromosome A2. Certainly, some tumors had greater variability than others.

Riccardi: Concerning malignancy in trisomy 8, I have two observations. First, of some 65 patients with *congenital* trisomy 8 known to me from a worldwide survey, one has developed a hematologic malignancy [*Clin. Genet.,* 9:134–142 (1976)]. Second, we studied a man in Denver who had acute myelogenous leukemia. His peripheral lymphocytes showed a reciprocal balanced translocation (7p;20p), which was also found in his brother, sister, and nephew. His bone marrow showed leukemic cells with trisomy 8. Skin fibroblasts showed the translocation, as anticipated, and, to our surprise, trisomy 8 as a mosaic line [*Am. J. Hum. Genet.,* 27:76a (1975)]. Both these observations caution us about drawing premature conclusions on the etiologic significance of the extra chromosome 8.

Rowley: I do not mean to imply that an additional chromosome 8 causes the leukemia. I do say there is an *association* that seems to be very important, although its significance is not presently understood. Further, one has to distinguish between trisomy 8 as a constitutional abnormality and the abnormalities we see in bone marrows that appear to be *somatic* mutations. In our trisomy 8 patients, we have not looked at skin fibroblast cultures, but phytohemagglutinin-stimulated peripheral lymphocytes from many cultures have had no additional chromosome 8 at 72 hr.

Genetics of Human Cancer, edited by J. J.
Mulvihill, R. W. Miller, and J. F. Fraumeni, Jr.
Raven Press, New York, 1977.

11

Genetic Repertory of Human Neoplasia

John J. Mulvihill

Clinical Epidemiology Branch, National Cancer Institute, Bethesda, Maryland 20014

Subsequent chapters discuss in detail selected single gene traits predisposing to
malignancy; however, it might be instructive first to consider the range of gene
loci that have been associated with neoplasia.

McKusick, in the fourth edition of his catalog of *Mendelian Inheritance in
Man* (14), enumerates 1,142 proved single gene traits and 1,194 others with
suggestive but inconclusive evidence of Mendelian behavior. From these, I have
extracted 200 (8.6%) conditions and added several others with neoplastic tendencies (Table 1). Traits included in Table 1 have benign or malignant neoplasia
or tumor as a sole feature, a frequent concomitant, or just a rare complication.
Because of their rarity, some traits are represented by only single case reports.
Certain entities may be contestable and others may be missing, e.g., not all
known reports of familial aggregation of neoplasms of the same or diverse cell
types are included.

One of several points to be made from Table 1 is its length; a substantial
portion of all known single gene traits in human beings can be manifested as
neoplasia. In many, neoplasia is only an occasional feature; therefore, other
factors, presumably in the environment, must be interacting to produce tumor.

Second, Table 1 is the mutant genetic repertory of neoplasia in human beings.
It emphasizes the large number of genes that might be involved in cancer
susceptibility, and, by inference, the number of normal genes contributing to
resistance to neoplasia. About one-half the traits are autosomal dominant; one-
third, autosomal recessive; and one-sixth, X-linked.

Third, nearly all histologic types of tumors are represented, including the
commonest malignancies—skin, breast, colon, and lung. These and other tumors
occurring in monogenic traits are often indistinguishable by morphology from the
sporadically occurring tumors. The hereditary tumors may be identified by recognizing other features of the trait or syndrome in the patient or his family. Thus,
the clinician who diagnoses the cancer but not the syndrome of which it is a
manifestation makes an incomplete diagnosis. Every surgeon who has a patient

TABLE 1. *Neoplasia as single gene traits or as a feature or complication of other Mendelian disorders*

Catalog no. or (ref)	Neoplasm or disorder	Inheri- tance	Associated neoplasms
	Phacomatoses		
16220	von Recklinghausen's neurofibromatosis	AD*	Fibrosarcoma, neuroma, schwannoma, meningioma, polyps, optic glioma, pheochromocytoma
19110	Tuberous sclerosis	AD*	Adenoma sebaceum, periungual fibroma, glial tumors, rhabdomyoma of heart, renal tumor, lung cysts
19330 23480	von Hippel-Lindau syndrome	AD* AR	Retinal angioma, cerebellar hemangio- blastoma, other hemangiomas, pheochro- mocytoma, hypernephroma, cysts
18530	Sturge-Weber syndrome	AD	Angioma of numerous organs
	Nervous System		
18020	Retinoblastoma, bilateral	AD*	Sarcoma
10100	Acoustic neuroma, bilateral	AD*	
25670	Neuroblastoma	AR	
(11)		AD	
15535	Megalencephaly	AD*	Ganglioneuroblastoma

Perhaps, meningioma, 15610-AD; glioma, 13780-AD; pseudoglioma, 26420-AR; pinealoma, 26220-AR; choroid plexus papilloma, 26050-AR; chordoma, 21540-AR; hypothalamic hamartoma, 21180-AR; congenital cerebral granulomas, 30630-XR

Catalog no. or (ref)	Neoplasm or disorder	Inheri- tance	Associated neoplasms
	Endocrine		
13110	Multiple endocrine neoplasia I (Wermer's syndrome, MEN I)	AD*	Adenomas of islet cells, parathyroid, pituitary and adrenal glands, malig- nant schwannoma, nonappendiceal carcinoid
17140	Multiple endocrine neoplasia II (Sipple's syndrome, MEN II)	AD*	Medullary carcinoma of thyroid, para- thyroid adenoma, pheochromocytoma
16230	Mucosal neuromas and endocrine adenomatosis (MEN III)	AD*	Pheochromocytoma, medullary carcinoma of the thyroid, neurofibroma, submucosal neuromas of tongue, lips, eyelids
16800	Paraganglioma (chemodectoma)	AD*	
17130	Pheochromocytoma	AD*	
14500	Hyperparathyroidism	AD	Parathyroid adenoma, chief cell hyperplasia
10390	Dexamethasone-sensitive aldosteronism	AD	Multiple adrenal cortical adenomas
13880 26070 27440- -90	Thyroid goiter and dyshormonogenesis, including Pendred's syndrome	AD AR AR*	Benign goiter

Perhaps, intestinal carcinoid, 11490-AD; amenorrhea-galactorrhea syndrome with pituitary adenoma, 10460-AD; Bartter's syndrome, 24120-AR*, arrheno- blastoma-thyroid adenoma, 10795-AD

TABLE 1 *(Continued)* 139

Catalog no. or (ref)	Neoplasm or disorder	Inheritance	Associated neoplasms
	Mesoderm (Soft Tissue)		
10940	Nevoid basal cell carcinoma syndrome	AD*	Basal cell carcinoma, medulloblastoma, jaw cysts, ovarian fibroma, and carcinoma
15835	Multiple hamartoma syndrome (Cowden's disease)	AD*	Papillomatosis of lip and mouth, hypertrophic and cystic breast with early cancer, thyroid adenoma and carcinoma, bone and liver cysts, lipoma, polyps, moningioma
15110	LEOPARD syndrome	AD*	Multiple lentigines
13530	Gingival fibromatosis ± hyper-	AD*	
13540	trichosis or other anomalies	AD	
13550			
22860	Juvenile fibromatosis	AR*	Multiple subcutaneous tumors
21660	Familial cutaneous collagenoma	AR	Multiple skin nodules
15080	Multiple leiomyomata	AD*	Cutaneous, uterine, and/or esophageal
24610		AR	leiomyomata
15070		AD	
15190	Multiple lipomatosis, some-	AD*	Skin cancer
15170	times site-specific, neck	AD	
15180	or conjunctiva		
11785			
25770	Goldenhar's syndrome	AR	Lipodermoid of conjunctiva, hemangioma
24810	Macrosomia adiposa congenita	AR	Obese soon after birth, eosinophilia, adrenal cortical adenoma
15740	Multiple eruptive milia	AD*	Carcinoma of colon
	Alimentary Tract		
17510	Familial polyposis coli	AD*	Intestinal polyps, carcinoma of colon
17530	Gardner's syndrome	AD*	Intestinal polyps, osteomas, fibromas, sebaceous cysts, carcinoma of colon, ampulla of Vater, pancreas, thyroid and adrenal
17520	Peutz-Jeghers syndrome	AD*	Intestinal polyps, ovarian (granulosa cell) tumor
(21)	Colorectal carcinoma	AD*	
16780	Hereditary pancreatitis	AD*	Carcinoma of pancreas
14850	Tylosis with esophageal cancer	AD*	Carcinoma of esophagus
11455	Hepatocellular carcinoma	AD	
24730		AR	
11890	Familial, juvenile, and	AD	Hepatocellular carcinoma
21160	neonatal cirrhosis	AR*	
21560		AR	
23520			
14160	Hemochromatosis	AD*	Hepatocellular carcinoma
23510		AR*	
23520			

Perhaps, solitary discrete polyps, 17540-AD; Turcot's syndrome, 27630-AR; polyposis-sarcoma, (8)-AD; esophageal cancer, (17)-AR; gastric cancer, (2)-AR; hepatoblastoma, (6)-AR; odontoma alone, 16435-AD, or with dysphagia, 16433-AD; hereditary bilateral parotidomegaly, 16880-AD

	Urogenital		
23330	Gonadal dysgenesis, her-	AR*	Gonadoblastoma, dysgerminoma
23560	maphroditism, Reifenstein's	AR	

TABLE 1 *(Continued)*

Catalog no. or (ref)	Neoplasm or disorder	Inheritance	Associated neoplasms
23340	syndrome, testicular	XR*	
31370	feminization	XR	
31230			
31210			
30610			
16695	Ovarian tumors	AD*	
16700		AD	
17645			
27780	Wilms' tumors	AR	
(12)		AD	
14340	Hydronephrosis, familial	AD	Congenital sarcoma of kidney

Perhaps, renal cell carcinoma, 14470-AD; ureteral cancer, 19160-AD; bladder cancer, (7)-AD; renal hamartomas, nephroblastomatosis, and fetal gigantism, 26700-AR

Pulmonary

13500	Fibrocystic pulmonary dysplasia	AD*	Bronchial adenocarcinoma
10834	Aryl hydrocarbon hydroxylase inducibility	AD*	Bronchogenic carcinoma

Vascular

13800	Multiple glomus tumors	AD*	
18730	Hereditary hemorrhagic telangiectasia of Rendu-Osler-Weber	AD*	Angioma
15340	Lymphedema with distichiasis	AD*	Lymphangiosarcoma of edematous limb

Perhaps, cardiac myxoma, 25595, 25597-AR; Kaposi's sarcoma, 14800-AD; blue rubber-bleb nevus, 11220-AD*; and various other angiomatous conditions, 10590, 14080, 14090, 14100, 15350, 18720, 20657, 27250, 30160-AD, AR*, AR, XR

Skeletal

13370	Multiple exostosis	AD*	Osteosarcoma, chondrosarcoma
13360		AD	
12830			
11840	Cherubism	AD*	Fibrous dysplasia of jaws, giant-cell tumor
11225	Fibro-osseous dysplasia	AD	Osteosarcoma, medullary fibrosarcoma
12390			
13560			
16725	Paget's disease of bone	AD	Osteosarcoma

Perhaps, osteosarcoma, 25950-AR, and chondrosarcoma, 21530-AR, isolated or complicating multiple enchondromatosis alone (Ollier's syndrome) or with hemangioma (Maffucci's syndrome), 16600-AD; Ewing's sarcoma, (9)-AD; metachondromatosis, 15625-AD; osteomas of mandible, 16640-AD, or middle ear, 25965-AR; osteoporosis-pseudoglioma, 25977-AR*

Skin and Appendages (Also refs. 3, 15, 18)

21200	Breast cancer	AR	
(1)		AD	
15480	Mastocytosis	AD	
15560	Malignant melanoma	AD	
15570			
24940	Neurocutaneous melanosis	AR	Malignant melanoma of skin and meninges
15580	Universal melanosis	AD*	
16290	Nevi (pigmented and halo)	AD*	Malignant melanoma
16300		AR	
16310			
23430			

TABLE 1 *(Continued)* *141*

Catalog no. or (ref)	Neoplasm or disorder	Inheri- tance	Associated neoplasms
20310 20320	Albinism	AR*	Skin cancer
27870 27880 19440	Xeroderma pigmentosum, xerodermoid pigmentosum (including DeSanctis-Cacchione syndrome)	AR* AD	Skin cancer
13170 22600	Epidermolysis bullosa dystrophica	AD* AR*	Skin cancer arising in scars
17590	Disseminated superficial actinic porokeratosis	AR*	Skin cancer
(10)	Multiple sebaceous gland tumors and visceral carcinoma (Torre's syndrome)	AR	Diverse gastrointestinal and urogenital cancers
10190 31450	Acrokeratosis verruciformis, van den Bosch's syndrome	AD* XR*	Warty hyperkeratosis
12420	Darier-White disease	AD*	Keratotic papules
18160	Scleroatrophy and keratosis of limbs	AD*	Skin and bowel cancer
12760	Pachyonychia congenita	AD*	Hyperkeratosis, cutaneous horns, leukoplakia
13270 31310 12385	Multiple trichoepithelioma (Spiegler-Brooke tumors; cylindromatosis)	AD* XD AD	
13280	Self-healing squamous epithelioma	AD*	
14415	Hyperkeratosis lenticularis perstans	AD	Skin cancer
18450 16720	Steatocystoma multiplex ± pachyonychia congenita	AD*	

Perhaps, epidermodysplasia verruciformis with basal cell carcinoma, 22640-AR; familial cutaneous papillomatosis, 16790, 16795-AD; pilomatrixoma, 13260-AD; multiple syringioma, 18660-AD; keloids alone, 14810-AD, or as part of syndrome with torticollis, cryptorchism, and renal dysplasia, 31430-XR; familial dyskeratotic comedones, 12045-AD; Kyrle's disease, 14950-AD

Lymphatic and Hematopoietic

24640 26770 24750 24760	Histiocytic reticulosis, generalized or neural only (Letterer-Siwe disease)	AR* AR	
23590	Familial lipochrome histiocytosis	AR*	
20270	Kostmann's infantile genetic agranulocytosis	AR*	Acute monocytic leukemia (chromosomal breaks)
26330	Polycythemia rubra vera	AR	Acute myelogenous leukemia (may have Philadelphia chromosome)
23190	Glutathione reductase deficiency	AR*	Leukemia (chromosomal breaks)

Perhaps, malignant reticuloendotheliosis, 31250-XR*; the four leukemias, 15140, 22335, 25470, (13,19)-AD, AR; Hodgkin's disease, 23600, (5)-AR, AD; mycosis fungoides, 25440-AR; multiple myeloma, 25450-AR; familial eosinophilia, 13140-AD*; hereditary leukemoid reaction, 15143-AD; thymoma, 27423-AR

Immunodeficiency

30030	Bruton's agammaglobulinemia	XR*	Leukemia, lymphoreticular
30100	Wiskott-Aldrich syndrome	XR*	Lymphoreticular
20890	Ataxia-telangiectasia	AR*	Lymphoreticular, leukemia, carcinoma of stomach, brain tumors (chromosomal breaks)

TABLE 1 *(Continued)*

Catalog no. or (ref)	Neoplasm or disorder	Inheri- tance	Associated neoplasms
21450	Chediak-Higashi syndrome	AR*	Pseudolymphoma
	Multiple System		
21090	Bloom's syndrome	AR*	Leukemia, intestinal cancer (chromosomal breaks)
22765 22785	Fanconi's anemia	AR*	Acute monomyelogenous leukemia, squamous cell carcinoma of mucocutaneous junctions, hepatic carcinoma, and adenoma (chromosomal breaks)
30500 12755	Dyskeratosis congenita (Zinsser-Cole-Engman syndrome)	XR* AD	Leukoplakia with squamous cell carcinoma, including of cervix
22560	Beckwith-Wiedemann syndrome	AR*	Visceromegaly, cytomegaly, macroglossia, adrenal cortical neoplasia, Wilms' tumor, hepatoma
26840	Rothmund-Thomson syndrome	AR*	Squamous cell carcinoma
27770	Werner's syndrome	AR*	Sarcoma
16670	Osteopoikilosis	AD*	Nevi
16395	Noonan's syndrome	AD*	Schwannoma
30560	Focal dermal hypoplasia (Goltz's syndrome)	XD*	Mucocutaneous papillomas
	Inborn Errors of Metabolism		
30150	Angiokeratoma diffusa (Fabry's syndrome)	XR*	
27670 23890 23040 27790 23250	Tyrosinemia, hypermethioni- nemia, galactosemia, Wilson's disease, glycogen storage disease-IV	AR* AR	Postcirrhotic hepatoma
(4)	Alpha$_1$-antitrypsin deficiency	Codomi- nant	Hepatoma
30780	Vitamin D-resistant rickets	XR*	Parathyroid adenoma
	Perhaps hyperprolinemia, type 1 with Wilms' tumor, 23950-AR*		

*Mode of inheritance is judged to be proved.
Abbreviations: (AD, autosomal dominant; AR, autosomal recessive; XD, X-linked dominant; XR, X-linked recessive. (Modified from ref. 14 with additions.)

with breast cancer should look for inconspicuous papillomas of the lips, gums, and palpebral fissures or hyperkeratotic papules of the hands, which would suggest Cowden's multiple hamartoma syndrome. Failure to recognize a rare syndrome is a disservice to the patient and perhaps relatives, who may be denied the possible benefits of counseling for prevention and early detection of cancer. Also, an opportunity for further research into pathogenesis is lost.

The conditions in Table 1 probably account for a small fraction of human cancer. A few, such as the polyposis and multiple endocrine neoplasia syndromes, have public health implications. When these dominant traits are discovered in a patient, the physician is responsible for alerting families to the hereditary nature of the disorders. The wider significance is the possibility that intense study of these conditions may help unravel the etiology and pathogenesis of cancers in general.

For example, as single gene traits, all presumably have simple changes or mutation in the DNA nucleotide sequence. If past experience holds, enzyme dysfunction could be predicted in many of the autosomal recessive traits, and have, indeed, been found in xeroderma pigmentosum (Chapter 32) and ataxia-telangiectasia (16,20).

REFERENCES

1. Anderson, D. E. (1974): Genetic study of breast cancer: Identification of a high risk group. *Cancer*, 34:1090–1097.
2. Creagan, E. T., and Fraumeni, J. F., Jr. (1973): Familial gastric cancer and immunologic abnormalities. *Cancer*, 32:1325–1331.
3. Dunham, L. J. (1972): Cancer in man at site of prior benign lesion of skin or mucous membrane: A review. *Cancer Res.*, 32:1359–1374.
4. Eriksson, S., and Hägerstrand, I. (1974): Cirrhosis and malignant hepatoma in alpha$_1$-antitrypsin deficiency. *Acta. Med. Scand.*, 195:451–458.
5. Fraumeni, J. F., Jr. (1974): Family studies in Hodgkin's disease. *Cancer Res.*, 34:1164–1165.
6. Fraumeni, J. F., Jr., Rosen, P. J., Hull, E. W., Barth, R. F., Shapiro, S. R., and O'Connor, J. F.: (1969): Hepatoblastoma in infant sisters. *Cancer*, 24:1086–1090.
7. Fraumeni, J. F., Jr. and Thomas, L. B. (1967): Malignant bladder tumors in a man and his three sons. *JAMA*, 201:507–509.
8. Fraumeni, J. F., Jr., Vogel, C. L., and Easton, J. M. (1968): Sarcomas and multiple polyposis in a kindred. A genetic variety of hereditary polyposis? *Arch. Intern. Med.*, 121:57–61.
9. Hutter, R. V. P., Francis, K. C., and Foote, F. W., Jr. (1964): Ewing's sarcoma in siblings. Report of the second known occurrence. *Am. J. Surg.*, 107:598–603.
10. Jakobiec, F. A. (1974): Sebaceous adenoma of the eyelid and visceral malignancy. *Am. J. Ophthalmol.*, 78:952–960.
11. Knudson, A. G., Jr., and Strong, L. C. (1972): Mutation and cancer: Neuroblastoma and pheochromocytoma. *Am. J. Hum. Genet.*, 24:514–532.
12. Knudson, A. G., Jr., and Strong, L. C. (1972): Mutation and cancer. A model for Wilms' tumor of the kidney. *J. Natl. Cancer Inst.*, 48:313–324.
13. Lundmark, K. M., Thilén, A., and Vahlquist, B. (1967): Familial leukaemia—three cases of acute leukaemia in four siblings. *Acta Paediatr. Scand. (Suppl.)*, 172:200–205.
14. McKusick, V. A. (1974): *Mendelian Inheritance in Man. Catalogs of Autosomal Dominant, Autosomal Recessive, and X-linked Phenotypes*, 4th ed. The John Hopkins Press, Baltimore.
15. Newbold, P. C. H. (1972): Pre-cancer and the skin. *Br. J. Dermatol.*, 86:417–434.
16. Paterson, M. C., Smith, B. P., Lohman, P. H. M., Anderson, A. K., and Fishman, L. (1976): Defective excision repair of γ-ray-damaged DNA in human (ataxia telangiectasia) fibroblasts. *Nature*, 260:444–446.
17. Pour, P., and Ghadirian, P. (1974): Familial cancer of the esophagus in Iran. *Cancer*, 33:1649–1652.
18. Reed, W. B., Boder, E., and Gardner, M. (1974): Congenital and genetic skin disorders with tumor formation. *Birth Defects*, 10(4):265–284.
19. Snyder, A. L., Li, F. P., Henderson, E. S., and Todaro, G. J. (1970): Possible inherited leukaemogenic factors in familial acute myelogenous leukaemia. *Lancet*, 1:586–589.
20. Taylor, A. M. R., Metcalfe, J. A., Oxford, J. M., and Harnden, D. G. (1976): Is chromatid-type damage in ataxia telangiectasia after irradiation at G_0 a consequence of defective repair? *Nature*, 260:441–443.
21. Wennstrom, J., Pierce, E. R., and McKusick, V. A. (1974): Hereditary benign and malignant lesions of the large bowel. *Cancer* 34:850–857.

Genetics of Human Cancer, edited by J. J.
Mulvihill, R. W. Miller, and J. F. Fraumeni, Jr.
Raven Press, New York, 1977.

12

Nosology Among the Neoplastic Genodermatoses

Marvin A. Lutzner

*Dermatology Branch, National Cancer Institute, National Institutes of Health,
Bethesda, Maryland 20014*

There are at least 50 inherited and congenital diseases that affect the skin and
are accompanied by benign or malignant tumors (57). Although classifications are
useful in understanding these diseases (1,57), only knowledge of the chemical
definition of the mutant gene product will permit an understanding of the role of
the gene in producing cancer. The emphasis here will be on those genodermatoses
accompanied by cancer in which current cell biology techniques have produced
insights into their pathogenesis.

TWO AUTOSOMAL RECESSIVE GENODERMATOSES IN WHICH SUNLIGHT CAUSES CANCER

Xeroderma pigmentosum (61)

The most exciting of the genodermatoses in which sunlight causes cancer is
xeroderma pigmentosum (XP). In patients with this autosomal recessive disease,
freckles of different shapes and sizes and different shades of black and brown,
occur on sun-exposed skin, along with dilated superficial blood vessels (telangiectasias) and white spots (Fig. 1). Eyelids and cornea are often damaged, even
to blindness, since they also intercept the sun's rays (Fig. 2). Hundreds of
malignant tumors (basal cell carcinomas, squamous cell carcinomas, and melanomas) occur, and frequently result in death at an early age. A small portion of
the ultraviolet (UV) light from the sun that strikes the human reaches the DNA
within nuclei of cells of the germinative layer of the epidermis producing thymine dimers which, if not removed, may produce mutations and cancer of the
skin (61). An important event was the discovery that cells of XP patients had a
defect in their ability to repair UV-induced damage (9). Within the clinical entity
of XP, cell fusion studies have shown five complementation groups, presumably
each with a different defective gene product (17,45,61). These groups, designated
A through E, were defined according to their characteristic rate of unscheduled

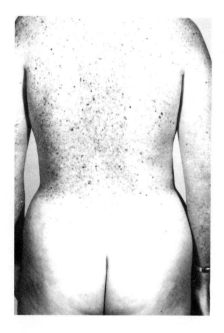

FIG. 1 Back of patient with XP showing heavily freckled sun-light exposed skin in contrast to areas protected against the sun in which there are no freckles.

DNA synthesis (UDS) (6,61), ranging from less than 2% of normal repair in the A group to greater than 50% repair in the E group. Our team at the National Institutes of Health (NIH) also discovered a patient who had a normal rate of DNA repair as measured by standard techniques, i.e., UDS, although he had classical XP; he was designated the XP variant (6,61). Other such patients have since been reported (11). It was found, using the method of viral host cell reactivation, that the variant's cells could repair UV-damaged virus but did so only at 70% of normal (14). Thus, although the variants seem to repair DNA at an almost normal rate, this repair must be error prone. Postreplication repair has been found to be defective in these variants (47).

Some families with XP, in addition to abnormal skin, have neurological abnormalities which may be severe—the so-called DeSanctis-Cacchione syn-

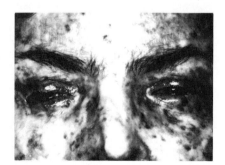

FIG. 2. Face of patient with XP showing freckles, depigmentation, blepharitis, and palpebral fissure deformity. Patient also had opacified cornea.

drome (61). Pathogenesis of the neurologic abnormalities presented an enigma for some time; however, recent work at NIH may shed light on this problem (2). At first, the neurologic abnormalities seemed to occur exclusively in group A patients, whose cells have almost zero repair. Then, members in this complementation group were found with no neurologic abnormalities; and, to complicate matters further, members of the D group, who have a fairly high rate of repair, were found with neurologic abnormalities. Thus, there seemed to be little correlation between neurologic abnormalities and rate of repair. Using the method of measuring colony-forming ability (CFA) of cells following UV-irradiation, which turns out to be a most sensitive method for measuring the ability of a cell to repair adequately enough for cells to survive and divide in culture, we found a close correlation between the ability of a cell to survive and form colonies in culture and the absence of neurologic abnormalities. Only those members of the D group with lowered CFA had neurologic abnormalities. The B, C, and E groups, which have almost normal survival following UV-irradiation, have no neurologic abnormalities. And most convincingly, those members of the A group with neurologic abnormalities have low CFA and those of the A group with no neurologic abnormalities have high CFA. In short, neurologic symptoms correlate best with post-UV-colony-forming ability (CFA), and not the rate of repair (UDS).

These results support the hypothesis that the neurologic abnormalities in XP result when functionally adequate DNA repair is below critical levels. Because UV light does not impinge on the nervous system, one might wonder about the importance of a DNA repair mechanism for neurologic tissue. Although neurons do not divide, they must last for the individual's lifetime; and at times neurons might be damaged by environmental DNA-toxic chemicals and might require a repair system. Such a theory of impaired DNA repair in XP suggests that, if errors are made during the lifetime of an individual and are not repaired, accumulating abnormalities might be one explanation for aging phenomena.

Albinism

Another genodermatosis that affects the ability of the skin to protect itself against sunlight is albinism. Patients with this autosomal recessive defect lack the ability to form pigment because of abnormalities in tyrosinase which ordinarily catalyses the formation of melanin pigment (23). There appears to be more than one genotype for albinism (23). Melanin granules form a protective cap on the sunny side of the nucleus and serve as an effective screen against the damaging UV rays. In albinism melanin granules are not fully formed and, therefore, the nucleus is more vulnerable to the effects of the sun's rays (23). It is of interest that although albinos develop malignancies of the skin (53) they are not as severely involved as patients with XP. Furthermore, black patients with XP have a much higher mortality than albinos even though both groups may be exposed to the tropical sun (40). This indicates that the more critical of the two protective mechanisms is not pigment but is the DNA repair system. Red-haired individuals with blue eyes have difficulty tanning after sun exposure and are able to form only freckles. These individuals, usually of Celtic ancestry, have an increased incidence of skin cancer (70). The inability of these individuals to tan is probably genetically determined. The heredity of red hair is not well understood, but the presence of red seems dominant to its absence and hypostatic to brown and black (60).

AN AUTOSOMAL RECESSIVE GENODERMATOSIS IN WHICH THE WART VIRUS MAY CAUSE SQUAMOUS CELL CARCINOMA

Epidermodysplasia Verruciformis (75)

Epidermodysplasia verruciformis is an autosomal recessive disease in which children develop multiple warts (Fig. 3). The common wart virus can be demonstrated in these warts by both electron and fluorescent microscopy (75). Warts appear to progress to squamous cell carcinoma at an estimated rate of about 10%. Within the cancers, no virus or viral antigens can be detected. This is reminiscent of other virus-induced tumors such as the Shope papilloma, in which the virus cannot be found in the neoplasms but can be found readily in the early precursor warts. The relationship of the common wart virus to squamous cell carcinoma in epidermodysplasia verruciformis deserves further study now that a method appears to have been developed for culturing the human wart virus (19).

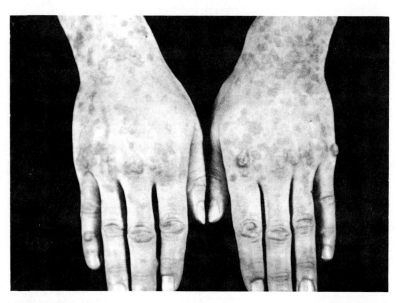

FIG. 3. Back of hands and forearms of patient with epidermodysplasia verruciformis showing many flat warts and a few raised warts. This patient also had squamous cell carcinomas of his forehead. (Photograph courtesy of Dr. Israel Zeligmann.)

THREE GENODERMATOSES WITH CHROMOSOMAL
INSTABILITY (29)

Ataxia-Telangiectasia

In ataxia-telangiectasia (AT) there are enlarged blood vessels of the face, ear lobes, and most prominently of the bulbar conjunctiva (Fig. 4). This autosomal recessive disease can be suspected in early childhood by recognition of cerebellar ataxia. Children have an abnormal immune system, often die of sino-pulmonary infections, are prone to lymphomas, leukemias, and other malignancies (29,41,71), and may be hypersensitive to standard doses of therapeutic irradiation. Clones of peripheral lymphocytes from AT patients are consistently marked by structural rearrangements of the long arm of chromosome 14 (51). There is report that AT fibroblasts have poor survival after *in vitro* irradiation (65) and little activity of an endonuclease necessary for repairing X-ray damage to DNA bases (54,67). The relationships between the predisposition to cancer and the abnormalities of chromosomes, cultured fibroblasts, the cerebellum, the blood vessels, and the immune system are not understood.

Bloom's Syndrome

In the autosomal recessive Bloom's syndrome, there is short stature recognizable even during infancy, sensitivity to the sun with resultant telangiectasias in a butterfly distribution over the face, and high risk of leukemia (4). Chromosomal abnormalities, especially quadriradials, are a hallmark of the disease (4,29,51). The DNA repair system functions normally in these patients (10,43,59). Minor

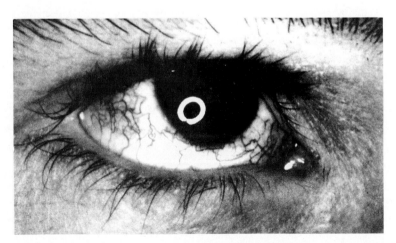

FIG. 4. Eye of patient with AT. Prominent telangiectatic blood vessels are seen in the bulbar conjunctiva.

abnormalities of the immune system correlate with a susceptibility to infection. An abnormality has been reported in the rate of DNA fiber elongation during DNA replication in Bloom's fibroblasts (5), i.e., there is a retardation in the rate of synthesis, which theoretically might explain the formation of the quadriradial chromosomes. This retardation might result from an abnormal enzyme involved directly with DNA replication.

Fanconi's Anemia

In Fanconi's anemia, an autosomal recessive disease, there is bone marrow hypoplasia, hemorrhage, and marrow failure leading to death. The skin shows petechiae, echymoses, and extensive brown pigmentation. Also common are skeletal and renal abnormalities. It has been found (69) that cultured fibroblasts from Fanconi's patients are more transformable by the SV-40 virus than are normal cells. This has not been found in XP cells (42). Increased frequency of chromosomal breaks and especially endoreduplications have been found in cells from these patients (29). Although one report noted normal DNA repair in cells from Fanconi's patients (59), another study indicated an abnormality in the exonuclease portion of the repair system (55). Compared to the general population, patients with Fanconi's anemia have a much greater risk of leukemia and other cancers (29).

IMMUNOLOGIC ABNORMALITIES RESULTING FROM SINGLE GENE DEFECTS, ASSOCIATED WITH NEOPLASMS

Ataxia-Telangiectasia

AT patients have deficiencies in both cellular and humoral immune systems. Ten percent of these patients have neoplasias mostly of the lymphoid system but also of the gastrointestinal system, brain, ovary, and skin (41,71). A defect in tissue differentiation has been hypothesized in AT (Fig. 5; ref. 71) specifically a defect in the interaction necessary for differentiation of gut-associated organs such as the thymus and liver. Consistent with this view is the finding of elevated alpha-fetoprotein in patients with AT, suggesting immaturity of the liver (71).

Wiskott-Aldrich Syndrome

Patients with this X-linked disorder often develop eczema of the atopic type, have thrombocytopenia with bleeding and multiple infections and may die at an early age (71). More than 10% of these patients develop malignancies, primarily lymphomas, astrocytomas, and reticuloendothelioses (41). They have a broad defect in the humoral and cellular immunity and a specific abnormality in the proximate, processing, or afferent limb of immunity, especially for polysaccharide antigens (71). It is also of interest that the BK papova virus has been found in a

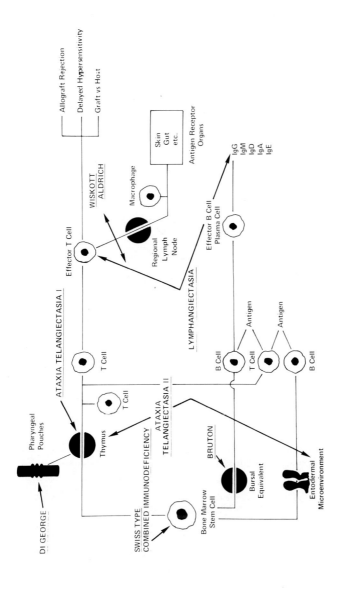

FIG. 5. Possible sites of defect for genetic immuno-deficiency diseases associated with neoplasms. [Modified from Waldmann et al.(71)].

reticulum cell sarcoma of the brain of a patient with the syndrome (64). The virus was also found in the urine of this patient and several others with the Wiskott-Aldrich syndrome. However, the same virus has also been found in immunosuppressed recipients of renal transplants (28).

Bruton's Disease, Swiss-Type Agammaglobulinemia, and Gastrointestinal Lymphangiectasia

Bruton's disease is considered to be an abnormality of the bursal analog; Swiss-type disease, a defect of the bone marrow stem cell; and gastrointestinal lymphangiectasia, a loss of T cells from the gut (Fig. 5; ref. 71).

Malignancies occur with increased frequency in these syndromes. Most tumors are lymphoreticular; however, 25% of tumors are of other varieties. It has been hypothesized that lymphoproliferative neoplasms in these patients result from intrinsic abnormalities of the lymphoid system plus an inability of immune mechanisms to destroy neoplastic cells (41). The association of malignancy with these immunologic disorders supports the concept that the immune system normally plays an important role in control of malignant disease by surveillance of tumor cells that possess new surface antigens and perhaps in preventing activation of latent viral genomes within the reticuloendothelial system (71).

A DISEASE WITH ABNORMAL GRANULES: CHEDIAK-HIGASHI SYNDROME

Patients with this autosomal recessive syndrome have a dilution of skin, hair, and eye pigment; their hair has a bluish sheen, patients suffer photophobia, and often die young from infection or a lymphoma-like "accelerated" phase (74). Leukocytes from these patients have giant granules that do not properly release their lysosomal enzyme. The disease has been considered to be an abnormality of lysosomes, but seems to be much more extensive, as melanin granules are also giant-sized. Indeed, huge granules can be found in most cells that produce granules (49), leading to the conclusion that Chediak-Higashi syndrome probably is a disease of granule formation (48), perhaps involving abnormal granule membranes. An abnormality in tubulin assembly has been indicated by some recent studies (76).

THE NEUROCRISTOPATHIES

In the past some of the diseases to be discussed under this new classification have been included in the neurocutaneous syndromes or phakomatoses. The term neurocristopathy has been introduced (Fig. 6; ref. 5) to include diseases which appear to result from abnormalities of the neural crest (46,73).

Nevoid Basal Cell Carcinoma Syndrome

This is an autosomal dominant disease that features multiple basal cell carcino-

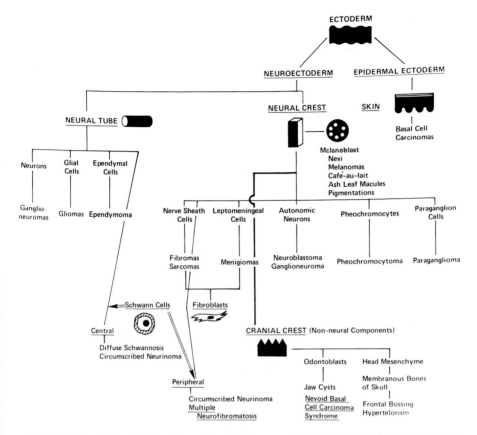

FIG. 6. Origin and derivations of neural crest tissue, neoplasms that might develop from these derivatives, and possible sites of defects in nevoid basal cell carcinoma syndrome and neurofibromatosis. [Modified from Kramer (46) and Weston (73)].

mas of the skin (Fig. 7; ref. 33). There is frontal bossing, hypertelorism, bone cysts especially in the jaw (invasive keratocysts), bifid ribs, agenesis of the corpus callosum, brachymetacarpalism, and palmar pits (Fig. 8). Calcification of the falx, nerve deafness, and endocrine abnormalities have all been reported. In addition, tumors may occur such as medulloblastomas, jaw fibrosarcomas, ameloblastomas, and ovarian fibromas.

A mechanism for this pleiotropic disease (Fig. 6) starts when the ectoderm in the early embryo forms neuroectoderm and epidermal ectoderm (46,73). The latter forms epidermis, except for the melanoblast, which is a neural crest derivative. The neuroectoderm generates both peripheral and cranial neural crests: The peripheral crest forms pheochromocytes, paraganglion cells, autonomic neurons, leptomeningeal cells, and nerve sheath cells (Schwann cells); the cranial neural crest, in addition, forms odontoblasts and head mesenchyme. The neural tube gives rise to neurons, glial cells, and ependymal cells, all with neoplastic potential. Fibroblasts and neuroblasts are thought to interact in producing sarcomas and

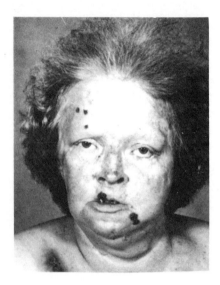

FIG. 7. Patient with nevoid basal cell carcinoma syndrome. Note frontal bossing and hypertelorism. The crusted lesions seen on the face, lip, chin, and shoulder are basal cell carcinomas.

meningiomas (44). Neural crest cells are multipotential (73) and disseminate widely throughout the body, migrating, dividing, differentiating during intrauterine life and even after birth. They seem to be prime targets for teratogenesis, mutagenesis, and oncogenesis. A possible explanation for the nevoid basal cell carcinoma syndrome is that some abnormal event occurs in the early ectoderm: Basal cell carcinomas might form from abnormal basal cells; frontal bossing and hypertelorism might result from abnormalities in membranous skull formation; jaw cysts may develop from abnormal odontoblasts, etc.

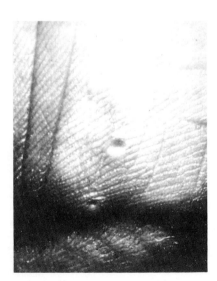

FIG. 8. Palmar pits in a patient with nevoid basal cell carcinoma syndrome. (Photograph courtesy of Dr. William Reed.)

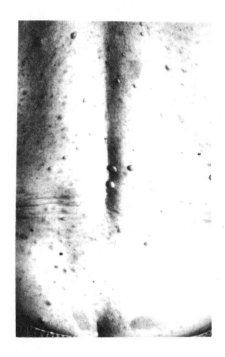

FIG. 9. Back of patient with neurofibroma-tosis. Cutaneous nodules and *café-au-lait* pigmentations can be seen. (Photograph courtesy of Dermatology Service, Walter Reed Army Hospital.)

NEUROFIBROMATOSIS (von RECKLINGHAUSEN'S SYN-DROME (5,44,46)

This autosomal dominant disease, sometimes included in the neurocristopathies, features multiple neuroid tumors of the skin, and abnormal skin pigmentations, primarily *café-au-lait* spots and axillary freckling (Fig. 9). Typical symptoms are not present at birth but begin around puberty. The disease may be exclusively of the peripheral or central type, or both. Skeletal erosions occur as does scoliosis. Ten to 30% of patients with this syndrome have been reported to develop malignant neurofibromas (44), and a small percentage have pheochromocytomas. Malignant melanomas and basal cell carcinomas have been reported. Any part of the central nervous system may have polymorphous lesions involving all three types of neural cells—neurons, glial cells, and supportive cells.

A possible pathogenesis of this disease (Fig. 6) may stem from an abnormality of the neural crest which affects melanoblasts, producing *café-au-lait* spots and axillary freckling, abnormal interactions between fibroblasts and Schwann cells producing neuroid tumors and sarcomas, and abnormal pheochromocytes forming pheochromocytomas, etc. Furthermore, neurofibromas are not of single cell origin, but evolve from multiple cells (22). A minimal estimate of the number of cells involved for each lesion is 150, but may be as high as several thousand, suggesting that the initial oncogenic event affects a relatively large number of cells simultaneously or that it affects one or a few cells, subsequently altering the

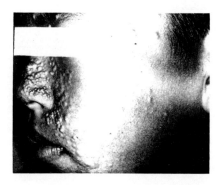

FIG. 10. Face of patient with tuberous sclerosis. Papules (adenoma sebaceum) can be seen clustered on the nose and nasolabial folds. (Photograph courtesy of Medcom.)

pattern of growth in adjacent cells. Such an event could take place in neural crest cells at an early time in the ontogeny of the patient with neurofibromatosis.

Finally, interesting new findings in von Recklinghausen's syndrome relate to nerve-growth factor. In affected patients, one laboratory reported increased nerve-growth stimulating activity (62), whereas another found it normal (68). A third group claimed that nerve-growth factor was increased, but only in the central form of this disease (63). The relationship of these findings to the neural crest remains to be determined.

Tuberous Sclerosis (Pringle's Disease, Epiloia, and Adenoma Sebaceum) (58)

In patients with this autosomal dominant syndrome, large nodules in the cerebral cortex develop, leading to mental deficiency, epilepsy, and other neurologic disorders. Death often occurs before the age of 20. Skin lesions include adenoma sebaceum, which are in reality, angiofibromas, appearing as papules and nodules mainly along the nasolabial folds (Fig. 10), and shagreen patches, namely flesh-colored plaques with a pigskin-like appearance, *café-au-lait* spots, freckles, and so-called "ash-leaf" depigmented spots, an important early finding, which is often predictively diagnostic (24) (Fig. 11). Subungual fibromas also occur (Fig. 12). Internal lesions include mulberry retinal tumors, rhabdomyosarcomas, and

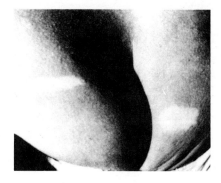

FIG. 11. "Ash leaf" depigmented macules on buttocks of patient with tuberous sclerosis. (Photograph courtesy of Dermatology Service, Walter Reed Army Hospital.)

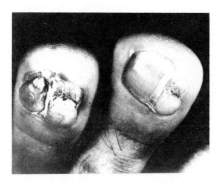

FIG. 12. Subungual fibromas and resultant dystrophic nails in patient with tuberous sclerosis. (Photograph courtesy of Dr. William Reed.)

various skeletal abnormalities, as well as tumors and cysts in the kidney and heart. Of the many cell types involved in this syndrome, fibroblasts, angioblasts, glioblasts, and neuroblasts, all derive from the neural crest or interact with it; hence, it is reasonable to include this disease with other neurocristopathies.

GENODERMATOSES WITH PREMATURE AGING

Progeria (Hutchinson-Gilford Syndrome)

Progeria is an autosomal recessive disease that is first manifested in infancy as a stunting of growth and precocious senility, resulting in early death because of coronary artery disease (15). The diminished number of cell turnovers in fibroblasts cultured from patients with this disease may reflect accelerated aging (31). Also, skin fibroblasts from progeric patients fail to show normal rejoining of DNA following X-radiation (21), whereas repair following UV-irradiation is normal (10). Progeric fibroblasts compared with normal fibroblasts contain a higher percentage of heat-labile enzymes (32); the authors postulate an error in the regulation of protein synthesis with improper functioning of the resulting denatured proteins; some postsynthetic modification of proteins has been hypothesized. Despite expectations, neoplasms have not been reported in progeria.

Werner's Syndrome

Premature aging is also part of the autosomal recessive disease, Werner's syndrome. Other characteristics are: shortness of stature with characteristic habitus, premature graying of the hair, premature baldness, scleropoikiloderma, trophic ulcers of the legs, juvenile cataracts, hypogonadism, tendency to diabetes, calcification of blood vessels, and osteosclerosis (20). There is a tendency toward tumor formation, especially noncarcinomatous neoplasia, such as fibroliposarcomas, osteogenic sarcomas, melanotic sarcomas, etc. Despite the chronic ulcerations and atrophic skin changes, skin cancers are uncommon (30). As in progeria,

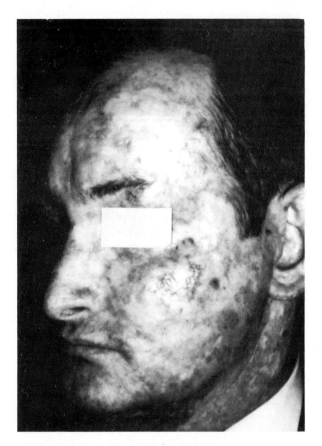

FIG. 13. Face of patient with the Rothmund-Thomson syndrome showing hyper- and depigmentation of skin along with atrophic areas (poikilodermatous), one of which shows a crusted ulceration. (Photograph courtesy of Dr. William Reed.)

abnormal heat-labile enzymes and decreased longevity of cultured fibroblasts have been found in Werner's syndrome (37,50).

Rothmund-Thomson Syndrome

This is an autosomal recessive disorder characterized by skin telangiectasias, scaling, and disorders of pigmentation (Fig. 13), juvenile cataracts, saddle nose, congenital bone defects, disturbances of hair growth, and hypergonadism (20). Multiple keratoses may develop on heavily involved skin followed by squamous cell carcinomas (57).

GENODERMATOSES WITH ABNORMAL KERATINIZATION

Keratinization is a process in which the outer layer of the skin forms specific intracellular proteins which serve as a protective fabric and barrier.

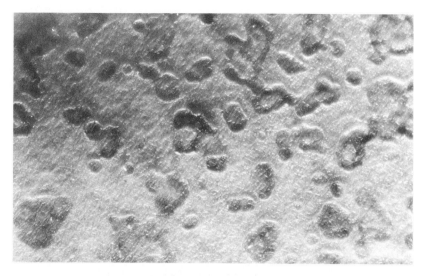

FIG. 14. Lesions of porokeratosis of the PPPD variety. Gyrate lesions show ridged borders. This patient also had two squamous cell carcinomas of the skin.

Porokeratosis

There are three types of porokeratosis, all autosomal dominant diseases: The Mibelli type (12), porokeratosis plantaris and palmaris disseminata (PPPD) (34) (Fig. 14), and disseminated superficial actinic porokeratosis (8). Squamous cell carcinomas have been reported in the Mibelli and PPPD types (12,34). Keratotic plaques, sharply delimited and raised with a horny ridge formed by a keratotic column of cells known as coronoid lamella, are characteristic of porokeratosis. Chromosome abnormalities have been found in cultured fibroblasts from lesions of a patient with the Mibelli type (66). Also, a clonal theory for formation of abnormal plaques has been recently set forth (56).

Tylosis

Tylosis (a Greek word for ''woody'') is an autosomal dominant disease characterized by symmetrical thickening of the skin of the hands and feet. Palms and soles show fissuring, flaking, and abnormalities of local sweating. There are two clinical types: One of early onset around the first year of life which is not involved with malignancies; and the second type, occurring around the age of 10 with a high risk of esophageal carcinoma (36). The late-onset type has been described in two Liverpool families. In 17 of 28 members with tylosis, well-differentiated squamous cell carcinomas of the esophagus developed at young ages. Since a portion of the mucosal lining of the esophagus is squamous epithelium like that of skin, it is tempting to speculate that these two fabrics, although derived from different germ layers, might be responding to a similar oncogenic stimulus directed by a gene defect. However, curiously enough carcinomas do not develop on the palms and soles.

POLYPOSIS ASSOCIATED WITH GENODERMATOSES

Gardner's Syndrome

Patients with Gardner's syndrome, an autosomal dominant syndrome (27), have epidermoid cysts, desmoid tumors, fibromas, and lipomas of both the skin and soft tissue and polyposis of the colon. The lesions of the colon are premalignant, almost always undergoing malignant transformation, primarily adenocarcinomas. Increased tetraploidy was noted in skin fibroblast cultures derived from patients with Gardner's syndrome (13).

Peutz-Jeghers' Syndrome

The skin pigmentations of Peutz-Jeghers' syndrome, an autosomal dominant syndrome, resemble freckles, especially around the lips, buccal mucosa, and digits (38). The associated polyps of the colon are hamartomatous and rarely undergo malignant transformation; polyps of the stomach and duodenum are more likely to become cancerous. Precocious puberty due to granulosa cell tumors of the ovaries has been reported. A suggested classification for intestinal polyposis syndromes labels the Peutz-Jeghers' syndrome as intestinal polyposis II and the Gardner's syndrome as intestinal polyposis III (52).

Cowden's Syndrome (Multiple Hamartoma Syndrome)

In Cowden's syndrome, an autosomal dominant syndrome, progressive wart-like lesions occur on the mucosa of the lips and mouth and other cutaneous surfaces (Fig. 15; ref. 72). Also, fibrocystic disease of the breast occurs, sometimes resulting in breast malignancy. Thyroid tumors, gastrointestinal polyps, ab-

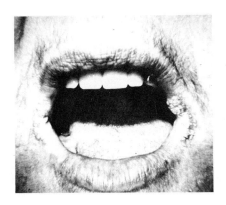

FIG. 15. Wart-like lesions on lips of patient with Cowden's syndrome. (Photograph courtesy of Dr. William Reed.)

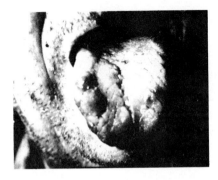

FIG. 16. Hemangiomas on tongue of patient with blue rubber bleb nevus syndrome. (Photograph courtesy of Dermatology Service, Walter Reed Army Hospital.)

normalities of the nervous system, fibromas, angiomas, and lipomas have been reported, along with high arched palate, scrotal tongue, and scoliosis.

The Blue Rubber Bleb Nevus Syndrome

An autosomal dominant disease, the blue rubber bleb nevus syndrome involves painful and depressible bladder-like cutaneous and mucosal hemangiomas (Fig. 16; ref. 26). Lesions in the gastrointestinal tract sometimes result in gastrointestinal hemorrhage (Fig. 17). Hemangiomas have also been reported in the liver, kidneys, spleen, lung, and central nervous system. Patients have been reported with medulloblastoma and enchondromatosis, requiring differentiation from Maffucci's syndrome (7).

EPIDERMOLYSIS BULLOSA

This is a complex entity with many different genotypes and phenotypes. In severely scarred lesions of skin, squamous cell carcinomas may develop (18).

CONGENITAL ANOMALIES OF THE SKIN ASSOCIATED WITH NEO-PLASIA

These anomalies are present at birth but are not single gene defects.

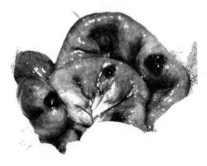

FIG. 17. Bowel hemangiomas in patient with blue rubber bleb nevus syndrome. (Photograph courtesy of Dr. William Reed.)

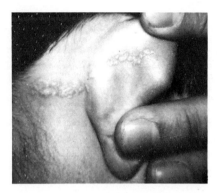

FIG. 18. Sebaceous nevus of Jadassohn. Appearing as a linear array of wax-like papules behind ear of patient. (Photograph courtesy of Dr. Israel Zeligmann.)

Giant Pigmented Nevus (Garment or Bathing-Suit Nevus)

Patients with giant pigmented nevi are prone to acquire neoplasms within the lesions; the risk has not been determined with certainty, ranging from 2 to 30% (16). Many of the developing tumors are melanomas; however, neuroblastomas, neurilemmomas, and undifferentiated neural tumors have been reported (39). Patients with these skin lesions may also have neuroblastomas of the kidney or cerebral melanomas.

Nevus Sebaceous of Jadassohn

These nevi occur exclusively on the face and scalp and may be associated with mental deficiency and epilepsy (Fig. 18; ref. 3). They are slightly raised yellowish-red plaques with a waxy surface. During puberty, lesions may become verrucous and may either undergo transformation or involute. Basal and squamous cell carcinomas are frequent.

Nevus of Ota (Oculodermal Melanosis or Melanocytosis)

These occur as pigmented lesions around the eye and on the sclera and are histologically blue nevi. Malignant melanomas have been reported to arise in these lesions (Fig. 19; ref. 25).

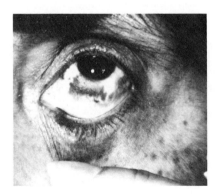

FIG. 19. Nevus of Ota. This patient has pigmented scleral lesions, and the periorbital skin is freckled. (Photograph courtesy of Dr. William Reed.)

SUMMARY

This review began with a description of cancer-associated genodermatoses for which molecular mechanisms are known, and then summarized some recent information of a novel nature in other genodermatoses. An attempt was made to classify and explain those syndromes which affect the immune system and those which might be derived from the neural crest. Finally, a brief description was given of some of the other well-described, but poorly understood, neoplastic genodermatoses. Hopefully, in this large group of genetic skin diseases associated with cancer, further inroads will be made into the molecular processes involved in human cancer.

REFERENCES

1. Anderson, D. E. (1969): Genetic varieties of neoplasia. In: *Genetic Concepts and Neoplasia,* pp. 85–109. Williams and Wilkins, Baltimore, Md.
2. Andrews, A. D., Barrett, S. F., and Robbins, J. H. (1975): Effects of DNA repair defects on the postultraviolet colony-forming ability of human fibroblasts *in vitro (Abstr). J. Cell. Biol.,* 67:10A.
3. Bianchine, J. W. (1970): Nevus sebaceous of Jadassohn. A neurocutaneous syndrome and a potentially premalignant lesion. *Am. J. Dis. Child.,* 120:223–228.
4. Bloom, D. (1966): Syndrome of congenital telangiectatic erythema and stunted growth. *J. Pediatr.,* 68:103–113.
5. Bolande, R. P. (1974): Neurocristopathies. A unifying concept of disease arising in neural crest maldevelopment. *Hum. Pathol.,* 5:409–429.
6. Burk, P. G., Lutzner, M. A., Clarke, D. D., and Robbins, J. H. (1971): Ultraviolet-stimulated thymidine incorporation in xeroderma pigmentosum lymphocytes. *J. Lab. Clin. Med.,* 77:759–767.
7. Carleton, A., Elkington, J. St. C., Greenfield, J. G., and Robb-Smith, A. H. T. (1942): Maffucci's syndrome (dyschondroplasia with hemangiomata). *Q. J. Med.,* 11:203–228.
8. Chernosky, M. E., and Freeman, R. G. (1967): Disseminated superficial actinic porokeratosis (DSAP). *Arch. Dermatol.,* 96:611–624.
9. Cleaver, J. E. (1968): Defective repair replication of DNA in xeroderma pigmentosum. *Nature,* 218:652–656.
10. Cleaver, J. E. (1970): DNA damage and repair in light-sensitive human skin disease. Special review article. *J. Invest. Dermatol.,* 54:181–195.
11. Cleaver, J. E. (1972): Xeroderma pigmentosum: Variants with normal DNA repair and normal sensitivity to ultraviolet light. *J. Invest. Dermatol.,* 58:124–128.
12. Cort, D. F., and Abdel-Aziz, A-H. (1972): Epithelioma arising in porokeratosis of Mibelli. *Br. J. Plast. Surg.,* 25:318–328.
13. Danes, B. S. (1975): Gardner syndrome—a study in cell culture. *Cancer,* 36:2327–2333.
14. Day, R. S., III, (1974): Studies on repair of adenovirus 2 by human fibroblasts using normal, xeroderma pigmentosum, and xeroderma pigmentosum heterozygous strains. *Cancer Res.,* 34:1965–1970.
15. DeBusk, F. L. (1972): Hutchinson-Gilford progeria syndrome. *J. Pediatr.,* 80:697–724.
16. Dellon, A. L., Edelson, R. L., and Chretien, P. B. (1976): Defining the malignant potential of the giant pigmented nevus. *Plast. Reconstr. Surg.,* 57:611–618.
17. DeWeerd-Kastelein, E. A., Keijzer, W., and Bootsma, D. (1972): Genetic heterogeneity of xeroderma pigmentosum demonstrated by somatic cell hybridization. *Nature* [*New Biol.*], 238:80–83.
18. Didolkar, M. S., Gerner, R. E., and Moore, G. E. (1974): Epidermolysis bullosa dystrophica and epithelioma of the skin. *Cancer,* 33:198–202.
19. Eisinger, M., Kucarova, O., Sarkar, N. H., and Good, R. A. (1975): Propagation of human wart virus in tissue culture. *Nature,* 256:432–434.

20. Epstein, C. J., Martin, G. M., Schultz, A. L., and Motulsky, A. G. (1966): Werner's syndrome: A review of its symptomatology, natural history, pathologic features, genetics and relationship to the natural aging process. *Medicine (Baltimore)*, 45:177–221.
21. Epstein, J., Williams, J. R., and Little, J. B. (1973): Deficient DNA repair in human progeroid cells. *Proc. Natl. Acad. Sci. USA*, 70:977–981.
22. Fialkow, P. J., Sagebiel, R. W., Gartler, S. M., and Rimoin, D. L. (1971): Multiple cell origin of hereditary neurofibromas. *N. Engl. J. Med.*, 284:298–300.
23. Fitzpatrick, T. B., and Quevedo, W. C., Jr. (1966): Albinism. In: *Metabolic Basis of Inherited Disease*, edited by J. B. Stanbury, J. B. Wyngarden, and D. S. Fredrickson, pp. 324–340. McGraw-Hill, New York.
24. Fitzpatrick, T. B., Szabó, G., Hori, Y., Simone, A. A., Reed, W. B., and Greenberg, M. H. (1968): White leaf-shaped macules. Earliest visible sign of tuberous sclerosis. *Arch. Dermatol.*, 98:1–6.
25. Font, R. L., Reynolds, A. M., Jr., and Zimmerman, L. E. (1967): Diffuse malignant melanoma of the iris in the nevus of Ota. *Arch. Ophthalmol.*, 77:513–518.
26. Fretzin, D. F., and Potter, B. (1965): Blue rubber bleb nevus *Arch. Intern. Med.*, 116:924–929.
27. Gardner, E. J., and Richards, R. C. (1953): Multiple cutaneous and subcutaneous lesions occurring simultaneously with hereditary polyposis and osteomatosis. *Am. J. Hum. Genet.*, 5:139–147.
28. Gardner, S. D., Field, A. M., Coleman, D. V., and Hulme, B. (1971): New human papovavirus (BK) isolated from urine after renal transplantation. *Lancet*, 1:1253–1257.
29. German, J. (1974): Genes which increase chromosomal instability in somatic cells and predispose to cancer. In: *Chromosomes and Cancer*, edited by J. German, pp. 61–101. Wiley, New York.
30. Gertler, H. (1964): Karzinombildung beim Werner-Syndrom. *Dermatol. Wochenschr.*, 150:606–616.
31. Goldstein, S. (1969): Lifespan of cultured cells in progeria. *Lancet*, 1:424.
32. Goldstein, S., and Moerman, E. (1975): Heat-labile enzymes in skin fibroblasts from subjects with progeria. *N. Engl. J. Med.*, 292:1305–1309.
33. Gorlin, R. J., and Sedano, H. O. (1972): Multiple nevoid basal cell carcinoma syndrome revisited. *Birth Defects*, 7(8):140–148.
34. Guss, S. B., Osbourn, R. A., and Lutzner, M. A. (1971): Porokeratosis plantaris, palmaris et disseminata. A third type of porokeratosis. *Arch. Dermatol.*, 104:366–373.
35. Hand, R., and German, J. (1975): Retarded rate of DNA chain growth in Bloom's syndrome. *Proc. Natl. Acad. Sci. USA*, 72:758–762.
36. Harper, P. S., Harper, R. M. J., and Howel-Evans, A. W. (1970): Carcinoma of the esophagus with tylosis. *Q. J. Med.*, 34:317–333.
37. Holliday, R., Porterfield, J. S., and Gibbs, D. D. (1974): Premature ageing and occurrence of altered enzyme in Werner's syndrome fibroblasts. *Nature*, 248:762–763.
38. Jeghers, H., McKusick, V. A., and Katz, K. H. (1949): Generalized intestinal polyposis and melanin spots of the oral mucosa, lips and digits. *N. Engl. J. Med.*, 241:993–1005.
39. Kaplan, E. N. (1974): Risk of malignancy in large congenital nevi. *Plast. Reconstr. Surg.*, 53:421–428.
40. Keeler, C. E. (1963): Albinism, xeroderma pigmentosum and skin cancer. *Natl. Cancer Inst. Monogr.*, 10:349–359.
41. Kersey, J. H., Spector, B. D., and Good, R. A. (1973): Primary immunodeficiency diseases and cancer: The Immunodeficiency-Cancer Registry. *Int. J. Cancer.*, 12:333–347.
42. Key, D. J., and Todaro, G. J. (1974): Xeroderma pigmentosum cell susceptibility to SV40 virus transformation: Lack of effect of low dosage ultraviolet radiation in enhancing viral-induced transformation. *J. Invest. Dermatol.*, 62:7–10.
43. Kleijer, W. J., and Bootsma, D. (1971): Repair of DNA damaged by UV- and X-irradiation in cultivated normal human, xeroderma pigmentosum and Bloom cells. *Proc. 1st. Eur. Biophys. Congr.* (Baden), 2:129–133.
44. Knight, W. A., III, Murphy, W. K., and Gottlieb, J. A. (1973): Neurofibromatosis associated with malignant neurofibromas. *Arch. Dermatol.*, 107:747–750.
45. Kraemer, K. H.; Coon, H. G., and Petinga, R. A. (1975): Genetic heterogeneity in xeroderma pigmentosum: Complementation groups and their relationship to DNA repair rates. *Proc. Natl. Acad. Sci. USA*, 72:59–63.
46. Kramer, W. (1971): Lesions of the central nervous system in multiple neurofibromatosis. *Psychiatr. Neurd. Neurochir.*, 74:349–368.
47. Lehmann, A. R., Kirk-Bell, S., Arlett, C. F., Paterson, M. C., Lohman, P. H. M., deWeerd-

Kastelein, E. A., and Bootsma, D. (1975): Xeroderma pigmentosum cells with normal levels of excision repair have a defect in DNA synthesis after UV-irradiation. *Proc. Natl. Acad. Sci. USA*, 72:219–223.

48. Lutzner, M. A., and Lowrie, C. T. (1972): Ultrastructure of the development of the normal black and giant beige melanin granules in the mouse. In: *Pigmentation: Its Genesis and Biologic Control*, edited by V. Riley, pp. 89–105. Appleton-Century-Crofts, New York.

49. Lutzner, M. A., Tierney, J. H., and Benditt, E. P. (1965): Giant granules and widespread cytoplasmic inclusions in a genetic syndrome of Aleutian mink. *Lab. Invest.*, 14:2063–2079.

50. Martin, G. M., Sprague, C. A., Epstein, C. J. (1970): Replicative lifespan of cultivated human cells. *Lab. Invest.*, 23:86–92.

51. McCaw, B. K., Hecht, F., Harnden, D. G., and Teplitz, R. L. (1975): Somatic rearrangement of chromosome 14 in human lymphocytes. *Proc. Natl. Acad. Sci. USA*, 72:2071–2075.

52. McKusick, V. A. (1975): *Mendelian inheritance in man. Catalogs of autosomal dominant, autosomal recessive, and x-linked phenotypes.* Johns Hopkins Univ. Press, Baltimore, Md. pp. 271–272.

53. Oettle, A. G. (1963): Skin cancer in Africa. *Natl. Cancer Inst. Monogr.*, 10:197–214.

54. Paterson, M. C., Smith, B. P., Lohman, P. H. M., Anderson, A. K., and Fishman, L. (1976): Defective excision repair of γ-ray-damaged DNA in human ataxia telangiectasia fibroblasts. *Nature*, 260:444–446.

55. Poon, P. K., O'Brien, R. L., Parker, J. W. (1974): Defective DNA repair in Fanconi's anemia. *Nature*, 250:223–225.

56. Reed, R. J., and Leone, P. (1970): Porokeratosis-A mutant clonal keratosis of the epidermis. *Arch. Dermatol.*, 101:340–347.

57. Reed, W. B., Boder, E., and Gardner, M. (1974): Congenital and genetic skin disorders with tumor formation. *Birth Defects*, 10(4):265–284.

58. Reed, W. B., Nickel, W. R., and Campion, G. (1963): Internal manifestations of tuberous sclerosis. *Arch. Dermatol.*, 87:715–728.

59. Regan, J. D., Sedow, R. B., Carrier, W. L., and Lee, W. H. (1970): Molecular events following the ultraviolet irradiation of human cells from ultraviolet-sensitive individuals. In: *Advances in Radiation Research*, edited by J. F. Duplan and A. Chapiro, pp. 119–126. Gordon and Breach Science Publ., New York.

60. Rife, D. C. (1967): The inheritance of red hair. *Acta. Genet. Med. Gemellol.* (Roma), 16:342–349.

61. Robbins, J. H., Kraemer, K. H., Lutzner, M. A., Festoff, B. W., and Coon, H. G. (1974): Xeroderma pigmentosum. An inherited disease with sun sensitivity, multiple cutaneous neoplasms and abnormal DNA repair. *Ann. Intern. Med.*, 80:221–248.

62. Schenkein, I., Bueker, E. D., Helson, L., Axelrod, F., and Dancis, J. (1974): Increased nerve-growth-stimulating activity in disseminated neurofibromatosis. *N. Engl. J. Med.*, 290:613–614.

63. Siggers, D. C., Boyer, S. H., and Eldridge, R. (1975): Nerve-growth factor in disseminated neurofibromatosis. *N. Engl. J. Med.*, 292:1134.

64. Takemoto, K. K., Rabson, A. S., Mullarkey, M. F., Blaese, R. M., Garon, C. F., and Nelson, D. (1974): Isolation of papovavirus from brain tumor and urine of a patient with Wiskott-Aldrich syndrome. *J. Natl. Cancer Inst.*, 53:1205–1207.

65. Taylor, A. M. R., Harnden, D. G., Arlett, C. F., Harcourt, S. A., Lehmann, A. R., Stevens, S., and Bridges, B. A. (1975): Ataxia telangiectasia: A human mutation with abnormal radiation sensitivity. *Nature*, 258:427–429.

66. Taylor, A. M. R., Harnden, D. G., and Fairburn, E. A. (1973): Chromosomal instability associated with susceptibility to malignant disease in patients with porokeratosis of Mibelli. *J. Natl. Cancer Inst.*, 51:371–378.

67. Taylor, A. M. R., Metcalfe, J. A., Oxford, J. M., and Harnden, D. G. (1976): Is chromatid-type damage in ataxia telangiectasia after irradiation at G_0 a consequence of defective repair? *Nature*, 260:441–443.

68. Tischler, A. S. (1974): Study of serum nerve growth stimulating activity in patients with neurofibromatosis utilizing a modified bioassay technique. *Exp. Neurol.*, 44:440–447.

69. Todaro, G. J., Green, H., Swift, M. R. (1966): Susceptibility of human diploid fibroblast strains to transformation by SV40 virus, *Science*, 153:1252–1254.

70. Urbach, F. (1969): Geographic pathology of skin cancer. In: *Biologic Effects of Ultraviolet Radiation*, edited by F. Urbach, pp. 635–650. Pergamon Press, Oxford.

71. Waldmann, T. A., Strober, W., and Blaese, R. M. (1972): Immunodeficiency disease and

malignancy. Various immunologic deficiencies of man and the role of immune processes in the control of malignant disease. *Ann. Intern. Med.,* 77:605–628.

72.   Weary, P. E., Gorlin, R. J., Gentry, W. C., Comer, J. E., and Greer, K. E. (1972): Multiple hamartoma syndrome (Cowden's Disease). *Arch. Dermatol.,* 106:682–690.
73.   Weston, J. A. (1970): Migration and differentiation of neural crest cells. *Adv. Morphol.,* 8:41–114.
74.   Windhorst, D. B., and Padgett, G. (1973): The Chediak-Higashi syndrome and the homologous trait in animals. *J. Invest. Dermatol.,* 60:529-537.
75.   Yabe, Y., and Sadakane, H. (1975): Virus of epidermodysplasia verruciformis: Electron microscopic and fluorescent antibody studies. *J. Invest. Dermatol.,* 65:324–330.
76.   Oliver, J. M., et al. (1976): *J. Cell. Biol.,* 69:205–210.

Discussion

Gorlin: Dr. Lutzner, in your unifying hypothesis for neurocristopathies (your Fig. 6), you correctly showed the odontoblast as a derivative of the neural crest. But that cell gives rise to dentin and *not* to the ectodermal component of the tooth. Yet, it is these ectodermally derived dentinal lamina remnants that produce the cysts of the nevoid basal cell carcinoma syndrome. So those cysts could not be derived from neural crest odontoblasts.

Blattner: Dr. Lutzner, would you care to interrelate the diverse features of Cowden's disease as you have for some other diseases?

Lutzner: The epidermal involvement, including lesions of the breast (which is an ectodermal derivative), could be explained by an abnormality occurring in embryonic ectoderm.

Li: What should the clinical oncologist do with patients who have cancer and a few scattered hamartomas that are not diagnostic for any syndrome? What studies can be made to identify whether the lesions are a part of a syndrome or just chance associations?

Meadows: To extend this line of reasoning: such hamartomas are really benign tumors that raise numerous questions. Are they harbingers of new malignancies elsewhere in the body? Do they have malignant potential? If so, is there a way to distinguish those with great malignant potential from those with little risk? Would such a distinction give clues to carcinogenic mechanisms? Is there any difference between tumors that arise *de novo* and those that arise in hamartomas?

Lutzner: The answers depend largely on the specific syndrome involved. Some hamartomas are always premalignant; some are occasionally malignant, and still others never become malignant. To prognosticate, one needs an encyclopedic knowledge of all these syndromes and the ability to diagnose the correct syndrome for each patient.

Gorlin: One answer would be that given by a man asked by a lost little boy walking the streets of New York City, "Mister, how do you get to Carnegie Hall?" The man responded, "Practice, practice, practice."

Seriously, Drs. Li and Meadows asked important but difficult questions. For example, Torre's syndrome at first looked like a chance association: a patient with cancer of the colon subsequently acquired multiple sebaceous adenomas of the skin, verrucal keratoacanthomas, and squamous cell carcinomas. It is now known as an autosomal dominant syndrome, partly because someone paid closer attention to an apparently chance event. The epidemiologists who keep careful records will have to set us straight.

Lynch: My answer would include taking a family history to determine the pattern of disease. For example, even fewer than five *café-au-lait* spots, insufficient to meet classic diagnostic criteria for von Recklinghausen's neurofibromatosis, may be associated with an increased risk for cancer in my experience. A few spots may be very significant clinically, particularly in context with a positive family history.

Motulsky: In short, many more observations are needed.

Sanford: With regard to your Fig. 5, is there any strong evidence that supports the notion that the risk of cancer in immunodeficiency disorders is related to faulty immunosurveillance and not to, for example, persistent antigenic stimulation of a faulty immune response system?

Lutzner: Although there are no hard data, it seems reasonable to view the immune system as playing an important role in controlling malignant disease by surveillance and elimination of exogenous oncogenic viruses and tumor cells that possess new surface antigens and perhaps in inactivating latent viral genomes within the reticuloendothelial system. There is some evidence to support your suggestions, though, of chronic antigenic stimuli producing lymphoma and leukemia.

Miller: In studying these rarities, what is the value with regard to preventing cancer?

Lutzner: Take xeroderma pigmentosum (XP) as an example. For some time, microbiologists knew much about the mechanisms of DNA repair, but no one had studied them in humans. For centuries, it was known that ultraviolet light caused skin cancers. Putting these two facts together, Cleaver postulated a faulty DNA repair mechanism in the so-called XP "night people." He studied these patients and proved his hypothesis. We still cannot do much for these rare patients beyond removing their tumors as they develop, alerting them to the hazards of sunlight, and suggesting protective measures. Still, the disorder has yielded much information on DNA repair in man and has, in turn, generated new hypotheses concerning neuronal death and the mechanisms of aging. Using XP as a model, Burnet has developed a mutational model for aging as well as carcinogenesis [*Lancet,* 2:495–498 (1974)].

Hecht: I should like to suggest that patients with XP could protect themselves from sunlight by moving to the Pacific Northwest. More seriously, I wonder whether XP associated with mental deficiency, the De Sanctis–Cacchione syndrome, is a discrete entity. The few affected families that I have seen were highly inbred. So, I raise the question as to whether they have two or more different autosomal recessive disorders at different loci; that is, one homozygous locus produces XP, and another mental retardation.

Lutzner: The De Sanctis–Cacchione syndrome is probably not a single disorder, but represents a spectrum. Among our 15 or so patients in a dozen kindreds, we have not seen in any one patient all the diverse neurologic deficiencies classically associated with De Sanctis–Cacchione. Nonetheless, the neurologic problems in general seem to correlate with the *in vitro* ability of fibroblasts to survive ultraviolet radiation, form clones, and divide.

Nance: I once observed a family with XP in which one grandparent on each side had senile keratoses and skin cancers, and I wonder if heterozygote carriers of the XP gene have a higher than expected frequency of such lesions?

Lutzner: This has not been carefully studied, but it seems from our observations that heterozygotes have no increased incidence of skin cancer. Heterozygotes cannot be detected chemically.

Swift: Our studies of families with XP suggest a remarkable frequency of skin malignancy; however, it is hard to evaluate because many of the families come not from the cloudy Northwest but from the southeastern and southwestern United States. Also, their ethnic origins seem to be concentrated among those populations with high rates of skin malignancy in general.

Genetics of Human Cancer, edited by J. J.
Mulvihill, R. W. Miller, and J. F. Fraumeni, Jr.
Raven Press, New York, 1977.

13

Monogenic Disorders Associated with Neoplasia

Robert J. Gorlin

Department of Oral Pathology, School of Dentistry, University of Minnesota, Minneapolis, Minnesota 55455

Many single-gene traits predispose to or are complicated by neoplasia (1). The better known of these syndromes—xeroderma pigmentosum, ataxia-telangiectasia, and Fanconi's syndrome—are mentioned throughout this volume; therefore, I have arbitrarily chosen seven monogenic disorders with neoplastic manifestations because they tend to be overlooked or because of recent developments.

NEVOID BASAL CELL CARCINOMA SYNDROME

Dr. Strong (Chapter 39) presents a typical case, and I have recently summarized (2) this autosomal dominant trait with multiple nevoid basal cell carcinomas, odontogenic keratocysts of the jaws, a characteristic facies, various skeletal anomalies, intracranial calcifications, medulloblastoma, ovarian fibroma, and lymphomesenteric cysts.

In addition, there have been reports of excessive chromosomal breaks in patients with the syndrome (3). We have been unable to verify this finding using standard techniques for counting chromosomal breaks and by studying sister chromatid exchange.

MULTIPLE CHEMODECTOMAS

Carotid body tumors or chemodectomas may be observed at any age, but are most common in middle age. They are usually sporadic and unilateral. Sporadic cases are rarely bilateral; bilateral cases are often familial. There is a marked female predilection (six females to every male) at high, but not low altitudes.

Chase (7) apparently first noted familial occurrence in reporting two sisters, one with bilateral carotid body tumors, the other with a unilateral tumor. Since then, numerous cases in two or more generations have been reported in clear autosomal dominant pattern (5-10, 15-23, 25-27). The report by Chedid and Jao (8) of chronic obstructive lung disease in three of four sibs with chemodectoma raises several interesting questions concerning the genetic origins of bilateral tumors.

The carotid body is a chemoreceptor organ that responds to changes in pO_2, pCO_2, and pH; any condition that chronically lowers oxygen pressure in the blood leads to carotid body enlargement. For example, hyperplastic carotid bodies are found in Quechua Indians living in the Peruvian Andes, but not in those living at sea level. The frequency of carotid body tumors is 10 times greater in individuals at high altitude than at sea level (4,24). Carotid body hyperplasia is also found in animals living at high altitudes (11). Hayes suggested that canine breeds at high risk of chemodectoma have craniofacial conformations that might, in theory, produce chronic hypoxia (13). Strength is given this argument because carotid bodies are enlarged in patients with cor pulmonale, Pickwickian syndrome, and emphysema (12,14). When emphysema is familial, it is often associated with a genetic deficiency of $\alpha_1$antitrypsin, which places homozygotes and some heterozygotes at high risk for emphysema. So, the family of Chedid and Jao raises the question of whether or not $\alpha_1$antitrypsin deficiency could be the genetic basis for some familial chemodectomas.

In short, chemodectomas may not be true neoplasms, but only hyperplasia produced by increased demand on its chemoreceptive and/or neuroendocrine function in genetically susceptible individuals. In the etiology of bilateral familial tumors, further analysis might reveal considerable heterogeneity of genetic and environmental factors.

MULTIPLE HAMARTOMA AND NEOPLASIA (COWDEN'S) SYNDROME

First described in 1963 (33), some 17 patients in 9 families have now been reported (29-32,35). Although every organ system can be involved, principal manifestations are in the skin, mucosae, thyroid, and breast.

Lichenoid and papillomatous lesions are frequent on the pinnas, lateral neck, nasal, periorbital, glabellar, and perioral areas, and dorsum of hands and forearms. On histologic examination, the lesions appear as hamartomas of hair follicle origin similar to inverted follicular keratoses. In addition, waxy punctate keratoderma and umbilicated hyperkeratotic papules develop on the palms and soles (34). Most patients have had papular lesions of the lips and gingiva and, to a lesser extent, palate, as well as papillomas of the buccal, faucial, and oropharyngeal mucosa. The tongue is pebbly and fissured (28).

In the female breast, fibroadenomatosis, virginal hypertrophy, and carcinoma have been described; in the thyroid, fetal adenoma, follicular adenocarcinoma, and "goiter."

Numerous, usually benign, soft-tissue neoplasms have been so common that Weary et al. (35), in reporting five additional cases, suggested the name "multiple hamartoma syndrome." The tumors include cysts of the ovary, acoustic neuromas, subcutaneous and retroperitoneal lipomas, angiomas of various tissues, and angiomyomas in the limbs. Gastric polyps have also been noted as well as a variety of colonic polyps including ganglioneuromas, retention and hyperplastic polyps, and adenomas which may contain adenocarcinoma. Hydronephrosis has been described; however, in one case (R. Lattes, S. Gellmani, and J. Zuflacht, *personal communication*), it was considered secondary to a retroperitoneal lipoma.

The syndrome is inherited as an autosomal dominant trait (30). Many aspects of this fascinating condition remain unknown; its frequency, spectrum of severity, and biologic and embryologic basis deserve study.

MULTIPLE SEBACEOUS ADENOMAS AND GASTROINTESTINAL AND OTHER CARCINOMAS

The association of multiple sebaceous adenomas and gastrointestinal carcinoma is sometimes called Torre's syndrome (43), although first described a year earlier by Muir et al. (40). Despite other case reports (36,37,39,41,42), the syndrome still needs sharper definition, partly because some features suggest Gardner's syndrome.

The sebaceous tumors most often involve the trunk, head, and neck, and may develop before or after the visceral carcinoma is diagnosed. Epidermal skin tumors (squamous cell carcinoma, keratoacanthoma, benign keratosis, and verrucae) are apparently part of the syndrome (38). The cancers tend to arise in the colon and be of low-grade malignancy.

Of 11 cases, 5 had relatives with colon cancer and 2 with breast cancer. One father and his three children are reportedly affected, making autosomal dominant inheritance possible but unconfirmed (38).

CUTANEOUS LEIOMYOMATA

Multiple cutaneous leiomyomata originating in the erector pili usually appear on the trunk, arms, or face around the age of 20 years (50). There may be only a few or literally hundreds of lesions which are firm, often grouped, and ranging from 1 to 15 mm in diameter. They are usually skin colored to reddish brown, mobile yet fixed to underlying tissues, tender to slight pressure, but exquisitely painful to sudden changes in the ambient temperature or on injection of epinephrine.

Microscopic identification is easy, especially with van Gieson, Masson trichrome, or reticulum stains. The leiomyoma is separated from the normal epithelium by a thin layer of normal connective tissue but is not encapsulated. Of considerable importance is the clear association with uterine leiomyomata (fibroids) or even leiomyosarcoma (47,49,52–55).

Although evidence is sparse, autosomal dominant inheritance with incomplete penetrance has been suggested (44). Concordant identical twins have been reported, which proves nothing (45,54). Early familial cases were reviewed by Kloepfer et al. (46) and Korn-Heydt (48). Affected sibs with normal parents have been noted (46,47,51,56); however, all members of the family were not examined. We have seen a single kindred of three affected generations.

HEREDITARY LIPOMATOSES

There are at least two different lipomatoses: multiple and symmetrical.

Multiple lipomatosis is inherited as an autosomal dominant trait (57,60,61,68,69,71-74). The tumors, first appearing in the third to fifth decades, tend to be soft, painless, and often scattered over the upper extremities, trunk, and neck. They vary in size from a few centimeters to as many as 25 cm in diameter, and may number from a few to hundreds. Elevated serum cholesterol has been found in a few cases (61,63).

Symmetrical lipomatosis is known as Fetthals, Madelung disease, or Launois-Bensaude syndrome. The term Fetthals (fat neck) is a poor one because the nonencapsulated, firm, nonpainful fat deposits, although often involving the neck, may be symmetrically distributed in the axilla and groin and submental, pre- and postauricular, supraclavicular, and paravertebral areas.

There is probably genetic heterogeneity. One emerging syndrome has been called "familial cervical lipodysplasia," a misleading name because the fat deposits may be around the neck, shoulders, buffalo hump area, and groin. The limbs are lean. Occasional features are phlebectasia, varices, coronary heart disease, type IV lipoproteinemia, hyperglycemia with insulin resistance, cirrhosis, hyperuricemia, and gouty arthritis. Of course, not all patients have all these signs or symptoms, or at least their presence has not been documented; therefore, the patient with telangiectasia reported by Kurzweg and Spencer (63) may be an additional example.

Inheritance is autosomal dominant (58,59,64-67,70,75,76). Kasish et al. (62) suggested that the fat had the distribution of brown (hibernation) fat and that the etiology was functional symmetrical denervation of adipose tissue.

MULTIPLE CUTANEOUS ANGIOLIPOMAS

Multiple cutaneous angiolipomas, usually developing after puberty, are painful and tender subcutaneous nodules of the trunk and extremities, sparing the face, scalp, palms, and soles. They are encapsulated, contain varying proportions of adipose and vascular tissue, and may be several hundreds in number (78). Clinical, pharmacologic, and pathologic studies have not revealed the cause of the pain (77). The lesions must be differentiated from the rare infiltrating angiolipoma which is capable of invading bone, muscle, nerve, and fibrous connective tissue and requires wide excision for removal (80).

Autosomal dominant inheritance of multiple cutaneous angiolipomas is possible, since two-generation families are recorded (77,79). The infiltrating angiolipoma has no familial predilection (80).

GLOMANGIOMA

Multiple glomus tumors are bluish to reddish masses, 0.1 to 4 cm in diameter, which resemble cavernous hemangiomas, both clinically and (to the uninitiated) microscopically. They may be congenital or appear in the first two decades of life, sometimes with over 50 separate lesions. Commonly found on the extremities, they may be generalized over the trunk and increase in size for a limited time. Usually they cannot be completely compressed. They may be asymptomatic, tender to palpation, remarkably painful even to light touch, or sensitive to an increase in ambient temperature. Microscopically, the multiple glomus tumor is unencapsulated, located in the deep corium or fat, and is composed of large, wide, irregularly shaped blood-filled cavities. Surrounding the endothelial lining is a two- to three-cell-thick layer of small polygonal cells with pale cytoplasm and homogeneous round nuclei.

Multiple glomus tumors are inherited as an autosomal dominant trait having been seen in several generations and with male-to-male transmission, but there is incomplete penetrance (81-95). Sibs with normal parents have also been reported (82,88).

In contrast, the nonhereditary, solitary glomus tumor is more painful and often appears in individuals over 30 years-of-age; about 25% are subungual in location. Other painful skin tumors include eccrine spiradenoma, angiolipoma, leiomyoma, traumatic neuroma, and blue rubber bleb nevus.

BLUE RUBBER BLEB NEVUS SYNDROME

Bean (96,97) defined this syndrome as multiple vascular, nipple-like, or bladder-like lesions of the skin, 1 to 20 mm in diameter, especially on the trunk, upper arms, and mucous membranes, sometimes accompanied by gastrointestinal bleeding and hepatic and pulmonary angiomas (100,102). The lesions may produce sweat and be painful. Microscopically, there are large numbers of dilated vascular spaces whose walls are often thrown into folds, separated by smooth muscle or fibrous connective tissue (99). Several families exhibit autosomal dominant inheritance of the syndrome (98,99,103,104). Medulloblastoma of the cerebellum has also been noted (101).

COMMENT

Further clinical and laboratory observations should clarify the heterogeneity of existing genetic syndromes (e.g., lipomatosis) and the possible overlap among others (e.g., Gardner's and Torre's syndromes). The recognition of hereditary cancer syndromes provides opportunities for insight into the origins of a wide variety of cancers. For example, the newly described multiple hamartoma syndrome may provide clues to developmental defects, hitherto unsuspected, in breast carcinogenesis. The role of environmental determinants also may be clarified by study of genetic syndromes, as illustrated by the suggestion that chronic hypoxia may be involved in familial occurrences of chemodectoma. The continuing delineation of cancer-prone syndromes by clinical investigators in the fields of genetics and oncology will not only enlarge the list of single-gene traits predisposing to cancer (1), but in a major way will help to uncover the susceptibility mechanisms and environmental interactions leading to cancer in the general population.

REFERENCES

1. Mulvihill, J. J. (1975): Congenital and genetic diseases, In: *Persons at High Risk of Cancer: An Approach to Cancer Etiology and Control,* edited by J. F. Fraumeni, Jr., pp. 3–37. Academic Press, New York.

Nevoid Basal Cell Carcinoma Syndrome
2. Gorlin, R. J., and Sedano, H. O. (1972): The multiple nevoid basal cell carcinoma syndrome revisited. *Birth Defects,* 7(8):140–148
3. Happle, R., and Hoehn, H. (1973): Cytogenetic studies on cultured fibroblast-like cells derived from basal cell carcinoma tissue. *Clin. Genet.,* 4:17–24.

Multiple Chemodectomas
4. Arias-Stella, J. (1969): Human carotid body at high altitude. *Am. J. Pathol.,* 55:82a.
5. Bartels, J. (1949): *De Tumoren Van Het Glomus Jugulare. Van Gorcum, Assen.*
6. Beard, M., and McQuarrie, D. G. (1968): Brotherly lumps. *Minn. Med.,* 51:79–82.
7. Chase, W. H. (1933): Familial and bilateral tumors of the carotid body. *J. Pathol. Bacteriol.,* 36:1–12.
8. Chedid, A., and Jao, W. (1974): Hereditary tumors of the carotid bodies and chronic obstructive pulmonary disease. *Cancer,* 33:1635–1641.
9. Del Fante, F. M., and Watkins, E., Jr. (1967): Chemodectoma of the heart in a patient with multiple chemodectomas and familial history. *Lahey Clin. Found. Bull.,* 16:224–229.
10. Desai, M. G., and Patel, C. C. (1961): Heredo-familial carotid body tumors. *Clin. Radiol.,* 12:214–218.
11. Edwards, C., Heath, D., Harris, P., Castillo, Y., Krüger, H., and Arias-Stella, J. (1971): The carotid body in animals at high altitude. *J. Pathol.,* 104:231–238.
12. Edwards, C., Heath, D., and Harris, P. (1971): The carotid body in emphysema and left ventricular hypertrophy. *J. Pathol.,* 104:1–13.
13. Hayes, H. M., Jr. (1975): An hypothesis for the aetiology of canine chemoreceptor system neoplasms, based upon an epidemiological study of 73 cases among hospital patients. *J. Small Anim. Pract.,* 16:337–343.
14. Heath, D., Edwards, C., and Harris, P. (1970): Postmortem size and structure of the human carotid body. *Thorax,* 25:129–140.
15. James, A. G., and Saleeby, R. (1953): The management of carotid body tumors—a case report of bilateral carotid body tumors. *Surgery,* 34:104–110.
16. Katz, A. D. (1964): Carotid body tumors in a large family group. *Am. J. Surg.,* 108:570–573.
17. Kroll, A. J., Alexander, B., Cochios, F., and Pechet, L. (1964): Hereditary deficiencies of clotting factors VII and X associated with carotid body tumors. *N. Engl. J. Med.,* 270:6–13.
18. Lahey, F. H., and Warren, K. W. (1947): Tumors of the carotid body. *Surg. Gynecol. Obstet.,* 85:281–288.
19. Lahey, F.H., and Warren, K. W. (1951): A long term appraisal of carotid body tumors with remarks on their removal. *Surg. Gynecol. Obstet.,* 92:481–491.
20. Lewison, E. F., and Weinberg, T. (1950): Carotid body tumors: a case report of bilateral carotid body tumors with an unusual family incidence. *Surgery,* 27:437–448.
21. Pratt, L. W. (1973): Familial carotid body tumors. *Arch. Otolaryngol.,* 97:334–336.
22. Resler, D. R., Snow, J. B., and Williams, G. R. (1966): Multiplicity and familial incidence of carotid body and glomus jugulare tumors. *Ann. Otol. Rhinol. Laryngol.,* 75:114–122.
23. Rush, B. F. (1963): Familial bilateral carotid body tumors. *Ann. Surg.,* 157:633–636.
24. Saldana, M. J., Salem, L. E., and Travezan, R. (1973): High altitude hypoxia and chemodectomas. *Hum. Pathol.,* 4:251–263.
25. Sprong, D. H., and Kirby, F. G. (1949): Familial carotid body tumors. *Ann. West. Med. Surg.,* 3:241–242.
26. Wilson, H. (1970): Carotid body tumors: familial and bilateral. *Ann. Surg.,* 171:843–848.

27. Wychulis, A. R., and Beahrs, O. H. (1965). Bilateral chemodectomas. *Arch. Surg.,* 91:690–696.

Multiple Hamartoma and Neoplasia Syndrome

28. Carlier, G., Larere, L., Carlier, C., and Houck, Mlle. (1971): Sclérose tubéreuse de Bourneville avec papillomatose de la muqueuse buccale. *Rev. Stomatol. Chir. Maxillofac. (Paris),* 72:607–614.
29. Burnett, J. W., Goldner, R., and Calton, G. J. (1975): Cowden disease. Report of two additional cases. *Br. J. Dermatol.,* 93:329–336.
30. Gentry, W. C., Eskritt, N. R., and Gorlin, R. J. (1974): Multiple hamartoma syndrome (Cowden's disease). *Arch. Dermatol.,* 109:521–525.
31. Gentry, W. C. (1975): Cowden disease. *Birth Defects.* 11(4):137–141.
32. Grupper, C., and Girard, J. (1974): Maladie des hamartomas multiples; maladie de Cowden. *Bull. Soc. Fr. Dermatol. Syphiligr.,* 81:578–584.
33. Lloyd, K. M., and Dennis, M. (1963): Cowden's disease. A possible new symptom complex with multiple system involvement. *Ann. Intern. Med.,* 58:136–142.
34. Rosenbluth, M. (1963): Multiple noduli manifestations. *Periodontics,* 1:81–83.
35. Weary, P. E., Gorlin, R. J., Gentry, W. C., Comer, J. E. and Greer, K. E. (1972): Multiple hamartoma syndrome (Cowden's disease). *Arch. Dermatol.,* 106:682–690.

Multiple Sebaceous Adenomas and Gastrointestinal Carcinoma

36. Bakker, P. M., Tjon A Joe, S. S. (1971): Multiple sebaceous gland tumours, with multiple tumours of internal organs. A new syndrome? *Dermatologica,* 142:50–57.
37. Bitran, J., and Pellettiere, E. V. (1974): Multiple sebaceous gland tumors and internal carcinoma: Torre's syndrome. *Cancer,* 33:835–836.
38. Jakobiec, F. A. (1974): Sebaceous adenoma of the eyelid and visceral malignancy. *Am. J. Ophthalmol.,* 78:952–960.
39. Leonard, D. D., and Deaton, W. R. (1974): Multiple sebaceous gland tumors and visceral carcinomas. *Arch. Dermatol.,* 110:917–920.
40. Muir, E. G., Bell, A. J. Y., and Barlow, K. A. (1967): Multiple primary carcinomata of the colon, duodenum, and larynx associated with kerato-acanthomata of the face. *Br. J. Surg.,* 54:191–195.
41. Rulon, D. B., and Helwig, E. B. (1973): Multiple sebaceous neoplasms of the skin: an association with multiple visceral carcinomas, especially of the colon. *Am. J. Clin. Pathol.,* 60:745–752.
42. Sciallis, G. F., and Winkelmann, R. K. (1974): Multiple sebaceous adenomas and gastrointestinal carcinoma. *Arch. Dermatol.,* 110:913–916.
43. Torre, D. (1968): Multiple sebaceous tumors. *Arch. Dermatol.,* 98:549–551.

Cutaneous Leiomyomata

44. Berendes, U., Kühner, A., and Schnyder, U. W. (1971): Segmentary and disseminated lesions in multiple hereditary cutaneous leiomyoma. *Humangenetik,* 13:81–82.
45. Fisher, W. C., and Helwig, F. B. (1963): Leiomyomas of the skin. *Arch. Dermatol.,* 88:510–520.
46. Kloepfer, H. W., Krafchuk, J., Derbes, V., and Burks, J. (1958): Hereditary multiple leiomyoma of the skin. *Am. J. Hum. Genet.,* 10:48–52.
47. Knoth, W., and Knoth-Born, R. C. (1964): Familiäre Utero-cutane Leiomyomatose. *Z. Hautkr.,* 37:191–206.
48. Korn-Heydt, G. E. (1966): Erbliche Aplasien, Hyperplasien und Tumoren. In: *Handbuch der Haut und Geschlechtskrankheiten,* Bd. 7, edited by A. Marchionini, pp. 585–587. Springer-Verlag, Berlin.
49. Mezzadra, G. (1965): Leiomioma cutaneo multiplo ereditario. *Minerva Dermatol.,* 40:388–393.
50. Montgomery, H., and Winkelmann, R. K. (1959): Smooth- muscle tumors of the skin. *Arch. Dermatol.,* 79:68–75.
51. Nair, B. K. H. (1973): Familial cutaneous leiomyoma. *Indian. J. Pathol. Bacteriol.,* 16:75–77.
52. Piredda, A. (1957): Leiomioma cutaneo e fibromiomatosi uterina. *Arch. Ital. Derm.,* 29:68–75.

53.   Reed, W. B., Walker, R., and Horowitz, R. (1973): Cutaneous leiomyomata with uterine leiomyomata. *Acta Dermatovener. (Stockh.)*, 53:409–416.
54.   Rudner, E. J., Schwartz, O. D., and Grekin, J. N. (1964): Multiple cutaneous leiomyoma in identical twins. *Arch. Dermatol.*, 90:81–82.
55.   Thomine, E., and Anzani, C. (1967): Métastases cutanées d'un léiomyome utérin. *Bull. Soc. Fr. Dermatol. Syphiligr.*, 74:170–172.
56.   Verma, K. C., Chawdhry, S. D., and Rathi, K. S. (1973): Cutaneous leiomyomata in two brothers. *Br. J. Dermatol.*, 90:351–353.

Lipomatosis

57.   Dietel, F. (1932): Lipome, Myome, Myxome, Chondrome, Osteome, Psammome und andere nichtepitheliale gutartige Neubildungen. In: *Handbuch der Haut und Geschlechtskrankheiten*, Bd. 12, T. 2, edited by J. Jadassohn, pp. 196–218. Springer-Verlag, Berlin.
58.   Greene, M. L., Glueck, C. J., Fujimoto, W. Y., and Seegmiller, J. E. (1970): Benign symmetric lipomatosis (Launois-Bensaude adenolipomatosis) with gout and hyperlipoproteinemia. *Am. J. Med.*, 48:239–246.
59.   Günther, H. (1920): Klinische Beobachtungen über Lipomatosis. *Z. Menschl. Vererb. Konstitutionel.*, 5:268–292.
60.   Hellier, F. F. (1935): Hereditary multiple lipomata. *Lancet*, 1:204–205.
61.   Humphrey, A. A., and Kingsley, P. C. (1938): Familial multiple lipomas. *Arch. Dermatol. Syph.*, 37:30–34.
62.   Kodish, M. E., Alsever, R. N., and Block, M. B. (1974): Benign symmetric lipomatosis: Functional sympathetic denervation of adipose tissue and possible hypertrophy of brown fat. *Metabolism*, 23:937–945.
63.   Kurzweg, F. T., and Spencer, R. (1951): Familial multiple lipomatosis. *Am. J. Surg.*, 82:762–765.
64.   Löwenstein, W. (1929): Über symmetrische, multiple lipomatosis. *Klin. Wochenschr.*, 8:1614–1618.
65.   Lyon, I. P. (1910): Adiposis and lipomatosis. *Arch. Intern. Med.*, 6:28–120.
66.   McKusick, V. A. (1962): Medical genetics. *J. Chron. Dis.*, 15:417–572.
67.   Michon, P. and Rose, F. (1935): Adénolipomatose symétrique familiale. *Bull. Soc. Fr. Dermatol. Syphiligr.*, 42:1005–1007.
68.   Miller, J. K. (1936): Multiple symmetrical lipomatosis. *JAMA*, 106:2059–2060.
69.   Muller, R. (1951): Observation sur la transmission héréditaire de la lipomatose circonscrite multiple. *Dermatologica*, 103:258–265.
70.   Ozer, F. L. Lichtenstein, J. R., Kwiterovich, P. O., and McKusick, V. A. (1973): A "new" genetic variety of "lipodystrophy." *Clin. Res.*, 21:533.
71.   Rauschkolb, J. E. (1931): Multiple lipomatosis. *Arch. Dermatol.*, 23:160.
72.   Shanks, J. A., Paranchych, W., and Tuba, J. (1957): Familial multiple lipomatosis. *Can. Med. Assoc. J.*, 77:881–884.
73.   Siemens, H. W. (1929): Die Vererbung in der Ätiologie der Hautkrankheiten. In: *Handbuch der Haut und Geschlechtskrankheiten*, edited by J. Jadassohn, pp. 1–165. Springer-Verlag, Berlin.
74.   Stephens, F. E., and Isaacson, A. (1959): Hereditary multiple lipomatosis. *J. Hered.*, 50:51–53.
75.   Strange, D. A., and Fessel, W. J. (1968): Benign symmetric lipomatosis. *JAMA*, 204:339–340.
76.   Taylor, L. M., Beahrs, O. H., and Fontana, R. S. (1961): Benign symmetric lipomatosis. *Proc. Mayo Clinic*, 36:96–100.

Multiple Cutaneous Angiolipomas

77.   Belcher, R. W., Czarnetzki, B. M., Carney, J. F., and Gardner, E. (1974): Multiple (subcutaneous) angiolipomas. *Arch. Dermatol.*, 110:583–585.
78.   Howard, W. R., and Helwig, E. B.(1960): Angiolipoma. *Arch. Dermatol.*, 82:924–931.
79.   Klem, K. K. (1949): Multiple lipoma-angiolipomas. *Acta Chir. Scand.*, 97:527–532.
80.   Lin, J. J., and Lin, F. (1974): Two entities in angiolipoma. A study of 459 cases of lipoma with review of literature on infiltrating angiolipoma. *Cancer*, 34:720–727.

Glomangioma
81. Berger, H., and Hundeiker, M. (1967): Multiple Glomustumoren als Phakomatose. *Dermatol. Wochenschr.*, 153:673–678.
82. Burford, C. (1974): Multiple glomus tumours. *Australas. J. Dermatol.*, 15:35.
83. Chasseuil, R., and Gautard, J. (1961): Tumeurs glomiques familiales: 6 cas en 4 générations. *Bull. Soc. Fr. Dermatol. Syphiligr.*, 68:635–636.
84. Conant, M. A., and Wiesenfeld, S. L. (1971): Multiple glomus tumors of the skin. *Arch. Dermatol.*, 103:481–485.
85. De Sablet, M., and Mascaro, J.-M. (1967): Tumeurs glomiques multiples et blue rubber bleb naevus. *Ann. Dermatol. Syphiligr. (Paris)*, 94:35–46.
86. Gorlin, R. J., Fusaro, R. M., and Benton, J. W. (1960): Multiple glomus tumor of the pseudocavernous hemangioma type. *Arch. Dermatol.*, 82:776–778.
87. Hollins, P. J. (1971): Multiple glomus tumours. *Proc. Roy. Soc. Med.*, 64:806.
88. Heuston, J. T. (1961): Multiple painless glomus tumours. *Br. Med. J.*, 1:1212–1213.
89. Kaufman, L. R., and Clark, W. T. (1941): Glomus tumors: report of four cases in the same family. *Ann. Surg.* 114:1102–1105.
90. Nödl, F. (1963): Multiple systematisierte Glomustumoren. *Arch. Klin. Exp. Dermatol.*, 217:405–416.
91. Reed, W. B. (1969): Multiple glomus tumors with a family history. *Arch. Dermatol.*, 100:496–497.
92. Reinhard, M., and Lüders, G. (1970): Zur Pathologie und Klinik multipler familiärer Glomustumoren. *Arch. Klin. Exp. Dermatol.*, 237:800–810.
93. Schnyder, U. W. (1965): Über Glomustumoren. *Dermatologica*, 131:83–88.
94. Sluiter, J. T. F., and Postma, C. (1959): Multiple glomus tumours of the skin. *Acta Dermatovener. (Stockh)*, 39:98–107.
95. Touraine, A., Renault, S. and Renault, P. (1936): Tumeurs glomiques multiples du tronc et des membres. *Bull. Soc. Fr. Dermatol. Syphiligr.*, 43:736–740.

Blue Rubber Bleb Nevus Syndrome
96. Bean, W. B. (1967): *Rare Diseases and Lesions.* Charles C. Thomas, Springfield, Illinois.
97. Bean, W. B. (1958): *Vascular Spiders and Related Lesions of the Skin.* Charles C. Thomas, Springfield, Illinois.
98. Berlyne, G. M., and Berlyne, N. (1960): Anemia due to "blue-rubber-bleb" naevus disease. *Lancet*, 2:1275–1277.
99. Fine, R. M., Derbes, V. J., and Clark, W. H. (1961): Blue rubber bleb nevus. *Arch. Dermatol.*, 84:802–805.
100. Fretzin, D. F., and Potter, B. (1965): Blue rubber bleb nevus. *Arch. Intern. Med.*, 116:924–929.
101. Rice, J. S., and Fischer, D. S. (1962): Blue rubber-bleb nevus syndrome. *Arch. Dermatol.*, 86:503–511.
102. Richter, G. (1965): "Blue rubber-bleb nevus syndrom" als Anämieursache. *Z. Haut-Geschlechtskr.*, 39:256–261.
103. Talbot, S., and Wyatt, E. H. (1970): Blue rubber bleb naevi. *Br. J. Dermatol.*, 82:37–39.
104. Walshe, M. M., Evans, C. D., and Warin, R. P. (1966): Blue rubber bleb naevus. *Br. Med. J.* 2:931–932.

Discussion

Hirschhorn: Since many of the conditions you mentioned are dominantly inherited, I see the opportunity to learn more about the genetics of each condition by comparing the frequencies of sporadic and familial occurrences, as Dr. Knudson has done for retinoblastoma, for example. Perhaps, the Klippel–Trenaunay–Weber syndrome could be studied with profit in this regard, since components of the syndrome can be inherited in some instances, although the syndrome itself is said not to be inherited.

Gorlin: Klippel–Trenaunay syndrome is by definition angioosteohypertrophy and is an angiomatous enlargement of the limbs. It probably is one end of a gaussian curve whose other extreme is represented by the Sturge–Weber anomalad. Certainly there are reported patients with both conditions [*Birth Defects,* 7(8):314 (1971)]; however, there is no evidence that genetic factors are involved anywhere in the spectrum. The report that claimed a heritable pattern relied on the presence of stork bites—occipital or glabellar angiomas—among relatives [*Acta Genet. Med. Gemellol.,* 5:326–370 (1956)]; I cannot accept these as evidence for a familial occurrence.

Hirschhorn: That's not really what I asked. Rather , do these sporadic conditions that involve enlargement or other anomalous development of blood vessels represent phenotypes of conditions with heritable tendencies that would be easily detected by comparing sporadic with familial occurrences?

Gorlin: There is not enough overlap in the conditions, beyond some arteriovenous aneurysms; I would look for a better pattern.

H. T. Lynch: Would not Dercum's disease be in your differential of patient with truncal adiposity, especially if it were painful?

Gorlin: Dercum's disease (adiposis dolorosa) seems to be disappearing; I have not seen any recent reports of it. To me, it is a vague term applied by some to any painful panniculus of truncal fat. Painful lipomas could also be angiolipomas.

Motulsky: Concerning multiple lipomatosis, I recall a hypothesis set forth that it was basically an error in metabolic regulation [*Lancet,* 1:1224–1226 (1975)].

Sanford: Is there any evidence that retinoblastoma is a polygenic trait rather than an autosomal dominant one with reduced penetrance?

Knudson: None whatsoever; having the single gene increases the probability of retinoblastoma about 100,000 times.

Genetics of Human Cancer, edited by J. J.
Mulvihill, R. W. Miller, and J. F. Fraumeni, Jr.
Raven Press, New York, 1977.

14

Tumors of the Neural Crest System

R. Neil Schimke

*The University of Kansas Medical Center, College of Health Sciences and Hospital,
Kansas City, Kansas 66103*

The neural crest has commanded intense interest among embryologists for more than a hundred years. There are few embryonic structures that account for as much morphogenetic and phenotypic diversity as does this tissue, since it is known to be responsible for pigment cells, sensory and autonomic ganglia, and even membranous bones of the face and skull. Certain supportive elements such as Schwann and glial cells probably are also derived from this source. More recent information would suggest that at least part of the endocrine system likewise originates in neural crest (Table 1).

It therefore should not be surprising that a number of neoplastic conditions might be pathogenetically related to maldevelopment of the neural crest; moreover, it might also be predicted that at least some of these malignancies would be heritable. Although the neural crest may contribute to a number of syndromes in which malignant changes have been described, this chapter will be concerned with those conditions in which the neoplastic tissue is solely derived from neural crest or in which this embryonic structure has been strongly incriminated in the pathogenesis of malignancy.

EMBRYOLOGY

The vertebrate neural crest appears coincidentally with the formation of the neural tube, a process that takes place in the third and fourth weeks of embryonic development. The component cells form bilateral, symmetrical ridges along the dorsal aspect of the primitive neural tube, extending the length of the embryonic axis. As Weston points out, the structure is transient and the constituent cells begin to emigrate almost immediately (86). Neural tube closure proceeds in a cephalad to caudad direction, and, even as caudal closure is occurring, migration of more anterior axial cells is well under way. During migration, the cells become separated from the overlying ectoderm and move in a ventral direction, initially following rather precise pathways. Differences between the cranial crest cells and those of the trunk have been suggested, largely based on the ultimate derivatives

TABLE 1. *Derivatives of the neural crest*

Pigment cells	Neurocytic elements	Supportive tissue	Endocrine cells
Melanoblasts	Spinal ganglia Cranial ganglia (V, VII, IX, X)	Schwann cells Some glial cells	Adrenal medulla Thyroid C cell
		Meningeal elements	Pancreatic islet cell
	Autonomic ganglia	Odontoblasts	? Enterochromaffin cells
		Membranous bones	? Argyrophilic cells

of each component. For example, whereas both contribute to cranial and spinal ganglia, the trunk crest appears to be largely responsible for pigment cells, and the cranial crest gives rise to head mesenchyme and, ultimately, membranous bones of the skull and face. These differences may be artifactual, since all the cells may be pluripotent when they begin to migrate, with the ultimate phenotype being related to local environmental factors (87). Alternatively, the cells may be developmentally restricted, necessitating the additional postulation of directed migration. Much of the difficulty in assessing the ultimate migratory and developmental potential of the neural crest cells comes about because of the lack of suitable, consistent histochemical markers to follow these cells during the various stages of embryogenesis. Probably for this reason, the more classic treatises of neural crest growth and differentiation make little mention of the endocrine system, save for the adrenal medulla. Using formaldehyde-induced fluorescence as a marker, Pearse and colleagues (55–57) have identified a further group of cells, the APUD series, likely also derived from the neural crest. The term APUD comes from the initial letters of their most typical cytochemical characteristics: *a*mine, *p*recursor, *u*ptake, and *d*ecarboxylation (Table 2). These workers have suggested that some

TABLE 2. *Histochemistry and ultrastructure of APUD cells*

1. Fluorogenic *a*mine content
2. A*mine p*recursor *u*ptake
3. Amino acid *d*ecarboxylase
4. α-Glycerophosphate dehydrogenase
5. Nonspecific esterases and cholinesterase
6. Side-chain carboxyl groups
7. Low level of rough and high levels of smooth endoplasmic reticulum
8. High content of free ribosomes
9. Electron-dense mitochondria
10. Prominent microtubules and centrosomes
11. Tendency to produce protein microfibrils
12. Membrane-bound secretory granules

From Pearse, refs. 55 and 56.

TABLE 3. *APUD series*

Organ	Cell	Secretory product
Pituitary	Corticotroph	ACTH
	Melanotroph	MSH
Thyroid	Parafollicular	Calcitonin
Pancreas	β	Insulin
	α_1	Glucagon
	α_2	Gastrin
	δ	HGH-release-inhibiting hormone
Adrenal medulla	A	Epinephrine
	NA	Norepinephrine
Stomach	Argyrophilic	Gastrin
	Enterochromaffin	Enteroglucagon
Intestine	S	Secretin
	D	Gastric inhibitory polypeptide
	Argyrophilic	Cholecystokinin-pancreozymin
	E	Enteroglucagon
	Argentaffin	Serotonin

From Pearse, ref. 55.

neural crest cells migrate into the primitive foregut and give rise to the amine and peptide-hormone producing part of the classical endocrine system.

The enterochromaffin system, so-called because the cells are located in the foregut and have an affinity for chromium salts similar to that of the adrenal medulla, has also been related to the neural crest, especially because enterochromaffin cells likewise produce biogenic amines such as serotonin and the polypeptide gastrointestinal hormones (84). The evidence relating the enterochromaffin system to the APUD series is not yet firm (3,58), however, and it is even less clear whether or not the argentaffin or argyrophilic cells often found in association with both the enterochromaffin and APUD cells in a single organ are precursors of, derived from, or are intimately related to either of these systems (58). It would be convenient to group all those cells together simply because of their capacity to produce amines and peptide hormones, the tinctorial differences notwithstanding (Table 3). However, cell-cell interaction (31) and even cell fusion (83) may also be potential mechanisms whereby secretory products are produced by cells from disparate embryonic origins. Nonetheless the unitary hypothesis for the origin of all foregut endocrine tissue remains intriguing.

NOSOLOGY WITHIN THE NEURAL CREST SYSTEM

Bolande has coined the inclusive term neurocristopathy to describe any disorder of development of the neural crest (10). A more precise word, referring to neoplastic alterations in this tissue was suggested by Pearse, who called such tumors *neurolophomas,* a construct developed from the Greek words for neural crest (58). He further subdivided the neurolophomas into four types: the neuro-cytomas, the melanomas, schwannomas, and so-called apudomas. Presumably neurocytomas would comprise neuroblastomas and possibly chemodectomas, melanomas would include all tumors derived from pigment cells, schwannomas might be composed of those syndromes whose main features are derived from supporting elements, and the apudomas would encompass endocrine tumor syn-dromes. Such a classification is somewhat arbitrary as neurofibromatosis could legitimately be included in both the neurocytic and supportive categories, and the mucosal neuroma syndrome might be considered part neurocytic and part endo-crine. Nonetheless, it provides a useful departure point for discussion purposes.

The *phacomatoses* are a group of disorders that feature tumors and cysts of various organs, especially the nervous system. The appellations *neurocutaneous* or, even more frequently, *neuroectodermal dysplasia* have been used synony-mously. Although it is true that ectoderm and neural crest are initially contiguous in the developing embryo, there is no good evidence that either tissue influences the other. Thus the words phacomatosis and neuroectodermal dysplasia are purely descriptive and, if they are to be retained, should be reserved for those disorders with both neural and cutaneous elements, without regard to embryogenesis. It is conceivable that the basic defect in some neuroectodermal dysplasias originates in a mutation occurring before either neural crest or overlying ectoderm have defini-tively appeared. Some so-called neuroectodermal disorders also feature abnormal-ities of mesodermally derived structures, such as vascular elements. A more proper name for these diverse conditions would be *hamartomatous syndromes.* Unfortunately, the list of such hamartomatous disorders appears to be ever length-ening, and there would seem to be little value in combining discrete entities like tuberous sclerosis and the Peutz–Jeghers' syndrome under the same heading. Table 4 lists a few of the conditions grouped as phacomatoses by various clinicians along with the tumors that have been described. Some of these disorders, such as xeroderma pigmentosum and incontinentia pigmenti probably have a neural crest component but are more properly considered as genodermatoses. The various types of partial and total albinism certainly also are neural crest diseases in the broadest sense, but the tumors occurring in these conditions are secondary. Another disorder, ataxia-telangiectasia, is probably better classified as an immune deficiency disease. Although a number of these syndromes includes develop-mental anomalies with the potential for malignancy, there is little evidence that the conditions are more than descriptively related. Some are chromosomal; others are not recognizably heritable. Whereas some facets of these conditions might be derived from the neural crest, it seems clear that based on present knowledge consideration of such a dysmorphic disorder as tuberous sclerosis simply as an abnormality in neural crest differentiation is quite likely fallacious. For this reason these conditions, save for a few pertinent exceptions, will not be considered further.

TABLE 4. *A partial list of the phacomatoses with associated tumors*

Disorder	Tumor type
Albinism	Skin (squamous cell)
Ataxia-telangiectasia	Lymphoreticular, central nervous system, other
Basal cell nevus	Basal cell, medulloblastoma
Blue rubber bleb nevus	Medulloblastoma
Cowden's syndrome	Thyroid, breast, colon
DeSanctis–Cacchione's syndrome	Skin (squamous cell, melanoma)
Facial hemihypertrophy	Hemangioblastoma
Goltz syndrome	—
Gruber's (Meckel's) syndrome	—
Incontinentia pigmenti	—
Klippel-Trenaunay's syndrome	? Wilms' tumor
LEOPARD syndrome	—
Linear sebaceous nevus	Ameloblastoma
Macrocephaly-cutaneous angiomatosis	—
Maffucci's syndrome	Bone (sarcoma)
Neurocutaneous melanosis	Melanoma
Neurofibromatosis	Glioma, neurofibrosarcoma, neuroma, meningioma, pheochromocytoma
Noonan's syndrome	Schwannoma, pheochromocytoma
Osler–Rendu–Weber's syndrome	—
Peutz–Jeghers' syndrome	Stomach, intestine, ovary (granulosa cell)
Sjögren–Larssøn's syndrome	—
Sturge–Weber's syndrome	—
Trichoepithelioma	Trichoepithelioma
Tuberous sclerosis	Glioma, cardiac rhabdomyoma, leiomyoma
Turner's syndrome	Numerous (ref. 85)
Von Hippel-Lindau's syndrome	Hemangioblastoma, hypernephroma
Waardenburg's syndrome	—
Xeroderma pigmentosum	Skin (squamous cell, melanoma)

ONCOGENESIS IN THE NEURAL CREST SYSTEM

The characteristics of familial tumors in general are equally applicable to heritable neurolophomas. The tumors tend to be multifocal, and in the case of paired organs, bilateral. They tend to occur at younger ages than the sporadic lesions and may even be congenital. In the case of dominantly inherited tumor syndromes, incomplete penetrance and variable expressivity is the rule, as in other nontumorous dominant conditions. A variety of theories have been proposed to explain this reduced penetrance including a two-stage mutational process, possible heritable chromosome breaks, unstable premutations, and delayed mutation. These various theories are discussed in detail elsewhere in this volume.

Neuroblastoma

One of the purest examples of malignancy in the various derivatives of the neural crest system is neuroblastoma. This tumor may be congenital or may become clinically evident anytime in the first 5 years of life (44). Although patients commonly present with an abdominal mass, more unusual initial symptoms have been described such as heterochromia and Horner's syndrome with mediastinal lesions (35), the polymyoclonia syndrome (52), and even profound hypoglycemia (77). Relatively few familial cases have been reported, and the mode of inheritance is not immediately clear (42,59). Both male and female sibs have been noted, and in three families there may have been an affected parent (44). Four other families had affected collateral relatives in the absence of any recognized consanguinity (42). A most interesting family has been described in which neuroblastoma occurred in a child of parents, each of whom had a child with neuroblastoma by a previous marriage (59). Taken in concert, these findings best argue for an autosomal dominant hypothesis, with decreased penetrance. The precise degree of penetrance may be difficult to determine for two opposing reasons: survival in most patients has been poor, but peculiarly, other patients may show maturation of the primitive tumor to more mature and hence benign types, e.g., ganglioneuroma (29), and thus may not be considered as a tumor suspect unless a residual mass or elevated catecholamine levels point toward the diagnosis (24).

Both sporadic and familial neuroblastoma show a preponderance of affected men (43). This phenomenon has been attributed to the more frequent maturation of neuroblastoma to ganglioneuroma in women considering both these tumors to be part of the same gene defect. The coexistence of these two tumor types in the same individual is quite rare, although again this might represent an age-related maturation sequence. Similarly, the presence of neuroblastoma or ganglioneuroma in patients with von Recklinghausen's disease is even more rare, having been reported on only three occasions (44,63,89).

Tumors of the Paraganglia (Chemodectomas)

The paraganglia comprise a number of different structures such as the carotid and aortic bodies, the glomus jugulare and the ganglion nodosum of the vagus nerve as well as a multiplicity of similar tissues throughout the body (10). The structures do not have an affinity for chromaffin stains, and their embryologic origin has been a source of some dispute. More recent ultrastructural and histochemical studies have shown evidence of catecholamine granules within the cells, thereby reinforcing the concept that these cells are derived from the neural crest.

Carotid body tumors or chemodectomas are more likely to appear in middle-aged individuals. Multiple instances of two generation transmission have been described, and inheritance of the familial lesion is clearly that of an autosomal dominant disorder (15,26). A most interesting family has been reported by Pollack who described two female sibs with bilateral carotid body tumors whose father had a glomus jugulare tumor. One of the sibs developed a unilateral pheochromocytoma 4 years after the successful resection of her carotid lesions (62). Revak et al. described a patient who had a pheochromocytoma at age

11, a mediastinal paraganglioma at age 13, a carotid body tumor at age 20, and bilateral carotid body tumors at age 36 (65).

Pigment-Cell Tumors

Cutaneous Melanoma

Virtually all authorities agree that the pigment-producing cell is derived from neural crest. Localized congenital hypermelanotic lesions are generally more common in pigmented races, tend to affect women more frequently than men, and can occur anywhere on the body, although some have a dermatome distribution; e.g., nevus of Ota. These lesions are not considered heritable and are only rarely malignant in the sense of being metastatic, although some are locally invasive (64). True melanomas may develop in genetic disorders in which the skin is predominantly involved such as xeroderma pigmentosum, but this disease is obviously more than a simple neurocristopathy (49).

Familial melanomas are more uncommon. The tumor follows the course of most familial cancers in that the lesions are generally multiple and of earlier onset than the sporadic type. Autosomal dominant inheritance is the generally accepted genetic mechanism but penetrance is incomplete (1). At least three families have been described in which two unrelated individuals living in the same household developed melanoma (67). Pseudodominant inheritance has been described in which maternal melanoma cells were transmitted to a fetus via the placenta (33).

Ocular Melanoma

Intraocular melanoma has been reported in families as an autosomal dominant trait (17). Bilaterality is the rule, as would be expected. A few familial examples of congenital ocular melanoma have been described, but it is unclear whether this condition is distinct from the hereditary form of ocular melanoma with later onset (64). Ocular lesions may be seen rarely in patients with cutaneous melanomas, and there is question whether or not ocular melanoma should be considered a separate, heritable entity.

Neurocutaneous Melanosis

Neurocutaneous melanosis is a rare variety of neural crest dysplasia comprising extensive, multiple pigmented nevi of the skin, brain, and meninges with obstructive hydrocephalus. The lesion is considered to be premalignant. Nevoid and nonnevoid pigmentation have been described in relatives without the full-blown syndrome (23), but the genetics of the condition remains in doubt.

Neurofibromatosis

Multiple neurofibromatosis or von Recklinghausen's syndrome is a well recognized autosomal dominant disorder with protean manifestations including skin lesions, disturbances in growth, often asymmetric, diverse neurologic symptoms, and endocrinologic abnormalities (12). Most, if not all, of the clinical symptoms in this condition are related to the neuromas or neurofibromas which anatomically disrupt normal growth and development. Some workers divide the condition into three subtypes—a peripheral form, a central form, and a mixed variety (34). This separation may be largely artifactual, as peripheral and central forms may be found in the same family. However, *bilateral acoustic neuroma* without any peripheral lesions has been suggested by Young et al. (92) to be a distinct entity, also inherited as an autosomal dominant disorder. In the more usual form of neurofibromatosis, peripheral sarcomatous degeneration can occur and central lesions such as neurinomas, gliomas with various degrees of malignancy, and meningiomas have been reported. Perhaps as many as 5% of patients with neurofibromatosis may also have one or more pheochromocytomas (25).

Although controversy exists concerning ultimate embryologic origin of the Schwann cell, most workers feel it is derived from the neural crest, and the entire syndrome should properly be considered a developmental anomaly of this tissue. Fialkow has shown that the neurofibromas are multicellular in origin (21). The germinal mutation may have simultaneously affected a large number of cells at a given stage of embryonic development, either primarily, or by rendering them unduly susceptible to tumorigenic viruses or other stimulatory factors. Another possibility is that the germinal event stimulated oncogenesis in only a single cell, but that this cell in some fashion influenced growth in surrounding cells perhaps by the elaboration of nerve-growth stimulating activity, a substance(s) that appears to have many characteristics of a hormone (71). Neurofibromas may be seen in some of the hamartomatous syndromes listed in Table 4, most notably tuberous sclerosis. *Café-au-lait* pigmentation is not uncommon in a host of disorders and indeed in the general population. Such findings should not be construed as being diagnostic of neurofibromatosis in adults unless the lesions are of such number and size to satisfy the criteria established by Crowe et al. nearly 20 years ago (16).

Pheochromocytoma

Pheochromocytoma may occur in individuals with a number of distinct heritable conditions, e.g., von Recklinghausen's and Sipple's syndromes, mucosal neuroma syndrome, and von Hippel-Lindau's syndrome. It may also occur in families independent of these other conditions. The incidence of pheochromocytoma in a random population has been estimated to be approximately 1 in 1000 (66). The prevalence of familial pheochromocytoma is more difficult to assess since some so-called sporadic cases may have asymptomatic relatives. Hermann and Mornex analyzed more than 500 cases of pheochromocytoma and found 6% of them to be familial (32). This figure is probably an underestimation. Bilateral and extraadrenal lesions are the rule, and true malignant degeneration is rare. The tumors tend to become symptomatic in the third and fourth decades of life, but childhood onset has been seen, albeit infrequently. The sexes are equally affected, and the tumor has been described in a variety of racial and ethnic groups.

In addition to the usual amines, pheochromocytomas have produced ectopic adrenocorticotropic hormone (ACTH) (54,58) and have been associated with hypercalcemia and high parathormone (PTH) levels which disappeared following adrenalectomy (79).

Review of the reported pedigrees of families with pheochromocytoma indicates the inheritance pattern is that of an autosomal dominant with a high degree of penetrance, once at-risk individuals are carefully evaluated (78).

Pheochromocytoma has been reported with various congenital heart defects of multifactorial origins (66), with incontinentia pigmenti (an X-linked dominant condition) (22), and with Noonan's syndrome (autosomal dominant) (6). In no case has more than one family member been affected, and pheochromocytoma in these conditions was probably coincidental (however, see p. 192).

Carcinoid Tumors

The term carcinoid was coined by Oberndorfer around the turn of the century to describe a distinctive gut tumor composed of uniform, oval nests of cells containing argyrophilic granules (10). Carcinoid tumors have been found at all levels of the gastrointestinal tract and in such other locations as the tracheobronchial tree, the thymus, parotid glands, and gonads. Tumors of the foregut and midgut differ somewhat with respect to basic histologic structure, staining reactions, and serotonin content, and the typical carcinoid syndrome is more likely to be associated with tumors of foregut origin (88). The histological and functional discrepancies between tumors in the two locations may reflect basic embryologic differences. Alternatively, the surrounding tissue may be responsible for the ultimate development of cells with a common origin and thus account for the above differences.

Weichert has suggested that both the enterochromaffin system and many components of the endocrine system are derived from the neural crest (84). Both systems are capable of secreting physiologic amines and peptide hormones. Considerable histologic similarity exists between carcinoid tumors and both islet cell and medullary thyroid carcinomas. The latter tumors are component parts of the multiple endocrine neoplasia syndromes, conditions felt by many to be due to faulty differentiation of the neural crest *(vide infra)* (72). Frank carcinoid tumors have been described in families with multiple endocrine neoplasia, type I (66), and have been reported to coexist with pheochromocytoma (82) and with neurofibromatosis (4). Foregut carcinoid tumors, in addition to producing those amines thought to be at least partly responsible for the carcinoid syndrome (serotonin, histamine, various kinins) have been implicated in ectopic secretion of insulin, glucagon, gastrin, ACTH, melanocyte-stimulating hormones, and calcitonin (70,84).

Pearse has argued that, despite the common secretory products, there is no firm data supporting the contention that all components of the endocrine system are derived from neural crest, and that although the hypothesis relating the enterochromaffin system to the endocrine system and hence to neuroectoderm is attractive, the evidence is circumstantial, and any relationship remains to be experimentally verified (58).

Familial examples of carcinoid tumors are rare, and only three reported instances have been found in the literature outside the confines of type I multiple endocrine neoplasia (2,20,53). One of the reported families had multiple members who suffered from other cancers, type and site unspecified. It is of interest that the carcinoid tumors in all these families were of hindgut origin, again raising the possibility that the enterochromaffin system is not a single, uniform entity.

Multiple Endocrine Neoplasia, Type I

Multiple endocrine neoplasia, type I (MEN I), or Wermer's syndrome is a well recognized autosomal dominant disorder (73). Whereas it is appropriate to consider this condition first on historical grounds, the neurocristopathic origin of the syndrome is perhaps less convincing than for the other endocrine adenoma syndromes. It comprises adenomas or adenocarcinomas of the pituitary, parathyroids, pancreas, and the adrenal cortex. Occasionally the various glands show diffuse hyperplasia of all endocrine elements, rather than frank adenoma formation. Less frequently, bronchial and intestinal carcinoid tumors, lipomas, schwannomas, and nonlymphoid thymomas have been reported in affected individuals (66). All of the tumors may be functional and produce the characteristic hormonal hypersecretion syndrome, e.g., pancreatic islet cell tumors may be insulinomas, glucagonomas, or gastrinomas with secretion of the latter hormone being responsible for perhaps 50% or more of the cases of Zollinger–Ellison's syndrome (73). Even the pancreatic delta or D cells, recognized first in 1931, have now been shown to contain growth-hormone release-inhibiting hormone, a substance previously detected only in the hypothalamus (61). The pituitary tumors may be nonfunctional with resultant target organ deficiency occasioned by compression and necrosis of normal cells.

Other amines and peptides may be secreted by any of the component tumor cells including serotonin, ACTH, and vasoactive intestinal polypeptide (VIP) and thus be responsible for some so-called ectopic hormone syndromes that occur in patients with MEN I.

There would appear to be little question that the pancreatic islet cells are of neural crest origin, and it is reasonable to assume that some of the other lesions, i.e., carcinoid tumors, schwannomas, etc., may be similarly derived (58). It is more difficult to relate the adrenal cortical lesion, which may be responsible for Cushing's syndrome or, less commonly, for hyperaldosteronism to neural crest for the following reasons: (a) the adrenal cortex is of mesodermal origin; (b) the hormones produced are not peptides but steroids, the synthesis of which requires a number of enzymatic steps; (c) the gonads, which are of similar embryologic origin and likewise synthesize steroids, are only rarely, and perhaps only coincidentally, involved in MEN I (30). This exception to the neural crest hypothesis may be more apparent than real since islet cell and carcinoid tumors have been shown to produce ectopic ACTH or at least an ACTH-like polypeptide, rendering the adrenal involvement secondary. ACTH excess may stimulate not only cortisol synthesis but in large quantities even aldosterone as well, in a relatively nonspecific manner. Although not yet detected within the diagnostic confines of MEN I, excess ectopic renin production could likewise result in aldosteronism. At least one case of hyperreninism has been found to be associated with an oat cell carcinoma (73), the cells of which are derived from Kulschitzky cells, an argyrophilic cell type that would appear to be of neural crest origin ('/).

APUD cells also have not definitely been found in the anterior pituitary, a tissue widely held to be of ectodermal origin (58). Hence, the neural crest origin of the pituitary component of MEN I becomes suspect. It is of interest that although the pituitary produces glycoprotein as well as peptide trophic hormones, no clear example of glycoprotein hormone excess in MEN I has been identified (81). It may be that the adenohypophysis contains two cell populations, one derived from neural crest, the other from ectoderm, and that the latter cell type is responsible for glycoprotein hormone synthesis. Present techniques may not be sophisticated enough to allow for the detection of neural crest cells within the anterior pituitary. Alternatively, the hypothalamus, which unquestionably contains neural crest derivatives, may be the primary structure involved in some cases of MEN I and may elaborate releasing hormones with the pituitary response being a secondary phenomenon. Following this line of reasoning, the absence of glycoprotein hormone-producing tumors in MEN I may be a technical phenomenon or may simply be fortuitous.

The parathyroid glands are involved in more than 80% of patients with MEN I. Although it is reasonable to assume that the parathyroid cells are of neural crest origin, they have not been rigorously established as being derived from this source. Vance et al. suggested that the MEN I syndrome was a nesidioblastosis, relating the primary event to abnormalities of pancreatic islet cell function with pituitary, parathyroid, and adrenal gland changes secondary to nonphysiologic stimulation of these glands, e.g., recurrent insulin-induced hypoglycemia leading to reactive hyperplasia of pituitary somatotrophic and corticotrophic cells, or glucagon stimulating parathormone secretion (81). This theory could account for the various glands being involved in MEN I and would relate the syndrome more closely to a primary neural crest abnormality, but it does not account for the fact that hyperparathyroidism occurs more commonly in MEN I than any islet cell lesion and in any event usually precedes, or at least is recognized before, the appearance of other endocrine neoplasia. If parathyroid hyperplasia is secondary in MEN I, the primary stimulus remains unknown. Ljunberg has found argentaffin cells in addition to clear cells and chief cells in the parathyroid glands of some patients with hyperparathyroidism (48). It is conceivable that these cells, which are quite likely neural crest derivatives, are actually the true "tumor" cells and are responsible for excess PTH excretion.

The thyroid, another branchial arch derivative, has been found to harbor some abnormality in approximately 20% of cases with MEN I (66). The pathologic lesion is diverse, comprising adenomas, colloid goiter, and thyroiditis, and there is some question about whether or not thyroid involvement is intrinsic to the MEN I syndrome, especially in view of the fact that these same thyroid abnormalities are not uncommon in the general population. Certainly the parafollicular cells of the thyroid are of neural crest origin, but no good evidence relates the follicular cells to this source.

Thus while it is attractive to relate all facets of MEN I ultimately to a genetic abnormality of neural crest development and differentiation, clear experimental verification of this hypothesis has not as yet been forthcoming (45,51,58).

Multiple Endocrine Neoplasia, Type II

Multiple endocrine neoplasia, type II (MEN II), or Sipple's syndrome includes pheochromocytoma, which is usually bilateral and/or extraadrenal, multifocal medullary thyroid carcinoma (MTC), and less commonly, parathyroid hyperplasia or adenomas (75). The condition is inherited as an autosomal dominant (78). A large body of histochemical, embryologic, and ultrastructural evidence supports the contention that the medullary thyroid tumor is derived from the thyroid parafollicular or C cell and thus ultimately from neural crest (58). The MTC produces calcitonin, and serum radioimmunoassay of this hormone either under basal conditions or after provocative testing with calcium, glucagon, pentagastrin, and even alcohol has proved to be extremely useful in diagnosis, particularly since the MTC may be otherwise asymptomatic. In addition to calcitonin, MTC has been found to produce ectopic amines such as serotonin, and hormones such as ACTH, with the presenting symptoms being related to the carcinoid syndrome or Cushing's syndrome, respectively. Whether the same cell that produces calcitonin also synthesizes these other substances is conjectural since Ljunberg (48) and Bussolati et al. (11) have found at least one other cell type in these tumors in addition to the C cell. This latter cell has histological features reminiscent of carcinoid tumor cells and may actually be the cell responsible for ectopic hormone synthesis. The amyloid deposits, characteristic of MTC, would appear to be derived from calcitonin (80). Diarrhea is a frequent accompanying feature of MEN II, and serotonin excess has been incriminated in its pathogenesis. Elevated levels of prostaglandin have been found in the MTC and in peripheral blood, and in at least one patient, the diarrhea ceased after the ingestion of nutmeg, a known potent inhibitor of prostaglandin synthesis (5). However, others have suggested a primary diarrheogenic role to calcitonin (28). Kallikrein and histaminase are also apparently synthesized by MTC and may be responsible for altered gut motility in some patients. Serum VIP levels have been found to be elevated in at least one patient with pheochromocytoma and could likewise be causally implicated (69).

There is some evidence the C cell hyperplasia precedes frank MTC development (91), just as diffuse adrenal medullary hyperplasia may be evident before the obvious development of pheochromocytoma (13). Baylin et al. (5a) have found that both the MTC and the pheochromocytoma are derived from a single clone. Frank tumor development may be dependent on an additional somatic event. In this regard it is interesting that fibroblasts from patients with MEN II have shown increased virus-induced transformation when compared to controls. An increased serologic reactivity to EB virus has also been found (46).

The pheochromocytoma seen in MEN II are quite typical histologically and may produce the classic symptoms of catecholamine excess. However, a surprising number of these tumors are found incidentally at autopsy. Some patients found to have pheochromocytomas showed no response to provocative histamine. The reasons for the absent pressor response are obscure but may be related to elaboration of potent smooth muscle relaxants such as prostaglandin by the MTC or by enhanced histamine degradation mediated by histaminase, an enzyme known to be present in large quantities in MTC. Malignant degeneration of pheochromocytoma is rare, but has occurred (13).

Parathyroid hyperplasia is often found in MEN II, whereas it is not generally seen with nonfamilial MTC (9). This factor has led some workers to postulate that the parathyroid lesion is a primary genetic feature of MEN II and not a consequence of excess calcitonin secretion by the thyroid tumor (38). As previously discussed, it has been difficult to prove that the parathyroid cells are of neural crest origin, whereas there is little question that the pheochromocyte and the C cell are so derived. If the parathyroid hyperplasia is primary and not secondary, the neurocristopathic origin of MEN II becomes suspect. However, calcitonin has been found to increase *in vitro* PTH production in porcine parathyroid slices directly (18), raising the possibility that small, local and early increases of calcitonin may stimulate the parathyroids to undergo hypertrophy before obvious MTC development occurs. Alternatively, the parathyroid cells may actually be of neural crest origin, although not demonstrable as such. A third possibility is that the argentaffin cells found in adenomatous parathyroid glands (48) in some fashion sensitize or stimulate the PTH-producing cells to undergo hyperplasia.

Although elevated plasma levels of calcitonin are one of the diagnostic hallmarks of MEN II, this hormone has been produced by a small cell tumor of the lung (14), by a pheochromocytoma (36), and by an islet cell tumor (19), although at least in the latter instance there were some immunologic differences between the ectopic and MTC-synthesized calcitonin.

Other tumors have been found in patients with MEN II such as gliomas, glioblastomas, and meningiomas (39). These tumors may logically be an additional potential consequence of abnormal neural crest differentiation. A breast carcinoma seen in one patient with MEN II was almost assuredly coincidental (47). Similarly, the discovery of a microscopic hypophyseal adenoma at autopsy in a single patient with MEN II does not constitute sufficient grounds for assuming identity of this syndrome with MEN I (90).

Multiple Endocrine Neoplasia, Type III

Multiple endocrine neoplasia, type III (MEN III), or the mucosal neuroma syndrome is sufficiently distinctive to warrant separate classification (40). In addition to medullary thyroid carcinoma and pheochromocytoma, affected patients have a pathognomonic facies (74). They have large, nodular "blubbery" lips, pseudoprognathism, enlarged corneal nerves, and neuromatous nodules on the tongue and within the labial, nasal, and laryngeal mucosa (76). Megacolon, probably secondary to intestinal neuromas, has been seen. Unexplained diarrhea occurs as in MEN II. Such patients are slender with a so-called Marfanoid habitus, and hypotonia is commonly seen along with a variety of musculoskeletal alterations such as kyphosis, lordosis, pes cavus, genu valgum, and generalized joint laxity (27). Peripheral neurofibromas, *café-au-lait* spots, and diffuse lentiginous pigmentation have been recorded, and an absent flare response to intradermal histamine is frequently present.

Although most reported cases are apparently sporadic, a recent review of 41 patients documents autosomal dominant inheritance of MEN III (40). The mucosal neuromas and other physical abnormalities should serve to differentiate this syndrome from MEN II. In addition, there would seem to be some endocrinologic differences; e.g., only one case of associated hyperparathyroidism has been seen and, at least thus far, none of the thyroid or adrenal medullary tumors has been responsible for ectopic hormone production. In view of the small number of cases described, this latter finding may be fortuitous. The range of phenotypic expression of MEN III has not been adequately defined, and it would be interesting to study the first degree relatives of patients with this condition in order to assess the frequency of underlying malignancy in those individuals with only minimal peripheral lesions.

This condition, of all the tumorous endocrinopathies, would best fit the category of a neurolophoma since all the major component elements, MTC, pheochromocytoma, and mucosal neuromas are derived from the neural crest.

Other Syndromes with Neural Crest Tumors

MTC has been reported in families in the absence of pheochromocytoma, and with and without parathyroid adenomas (8,50). Because the adrenal medullary tumor may be chemically quiescent and in view of the fact that the age of onset of the component tumors of the MEN II syndrome is so variable, it is difficult to determine whether or not sufficient grounds exist to catalog these endocrinopathies separately.

Similarly, hyperparathyroidism has been seen in familial aggregates as an autosomal dominant disorder. However, most workers consider this condition merely a limited expression of MEN I (66). The rare familial occurrences of pituitary adenomas also can best be considered in this light.

A number of patients with Turner's syndrome have been found to harbor nongonadal neoplasias, and some of these tumors are of neural crest origin (60,85). Similarly, Noonan's syndrome, a dominantly inherited disorder that phenotypically resembles Turner's syndrome, has been associated with tumors of neural crest origin such as a schwannoma and a pheochromocytoma (6,37,41).

Medulloblastoma is considered by some to be a central counterpart of peripheral neuroblastoma (68). Two other hamartomatous conditions feature this neoplasm, the blue rubber bleb nevus syndrome and the nevoid basal cell carcinoma syndrome. These few cases hardly constitute *prima facie* evidence for these syndromes being neurocristopathies, but the associations are noteworthy.

Families have also been described in which multiple members suffered from a variety of different brain tumors (34). Some of these tumors may be derived solely from neural crest, but such a contention is essentially unprovable.

SUMMARY AND CONCLUSIONS

The neural crest is a most fascinating tissue. Even today the destiny of all its component cells has not been definitively established. The possible influences exerted on these cells by the overlying ectoderm or the surrounding mesenchymal milieu through which they migrate remains enigmatic. More knowledge will be required before we can be certain of the relationship between the neural crest and various endocrine organs, both the classic ones and the more recently discovered, but perhaps more phylogenetically atavistic, gastrointestinal hormone-producing tissues. The neural crest may be the ultimate source of further cell types, notably the oat cell, and perhaps other cells that produce ectopic peptide hormones. Neoplasia in this system is not uncommon, and many of these tumors are heritable. It is apparent that study of the neural crest and its malignant derivatives may have tremendous genetic and therapeutic implications. A practical consequence of such investigation might be the development of chemotherapeutic agents effective against a host of malignancies that develop in what are seemingly diverse tissues, but which are in reality embryonically related. Although much is known about the ubiquitous neural crest and its derivatives, it is likely that we are merely on the frontiers of even greater knowledge of this system and ultimately its contribution to a more comprehensive understanding of basic mechanisms of hereditary oncogenesis.

ACKNOWLEDGMENT

This work was supported in part by a grant (RR-828) from the General Clinical Research Centers Program of the Division of Research Resources, National Institutes of Health.

REFERENCES

1. Anderson, D. E. (1971): Clinical characteristics of the genetic variety of cutaneous melanoma in man. *Cancer,* 28:721–725.
2. Anderson, R. E. (1966): A familial instance of appendiceal carcinoid. *Am. J. Surg.,* 111:738–740.
3. Andrew, A. (1963): A study of the developmental relationship between enterochromaffin cells and the neural crest. *J. Embryol. Exp. Morphol.,* II:307–324.
4. Arnesjö, B., Idvall, I., Ihse, I., Telenius, M., and Tylen, V. (1973): Concomitant occurrence of neurofibromatosis and carcinoid of the intestine. *Scand. J. Gastroenterol.,* 8:637–643.

5. Barrowman, J. A., Bennett, A., Hillenbrand, P., Rolles, K., Pollock, D. J., and Wright, J. T. (1975): Diarrhoea in thyroid medullary carcinoma: Role of prostaglandins and therapeutic effect of nutmeg. *Br. Med. J.*, 3:11–12.

5a. Baylin, S. B., Gann, D. S., and Hsu, S. H. (1976): Clonal origin of inherited medullary thyroid carcinoma and pheochromocytoma. *Science,* 193:321–323.

6. Becker, C. E., Rosen, S. W., and Engleman, K. (1969): Pheochromocytoma and hyporesponsiveness to thyrotrophin in a 46,XY male with features of the Turner phenotype. *Ann. Intern. Med.,* 70:325–333.

7. Bensch, K. G., Corrin, B., Pariente, R., and Spencer, H. (1968): Oat-cell carcinoma of the lung. *Cancer,* 22:1163–1172.

8. Block, M. A., Horn, R. C., Miller, J. M., Barrett, J. L., and Brush, B. E. (1967): Familial medullary carcinoma of the thyroid. *Ann. Surg.,* 166:403–412.

9. Block, M. A., Jackson, C. E., and Tashjian, A. H. (1975): Management of parathyroid glands in surgery for medullary thyroid carcinoma. *Arch. Surg.,* 110:617–622.

10. Bolande, R. P. (1974): The neurocristopathies. *Hum. Biol.,* 5:409–428.

11. Bussolati, G., Van Noorden, S., and Bordi, C. (1973): Calcitonin and ACTH-producing cells in a case of medullary carcinoma of the thyroid. *Virchows Arch. [Pathol. Anat.]*, 360:123–127.

12. Canale, D. J., and Bebin, Jr. (1972). Von Recklinghausen disease of the nervous system. In: *Handbook of Clinical Neurology,* Vol. 14, edited by P. J. Vinken and G. W. Bruyn, pp. 132–162. American Elsevier, New York.

13. Carney, J. A., Sizemore, G. W., and Tyce, G. M. (1975): Bilateral adrenal medullary hyperplasia in multiple endocrine neoplasia, type 2. *Mayo Clin. Proc.,* 50:3–10.

14. Cattan, D., Belaiche, J., Milhaud, G., Kalifat, R., Rougier, P., Vesin, P., Pappo, E., and Parrot, M. (1974): Cancer bronchique à petites cellules, syndrome de Schwartz-Bartter et hyperthyrocalcitonémie. *Nouv. Presse Med.,* 3:2391–2394.

15. Chedid, A., and Jao, W. (1974): Hereditary tumors of the carotid bodies and chronic obstructive pulmonary disease. *Cancer,* 33:1635–1641.

16. Crowe, F. W., Schull, W. J., and Neel, J. V. (1956): *Multiple Neurofibromatosis.* Charles C. Thomas, Springfield, Ill.

17. Davenport, R. C. (1927): Familial history of choroidal sarcoma. *Br. J. Ophthalmol.,* 11:443–445.

18. Deftos, L. J., and Parthemore, J. G. (1974): Secretion of parathyroid hormone in patients with medullary thyroid carcinoma. *J. Clin. Invest.,* 54:416–420.

19. Deftos, L. J., Roos, B. A., Bronzert, D., and Parthemore, J. G. (1975): Immunochemical heterogeneity of calcitonin in plasma. *J. Clin. Endocrinol. Metab.,* 40:409–412.

20. Eschbach, J. W., and Rinaldo, J. A. (1962): Metastatic carcinoid. *Ann. Intern. Med.,* 57:647–650.

21. Fialkow, P. J. (1974): The origin and development of human tumors studied with cell markers. *N. Engl. J. Med.,* 291:26–35.

22. Fischbein, F. I., Schub, M., and Lesko, W. S. (1972): Incontinentia pigmenti, pheochromocytoma and ocular abnormalities. *Am. J. Ophthalmol.,* 73:961–964.

23. Fox, H. (1972): Neurocutaneous melanosis. In *Handbook of Clinical Neurology,* Vol. 14, edited by P. J. Vinken and G. W. Bruyn, pp. 132–162. American Elsevier, New York.

24. Gerson, J. M., Chatten, J., and Eisman, S. (1974): Familial neuroblastoma—a follow-up. *N. Engl. J. Med.,* 290:1487.

25. Glushien, A. S., Mansuy, M. M., and Littman, D. S. (1953): Pheochromocytoma. *Am. J. Med.,* 14:318–327.

26. Gorlin, R. J. (1976): Some soft tissue heritable tumors. *Birth Defects,* 12(1):7–14.

27. Gorlin, R. J., Sedano, H. O., Vickers, R. A., and Cervenka, J. (1963): Multiple mucosal neuromas, pheochromocytoma and medullary carcinoma of the thyroid—a syndrome. *Cancer,* 22:293–299.

28. Gray, T. K., Bieberdorf, F. A., and Fordtran, J. S. (1973): Thyrocalcitonin and the jejunal absorption of calcium, water and electrolytes in normal subjects. *J. Clin. Invest.,* 52:3084–3088.

29. Griffin, M. E., and Bolande, R. P. (1969): Familial neuroblastoma with regression and maturation to ganglioneurofibroma. *Pediatrics,* 43:377–382.

30. Griffin, P. E. (1972): Multiple endocrine adenomatosis. *Rocky Mt. Med. J.,* 69:64–65.

31. Grzeschik, K. (1973): Utilization of somatic cell hybrids for genetic studies in man. *Humangenetik,* 19:1–40.

32. Hermann, H., and Mornex, R. (1964): *Human Tumors Secreting Catecholamines.* MacMillan, New York.

33. Holland, E. (1949): A case of transplacental metastasis of malignant melanoma from mother to fetus. *J. Obstet. Gynaecol. Br. Commonw.*, 56:529–536.
34. Horton, W. A. (1976): Genetics of central nervous system tumors. *Birth Defects*, 12(1):91–97.
35. Jaffe, N., Cassady, R., Filler, R. M., Petersen, R., and Traggis, D. (1975): Heterochromia and Horner syndrome associated with cervical and mediastinal neuroblastoma. *J. Pediatr.*, 87:75–77.
36. Kaplan, E. L., Hill, B. J., and Peskin, G. W. (1970): A calcitonin-like factor from the adrenal medulla. *Clin. Res.*, 18:362.
37. Kaplan, M. S., Opitz, J. M., and Gosset, F. R. (1968): Noonan's syndrome. *Am. J. Dis. Child.*, 116:359–366.
38. Keiser, H. R., Beaven, M. A., Doppman, J., Well, S., and Buja, L. M. (1973): Sipple's syndrome. *Ann. Intern. Med.*, 78:561–579.
39. Keynes, W. M., and Till, A. S. (1971): Medullary carcinoma of the thyroid gland. *Q. J. Med.*, 40:443–456.
40. Khairi, M. R., Dexter, R. N., Burzynski, N. J., and Johnston, C. C. (1975): Mucosal neuroma, pheochromocytoma and medullary thyroid carcinoma: Multiple endocrine neoplasia, type 3. *Medicine*, 54:89–112.
41. Khodadonst, A., and Paton D. (1967): Turner's syndrome in a male. *Arch. Ophthalmol.*, 77:630–634.
42. Klein, H., and Plöchl, E. (1974): Familiäres Neuroblastom der Nebennieren beim neugeborenen. *Munch. Med. Wochenschr.*, 116:1163–1168.
43. Knudson, A. G., and Amromin, G. D. (1966): Neuroblastoma and ganglioneuroma in a child with multiple neurofibromatosis. *Cancer*, 19:1032–1037.
44. Knudson, A. G., and Strong, L. C. (1972): Mutation and cancer: Neuroblastoma and pheochromocytoma. *Am. J. Hum. Genet.*, 24:514–532.
45. Levine, R. J., and Metz, S. A. (1974): A classification of ectopic hormone-producing tumors. *Ann. N.Y. Acad. Sci.*, 230:533–546.
46. Li, F. P., Melvin, K. E. W., Tashjian, A. H., Levine, P. H., and Fraumeni, J. F. Jr. (1974): Familial medullary thyroid carcinoma and pheochromocytoma: Epidemiologic investigations. *J. Natl. Cancer Inst.*, 52:285–287.
47. Lima, J. B., and Smith, P. D. (1971): Sipple's syndrome with bilateral breast carcinoma. *Am. J. Surg.*, 121:732–735.
48. Ljunberg, O. (1972): Argentaffin cells in human thyroid and parathyroid and their relationship to C-cells and medullary carcinoma. *Acta Pathol. Microbiol. Scand. A.* 80:589–599.
49. Lynch, H. T., Anderson, D. E., Smith, J. L., Howell, J. B., and Krush, A. J. (1967): Xeroderma pigmentosum, malignant melanoma, and congenital ichthyrosis. *Arch. Dermatol.*, 96:625–635.
50. Markey, W. S., Ryan, W. G., Economou, S. G., Sizemore, G. W., and Arnaud, C. D. (1973): Familial medullary carcinoma and parathyroid adenoma without pheochromocytoma. *Ann. Intern. Med.*, 78:898–901.
51. Metz, S. A. (1975): Ectopic hormones from tumors. *Ann. Intern. Med.*, 83:117–118.
52. Moe, P. G., and Nellhaus, G. (1970): Infantile polymyoclonia-opsoclonus syndrome and neural crest tumors. *Neurology (Minneap.)*, 20:756–764.
53. Moertel, C. G., and Dockerty, M. B. (1973): Familial occurrence of metastasizing carcinoid tumors. *Ann. Intern. Med.*, 78:389–390.
54. O'Neal, L. W., Kipnis, D. M., Luse, S. A., Lacy, P. E., and Jarett, L. (1968): Secretion of various endocrine substances by ACTH-secreting tumors. *Cancer*, 21:1219–1232.
55. Pearse, A. G. E. (1968): Common cytochemical and ultrastructural characteristics of cells producing polypeptide hormones (the APUD series) and their relevance to thyroid and ultimobranchial C cells and calcitonin. *Proc. R. Soc. Med.*, 170:75–80.
56. Pearse, A. G. E. (1969): The cytochemistry and ultrastructure of polypeptide hormone-producing cells of the APUD series and the embryologic, physiologic and pathologic implications of the concept. *J. Histochem. Cytochem.*, 17:303–313.
57. Pearse, A. G. E., and Polak, J. M. (1971): Neural crest origin of the endocrine polypeptide (APUD) cells of the gastrointestinal tract and the pancreas. *Gut*, 12:783–788.
58. Pearse, A. G. E., and Polak, J. M. (1974): Endocrine tumors of neural crest origin. *Med. Biol.*, 52:3–18.
59. Pegelow, C. H., Ebbin, A. J., Powars, D., and Towner, J. W. (1975): Familial neuroblastoma. *J. Pediatr.*, 87:763–765.
60. Pendergrass, T. W., Fraumeni, J. F., Jr., and Fagan, E. L. (1974): Brain tumors in sibs, one with the Turner syndrome. *J. Pediatr.*, 85:875.

61. Polak, J. M., Grimelius, L., Pearse, A. G. E., Bloom, S. R., and Arimura, A. (1975): Growth-hormone release-inhibiting hormone in gastrointestinal and pancreatic D cells. *Lancet*, 1:1220–1222.
62. Pollack, R. S. (1973): Carotid body tumors—idiosyncracies. *Oncology*, 27:81–91.
63. Potter, E. L., and Parrish, J. M. (1942): Neuroblastoma, ganglioneuroma and fibroneuroma in a stillborn fetus. *Am. J. Pathol.*, 18:141–151.
64. Reese, A. B. (1974): Congenital melanomas. *Am. J. Ophthalmol.*, 77:798–808.
65. Revak, C. S., Morris, S. E., and Alexander, G. H. (1971): Pheochromocytoma and recurrent chemodectomas over a twenty-five year period. *Radiology*, 100:53–54.
66. Rimoin, D. L. and Schimke, R. N. (1971): *Genetic Disorders of the Endocrine Glands*. Mosby, St. Louis, Mo.
67. Robinson, M. J., and Manheimer, L. (1972): Familial melanomas. *JAMA*, 220:277.
68. Rubinstein, L. J. (1972): Cytogenesis and differentiation of primitive central neuroepithelial tumors. *J. Neuropathol. Exp. Neurol.*, 31:7–26.
69. Said, S. I., and Faloona, G. R. (1975): Elevated plasma and tissue levels of vasoactive intestinal polypeptide in the watery-diarrhea syndrome due to pancreatic, bronchogenic and other tumors. *N. Engl. J. Med.*, 293:155–160.
70. Samaan, N. A., Hickey, R. C., Bedner, T. D., and Ibanez, M. L. (1975): Hyperparathyroidism and carcinoid tumor. *Ann. Intern. Med.*, 82:205–207.
71. Schenkein, I., Bueker, E. D., Helson, L., Axelrod, F., and Dancis, J. (1974): Increased nerve-growth-stimulating activity in disseminated neurofibromatosis. *N. Engl. J. Med.*, 290:613–614.
72. Schimke, R. N. (1971): Familial tumor endocrinopathies. *Birth Defects*, 76:55–65.
73. Schimke, R. N. (1976): Multiple endocrine adenomatosis syndromes. *Adv. Intern. Med.*, 21:249–265.
74. Schimke, R. N. (1973): Phenotype of malignancy; mucosal neuroma syndrome. *Pediatrics*, 52:283–284.
75. Schimke, R. N., and Hartmann, W. H. (1965): Familial amyloid-producing medullary thyroid carcinoma and pheochromocytoma. *Ann. Intern. Med.*, 63:1027–1039.
76. Schimke, R. N., Hartmann, W. H., Prout, T. E., and Rimoin, D. L. (1968): Syndrome of bilateral pheochromocytoma, medullary thyroid carcinoma and multiple neuromas. *N. Eng. J. Med.*, 279:1–7.
77. Shuangshoti, S., and Ekaraphanich, S. (1972): Congenital neuroblastoma and hyperplasia of islets of Langerhans in an infant. *Clin. Pediatr. (Phila.)*, 11:241–243.
78. Steiner, A. L., Goodman, A. D., and Powers, S. R. (1968): Study of a kindred with pheochromocytoma, medullary thyroid carcinoma, hyperparathyroidism and Cushing's disease: Multiple endocrine neoplasia, type 2. *Medicine (Baltimore)*, 47:371–409.
79. Swinton, N. W., Clerkin, E. P., and Flint, L. D. (1972): Hypercalcemia and familial pheochromocytoma. *Ann. Intern. Med.*, 76:455–457.
80. Tashjian, A. H., Wolfe, H. J., and Voelkel, E. F. (1974): Human calcitonin. *Am. J. Med.*, 56:840–849.
81. Vance, J. E., Stoll, R. W., Kitabchi, A. E., Buchanan, K. D., Hollander, D., and Williams, R. H. (1972): Familial nesidioblastosis as the predominant manifestation of multiple endocrine adenomatosis. *Am. J. Med.*, 52:211–227.
82. Warner, R. R. P., and Blaustein, A. S. (1970): Coexistence of pheochromocytoma and carcinoid syndrome produced by metastatic carcinoid of the ileum. *Mt. Sinai Med. J.*, 36:536–548.
83. Warner, T. F. (1974): Cell hybridization in the genesis of ectopic hormone-secreting tumors. *Lancet*, 1:1259–1260.
84. Weichert, R. F. (1970): The neural ectodermal origin of the peptide-secreting endocrine glands. *Am. J. Med.*, 49:232–241.
85. Wertelecki, W., Fraumeni, J. F., Jr., and Mulvihill, J. J. (1970): Nongonadal neoplasia in Turner's syndrome. *Cancer*, 26:485–488.
86. Weston, J. A. (1970): The migration and differentiation of neural crest cells. *Adv. Morphol.*, 8:41–114.
87. Weston, J. A. (1971): Neural crest cell migration and differentiation. *UCLA Forum Med. Sci.*, 14:1–22.
88. Williams, E. D., and Sandler, M. (1963): The classification of carcinoid tumors. *Lancet*, 1:238–239.
89. Witzleben, C. L., and Landy, R. A. (1974): Disseminated neuroblastoma in a child with von Recklinghausen's disease. *Cancer*, 34:786–790.

90. Wolf, L. M., Duduisson, M., Schrub, J. C., Metayer, J., and Laumonier, R. (1972): Syndrome de Sipple associé à des adenomes hypophysaires et parathyroidiens. *Ann. Endocrinol. (Paris),* 33:455–463.
91. Wolfe, H. J., Melvin, K. E. W., Cervi-Skinner, S. J., Saadi, A. A., Juliar, J. F., Jackson, C. E., and Tashjian, A. H. (1973): C-cell hyperplasia preceding medullary thyroid carcinoma. *N. Engl. J. Med.,* 289:437–441.
92. Young, D. F., Eldridge, R., and Gardner, W. J. (1970): Bilateral acoustic neuroma in a large kindred. *JAMA,* 214:347–353.

Discussion

Gorlin: One weakness of the concept of neurocristopathy is the fact that enterochromaffin cells are detectable *before* any migration of neural crest tissue.

Schimke: Yes, as Pearse has pointed out, the proposal of Weichert [*Am. J. Med.,* 49:232–241 (1970)] is a broad generalization synthesizing some statements that are not well verified by experimentation.

Gerald: Turning to the genetics of the neurocristopathies, could you report on any phenomena suggesting premutation and any studies of linkage?

Schimke: I know of no one who has made a statistical analysis of premutation. However, with regard to mutational models, it does appear that the thyroid neoplasm, in fact, starts out as C cell hyperplasia. By this criterion, which requires assays of calcitonin or even thyroidectomy, the gene seems highly penetrant. Dr. Stephen Baylin has recently reported a single, black woman with medullary thyroid carcinoma and pheochromocytoma (MEN II) in whom both tumors seemed to arise from a single clone according to G-6-PD markers [*Science,* 193:321–323 (1976)]. Although intriguing, such concordance would be expected half the time by chance. Perhaps Dr. Jackson would report his linkage data.

Jackson: Our study suggested that the locus for MEN II may be linked to that for the P antigen and *not* to the *HLA-A* locus [*Birth Defects,* 12(1):159–164 (1976)].

Riccardi: In studying many markers in two large kindreds with neurofibromatosis in the Denver area, we detected no significant linkages.

Schimke: It would certainly be worthwhile to investigate linkage with common markers. Such data would be useful because of occasional difficulty in identifying which young people in an affected family actually have the gene. The thyroid carcinoma may be only slowly progressive—a late manifestation of the presence of the gene.

Gorlin: At one institution, thyroidectomy was done on a 4-year-old child because of the presence of the phenotype of MEN III, although the thyroid gland was clinically normal. The surgical specimen included a C cell adenoma, which, I suppose, may have remained latent until puberty.

Regarding early diagnosis, I have two comments on the histamine test, the reaction to intradermal injection of 1:1,000 histamine. The positive reaction was at first attributed to increased amounts of histaminase elaborated by the medullary thyroid carcinoma. Yet, we have found this test positive in some individuals who have already had thyroid surgery. Also, we have seen positive tests in 3- and 4-year-old children even though medullary thyroid carcinoma was not present.

Schimke: I would hope those people have no metastases. It is a strange tumor; it can remain silent for a long time. I have seen people survive for 10 to 15 years with obvious metastases at operation.

Bolande: There have been four reported cases of diffuse C cell hyperplasia with metastases; we had another recently. As for the value of the serum levels of calcitonin, you know that the current radioimmunoassays will not pick up fragments of the molecule. We have had frank cases with ostensibly normal calcitonin levels, although the normal range is difficult to determine. Because of these falsely negative values, one can almost make a case for prophylactic thyroidectomy in a patient with the phenotype of MEN III.

Schimke: If a typical facies is present, there is no question that thyroid probably belongs in a jar on your shelf. I have concerns about the many problems of the calcitonin assay reminiscent of the parathormone assays. Different laboratories have different antisera that detect different ends of the molecule, as it were. There seems to be immunologic heterogeneity even with proved medullary thyroid carcinoma. An immunologically distinct calcitonin has been found elevated in patients with oat cell carcinoma of the lung. There is the additional question of the place for provocative testing, for example, following administration of alcohol or gastrin. For diagnosing MEN II, we must rely on all these approaches, despite the difficulties. But, with the pathognomonic facies of MEN III, I think, the thyroid gland should definitely be removed as soon as possible.

Gorlin: Are not elevated calcitonin levels found locally in the multiple mucosal neuromas of the tongue and buccal mucosa in patients with MEN III?

Schimke: Yes, I understand they are, although I have not had personal experience.

Nance: Have you calculated the public health impact of removing thyroid glands from all patients with MEN II or III across the nation?

Schimke: To my knowledge, no calculations have been done. Of course, only 41 cases of MEN III have been compiled in the literature to date; it is obviously not a big public health menace. Also, there are certainly sporadic patients with medullary thyroid carcinoma that is not familial. Of course, these patients may have new dominant mutations, especially since familial medullary thyroid carcinoma can occur without pheochromocytoma.

Bolande: I believe medullary thyroid carcinoma is notoriously underdiagnosed. I have seen it misdiagnosed as follicular carcinoma, as you mentioned, and as Hürthle cell adenomas, oncocytoid tumors, and in lymph nodes as metastatic from chemodectomas or carotid body tumors. If you go back through records with specific features in mind, you find a significant number of cases.

Schimke: In fact, I did just that. I reviewed tumors diagnosed as oat cell, round cell, or undifferentiated tumors and found three or four medullary thyroid carcinomas in a recent 10-year period. The clinical pathologist at that time was uncertain about the existence of the pathologic entity and obviously would not make the diagnosis.

Minna: I have two points concerning small or oat cell carcinoma of the lung, which has been mentioned several times but only in passing. First, some 20,000 to 25,000 cases occur a year in the United States. As for impact on health, if this cell type represents a neurocristopathy—and I think it most certainly does—it has *the* greatest public health impact of all neural crest tumors. Secondly, it is interesting that the tumor has metastatic behavior that recapitulates its embryologic origins. In a fashion distinct from most other cancers, it migrates in a large number of cases as metastases to the pituitary, thyroid, adrenal, and pancreas. This pattern is important clinically in anticipating and interpreting symptoms, and probably gives some clue about basic biology.

Schimke: That is intriguing. Along the same line, I have been waiting for examples of familial oat cell carcinoma. I suspect sooner or later they will occur.

Minna: We have had several instances already.

Schimke: I am not at all surprised.

Genetics of Human Cancer, edited by J. J.
Mulvihill, R. W. Miller, and J. F. Fraumeni, Jr.
Raven Press, New York, 1977.

15

Phacomatoses, Hamartoses, and Neurocristopathies: A Personal View

J. Warkany

Children's Hospital Research Foundation, Cincinnati, Ohio 45229

PHACOMATOSES

The term "phacomatosis" has become a purely descriptive name that could be replaced by a better one. J. van der Hoeve, a farsighted ophthalmologist, recognized in 1932 that Recklinghausen's neurofibromatosis, tuberous sclerosis, and Hippel-Lindau's disease are disorders of a special kind (1). He perceived that certain skin malformations often associated with eye defects lie somewhere between congenital anomalies and tumors, and may be called phacomata (mother spots or birth marks); they differ from nevi since they may be free of nevus cells and located in many parts of the body besides the skin. Van der Hoeve knew that such disorders were hereditary and varied greatly in their expression in different individuals. Unfortunately, in 1936 he added encephalofacial angiomatosis (Sturge-Weber) as a fourth entity to the phacomatoses (2). Transmission comparable to that of the earlier disorders is not known to occur with Sturge-Weber's disease which may have a different etiology. From then on a number of disorders of heterogeneous origin have been added to the phacomatoses (3) so that the term has lost its value; but it remained in use in the French and German literature. In English articles names such as neuroectodermal dysplasias, neuroectodermoses, neurocutaneous syndromes, and neuroophthalmic genopathies were used for diseases which are, however, not limited to the nervous system, skin, or tissues of ectodermal origin. Often derivatives of all germ layers are involved.

HAMARTOSES

The term "hamartoses" is recommended. The lesions begin as tissue malformations; they are systemic and tend to tumor formation. Most important, they usually are transmitted from a parent to some of the children and act like dominant traits. Whether they are transmitted by a dominant gene or another mechanism

199

may be questioned; they differ greatly clinically and the expressivity or penetrance varies for each entity. We do not know what is inherited and causes malformations or tumors. The idea of increased amounts of nerve growth factor as the cause of the many manifestations of Recklinghausen's neurofibromatosis is a good one but the findings published may be dealing with the results and not the actual cause of the disease.

There exists a long list of these peculiar diseases that we consider "hamartoses" and their number is growing (Table 1). The table is incomplete according to some clinicians; several phacomatoses are intentionally omitted. I believe that Sturge-Weber's disease and Klippel-Trenaunay's syndrome are nonfamilial disorders of a different kind; they show preference for one side and may belong with other "hemisyndromes." Xeroderma pigmentosum and Meckel-Gruber's splanchnocystic dysencephaly are left out because they are recessive heritable traits. Thus rather well-defined (4), the term "hamartoses" can be recommended.

NEUROCRISTOPATHIES

This large and overwhelming concept is rather new to me. It may be wise to keep it circumscript and unwise to put too much into it. I remember the term "dysraphia" which flourished about 40 years ago; it dealt with disorders that were blamed on faulty formation of the midline structures of the central nervous system. It was and is a useful concept, but some enthusiasts put too much into it, made it meaningless, and brought it into disrepute.

As has been pointed out, in the present group of neurocristopathies there are many unknowns and many assumptions. I wonder if an experimental approach could be helpful. The neural crest is formed from cells which split off from the margins of the neural folds as they unite to form the neural tube. What happens to the neural crest in congenital malformations where the neural folds do not unite

TABLE 1. *The hamartoses*

Neurofibromatosis (Recklinghausen)
Tuberous sclerosis (Bourneville)
Ocular-cerebellar angiomatosis (Hippel-Lindau)
Nevoid basal cell carcinoma syndrome
Multiple trichoepitheliomas (Brooke)
Multiple dermal cylindromas or turban tumors (Spiegler)
Multiple hamartoma syndrome (Cowden)
Hereditary polyposis of the colon
Hereditary polyposis of the colon with osteomas, fibromas, and epidermal cysts (Gardner)
Gastrointestinal polyposis with perioral pigmentations (Peutz-Jeghers)
Hereditary hemorrhagic telangiectasis (Rendu-Osler-Weber)
Blue rubber-bleb nevus syndrome
Glomus tumors
Multiple lipomas (Krabbe-Bartels)
Familial glioma-gliomatosis (Hallervorden-Spatz)

and the neural tube is not formed? The neural crest should be adversely affected in spina bifida aperta and destroyed as the dorsal parts of the neural plate deteriorate in intrauterine life. Nerve cells, nerves, and meninges are destroyed in these malformations. What about the chromaffin cells, the melanoblasts and the more hypothetical derivatives of the neural crest? There are survivors with some of these "dysraphias," and they could be examined for symptoms attributed to neural crest deficiencies. Spina bifida, including craniorachischisis, can be produced experimentally and the cells and the organs under indictment could be examined in experimental specimens. If there are new fluorescent methods available which can identify neural crest cells during migration, one could possibly prove or disprove some of the assumptions now made in the concept of the neurocristopathies.

REFERENCES

1. Van der Hoeve, J. (1932): The Doyne memorial lecture: Eye symptoms in phakomatoses. *Trans. Ophthalmol. Soc. U. K.,* 52:380–403.
2. Van der Hoeve, J. (1936): Eine vierte Phakomatose. *Ber. Dtsch. Ophthalmol. Ges.,* 51:136–148.
3. Vinken, P. J., and Bruyn, G. W. (eds.) (1972). The Phakomatoses. In: *Handbook of Clinical Neurology, Vol. 14,* American Elsevier, New York.
4. Warkany, J., and Miller, R. W. (1975): Book review: The Phakomatoses. In: *Handbook of Clinical Neurology, Vol. 14,* edited by P. J. Vinken and G. W. Bruyn. American Elsevier, New York.

Discussion

Bolande: The neurocristopathies have thus far been presented as dysplastic, neoplastic, or hamartoid disorders. I think the term has a broader meaning, however, and should include deficiencies, the most obvious being aganglionic megacolon. Dr. Warkany, what do the myenteric plexuses look like in your experimental models?

Warkany: We never went into that. I am a neo-neuro-christian and haven't tried anything of the kind. It could be approached experimentally however.

Gorlin: We have not lacked tools to investigate the neural crest. Experiments date back for decades. When salamander (urodele) eggs are placed in tritiated water and segments from their neural crests inserted into the neural crests of eggs not placed in tritiated water, migration from the transplant can be observed. A similar substitution can be made from a chicken egg into the neural crest of a Japanese quail with its characteristic giant nucleolus. The neural crest of a mouse can be labeled with tritiated thymidine, using a sable's hair brush to make the inoculation through the amnion [*J. Embryol. Exp. Morphol.* 24:479–496 (1970)].

With respect to extending the range of neurocristopathy, it is of interest that Poswillo has given rats very high doses of vitamin A and demonstrated selective killing of certain neural crest cells. He has produced facial dysmorphology and now speaks of Treacher–Collins' syndrome as a neurocristopathy [*Br. Med. Bull.,* 31:101–106 (1975)]. The term has thus been warped and distorted to apply to facial dysmorphologic disorders, because, after all, the ectomesenchyme, anterior to the ears, is a derivative of the neural crest.

Warkany: May I again warn that the concept will be harmed if everything is squeezed into it.

Knudson: In speaking of neural disorders, it is well to raise again the question asked earlier: why are we interested in the implications for carcinogenesis of these genetic disorders that are not cancers? What can we learn from them?

We must be mindful of several kinds of genetic disorders. First, some are due to the effects of dominant genes. We have several examples of neuroblastoma that can be dominantly inherited. It is worthy of note that Dr. Meadows and I have reported on the occurrence of aganglionic megacolon in several families with neuroblastoma, possibly another manifestation of mutation [*J. Natl. Cancer Inst., in press* (1976)].

Isolated pheochromocytoma is a dominantly inherited disorder in 20 to 25% of all cases, according to an estimate by Dr. Strong and myself. The gene responsible affects any part of the sympathetic nervous system, whereas in the medullary thyroid carcinoma-pheochromocytoma syndromes (MEN II and III), only the adrenal medulla—and no other part of the sympathetic nervous system—is affected. Each of these genes, then, produces a specific kind of tumor in the sympathetic nervous system, and at a particular level of differentiation. One must take this concept into account to understand what these genes are doing.

Other actions of the genes provide important clues to mechanisms. If medullary carcinoma of the thyroid is induced, for example, the gene must somehow influence this organ in addition to its neural effect. Von Recklinghausen's disease presents more of a problem, because it is associated with ganglioneuroma and, in a few instances, with neuroblastoma. Dr. Fialkow's group has found that the neurofibromas in von Recklinghausen's disease have multicellular origin [see chapter 41]. As we have heard in the discussion today, medullary tumors arising in the thyroid have unicellular origin, even though the affected persons have already inherited one gene as the first step in the development of their tumor. The unicellular origin of medullary carcinoma of the thyroid suggests that, in contrast to von Recklinghausen's disease, the second step is a somatic mutation. In this group of diseases we do not have examples like xeroderma pigmentosum, which teaches us that we inherit not a gene on the carcinogenic pathway but a gene that affects the rate at which mutations occur on that pathway.

It is unclear whether the neurofibromatosis gene, with respect to pheochromocytoma, causes proliferation of target cells (i.e., a wider target for mutation) or promotes their growth once they mutate. I wonder if Dr. Warkany would comment on the discontinuous and qualitative differences in the kinds of genes that affect neural crest derivatives.

Warkany: I? No! Perhaps others would.

Gerald: I wish to emphasize some distinctions. I worry when we mix autosomal recessively inherited diseases with the dominantly inherited hamartomatous syndromes. I think the basic mechanisms are very different. At least five different enzyme defects can produce xeroderma pigmentosum. A similar circumstance may apply to ataxia-telangiectasia, among other recessively inherited diseases. With respect to dominantly inherited diseases, the only one for which we have any knowledge about its mechanism is Type II hyperlipoproteinemia, in which a receptor on the surface of the affected cell is involved. I suspect that the mechanisms of action are going to differ in relation to the genetic mode of transmission—and I worry about lumping together all genetic disorders that carry an increased risk of cancer.

Bolande: A basic feature in the embryogenesis of the neural crest in explaining its rapid dissemination, acting like a fourth germ layer as some people refer to it, is contact inhibition. It has been suggested that the cellular expression of the von Recklinghausen gene is, in effect, loss of contact inhibition of migrating neural crest cells, which allows development of hamartoid aggregations—of neurofibromas, melanoblasts, glial cells, and pheochromoblasts—thus accounting for the various manifestations of the disease. I do not know if anyone is examining this hypothesis experimentally, but it could be done.

Eldridge: In 1930, Dr. W. James Gardner described a kindred that we reexamined 6 years ago, and found over 100 persons with definite or possible central neurofibromatosis, that is, bilateral acoustic neuromas often associated with meningiomas and other tumors of the central nervous system, but with minimal involvement of peripheral nerves or skin [*JAMA*, 214:342–353 (1970); *Birth Defects*, 10 (10):171–184 (1974)].

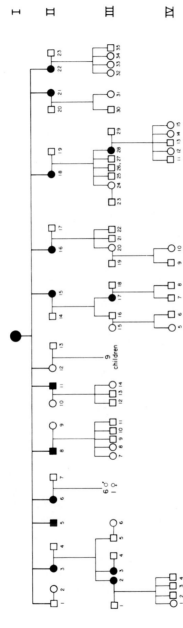

FIG. 1. Record linkage studies showing an unusual aggregation of several cancer cases in one Hawaiian family due to von Hippel-Lindau syndrome. (*Black area*, affected individuals.)

Careful scrutiny showed that the majority had only one or two *café-au-lait* spots. One possibly affected member had three spots, and four affected had one to three subcutaneous nodules suggestive of neurofibromas. In preliminary study of another kindred, we found increased nerve growth factor in the sera of three persons with acoustic neuromas and in two at-risk members of the family who had large *café-au-lait* spots. In five individuals with peripheral neurofibromatosis, by contrast, increased levels of nerve growth factor were not found [*N. Engl. J. Med.*, 292:1134 (1975)].

On a practical note: There are now screening techniques to detect tumors early in persons at high risk either because of family history or because of the presence of *café-au-lait* spots, or both. The onset of tumors is usually at about 20 years of age. Computer assisted tomography, and possibly assay for nerve growth factor in serum, provide noninvasive methods for evaluation. Diagnosis of acoustic neuroma does not automatically mandate surgery. We have a number of persons under observation who have had tumors and functioned normally for 20 to 30 years. Others have rapid spread that does require surgical intervention. Drowning sometimes occurs because the patient may lose his sense of direction when underwater, and those affected or at risk should be warned about this.

Rashad: Record linkage studies demonstrated an unusual aggregation of several cancer cases in one family in Hawaii due to von Hippel–Lindau syndrome (see Fig. 1). The first generation begins with Case I.1 who died of pancreatic carcinoma in 1940 at 47 years of age. She had 12 children, 10 of whom were affected with the disease: II.3 and II.11 died of cerebellar tumor, case II.21 of polycystic kidney. Postmortem examination confirmed the diagnosis. Of those persons in the third generation over the age of 25, only four of 13 persons were affected. The earliest age of onset of symptoms occurred at age 19 (II.11) and the latest at age 54 (II.18). Over two generations, 11 of 14 women over 25 had the disease, whereas three of 11 men were affected.

Genetics of Human Cancer, edited by J. J.
Mulvihill, R. W. Miller, and J. F. Fraumeni, Jr.
Raven Press, New York, 1977.

16

Prevalence of
Endocrine Neoplasia Syndromes
in Genetic Studies of Parathyroid Tumors

Charles E. Jackson, Boy Frame, and Melvin A. Block

Departments of Medicine and Surgery, Henry Ford Hospital, Detroit, Michigan 48202

In a study of the families of 100 consecutive patients with parathyroid tumors, we have encountered 10 individuals in whom other family members are affected. Evidence of multiple endocrine neoplasia type I (MEN I) was found in three families (Fig. 1), multiple endocrine neoplasia type II (MEN II) in two families (Fig. 2), and familial hyperparathyroidism alone in five kindreds. In this study it was possible to study 319 of 426 available first degree relatives. No relatives of nine individuals could be studied, so that it can be stated that 10 of 91 individuals (11%) had evidence that others within their families were affected. In other series of hyperparathyroidism, 14 to 18% of the patients had affected family members (1–3). The evidence of other endocrine involvement in hyperparathyroid families has suggested that many cases of hereditary hyperparathyroidism are actually part of MEN I (3,4,8). Two cases of parathyroid carcinoma were encountered in the present series of 100 cases; however, the limited studies possible in these two families revealed no other cases of hyperparathyroidism. Parathyroid carcinoma has been reported by Mallette et al. (6) in a patient whose other glands were hyperplastic; two sibs had parathyroid hyperplasia and their mother died of an uncertain type of pancreatic tumor (Fig. 3). Combinations of hyperplasia, adenoma, and carcinoma of the parathyroid glands may occur in a single individual and in different members of the same family. This suggests a close relationship between these parathyroid conditions similar to that seen in the pancreatic islets (7) and C cells of the thyroid (9) in which hyperplasia, adenoma, and carcinoma also appear to form a continuous spectrum. The hyperplasia may result from the initial mutation, either genetic or somatic, which may be followed by a second mutational event (5) leading to malignant change.

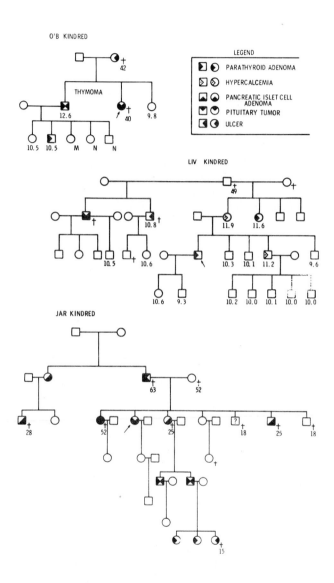

FIG. 1. Pedigrees of the three families of multiple endocrine neoplasia type I encountered in genetic studies of 100 consecutive patients with parathyroid tumors. Serum calcium levels (in mg%) are listed under the symbols for individuals in the O'B and LIV kindreds. The JAR kindred has been published in part by Ballard, Frame, and Hartsock in *Medicine (Baltimore),* 43:481 (1964).

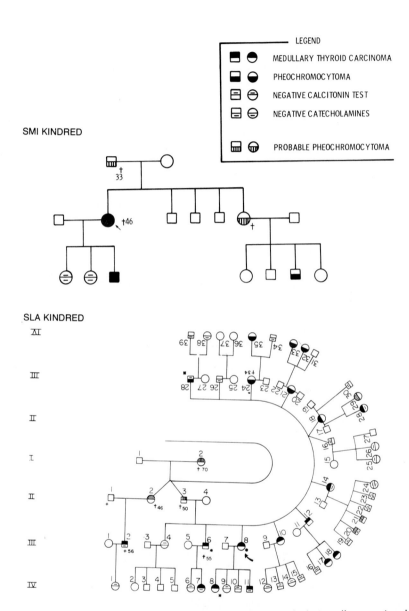

FIG. 2. Pedigrees of the two families of multiple endocrine neoplasia type II encountered. The propositi of both kindreds had parathyroid adenomas, as did those indicated by the asterisks in the SLA kindred. These pedigrees were modified from those reported by Jackson, Tashjian, and Block. *Ann. Intern. Med.,* 78:845 (1973). Medullary thyroid cancers in most instances were detected by calcitonin determinations after calcium or pentagastrin provocative procedures.

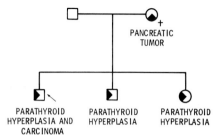

PANCREATIC
TUMOR

FIG. 3. Pedigree of family with hereditary hyperparathyroidism in which one member had parathyroid carcinoma. From the report by Mallette et al. (6).

PARATHYROID
HYPERPLASIA AND
CARCINOMA

PARATHYROID
HYPERPLASIA

PARATHYROID
HYPERPLASIA

ACKNOWLEDGMENT

The work represented in this report was supported in part by U. S. Public Health Service Grant # AM14876.

REFERENCES

1. Boey, J. H., Cooke, T. J. C., Gilbert, J. M., Sweeney, E. C., and Taylor, S. (1975): Occurrence of other endocrine tumours in primary hyperparathyroidism. *Lancet,* 2:781–784.
2. Boonstra, C. E., and Jackson, C. E. (1971): Serum calcium survey for hyperparathyroidism: Results in 50,000 clinic patients. *Am. J. Clin. Pathol.,* 55:523–526.
3. Jackson, C. E., and Boonstra, C. E. (1967): The relationship of hereditary hyperparathyroidism to endocrine adenomatosis. *Am. J. Med.,* 43:727–734.
4. Jackson, C. E., and Frame, B. (1971): Relationship of hyperparathyroidism to multiple endocrine adenomatosis. *Birth Defects,* 7(6):66–68.
5. Knudson, A. G., Jr., and Strong, L. C. (1972): Mutation and cancer. Neuroblastoma and pheochromocytoma. *Am. J. Hum. Genet.,* 24:514–532.
6. Mallette, L. E., Bilezikian, J. P., Ketcham, A. S., and Aurbach, G. D. (1974): Parathyroid carcinoma in familial hyperparathyroidism. *Am. J. Med.,* 57:642–648.
7. Ptak, T., and Kirsner, J. B. (1970): The Zollinger–Ellison syndrome, polyendocrine adenomatosis and other endocrine associations with peptic ulcer. *Adv. Intern. Med.,* 16:213–242.
8. Steiner, A. L., Goodman, A. D., and Powers, S. R. (1968): Study of a kindred with pheochromocytoma, medullary thyroid carcinoma, hyperparathyroidism, and Cushing's disease: Multiple endocrine neoplasia type 2. *Medicine (Baltimore)* 47:371–409.
9. Wolfe, H. J., Melvin, K. E. W., Cervi-Skinner, S. J. AlSaadi, A. A., Juliar, J. F., Jackson, C. E., and Tashjian. A. H. (1973): C-cell hyperplasia preceding medullary thyroid carcinoma. *N. Engl. J. Med.,* 289:437–441.

Genetics of Human Cancer, edited by J. J. Mulvihill, R. W. Miller, and J. F. Fraumeni, Jr. Raven Press, New York, 1977.

17

Malignant Neoplasms in Heterozygous Carriers of Genes for Certain Autosomal Recessive Syndromes

Michael Swift

Department of Medicine and the Biological Sciences Research Center, University of North Carolina, Chapel Hill, North Carolina 27514

Is there a relationship between rare single gene syndromes and the cancers which account for so much illness and death in the general population? Our research group has employed a particular strategy to identify and study genes which may predispose in subtle fashion a substantial proportion of the population to malignant disease (9-11).

Associations between specific autosomal recessive syndromes and cancer have been recognized through case reports which, taken together, showed that the homozygous affected individuals were extraordinarily likely to die from a malignancy (1-8,12). Some of the reports of malignant neoplasms in patients with Fanconi anemia (FA) or ataxia telangiectasia (AT) also noted similar tumors in close relatives (3,5,6,12). These relatives had no signs of the particular recessive syndrome and had to be heterozygous for the FA or AT gene if they carried it at all.

ESTIMATES OF HETEROZYGOTE FREQUENCY

Heterozygotes for rare autosomal recessive syndromes are, according to the Hardy-Weinberg principle, relatively common in the general population. Homozygotes with AT may occur as often as one in 40,000 births (8); from this, heterozygotes are estimated to be 1% of the population. Homozygotes with the Werner syndrome may be as rare as one in a million (2), but heterozygotes for the Werner syndrome gene would still be about 0.2% of the population. Thus, if a gene for an autosomal recessive syndrome predisposed the heterozygote to cancer, this gene would be, on a numerical basis alone, an important neoplasia-predisposing gene.

FAMILY STUDIES OF HETEROZYGOTE RISK

It is not yet possible to measure directly the risk of cancer and leukemia for heterozygous carriers of the genes under consideration. There are no tests to identify heterozygotes for these genes among cancer patients or among members of the general population. Since such heterozygotes are, however, common along close relatives of homozygous probands, we chose to compare the incidence of malignant neoplasms in families of patients with recessive syndromes associated with carcinoma, lymphoma, and leukemia in the homozygote to the incidence in the general population. We developed statistical methods which gave each relative a proper weight according to his or her relationship to the homozygous proband. These methods extract from the family data an estimate of the cancer risk associated with the gene under study (10).

DEATHS FROM MALIGNANT NEOPLASMS IN FAMILIES OF PATIENTS WITH FA OR AT

FA is a multisystem disease occurring about once in 350,000 births. In eight families of patients with FA, we found 25 deaths from malignancy among 102 deaths, significantly more than the 15.6 expected (9). For blood relatives of patients with AT (11), we found an increase in deaths from all types of malignancy, primarily in younger persons (Table 1). There were 329 deaths from all causes in 27 AT families. Below age 75, there were 59 deaths from malignant neoplasms (42.6 expected); below age 45, 15 of the deaths were from malignancy (5.2 expected). There were actually fewer deaths from cancer than expected in persons dying after 75 years of age.

ARE DEATHS FROM CANCER ASSOCIATED WITH THE AT GENE?

The increased proportion of deaths from malignant neoplasm among FA or AT families could have come from familial factors apart from the gene on which we focus. The AT family data provide some evidence, however, that the increased risk of cancer is associated with the AT gene. First, we found fewer deaths than expected from malignant neoplasms among spouse controls, persons who are not blood relatives but share the same ethnic, social, and environmental settings as the

TABLE 1. *Deaths from malignant neoplasms in 27 families of AT patients*[a]

	From all causes		From malignant neoplasms	
	Observed	Expected	Observed	Expected
All ages	329	330.3	67	52.6
≤75 years	—	—	59	42.6 ($p<0.02$)
≤45 years	—	—	15	5.2 ($p<0.001$)

[a] From ref. 11.

TABLE 2. *The distribution of deaths from malignant neoplasms in AT families by probability of heterozygosity*[a]

	Probability of heterozygosity						
	1.0		0.5		0.25		0.00 (Spouse controls)
	O	E	O	E	O	E	O	E
	3	1.2	25	14.5	39	37.0	11	20.5
O/E	2.5		1.72		1.05		0.54	

[a]O, observed deaths from malignant neoplasms; E, expected deaths.

blood relatives (Table 2). Second, the ratio of observed to expected deaths from malignant neoplasms increased along with increasing probability of heterozygosity for the AT gene. Goodness-of-fit tests showed that a model which assumes an increased risk associated with the AT gene fits the observed data much better than does a model which assumes that the entire population sample had an increased risk of dying from cancer or leukemia.

PROPORTION OF FA OR AT HETEROZYGOTES AMONG ALL PERSONS DYING FROM CANCER

Estimates of relative risk (Table 3) are useful for estimating what proportion of all cancer and leukemia patients carry either the FA or AT genes. For a particular

TABLE 3. *Estimates of relative risk and of the proportion of FA or AT heterozygotes among all persons dying from cancer or leukemia*[a]

Type of malignancy	Estimate of relative risk	Estimated proportion of FA or AT heterozygotes among all persons with that malignancy
Fanconi anemia (estimated heterozygote frequency 0.0033)		
All	3	0.01
Acute leukemia	12	0.04
Ataxia-telangiectasia (estimated heterozygote frequency 0.01)		
All	2	0.02
All (<45 years)	5.5	0.055
Ovarian (≤55 years)	10	0.1
Lymphopoietic (≤45 years)	7	0.07
Gastric (≤75 years)	8	0.08
Biliary system	6	0.06
Other autosomal recessive syndromes associated with malignancy (heterozygote frequencies 0.001—0.01)		
All	?	?

[a] From refs. 9-11.

gene this proportion is estimated by the product of the relative risk and the heterozygote frequency. If our interpretation of the AT family data is correct, over 5% of all persons dying before age 45 from any malignancy may carry the AT gene. Perhaps 3% of persons dying from a malignancy at any age carry either an FA or AT gene.

INDIVIDUAL NEOPLASMS ASSOCIATED WITH THE AT OR FA GENE

Our family studies may detect associations between a gene and a particular type of neoplasm. It is important, however, to be cautious in accepting such associations, not only because of the small number in each tumor category but also because most of these possible associations were detected in a retrospective examination of the family data. For certain neoplasms—those noted in the FA or AT homozygotes, for example—an association may be hypothesized in advance and, if the data support it, accepted with greater confidence. The association of a particular type of neoplasm with a given gene may also be suspected if that neoplasm occurred unusually frequently in obligatory heterozygotes or in blood relatives who died at an early age.

In the original survey of FA families (9), the incidence of gastrointestinal malignancies and leukemias was higher than expected and, although the sample was small, we found three carcinomas of the base of the tongue. AT heterozygotes seemed to be predisposed to lymphoproliferative and ovarian malignancies in younger persons and to gastric carcinomas at all ages. It is notable that, among 329 total deaths in the AT families, five blood relatives died from biliary system carcinomas (11). The AT gene may also predispose to breast, cervical, uterine, and colonic carcinomas. Persons with the AT or FA gene may constitute 5 to 10% of all individuals who develop a specific type of malignancy.

Although over 90% of the data from 30 xeroderma pigmentosum (XP) families has been collected, no final statement can be made about the incidence of malignant neoplasms in these families. Based on a preliminary analysis, there is no evidence for an overall increase in risk of cancer deaths for XP heterozygotes. There are a large number of skin cancers in these 30 families—I am not aware of previous reports commenting on this—but our evaluation of the skin cancer risk for XP heterozygotes will depend on a careful consideration of the epidemiological characteristics of the families (e.g., ethnic origin, place of residence) and on a comparison of the incidence of skin cancers in the spouse controls with that of the blood relatives.

We have begun collecting data from a new group of 30 FA families in order to validate our method and to test the conclusions of the original small scale FA family study. While only a small proportion of the death certificates have been collected in the new study, we have already found two additional deaths from pharyngeal carcinomas in blood relatives of FA patients. Appreciation of the relationship between a particular gene and neoplasm may add a needed dimension to laboratory and epidemiological studies of the pathogenesis of that neoplasm.

Although the hypothesis that heterozygous carriers of genes for certain autosomal recessive syndromes comprise a substantial proportion of all persons genetically predisposed to cancer is supported by the family studies reported here, it is important to try to measure more directly the cancer risk associated with each of these genes. For FA and AT, homozygous fibroblast cultures probably provide the best tool for elucidating the biochemical abnormality determined by each of these genes. We do not yet understand the action of the AT or FA genes well enough to devise a reliable test for heterozygous carriers or to determine how these genes predispose to specific neoplasms.

The usefulness of our conjecture that certain autosomal recessive syndromes identify important neoplasia-predisposing genes depends, in part, on the number of these syndromes. Our research group is currently developing methods for identifying the recessive syndromes most promising for future study. We are continuing family studies of syndromes already known to be associated with leukemia and other cancers in homozygotes, and have begun metabolic investigations of genes which, based on family data, are important in predisposing a substantial proportion of the general population to malignant disease.

REFERENCES

1. Dunn, H. G., Meuwissen, H., Livingstone, C. S., and Pump, K. K. (1964): Ataxia-telangiectasia. *Can. Med. Assoc. J.*, 91:1106–1118.
2. Epstein, C. J., Martin, G. M., Schultz, A. L., and Motulsky, A. G. (1966): Werner's syndrome: A review of its symptomatology, natural history, pathologic features, genetics and relationship to the natural aging process. *Medicine*, 45:177–221.
3. Garriga, S., and Crosby, W. H. (1959): The incidence of leukemia in families of patients with hypoplasia of the marrow. *Blood*, 14:1008–1014.
4. German, J. (1969): Bloom's syndrome. I. Genetical and clinical observations in the first twenty-seven patients. *Am. J. Hum. Genet.*, 21:196–227.
5. Haerer, A. F., Jackson, J. F., and Evers, C. G. (1969): Ataxia-telangiectasia with gastric adenocarcinoma. *JAMA*, 210:1884–1887.
6. Reed, W. B., Epstein, W. L., Boder, E., and Sedgwick, R. (1966): Cutaneous manifestations of ataxia-telangiectasia. *JAMA*, 195:746–753.
7. Robbins, J. H., Kraemer, K. H., Lutzner, M. A., Festoff, B. W., and Coon, H. G. (1974): Xeroderma pigmentosum: An inherited disease with sun sensitivity, multiple cutaneous neoplasms, and abnormal DNA repair. *Ann. Intern. Med.*, 80:221–248.
8. Sedgwick, R. P., and Boder, E. (1972): Ataxia-telangiectasia. In: *Handbook of Clinical Neurology*, Vol. 14, edited by P. J. Vinken and G. W. Bruyn, pp. 267-339. American Elsevier, New York.
9. Swift, M. (1971): Fanconi's anemia in the genetics of neoplasia. *Nature*, 230:370–373.
10. Swift, M., Cohen, J., and Pinkham, R. (1974): A maximum likelihood method for the disease predisposition of heterozygotes. *Am. J. Hum. Genet.*, 26:304–317.
11. Swift, M., Sholman, L., Perry, M., and Chase, C. (1976): Malignant neoplasms in the families of patients with ataxia-telangiectasia. *Cancer Res.*, 36:209–215.
12. Swift, M. R., Zimmerman, D., and McDonough, E. R. (1971): Squamous cell carcinomas in Fanconi's anemia. *JAMA*, 216:325–327.

Discussion

Gerald: Are you making use of those areas of the world where there is a high incidence of certain rare recessive disorders, such as xeroderma pigmentosum (XP) in North Africa, and ataxia-telangiectasia (AT) in Israel?

Swift: We are in touch with Dr. Maimon Cohen about studying AT in Israel. We have had a hard time finding XP families in the United States; if the risk of noncutaneous tumors is unremarkable here, it would probably not be worth going abroad.

Gerald: Would Egypt, with its tropical climate, be a better place to study XP?

Swift: It would be good for studying skin cancer, but not for studying other malignancies. Also, foreign travel is costly.

Littlefield: What is the status of chromosome studies in the heterozygotes for Bloom's and Fanconi's syndromes and for AT?

Swift: There are no conclusive data for Fanconi's anemia heterozygotes. Dr. Cohen has some data that indicate that the chromosomes of AT heterozygotes have clear-cut aberrations in fibroblast and leukocyte cultures [*Am. J. Hum. Genet.,* 27:27a (1975)]. Dr. German has the most extensive experience with chromosome preparations from Bloom's syndrome heterozygotes. Perhaps he will comment on his findings.

However, we should not limit our interest to the chromosome fragility syndromes. Those are the obvious ones to start with, but there may be a host of recessively inherited syndromes to which we should pay attention. I wish also to stress that we are informing the families with AT in our studies of our results. The close relatives of AT patients can decide for themselves whether our data are sufficient for their purpose.

Knudson: I greatly admire your work, Dr. Swift, and I think it is very important. However, I wonder if the risk of cancer is even greater among AT heterozygotes because of the generally young age at which they develop cancer. If an age-specific incidence curve for all cancers were constructed for a large enough group of first degree relatives of the proband and then compared at given ages with that of a normal population, the risk in relatives should be greater.

Swift: All our data are age-corrected. Dr. Mary Daly analyzed the age patterns in incidence and found that the usual childhood peak is most exaggerated in the AT families and that another peak develops at about age 35 to 50. Although our data are barely sufficient to subdivide by age, we found that below age 45 the risk appeared to be 5.5 times normal, whereas above it the risk was about twice normal. Beyond age 75 there were actually fewer deaths than expected. The only exception was for cancer of the biliary system, where deaths occurred in the usual age range, that is, in the late 60s and 70s. The other tumors developed at a younger age.

Nance: How do you account for the markedly decreased incidence of cancer among spouse controls in the AT study? Is it an ascertainment problem?

Swift: We failed to get only four out of 329 death certificates from the blood relatives, but the recovery of data was slightly poorer for the spouse controls. This may account for the apparent decreased risk for cancer in the spouses. The other possibility is that our sample was derived from a group that had base-line cancer rates lower than the standard population rates. If this is the case, we may be underestimating the relative risk for the AT heterozygote.

Nance: Could it also result from overreporting in the AT relatives? This is certainly a common source of bias in family studies.

Swift: We were able to use 325 of 329 death certificates, and our control data are based on death certificates, so I cannot see how we could be overreporting.

Hirayama: How did you calculate the expected numbers?

Swift: We simply applied the age-, sex-, race-, and time-specific death rates to the study population to obtain expected mortality experience for various causes of death.

Hirayama: You mentioned race-specific rates, but how do you account for migration and ethnic differences?

Swift: Dr. Mary Daly has investigated that important question. She found, for example, that a number of deaths from gastric carcinoma occurred in people from Scandinavia. In that part of the world the risk of gastric carcinoma is increased; this trend is maintained even among individuals who migrate to the United States. Dr. Daly showed that, even if our entire study group had been Scandinavian, this variable could not explain the increase in risk.

Genetics of Human Cancer, edited by J. J.
Mulvihill, R. W. Miller, and J. F. Fraumeni, Jr.
Raven Press, New York, 1977.

18

A Statistician's Viewpoint of Familial Cancer

Edmond A. Murphy

*Department of Medicine, Johns Hopkins University School of Medicine, Baltimore,
Maryland 21205*

My point of departure is genetics, and my concern is to find how statistics may help our endeavor. Those of us who have data to publish are perpetually concerned with two questions. What can be inferred from the data? And how much detail should be published? There is no answer to either question which is universally applicable: I propose to discuss briefly why not, and how to approach the individual case. I want to deal with two related matters.

MOMENT, PARAMETER, AND BIOLOGIC HYPOTHESIS

First, I shall discuss the distinction between a moment and a parameter. It is an unfortunate coincidence that for the three most widely used distributions—the normal, the binomial and the Poisson—the moments usually computed are direct sample estimates of the parameters, i.e., of the distinctive constants of the distribution. It so happens that, for the normal, the mean and the variance are exactly equal to the centrality and dispersion parameters; for the binomial, the expected proportion of successes is exactly equal to the probability of success. A colleague and I wrote a paper designed to solve a paradox arising from a confusion between a parameter and a moment (2) which was rejected by one journal with the comment that the distinction was "captious," although failure to recognize the difference had led to a great deal of confusion in genetic counseling. Those who never have occasion to use other than those three distributions may fail to grasp the distinction between moment and parameter altogether. Yet such identity of moments and parameters is exceptional; and in general, constructing estimates of parameters may be much more demanding.

To those who suppose all dichotomous data to follow a binomial distribution, it comes as a shock to find that there can be any more to analysis than finding the proportion affected, complete with standard errors which have been incorrectly calculated. This simplistic attitude is distressingly common even among epidemiologists. Despite the existence of an elaborate theory of epidemics, most reports dealing with infectious diseases are based on the idea that proportions are all that is needed. This error is most obvious in analyses of data on the evidence of cancer such as that of the uterine cervix in which the writer attempts to defend the theory of an infectious etiology. If true, the claim would show that the method of proof is invalid.

Those of us who view familial aggregation from a *genetic* standpoint are appalled by reports which deal promiscuously with recurrence risks in something called "first degree relatives." It is as if there were no such thing as sex-linkage or as if the differences did not exist between parent-child and sib-sib covariance which were so carefully laid out by Fisher (1) nearly 60 years ago.

However, these are technical matters. There is a deeper, more subtle issue. Whether the ultimate components of the universe are dichotomous we may never know; but it is clear that the crude enumerations used in the study of familial cancer are certainly not these ultimate components. The outcomes represent complicated processes, and an analysis implying that all we should be considering is presence or absence of a result is archeology, not science. A merely enumerative approach to familial occurrence of erythroblastosis fetalis would have squandered almost all the useful information. Variance among families may be at least as enlightening as the overall mean. If we conceive cancer as a multiple-hit process or an intricate conjunction of somatic mutation and a lapse in immunological surveillance, little will come of trying to contain the empirical data in any such naive statistic. One would expect much more interest than there is in age of onset of manifest disease, for example, not only because it is indispensable for segregation analysis or even the crudest epidemiological enquiry, but because there may be significant information in the components of variance within and among families. Veale's surmise that there may be a modifier gene affecting the age of onset of Gardner's syndrome (3) is an excellent example.

Finally, one may note that there are distributions with well-defined parameters but with no moments whatsoever. If there are no true moments, it seems to make no sense whatsoever trying to estimate them.

Thus, I see a major endeavor in an analysis to be the development of *biological* hypotheses which lead to their own distinctive procedure for estimation and confirmation or disproof. If the biostatistician will not at least collaborate in this task, his position will be usurped by those who will; and in my opinion this is as it should be, even if the quality of the statistical analysis has to suffer.

THE SUFFICIENT STATISTIC AND THE BIOLOGIC MODEL

We come then to the second question. What detail should be furnished about the results of a study? The problem is complicated. Statistical theory has developed the notion of what are called sufficient statistics which are a pure distillation of all the pertinent information contained in the sample. For instance, suppose there were doubts about the fairness of a coin, and we wished to estimate the probability of heads by tossing the coin a thousand times. The *number* of times the coin came up heads would be a sufficient statistic: it would be irrelevant *which* tosses came up heads. Therefore, it would be unnecessary to publish the results of each toss in the *Journal of Numismatics*.

The example I quote is a binomial process and so long as we are assured or are prepared to assume that this model is sound, we can, in many cases, find sufficient statistics. If we conjecture that a trait is an autosomal dominant and the object is to test it formally, then the proportion of children at risk who are affected is a sufficient statistic, and sex, birth order, and age are irrelevant and need not be recorded. But for an X-linked disorder, this would not do: We would have need of four sufficient statistics according to the sex of the parent with the mutant gene and the sex of the child. However, birth order and family size would be irrelevant. Birth order would matter if there is maternal-fetal interaction, family size if there is ascertainment bias, age in an abiotrophy, ethnic background is relevant in linkage analysis where genotypes are ambiguous, and so forth.

The geneticist does well to know both the advantages and the limitations of the idea of the sufficient statistic. The theoretical advantages are expounded in textbooks on statistical theory; the practical disadvantages are not. For example, a statistic sufficient under one model will not in general be sufficient under another. The sample mean is sufficient for the centrality parameter of the normal distribution, but not of the log-normal. The two most extreme values are of little importance for a multiple-hit model but are the only quantities of any importance for the rectangular distribution.

Thus, the analyst who presumes to use and publish sufficient statistics rather than the entire data must take responsibility for the aptness of the model for which the sufficient statistics were prescribed. The problem is that some geneticist may subsequently set up a conjecture for which the published statistics are not sufficient. For example, there is some discussion about familial aggregation of common cancers. If it is a true bill, it might be Mendelizing but with hypostasis, or low penetrance; it might be autosomal or X-linked, cytoplasmic, multilocal, or even cultural. I need hardly point out that conformity of the data to a model is not enough to constitute final proof of the model's aptness. The same data may fit a dozen quite different models adequately. The point is that as the model changes the moments will remain the same, but the parametrization will change and therefore, the sufficient statistics. A publication which is narrowly focused on one model may furnish a limited set of moments which are incidentally sufficient for that model but not for others. It may then be difficult or impossible to reconstruct the information in the sample which is pertinent to some other model.

What, then, should be published? In brief, as much as the editors will allow, and the rest should be made available, in the National Archives if necessary. Editors, so disposed, can have their contributors both ways. If they furnish much detail, the editor can reject a paper because of length. If they furnish little, the editor may reject it because of ellipsis. I have never discovered any rational policy on the point which editorial policies pursue. Perhaps we should try to educate them.

REFERENCES

1. Fisher, R. A. (1918): The correlation between relatives on the supposition of Mendelian inheritance. *Trans. R. Soc. Edin.*, 52:399.

2. Murphy, E. A., and Chase, G. A. (1975): *Principles of Genetic Counseling.* Year Book Medical Publishers, Chicago, Ill.

3. Veale, A. M. O. (1960): Clinical and genetic problems in familial intestinal polyposis. *Gut,* 1:285–290.

Discussion

Miller: How would you evaluate the material on cancer-prone families that Dr. Fraumeni describes [*this volume*]? Is it worth publishing?

Murphy: I think information of this kind is highly important and may be extremely enlightening. It is very difficult in many instances to come up with formal tests of any genetic hypothesis on the basis of this type of data unless there is an unusually carefully documented procedure by which the cases are actually ascertained. For example, if you are dealing with autosomal recessive inheritance, there is a widely used, well-established theory, which was worked out a long time ago, that adjusts for ascertainment bias in these cases. However, when you are dealing with dominant inheritance, the situation is much more complicated. I think there is general agreement that it is best to collect the data systematically. But if you cannot do so, at least keep track of how it was collected and do plastic surgery afterward.

Skolnick: To solve the problems of knowing how a family was ascertained (because sometimes one hears of a number of cases at once), we are trying to put together the genealogy of the entire state of Utah which we hope to link to a tumor registry so that the familial cancer cases can be studied in the context of the other cancer cases in the population [see chapter 3, *this volume*]. I think only in this fashion can we relate such cancer families to the etiology of, say, breast or colon cancer in general.

Murphy: When you have total ascertainment of cases in the population, the problem of handling bias is more simple than when you only have a sample of the population for which the ground rules of sampling have not been clearly spelled out. Even in the first situation, many problems will exist, but they will be logical problems rather than uncertainties as to what has been left out and what precisely the biases are.

Miller: May I ask Dr. Fraumeni, now that he has heard the perfect scientific design described by Dr. Murphy, what good are his own studies?

Fraumeni: There is one other population-based data resource linking genealogic and cancer information that Dr. Murphy would probably agree should be pursued. In Iceland, studies are underway by the International Agency for Research on Cancer, which ordinarily focuses on environmental studies of cancer, to assess the risk of cancer in families. A preliminary communication suggests confirmation of Dr. Anderson's estimates of increased familial risk of breast cancer that had been determined from a hospital-based series. So perhaps the biases and artifacts that are involved in the sampling of hospital-based patients are not so serious after all.

Miller: Yes, but what good comes of studying catch-as-catch-can families that are referred by mail or phone, without any population or hospital base?

Fraumeni: We are concerned primarily with striking family aggregations of cancer, and these events are infrequent in the experience of a single physician or hospital. Despite the absence of a population base, it is possible to identify syndromes in which different tumors appear together in families. This is especially true if the tumors are ordinarily rare, such as sarcomas and adrenocortical neoplasms. By identifying meaningful associations between tumors, we may learn something about common susceptibility mechanisms.

In addition, these families provide a resource to identify mechanisms of susceptibility by interdisciplinary laboratory studies [W. A. Blattner, *this volume*]. If we were to limit ourselves to the patient experience of a given hospital or area, we might have to wait quite a while to identify a cancer family syndrome for study.

Nance: I wonder whether you have observed an increased incidence of congenital malformations or abnormal pregnancy outcome in these multiple-case families?

Fraumeni: In some family aggregations of cancer, particularly the ones that have involved children, we have seen some minor but tantalizing birth defects in the form of hamartomatous lesions. At present, these defects are ill defined, and we cannot put them together into any previously defined syndrome. We have not noted a tendency to pregnancy wastage in these families.

Genetics of Human Cancer, edited by J. J. Mulvihill, R. W. Miller, and J. F. Fraumeni, Jr. Raven Press, New York, 1977.

19

Clinical Patterns of Familial Cancer

Joseph F. Fraumeni, Jr.

Environmental Epidemiology Branch, National Cancer Institute, Bethesda, Maryland 20014

The epidemiologic patterns of cancer have suggested to many observers that the environment contributes more to cancer risk than do genetic factors. Perhaps in most patients, the role of inherited susceptibility and the interactions with environmental influences are too subtle or complex to be detected by ordinary epidemiologic means. On occasion, when susceptibility is conspicuous as in cancer-prone families, research opportunities are provided that may clarify the role of genetic mechanisms in carcinogenesis.

MONOGENIC SYNDROMES

A small but increasing percentage of cancers are being recognized which exhibit Mendelian patterns of inheritance. Mulvihill (31; Chapter 11) recently identified 161 single-gene traits with neoplastic or preneoplastic manifestations.

Hereditary Neoplasms

The hereditary neoplasms are autosomal dominant traits which seem to be the direct expression of an inherited defect (2,7,21,31). As a rule, the hereditary neoplasms are less common than are nonfamilial occurrences of the same tumor, and they tend to develop earlier in life and from multiple foci within affected organs. The tumors may be the sole manifestation of the gene defect, such as in retinoblastoma, intestinal polyposis, and chemodectoma; or part of a wider biologic disturbance, such as the nevoid basal cell carcincoma sydrome, medullary thyroid carcinoma with pheochromocytoma, Gardner syndrome, and esophageal carcinoma with tylosis.

Hamartomatous Syndromes

In other Mendelian syndromes, the gene defect results in a preneoplastic state which in turn carries a high risk of cancer. Some fall into the category of the phacomatoses or hamartomatous syndromes (37). In affected individuals several organs show structural defects of development which lead to benign growths (hamartomas) and occasionally to cancer. Like the hereditary neoplasms, these syndromes are dominantly inherited and may underlie familial occurrences of cancer. They include multiple neurofibromatosis and tuberous sclerosis, which are associated with tumors of the nervous system; von Hippel-Lindau syndrome, with hypernephroma or pheochromocytoma; multiple exostoses, with chondrosarcoma; and Peutz-Jeghers syndrome, with granulosa-cell tumors of the ovary. Recently described is the "multiple hamartoma syndrome" of Cowden, which consists of oral papillomas, cystic mastopathy with breast cancer, thyroid adenoma and carcinoma, colonic polyps, lipomas, and other lesions (3).

In some families, the usual stigmata of hamartomatous disorders may be inconspicuous, while the associated cancer is prominent. For example, hypernephroma-prone families may show limited signs of the von Hippel-Lindau syndrome (35), and families prone to glioma (22) or acoustic neuroma (38) may have barely discernible manifestations of neurofibromatosis. These observations suggest that some family aggregations of cancer are due to variants of the genes for hamartomatous disorders, with malignant tumors expressed instead of the benign growths that are usually seen.

Immunodeficiency Syndromes

In another group of preneoplastic disorders, the common feature is primary immunodeficiency (19). Three recessively inherited syndromes are well known— X-linked (Bruton) agammaglobulinemia, ataxia telangiectasia (AT), and Wiskott-Aldrich syndrome. These disorders predispose to cancer, primarily lymphoma, which may aggregate in siblings. Familial occurrence of lymphoid tumors may also be linked to immune defects of a more subtle nature, as suggested by laboratory studies of clinically normal individuals from high-risk families (15,16). The abnormalities may represent a subclinical counterpart of the syndrome "common variable immunodeficiency." Immunologic impairment and susceptibility to lymphoid neoplasms occur in a variety of familial patterns, some of which are compatible with dominant (16) and others with recessive (34) inheritance.

Families at high risk of nonlymphoid neoplasms have shown no consistent evidence of defective immunity. An exception may be stomach cancer; cellular immune defects and antibodies to gastric parietal cells were unusually common in an inbred family prone to this cancer (5), and an apparent excess of stomach cancer has been reported (Chapter 30, *this volume*) in patients with primary immunodeficiency who survive beyond childhood.

FAMILIAL CANCER

Tumor-Specific Aggregation

While the rare hereditary neoplastic syndromes have striking patterns of Mendelian inheritance, the common cancers of man have small familial tendencies. In general, the risk of the same neoplasm developing in a close relative of a cancer patient is about three times greater than would be expected in the general population (2,7). This estimate is based on surveys of empiric risk for cancers of the breast, stomach, colon, endometrium, prostate and lung, and for leukemia. Recent studies have provided evidence of even greater familial risk among subgroups of patients with various cancers, particularly embryonal tumors of childhood and cancers of the breast and colon (2). In families in which tumors develop at a younger-than-usual age or at multiple foci, the risk for unaffected relatives may be 20 to 30 times greater than in the general population.

Occasionally, the familial clusters of specific cancers are pronounced and segregate in a pattern matching or exceeding expectations of autosomal dominant inheritance. Usually there is no evidence of an underlying monogenic syndrome; this is illustrated by several families in which colorectal carcinoma developed in the absence of multiple polyposis (11). We have reported on a number of families with tumor-specific aggregation, including cancers of the bladder (13), ovary (25), stomach (5), and male breast (6), and hepatoblastoma (12), acute myelogenous leukemia (33), chronic lymphocytic leukemia (15), and Hodgkin's disease (4). Sometimes the familial aggregation affords an opportunity to detect and treat early cancer in high-risk individuals; it also provides a resource for etiologic studies that may give insights into the mechanisms of cancer susceptibility and pathogenesis.

Multiple Cancer Syndromes

In statistical surveys of familial risk, the data have been insufficient to determine whether certain cancers coexist excessively in close relatives. Pedigree studies of high-risk families, however, have provided mounting clinical evidence for familial syndromes of multiple cancers.

Familial Adenocarcinomatosis

Lynch and his colleagues (28) reported on a series of families prone to adenocarcinomas arising from various sites, particularly the colon and endometrium. The tumors tend to occur at an early age in adults and to develop as multiple primaries in certain individuals. Our experience with this syndrome includes a pedigree (Fig. 1) in which stomach cancer was part of the aggregation. This observation is consistent with reports linking gastric and colon adenocarcinomas in some families (27).

In other adenocarcinoma-prone families, involvement of the ovary and breast is common. After the report of a family aggregation of ovarian adenocarcinoma (25), six similar families were brought to light, including three with a concurrent cluster of breast cancer (9). The exceptional risk of ovarian cancer in such families has prompted prophylactic oophorectomy, and in some cases the microscopic sections of ovary indicated epithelial and mesothelial abnormalities that may portend neoplastic change.

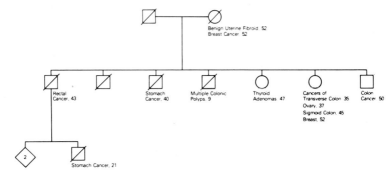

FIG. 1. Pedigree of family prone to multiple adenocarcinomas with ages at diagnosis.

No family syndromes have been identified that link other cell types of carcinoma. In general, it seems that familial concentrations of cancer—at single or multiple sites—are much more pronounced for adenocarcinomas (e.g., breast, ovary, endometrium, stomach, and colon) than for squamous or transitional-cell carcinomas (e.g., lung, cervix, esophagus, and bladder). This may reflect differences in the relative contributions of genetic and environmental determinants, or in the mechanisms by which these factors interact to produce various cell lines of carcinoma.

Familial Cancer of Diverse Cell Types

The concept of "cancer families" has been broadened recently to encompass familial occurrences of neoplasms of very dissimilar cell types, including childhood cancers. Our first encounter with such a family occurred in 1966 when a boy was admitted to the National Cancer Institute with histiocytic lymphoma and a history of rectal bleeding (14). A sister had retroperitoneal liposarcoma, a brother had multiple adenomatous polyps with carcinoma of the large bowel, and the father had an osteogenic sarcoma arising in the lung. Sigmoidoscopy and barium enema revealed scattered polyps in the patient with lymphoma. Although we speculated about some variant of intestinal polyposis or Gardner syndrome, the significance of the family aggregation was unclear at the time.

In 1969, studies of childhood rhabdomyosarcoma, reviewed by Li (*this volume*), identified a familial syndrome of soft-tissue sarcomas, breast cancer and other neoplasms affecting children and young adults (23,24). In some families the children were prone not only to soft-tissue sarcomas but also to brain tumors, adrenocortical neoplasms, and osteosarcoma (Fig. 2). The familial tendency to multiple cancer was seen to a lesser degree in a study of childhood osteosarcoma (17). Figure 3 shows two pedigrees in which osteosarcoma in a child occurred in association with other tumors, particularly of the nervous system, in siblings and parents. Further insight into multiple cancer syndromes in children was provided by Miller (30) from a national survey of cancer deaths. The sibs of children with brain tumors had not only an increased risk of the same tumors, but also an excess of sarcomas originating from the bone or muscle.

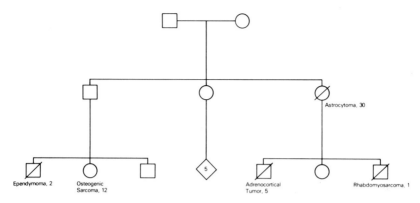

FIG. 2. Pedigree of family prone to sarcomas and other cancers with ages at diagnosis.

Recent experience suggests that some families are prone to diverse childhood cancers in the absence of sarcoma (26). Figure 4 shows the pedigrees of two families with sib aggregations of brain tumor, lymphoma, and other tumors. Various benign lesions of a hamartomatous nature were seen in certain affected children. No known hereditary syndromes have been identified, although some manifestations suggest possible variants of neurofibromatosis, AT, or the multiple hamartoma syndrome. These preliminary observations suggest that in these families the predisposition to certain cancers is associated with a generalized developmental disorder that includes hamartomatous manifestations. Additional studies are needed to delineate the syndrome.

Relation to Multiple Primary Neoplasia

Among 62 children with adrenocortical neoplasms reported in 1967, two had second primaries originating in the brain (10). Subsequently, a third child in the original survey was found who had survived the adrenocortical neoplasm but later died at age 19 of glioblastoma multiforme. One sib of this child had osteosarcoma, a second had chondrosarcoma, and the mother had bilateral breast cancer (Fig. 5). Thus, adrenocortical and brain tumors represent a tumor complex that is expressed in individuals as multiple primaries, and in families as part of a genetically regulated constellation of related neoplasms.

In adults also, multiple cancers may aggregate in one person or appear separately in different family members. This is seen, for example, in associations between cancers of the breast and ovary, or cancers of the colon and endometrium (8). A new syndrome of multiple tumors was suggested recently by the excessive concurrence of thyroid adenoma in a series of young women with ovarian arrhenoblastoma and in families predisposed to arrhenoblastoma (18). Perhaps on the basis of a common genetic predisposition, various combinations of cancers that occur excessively as double primaries also seem to aggregate excessively in close relatives (Fig. 6). Surveys of multiple primary neoplasms complement family studies as

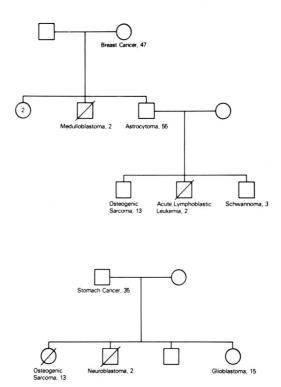

FIG. 3. Pedigrees of two families prone to osteosarcoma, tumors of nervous system and other sites with ages at diagnosis.

means of identifying etiologic relationships between cancers, and also extend opportunities for diagnostic surveillance and etiologic research in cancer.

CONCLUSIONS

Familial occurrences of cancer usually suggest genetic susceptibility, but with such a common disease the role of chance must always be considered as an explanation. This becomes less likely, of course, when families have an exceptional concentration of tumors on a line of descent, or conform to the known clinical syndromes of familial cancer. In the absence of these situations, however, it is often difficult to determine if a given family with multiple tumors has biologic meaning or represents a coincidence. Nevertheless, such families should be reported in some manner with the hope of encouraging related observations.

Consideration should be given also to the role of environmental factors in familial cancer. Some aggregations may be due to common exposures to chemicals, as illustrated by a report of familial leukemia following occupational contact with benzene (1). Infectious agents are suspected in families prone to liver cancer and with serological evidence of hepatitis B infection (32), and in families in

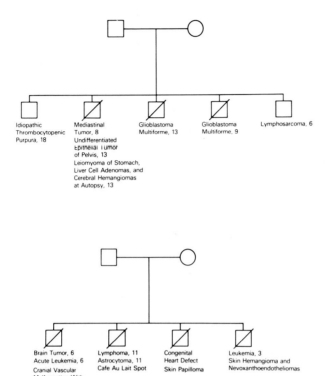

FIG. 4. Pedigrees of two families prone to childhood neoplasms arising from the brain, lymphoid and hematopoietic system, and to harmartomatous growths, with ages at diagnosis.

which two or more members develop Hodgkin's disease within a brief time period (29). It seems likely that interactions between genetic and environmental factors are involved in the familial susceptibility to many cancers. This is suggested by a study of lung cancer that showed a synergism in risks from familial predisposition and cigarette smoking (36). Although most family cancer syndromes are transmitted vertically in a pattern compatible with autosomal dominant

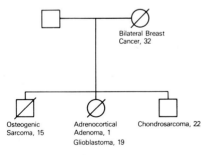

FIG. 5. Pedigree of family prone to bone sarcomas, breast cancer, and tumors of adrenal cortex and brain, with ages at diagnosis.

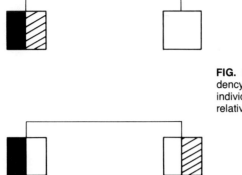

FIG. 6. Diagrammatic illustration of the tendency for the same multiple primary cancers in individuals *(above)* to arise separately in close relatives *(below)*.

inheritance (20), the frequency of cancer sometimes seems to exceed the number expected by this genetic mechanism. Although extranuclear inheritance, virus transmission, or other factors may be involved, these unusual concentrations of cancer are probably related to the selection bias of investigators who are drawn toward the exceptional pedigrees.

Genetic factors may contribute not only to familial tendencies but also to single occurrences of cancer in a family. This point is worth emphasizing with the growing trend toward smaller families in our society. In the absence of familial aggregation, genetic predisposition to cancer may be suspected among patients with early onset of cancer or with multiple primary neoplasms, but recognition of a susceptibility state will not be precise until appropriate biological markers are developed in the laboratory.

REFERENCES

1. Aksoy, M., Erdem, S., Erdogan, G., and Dincol, G. (1974): Acute leukaemia in two generations following chronic exposure to benzene. *Hum. Hered.,* 24:70-74.
2. Anderson, D. E. (1975): Familial susceptibility. In: *Persons at High Risk of Cancer: An Approach to Cancer Etiology and Control,* edited by J. F. Fraumeni, Jr., pp. 39-54. Academic Press, New York.
3. Burnett, J. W., Goldner, R., and Calton, G. J. (1975): Cowden disease. Report of two additional cases. *Br. J. Dermatol.,* 93:329-336.
4. Creagan, E. T., and Fraumeni, J. F., Jr. (1972): Familial Hodgkin's disease. *Lancet,* 2:547.
5. Creagan, E. T., and Fraumeni, J. F., Jr. (1973): Familial gastric cancer and immunologic abnormalities. *Cancer,* 32:1325-1331.
6. Everson, R. B., Fraumeni, J. F., Jr., Wilson, R. E., Li, F. P., Fishman, J., Stout, D., and Norris, H. J. (1976): Familial male breast cancer. *Lancet* 1:9-12.
7. Fraumeni, J. F., Jr. (1973): Genetic factors. In: *Cancer Medicine,* edited by J. F. Holland and E. Frei, III, pp. 7-15. Lea and Febiger, Philadelphia.
8. Fraumeni, J. F., Jr. (1975): Multiple primary neoplasms: Relationship to familial cancer. In: *Multiple Primary Malignant Tumours,* edited by L. Severi, pp. 177-184. Division of Cancer Research, Perugia, Italy.
9. Fraumeni, J. F., Jr., Grundy, G. W., Creagan, E. T., and Everson, R. B. (1975): Six families prone to ovarian cancer. *Cancer,* 36:364-369.
10. Fraumeni, J. F., Jr., and Miller, R. W. (1967): Adrenocortical neoplasms with hemihypertrophy, brain tumors, and other disorders. *J. Pediatr.,* 70:129-138.
11. Fraumeni, J. F., Jr., and Mulvihill, J. J. (1975): Who is at risk of colorectal cancer? In: *Cancer*

Epidemiology and Prevention, edited by D. Schottenfeld, pp. 404-415. Charles C Thomas, Springfield, Ill.

12. Fraumeni, J. F., Jr., Rosen, P. J., Hull, E. W., Barth, R. F., Shapiro, S. R., and O'Connor, J. F. (1969): Hepatoblastoma in infant sisters. *Cancer,* 24:1086-1090.

13. Fraumeni, J. F., Jr., and Thomas, L. B. (1967): Malignant bladder tumors in a man and his three sons. *JAMA,* 201:507-509.

14. Fraumeni, J. F., Jr., Vogel, C. L., and Easton, J. M. (1968): Sarcomas and multiple polyposis in a kindred. *Arch. Intern. Med.,* 121:57-61.

15. Fraumeni, J. F., Jr., Vogel, C. L., and De Vita, V. T. (1969): Familial chronic lymphocytic leukemia. *Ann. Intern. Med.,* 71:279-284.

16. Fraumeni, J. F., Jr., Wertelecki, W., Blattner, W. A., Jensen, R. D., and Leventhal, B. G. (1975): Varied manifestations of a familial lymphoproliferative disorder. *Am. J. Med.,* 59:145-151.

17. Glass, A. G., and Fraumeni, J. F., Jr. (1970): Epidemiology of bone cancer in children. *J. Natl. Cancer Inst.,* 44:187-199.

18. Jensen, R. D., Norris, H. J., and Fraumeni, J. F., Jr. (1974): Familial arrhenoblastoma and thyroid adenoma. *Cancer,* 33:218-223.

19. Kersey, J. H., Spector, B. D., and Good, R. A. (1973): Primary immunodeficiency diseases and cancer: The Immunodeficiency-Cancer Registry. *Int. J. Cancer,* 12:333-347.

20. Knudson, A. G., Jr. (1975): Genetic influences in human tumors. In: *Cancer, Vol. 1,* edited by F. F. Becker, pp. 59-74. Plenum, New York.

21. Knudson, A. G. Jr., Strong, L. C., and Anderson, D. E. (1973): Heredity and cancer in man. *Prog. Med. Genet.,* 9:113-158.

22. Lee, D. K., and Abbott, M. L. (1969): Familial central nervous system neoplasia. Case report of a family with von Recklinghausen's neurofibromatosis. *Arch. Neurol.,* 20:154-160.

23. Li, F. P., and Fraumeni, J. F., Jr. (1969): Rhabdomyosarcoma in children: Epidemiologic study and identification of a familial cancer syndrome. *J. Natl. Cancer Inst.,* 43:1365-1373.

24. Li, F. P., and Fraumeni, J. F., Jr. (1969): Soft-tissue sarcomas, breast cancer, and other neoplasms. A familial syndrome? *Ann. Intern. Med.,* 71:747-752.

25. Li, F. P., Rapoport, A. H., Fraumeni, J. F., Jr., and Jensen, R. D. (1970): Familial ovarian carcinoma. *JAMA,* 214:1559-1561.

26. Li, F. P., Tucker, M. A., and Fraumeni, J. F., Jr. (1976): Childhood cancer in sibs. *J. Pediatr.,* 88:419-423.

27. Lindberg, B., and Kock, N. G. (1975): A family with atypical colonic polyposis and gastric cancer: A three-decade followup. *Cancer,* 35:255-259.

28. Lynch, H. T., Krush, A. J., Thomas, R. J., and Lynch, J. (1976): Cancer family syndrome. In: *Cancer Genetics,* edited by H. T. Lynch, pp. 355-388. Charles C. Thomas, Springfield, Ill.

29. MacMahon, B. (1966): Epidemiology of Hodgkin's disease. *Cancer Res.,* 26:1189-1200.

30. Miller, R. W. (1971): Deaths from childhood leukemia and solid tumors among twins and other sibs in the United States, 1960-67. *J. Natl. Cancer Inst.,* 46:203-209.

31. Mulvihill, J. J. (1975): Congenital and genetic diseases. In: *Persons at High Risk of Cancer: An Approach to Cancer Etiology and Control,* edited by J. F. Fraumeni, Jr., pp. 3-37. Academic Press, New York.

32. Ohbayashi, A., Okochi, K., and Mayumi, M. (1972): Familial clustering of asymptomatic carriers of Australia antigen and patients with chronic liver disease or primary liver cancer. *Gastroenterology,* 62:618-625.

33. Pendergrass, T. W., Mann, D. L., Stoller, R. G., Halterman, R. H., and Fraumeni, J. F., Jr. (1975): Acute myelocytic leukaemia and leukaemia-associated antigens in sisters. *Lancet,* 2:429-431.

34. Purtilo, D. T., Yang, J. P. S., Cassel, C. K., and Harper, R. (1975): X-linked recessive progressive combined variable immunodeficiency (Duncan's disease). *Lancet,* 1:935-940.

35. Schimke, R. N., Mebust, W. K., and Richards, R. D. (1974): Multiple hypernephromas in a family with the von Hippel-Lindau syndrome. *Birth Defects,* 10(4):179-180.

36. Tokuhata, G. K., and Lilienfeld, A. M. (1963): Familial aggregation of lung cancer in humans. *J. Natl. Cancer. Inst.,* 30:289-312.

37. Vinken, P. J., and Bruyn, G. W. (eds.) (1972): The Phakomatoses. In: *Handbook of Clinical Neurology, Vol. 14.* North-Holland, Amsterdam.

38. Young, D. F., Eldridge, R., and Gardner, W. J. (1970): Bilateral acoustic neuroma in a large kindred. *JAMA,* 214:347-353.

Discussion

Rashad: Family history of cancer of all anatomic sites was evaluated in 1,054 consecutive patients attending the chemotherapy clinic for treatment of cancer. There were 131 probands (12.4%) with histories of cancer in first- or second-degree relatives. Breast cancer occurring on a site-specific basis and not associated with an excess of malignant neoplasm of other anatomic sites was observed in eight families—six caucasians, one Korean, and one Japanese.

Other site-specific familial aggregations were observed for stomach cancer in one Caucasian family and for cancer of the lung in one Japanese family. Family history of cancer in other sites was obtained from seven patients with cancer of the lung, nine cases with cancer of the colon, eight cases with cancer of the stomach, and 19 cases with cancer of the breast. Familial aggregations of cancer cases were more common in caucasian families than in other ethnic groups studied.

These observations illustrate the importance of racial variation in familial clustering. They also confirm earlier findings that familial clustering of cancer may be site-specific, particularly for breast cancer, and may also involve other sites.

Lynch: I think that your presentation shows well the importance of extended family studies in looking beyond tumors of a single site and identifying syndromes of related cancers. One tumor that we are finding in the syndrome that you first described with Dr. Li—the association of breast cancer, sarcomas, brain tumors, and adrenocortical neoplasms—is laryngeal carcinoma in nonsmokers. We have found a number of these occurrences. The proband in one family was a nonsmoker who developed laryngeal carcinoma followed by an adenocarcinoma of the lungs at autopsy he had a third primary, namely gastric carcinoma. I wonder if you have encountered laryngeal carcinoma, and whether you think this might be an integral component of the syndrome?

Fraumeni: Yes, we have seen laryngeal carcinoma in a couple of families [See also the chapter by Li, *this volume*]. This tumor was brought to our attention in a family in which two cousins had rhabdomyosarcoma. A 35-year-old man on the line of descent seemed to us to be at very high risk. We called him up, but he refused to talk, being uninterested in participating in the survey. Two months later, his wife called back and said he would now be willing to talk, but could not because he had a tumor on the vocal cords. It turned out to be squamous cell carcinoma; the patient subsequently developed a primary carcinoma of the lung and died.

Gatti: Have you or anyone else tried to look at children who have been adopted either into or out of any of these high-risk families?

Fraumeni: I cannot recall any families we have studied in which there were adopted children; and I am not aware of cancer-prone families in the literature in which adopted individuals were part of the familial aggregation. I should stress that some of our cancer-prone families are scattered throughout the country; consequently very little contact occurs between certain branches of the family. Since the predisposition to cancer affects geographically separated branches and does not extend to spouses, it seems unlikely that extrinsic environmental factors are primarily involved.

Yerganian: During the course of inbreeding wild hamsters, the tumor spectra of both the Chinese and Armenian hamsters altered dramatically. After 25 generations of full-sib matings, uterine tumors of the Chinese hamster changed from the monotonous series of pre-inbred fibrosarcomas to various forms of adenocarcinomas. Similarly, cirrhotic liver altered to hepatocarcinoma. In a related study, the Armenian hamsters remained tumor-free for 10 years until the 17th generation was attained, and lymphoreticular proliferations developed suddenly among the offspring and sublines linked to one particular male parent. Related tumor-free sublines failed to withstand the detrimental aspects of inbreeding and were lost soon thereafter. Although the tumor-prone sublines continue to breed readily, they do so with the elevated risk of developing myeloproliferative disorders and reticular cell neoplasms. [*Proc. Am. Assoc. Cancer Res.*, 15:135 (1974); *Proc. XIth Int. Cancer Congr.*, 80 (1974).]

Genetics of Human Cancer, edited by J. J.
Mulvihill, R. W. Miller, and J. F. Fraumeni, Jr.
Raven Press, New York, 1977.

20

Management and Control of Familial Cancer

Henry T. Lynch, Jane Lynch, and
Patrick Lynch

*Department of Preventive Medicine and Public Health, Creighton University School of
Medicine, Omaha, Nebraska 68178*

Cancer control is a two-way street involving both the patient and physician (8,13,36). It suffers when the family physician fails to involve the patient fully. In the area of familial cancer the patient may significantly enhance cancer control by supplying the physician with as detailed a family history as possible, relevant to all major causes of morbidity and mortality, with particular attention given to cancer (14). The physician may in turn be able to identify particular patterns of tumor transmission, and in some cases he will be able to determine the patient's risk for manifesting a component of a specific hereditary cancer syndrome (29).

Thus armored with specific information about cancer risk for particular anatomic sites, the doctor can focus his attention upon those target organs in his patient(s) that harbor an inordinately high risk for malignant transformation. The product of such an approach could be early cancer detection that may result in significantly improved prognosis. Cancer prevention may also be accomplished such as in colectomy for familial polyposis coli.

The purpose of this chapter will be to provide insights into improved management and control of familial cancer through the application of family history to knowledge of cancer genetics and hereditary cancer syndrome identification. Alternative procedures for acquisition and evaluation of family history will be discussed, including evaluation by the family physician himself, referral to familial cancer researchers for work up, or implementation of a nationwide registry of cancer prone families. Several familial cancer problems will be emphasized in order to demonstrate clearly how these objectives can best be achieved.

FAMILIAL BREAST CANCER

Cancer control programs in familial breast cancer must take into consideration the variety of clinical settings in which this malignant neoplasm might occur (Table 1) (9,12,26,30,33,38,39). The site-specific variety accounts for about one-half of all the familial occurrences of this disease (28). As in all familial occurrences of breast cancer, an early age of onset and an excess of bilateral disease is often encountered (1,27). In some families the age of onset may be extraordinarily early. For example, in one of our breast cancer-prone families, two sisters had histologically verified breast cancer at ages 22 and 29, respectively. Their mother had verified breast cancer at age 42, their maternal grandmother had breast cancer at age 48, and several maternal aunts and cousins had breast cancer in their early forties and fifties. These two affected sisters had a 19-year-old sister who was greatly concerned about her own risk for eventual development of breast cancer. Her physician consulted me about performing a bilateral prophylactic mastectomy. I recommended bilateral reduction mammoplasty with subcutaneous prosthesis. The alternative to this procedure would be meticulous surveillance with monthly self-breast examination by the patient, semiannual examination by her physician, with annual thermography, mammography, or xeroradiography, Here, as in other contexts, the problem of the fearful, unmotivated, or impoverished patient must be contended with. If mammography were to be effective, the patient would have to begin this procedure at her current youthful age of 19, and in order to assure maximum effectiveness, this procedure would have to be done annually. Thus the patient would receive significant cumulative radiation exposure because of the large number of procedures that such a plan would call for throughout the patient's lifetime. There is also the theoretical possibility that host susceptibility to breast cancer would interact with the radiation exposure, and possibly cause a heightened risk for malignant transformation. There are no clinical studies demonstrating an increased risk of radiation carcinogenesis in patients prone to familial breast cancer, though we certainly cannot exclude this as a possibility, since even the normal breast is susceptible to radiogenic cancer. Indeed, Bailar (3) has recently questioned the wisdom of mammography screening in general because of the radiation hazard.

TABLE 1. *Breast cancer genotypes*

1. Site-specific breast cancer, early age of onset, and excess of bilaterality
2. Breast cancer in familial association with carcinoma of the ovary and endometrium
3. Breast cancer in familial association with cancer of the gastrointestinal tract
4. Breast cancer in familial association with sarcoma, leukemia, brain tumor, and laryngeal and adrenal cortical carcinoma
5. Breast cancer in familial association with cutaneous malignant melanoma, and other histologic varieties of cancer
6. Breast cancer in Klinefelter's syndrome
7. Breast cancer in Cowden's disease
8. Possible association of breast cancer and Sipple's syndrome

Knowledge of tumor associations in familial breast cancer could be of extreme benefit to cancer control programs. For example, the familial association between carcinoma of the breast and the ovary suggests that physicians should be concerned with the patient's risk for *both* of these malignant neoplasms (9,33). In the case of carcinoma of the ovary, the diagnostic techniques available for early detection of this disease are poorly developed. Fraumeni and associates (9) reported six families prone to ovarian cancer, three of which showed the familial association of breast and ovarian carcinoma. Because of the exceptional risk for ovarian cancer in these families, prophylactic oophorectomy was performed in 14 asymptomatic women from four of the families. Ovarian tissue from three of the eight cases of prophylactic oophorectomy, in which slides were available for review, showed evidence of histologic aberrations (hyperplastic foci of epithelial and mesothelial tissue) although the women were asymptomatic. The authors reviewed the current status of diagnostic studies capable of detecting this disease at an early stage. They suggested that several approaches might be beneficial. These include: urinary estrogen and pregnanediol levels; vaginal cornification index, particularly in postmenopausal women; analysis of peritoneal fluid obtained by culdocentesis for biochemical and cytologic abnormalities. For the most susceptible cases they suggested culdoscopy or peritoneoscopy for direct visualization of the ovaries. However, because of the overall ineffectiveness of present techniques for early diagnosis of ovarian cancer, these investigators suggested that patients who are at exceptional risk for this disease undergo prophylactic oophorectomy. They further suggest that the timing of surgery could be individualized so that in most instances it could be performed after the woman had completed her family. We concur fully with these suggestions and indeed we have studied several families that showed striking similarities to those reported by Fraumeni et al. (9), and in each one we have advised prophylactic oophorectomy for those women at exceptionally high cancer risk.

In families showing a familial association between carcinoma of the breast and gastrointestinal tract cancer, particularly colon cancer, we strongly advise that such patients begin having routine proctosigmoidoscopies performed beginning in their early thirties because cancer of the colon occurs at a significantly earlier age in such patients (37). Men as well as women in these families have been shown to be at risk for gastrointestinal tract cancer. Women members from these families should also be followed carefully for carcinoma of the breast.

In the syndrome showing familial association between carcinoma of the breast, brain tumors, sarcoma, leukemia, laryngeal carcinoma, and adrenocortical carcinoma, extremely early occurrences of carcinoma of the breast have been observed (12,38,41). In one such family currently under investigation, four women manifested breast cancer at ages 23, 29, 36, and 43. This syndrome appears to be inherited via a single autosomal dominant gene (14,41), permitting the physician to identify patients who show an extraordinary cancer risk (50%) for any of these several designated malignant neoplasms. Patients are also in jeopardy for development of multiple cancers. For example, the male proband from the above family was a nonsmoker, nondrinker in whom laryngeal carcinoma (squamous cell) nevertheless developed at age 50. Subsequently adenocarcinoma of the lung developed at age 55, and an autopsy revealed a possible third primary cancer, namely, cancer of the stomach. Significantly, the proband had a long occupational history of exposure to varnish and wood dust as a cabinetmaker. Nasal sinus carcinoma has been found in excess among woodworkers.

Because the only hope for control of malignant neoplasms such as brain tumors, sarcomas, and leukemias lies in the earliest possible diagnosis, it would be prudent to follow such patients very carefully. However, the physician must walk a tightrope as undue attention could lead to cancer phobia and more generalized psychological distress. This often manifests itself in the form of a paradoxical delay in attending to early signs or symptoms of cancer. Thus the physician must proceed with cautious deliberation in the management of such cancer-prone families (8,13,14,31,36).

CANCER FAMILY SYNDROME

The cancer family syndrome is characterized by an excess of adenocarcinomas of all types, but in particular adenocarcinoma of the colon and endometrium, early age of onset of cancer (compared to the corresponding histologic variety occurring in the general population), an excess of multiple primary malignant neoplasms (more than 20%), and a vertical transmission of cancer consistent with an autosomal dominant inheritance pattern (14,16,17,32,34,36,42). It should be noted again that definition and classification of this syndrome and others described here are operational, simply reflecting the patterns observed thus far in known families. As families are followed in prospective studies, description of further tumor associations comprising a given syndrome will occur, also yielding more reliable classification.

The cancer family syndrome has now been confirmed in more than 15 families by Lynch and associates (14), and it has been described by others in the United States and other parts of the world (17). This hereditary cancer syndrome provides the physician with an excellent opportunity to identify patients at an inordinately high risk (50%) for cancer of the colon, endometrium, and other anatomic sites in members of cancer-prone lines from these families. In one such family identical twin sisters showed concordance for this syndrome (36). A unique factor in this family was the manner in which increased suspicion for cancer of site-specific organs, namely, endometrium and colon, led to early cancer diagnosis. The context was *patient awareness* of family history of cancer which prompted them to request that their physician perform specific diagnostic evaluations. Specifically, the proband was a 51-year-old white woman who in 1958 had received a diagnosis of endometrial carcinoma at the age of 40 years. In 1968, because of the occurrence of adenocarcinoma of the colon in her 52-year-old brother, this patient requested that her physician perform appropriate diagnostic studies on her colon even though she was completely asymptomatic. Findings on proctosigmoidoscopy and barium enema revealed the presence of an early adenocarcinoma of the transverse colon. A colectomy was successfully performed. The identical twin sister of the proband had been completely asymptomatic at the age of 40 years in 1958. Yet she requested an evaluation of her uterus because of the occurrence of endometrial carcinoma in her co-twin. Diagnosis of early endometrial carcinoma was established, and a hysterectomy was successfully performed. When adenocarcinoma of the colon developed in her twin sister in 1968, this patient requested that her physician perform a sigmoidoscopic examination. This examination was negative, and she continues to receive follow-up rectal examinations (Fig. 1).

In summary, a first degree relative of a cancer proband from a family manifesting the cancer family syndrome has an approximate 50% risk for the development of cancer, and the likelihood is that the cancer will be of the colon or endometrium, although other anatomic sites may be affected. The patient will be at risk for the development of subsequent additional primary adenocarcinomas and therefore should be followed carefully for the rest of his or her life. When undergoing laparotomy, meticulous evaluation of abdominal organs should be carried out, particularly of the corpus uteri and the colon. The patient should undergo careful cancer-screening tests early in life because cancer may have its onset significantly earlier than for the same histologic variety occurring in the general population.

XERODERMA PIGMENTOSUM

Xeroderma pigmentosum (XP) is an exceedingly rare, autosomal excessively inherited, chronically progressive, multisystem disease (19,22). The skin is the major target organ, with malignant skin tumors, most commonly of the basal and squamous cell variety, occurring in practically all of these patients at a very early age. Malignant melanoma occurs in at least 3% of these patients (2,20). XP patients rarely survive beyond the first two decades of life, typically succumbing to multiple skin cancers and inanition (43). This disease is unique in cancer genetics because of the rather striking interaction between host and environmental factors (solar radiation exposure) in the production of skin cancer. A major breakthrough in comprehension of the etiology of XP at the molecular level occurred in 1968 when Cleaver demonstrated defective repair replication of DNA in fibroblasts from the skin of affected patients following exposure of these cells to ultraviolet light (5–7).

We first studied a family with this disease wherein five of nine siblings showed clinically and histologically verified evidence of XP (22). Two of these siblings were identical twin brothers in whom increased pigmentation was apparent almost at birth, and later progressed. The diagnosis of XP was made in the proband prior to the birth of the identical twins. The proband and two other affected sisters each

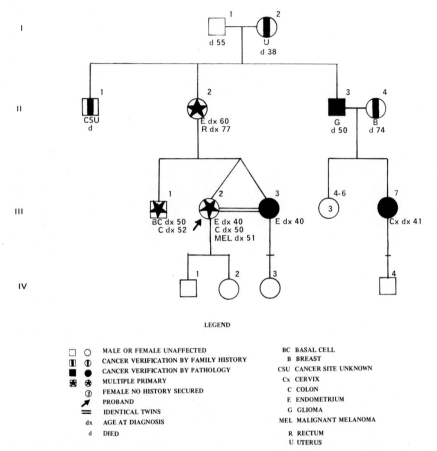

LEGEND

□ ○	MALE OR FEMALE UNAFFECTED	BC BASAL CELL
◨ ◑	CANCER VERIFICATION BY FAMILY HISTORY	B BREAST
■ ●	CANCER VERIFICATION BY PATHOLOGY	CSU CANCER SITE UNKNOWN
▨ ✸	MULTIPLE PRIMARY	Cx CERVIX
③	FEMALE NO HISTORY SECURED	C COLON
↗	PROBAND	E ENDOMETRIUM
=	IDENTICAL TWINS	G GLIOMA
dx	AGE AT DIAGNOSIS	MEL MALIGNANT MELANOMA
d	DIED	R RECTUM
		U UTERUS

FIG. 1. Pedigree of a family manifesting the cancer family syndrome with affected identical twins. [From H. T. Lynch, and A. J. Krush: *Surg. Gynecol. Obstet.,* 132:247 (1971), with permission of the publisher.]

had more than 25 skin cancers. Malignant melanoma with metastases occurred in the proband and one of these sisters. Interestingly, in spite of the absence of specific therapy for metastatic malignant melanoma, the proband and his affected sister have fully recovered and fail to show any evidence of malignant melanoma, 8 and 5 years later, respectively.

The highly motivated parents have provided a program of protection from solar radiation exposure for all five of the affected children. This program was instituted almost at birth for the identical twins. We began our study in 1967 when the twins were only 8 years old. Examination of the twins at the time showed classical clinical findings for XP though there was no evidence of any skin cancer. In 1974, we restudied the family in collaboration with a dermatologist (24). The twins were healthy and intelligent, having been consistently on the honor roll at their high school. Their cutaneous findings were identical, including mild conjunctivitis, pigmented mascules of the face, "V" of the neck, upper back, forearms, hands, and dorsa of the feet. Keratosis pilaris was present on the extensor aspects of the upper arms. Neither twin had any clinical evidence of actinic keratoses, basal or squamous cell carcinoma, nor malignant melanomas. The cancer control program instituted at birth included use of an ester of para-aminobenzoic acid applied topically for photoprotection. Their classroom at school had fluorescent lighting with plastic covers over the bulbs. The home was lit by incandescent bulbs. The twins wear long trousers, long-sleeved shirts, wide-brimmed hats, and dark glasses. Physical activities such as swimming and playing tennis are accomplished at night under artificial lighting. This lifelong regimen has been well accepted by them. The twins are popular with their friends and appear well adjusted. The success of this program, particularly as it has met the psychological needs of the participants, has been primarily due to the motivation and compassionate attention of their parents (21). This is an example of cancer control that has been well planned and meticulously executed by all parties concerned.

SIPPLE'S SYNDROME OR MULTIPLE ENDOCRINE NEOPLASIA II (MEN II)

The association of thyroid carcinoma and pheochromocytoma was first described by Sipple in 1961 (45). The thyroid cancer was described as medullary or solid type with amyloid stroma by Williams in 1965 (47). (Parathyroid hyperplasia is also recognized as a component of the syndrome.) Since these reports, more than 250 cases of medullary thyroid carcinoma have appeared in the literature. Several families have been described wherein transmission of the disease has been consistent with an autosomal dominant mode of inheritance.

Sipple's syndrome can be diagnosed by biochemical means through assay of calcitonin (10). Thus, a patient at risk for Sipple's syndrome who may not have palpable disease in his thyroid but who has an elevated serum calcitonin, should be surgically explored for the presence of medullary thyroid carcinoma. Keiser and associates (10) coordinated a screening program for available members of a large kindred with Sipple's syndrome. The screening included medical history, blood pressure, palpation of the neck, and venipuncture for measurement of calcitonin, calcium, phosphorus, alkaline phosphatase, and histaminase. They also collected a 24-hr urine sample for catecholamine metabolites. Through this screening program they diagnosed medullary carcinoma of the thyroid in 16 patients, 10 of whom had palpable thyroid nodules, whereas six did not show evidence of thyroid disease on neck palpation. Radioscopic scans identified nodules in nine of the 10 patients. Eleven of the 12 patients with preoperative measurements had elevated calcitonin levels (i.e., greater than 0.38 ng/ml). Of the 11 patients with elevated calcitonin, four had thyroid nodules whereas seven had no palpable disease and therefore would ordinarily not have undergone operation. One of the patients had a normal basal level of calcitonin which remained normal following a calcium infusion test. Nevertheless, this patient had a palpable thyroid nodule that proved to be medullary thyroid carcinoma. Therefore, patients having palpable thyroid nodules from families with this disorder, despite a normal calcitonin level, should undergo biopsy of their nodular thyroid gland. Since these patients are also at increased risk for development of pheochromocytoma, it is important that they be evaluated for this tumor through periodic monitoring of their blood pressure and catecholamines. Should pheochromocytoma be suspected, both adrenal glands should be carefully examined at surgery because of the increased frequency of bilateral occurrence of this disease. Surgical management of the thyroid should involve total thyroidectomy because the carcinoma is or will become bilateral in virtually all cases. The parathyroid glands are removed only if the patient is hypercalcemic or if tissue is grossly abnormal (10).

Each of these familial cancer problems could benefit immensely through specific surgical cancer control practices since the particular lesions are readily resectable and when detected early an excellent prognosis can be provided the patient.

Genetic pleiotropism was originally suggested to explain the three components of the syndrome (medullary thyroid carcinoma, pheochromocytoma, parathyroid hyperplasia). However, the finding of DOPA decarboxylase, an enzyme present in pheochromocytoma, but now observed in medullary thyroid carcinoma, provides a new biochemical link bridging the thyroid carcinoma and the pheochromocytoma components of the syndrome. It is likely that a single gene is involved; and recent evidence of neural crest origins of the parafollicular C cell suggests that this gene may be affecting the neural crest (44).

In the differential diagnosis of Sipple's syndrome one must consider the multiple mucosal neuroma syndrome (MEN III) (19). In this syndrome the same cancers occur, namely medullary thyroid carcinoma and pheochromocytoma. Calcitonin also serves as a marker with serum elevations indicating the presence of medullary thyroid carcinoma. The disease is distinguished readily from Sipple's syndrome by physical characteristics of these patients, including multiple mucosal neuromas of the lips, the anterior part of the tongue, and occasionally the buccal, gingival, nasal, or conjunctival mucosa. The age of onset of neuromas varies with some being present at birth. The corneal nerves may be strikingly enlarged. Patients may show a Marfanoid habitus. Multiple ganglioneuromas may occur in the large bowel where the radiologic findings may suggest ulcerative colitis. Patients may occasionally have *café-au-lait* spots, suggesting a relationship with the autosomal dominantly inherited neurofibromatosis. Recall that in neurofibromatosis, pheochromocytomas also occur in excess. Pheochromocytoma also occurs in excess in the autosomal dominantly inherited von Hippel–Lindau's disease. Families have also been observed with isolated pheochromocytomas showing autosomal dominant inheritance. Familial aggregates of isolated thyroid carcinoma have also been described. Wermer's syndrome, multiple endocrine neoplasia, type I (MEN I) (autosomal dominant) must also be considered in the differential diagnosis of Sipple's syndrome. This disorder involves tumors of the pituitary, pancreas, and adrenal cortex, as well as parathyroid adenomas. However, pheochromocytoma has not been reported in Wermer's syndrome, and thyroid carcinoma is uncommon. When it does occur it is not of the medullary type (19).

In summary, patients at risk for Sipple's syndrome or MEN III should be monitored through neck palpation and calcitonin assay. When calcitonin is elevated, the neck should be explored for the presence of thyroid carcinoma. The patient should also be monitored for the possibility of pheochromocytoma, and if it is suspected, both adrenals should be evaluated because of the increased frequency of bilaterality of this lesion. If the pheochromocytoma component is recognized, then the patient must be considered at extremely high risk for medullary thyroid carcinoma, and vice versa.

FAMILIAL MALIGNANT MELANOMA

The first familial occurrence of cutaneous malignant melanoma was described by Cawley in 1951 (4). He described the disease in a father and two of his three children. Since this report several other investigators have confirmed the existence of a hereditary etiology for this disease in certain families (19). Anderson has described the familial variety as showing an early age of onset and multiple primary malignant melanomas (2). He suggested that the frequency of the hereditary form of this disease may be approximately 3%. However, this determination was limited to occurrences of melanoma and did not consider associated family cancers. This figure may therefore underestimate the total clinical pool of familial melanoma. Lynch (19) has suggested that melanoma, like an increasing number of putative site-specific cancers, may be associated with other histologic varieties of cancer and thus may occur more frequently as a component of a broader tumor spectrum (14,18,25). For example, in the study of five melanoma-prone families (25; summarized in Table 2), an excess of several varieties of cancer occurred. It was also of interest that in one of these families, two sisters (III-17, III-19) had multiple primaries consisting of breast carcinoma and malignant melanoma (Fig. 2). Similar multiple primary combinations of carcinoma of the breast and malignant melanoma were found in two patients from two other melanoma-prone families. It is possible that this particular combination may be biologically meaningful, though further studies will be required (25).

Figure 3 shows the pedigree of a family with malignant melanoma (Family 5 from Table 2). The proband had advised her son (III-1) to consult me for medical evaluation and genetic counseling. This 26-year-old white man had previously had four melanomas excised from his skin. Pathologically, each was considered to represent a separate primary melanoma. Physical examination of his skin revealed multiple moles, none of which appeared to be suspicious for malignant melanoma. At the completion of the examination the patient expressed relief in the fact that I did not find any cutaneous abnormalities. As he was ready to leave he thanked me and told me that he would be able to relieve his wife's anxiety because she had

TABLE 2. *Cancer sites and number in the five families*

Cancer	Family 1 (MM5)	Family 2 (C49)	Family 3 (B35)	Family 4 (MM1)	Family 5 (C100)
Malignant melanoma	3	4	2	2	3
Breast	—	2	3	—	1
Stomach	2	1	—	3	—
Lung	3	2	—	1	—
Colon	—	—	2	—	—
Ovary	1	—	1	—	—
Lymphoma	1	—	—	—	—
Pancreas	1	—	—	—	2
Hodgkin's disease	1	—	—	—	—
Throat	—	1	—	—	—
Urinary bladder	—	1	—	—	—
Skin	—	2	—	—	—
Larynx	—	1	—	—	—
Gallbladder	—	—	1	—	—
Endometrium	—	—	—	—	—
Kidney	—	—	—	—	—
Liver	—	—	—	1	—
Leukemia	—	—	1	—	—
Cancer site unknown	—	5	—	1	—
Cervix	—	—	—	—	1

noticed an area on his back which had been increasing in size and darkening in color. I then had him undress again and reexamined his back. The area still did not appear to be suspicious, but on the strength of the family history and the occurrence of multiple melanomas in this patient, coupled with the fact that his wife had observed a change in a specific mole, he was referred to a plastic surgeon. The plastic surgeon also believed the area to be normal but agreed to excise this mole widely. The diagnosis was cutaneous malignant melanoma, the patient's fifth primary malignant melanoma (35).

Malignant melanoma may occur in other hereditary diseases including XP and von Recklinghausen's neurofibromatosis. Malignant melanoma may also complicate giant pigmented nevi of congenital origin (25).

Pedigrees of families with familial melanoma suggest autosomal dominance. However, the inheritance pattern may be more complex (2), with one explanation being reduced penetrance of the gene. It is also possible that more than one gene is involved (25).

The association of malignant melanoma with other histologic varieties of cancer harbors important cancer control implications (25). Thus it will be important to consider patients from families with malignant melanoma as being at risk for other histological varieties of cancer. In addition, such patients should have lifelong surveillance for multiple primary malignant melanomas. The error involved in such diagnosis may be great. In some series, highly trained physicians have failed to make the diagnosis as often as 50% of the time. Some recent evidence suggests that the accuracy may be slightly better (11). Nevertheless, as attested to by

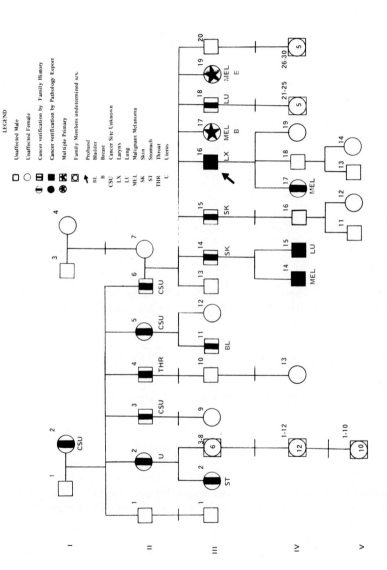

FIG. 2. Pedigree of a family (Table 2, No. 2) prone to malignant melanoma wherein two sisters (III-17, III-19) each manifested the combination of malignant melanoma and adenocarcinoma of the breast, histologically verified. [From H. T. Lynch, et al.: *Surg. Gynecol. Obstet.*, 141:517 (1975), with permission of the publisher.]

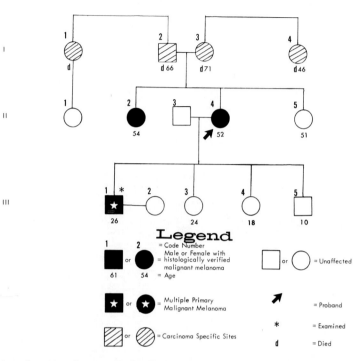

FIG. 3. A malignant melanoma family (Table 2, No. 5) in which the proband had multiple primary malignant melanoma. [From H. T. Lynch, and A. J. Krush: *Can. Med. Assoc. J.,* 99:17 (1968), with permission of the publisher.]

patient III-1 (Fig. 3), a lesion that is changing in character in any patient, but particularly in one with a past history of melanoma or who is at high familial risk for this disease, should be biopsied. All nevi in relatives at risk should be examined periodically, and of course suspicious lesions should be biopsied. Again the physician should avoid provoking apprehension and anxiety in the patient since this could paradoxically cause them to repress the entire issue. We have already mentioned that this may be one of the most difficult problems encountered in the management of individuals at high genetic risk for cancer. In the case of familial melanoma, the physician has an excellent opportunity to educate his patients about the skin changes that could be consistent with this disease. We have provided our patients with a card (Table 3) that characterizes some of the features of cutaneous malignant melanoma. This card is laminated in plastic so that it can be carried in a wallet or purse and is given to all members of melanoma-prone families. In turn, we counsel each patient about the significance of cutaneous signs of this disease and concurrently show them color photographs of a variety of melanomas. Our patients appear to accept this educational exercise with objectivity and equanimity.

TABLE 3. *Signs for malignant melanoma*

A.	Change in size of a mole, especially sudden enlargement
B.	Change in the surface characteristics such as oozing, scaling, (flaking), erosion (as when a scab comes off), or bleeding
C.	Change in consistency (becoming lumpy or hard)
D.	Change in shape (outline changes)
E.	Color (red, white, and blue)
F.	Pigment leaking (any change in color around mole)
G.	Mole becomes itchy

If any of these conditions arise in you or a family member, consult your family physician.

DISCUSSION

Limited physician manpower, cost, logistical considerations relevant to patient and physician accessibility, education, socioeconomic background, as well as emotional and motivational problems make it impractical to perform cancer screening examinations successfully on the entire adult population in order to achieve the goal of early cancer detection. These problems are further compounded by the lack of a single test for detection of cancer of all anatomic sites. Needed, therefore, are programs utilizing a cancer risk factor approach. Genetics is an important risk factor which could be employed effectively to improve the efficiency and hence the cost-benefit balance of cancer screening programs.

Data from our Mobile Cancer Detection Unit study (29,40) strengthen the hypothesis that for a given patient, cancer risk increases as family history of cancer becomes stronger. Specifically, we found that 9.8% of the patients with one cancer in the family had cancer themselves; 16.3% of those patients with two cancers in their first degree relatives had cancer themselves; finally, 22% of those patients with three or more affected first degree relatives had cancer themselves (23). We have estimated that approximately 47% of patients do not have any first degree relatives with cancer; about 30% of the patients in the general population will have one first degree relative with cancer; about 20% will have two or more first degree relatives with cancer, and approximately 7% will have three or more first degree relatives with cancer (26). It is primarily this 7% category which contributes to the familial cancer problem in general and the many hereditary cancer syndromes in particular.

These statistics are a gross estimate of the magnitude of the problem; however, they do not shed light on etiology since family history of cancer may well reflect nongenetic (environmental) as well as genetic factors. Of course, increased cancer risk is the crucial variable of concern to the family physician. Whether such risk stems from strictly genetic factors or is the result of shared environmental exposures or a combination of the two would not markedly affect the fact of increased risk to the individual patient.

The starting point in identifying those family members at highest risk is necessarily the acquisition and evaluation of the family history. Developing the family history consists of constructing a rough pedigree, identifying at least the patient's first- and second-degree relatives, specifying those who have been affected by cancer, and verifying the nature of the cancers. If at this point a known cancer syndrome is recognized, relatives at risk can be identified. This can typically be accomplished by the family physician if his search is expedited by a patient and family who are diligent in tracing relatives and their hospital records. We have had experience with this approach in our cancer screening activities in a multiphasic mobile cancer detection unit (29). The patients were given a questionnaire designed to elicit detailed medical and family history to be completed in advance of their appointment in the unit. The overwhelming majority of these patients were able to bring forth a remarkably accurate family history. This was used successfully as part of our risk factor assessment as the patients moved through the unit for their examinations (23).

If the family is less cooperative, or further investigation into a less well defined tumor association pattern is indicated, or if for any other reason the demands on the physician's time prevent his being able to obtain and evaluate the family history to his satisfaction, he may refer the family to individuals who are more accustomed to family history acquisition and evaluation, including risk assessment.

In most of the families described above, a remarkable synergy has occurred between the family doctor and ourselves. In these situations, the physician will generally have seen a patient who presented with a strong family history of cancer. This patient may or may not be affected. The physician recognizes that the history had potential cancer control significance; yet despite his careful cataloging of familial cancer occurrences, he would feel unable to assess the full cancer risk for his patient(s) and their relatives. Lacking the time and expertise to pursue the matter, he would then send us a letter describing the situation that confronted him, requesting that we pursue the matter and inform him about our results and suggestions. Our detailed family investigation would then follow.

The described procedure has worked well. In many cases the referring physician would be able to provide a cancer control program for family members with confidence since he has been fully informed of the results of the study. The family members are often convinced that as thorough an inquiry as possible has been conducted. Education about their cancer risk, including specific signs, symptoms, and diagnostic procedures are provided them in detail. They are encouraged to work closely with their family physician toward their mutual goal of the best possible control of high-risk cancer problems. In turn the research team is provided with many opportunities to design studies on cancer etiology and carcinogenesis on subjects through the same type of referral mechanism that we utilize. In the future, more institutionalized processes will be required.

NATIONAL FAMILIAL CANCER REGISTRY SYSTEM

In the United States, we should strive for the establishment of a National Familial Cancer Registry System designed to record genealogic and medical data on cancer-prone families. The National System would include and be serviced by Regional Centers, selected on the basis of population density and geography. The main focus of attention would be compilation of pedigrees, followed by estimation of cancer risks to all members of these cancer-prone families.

The network of Regional Centers dispersed throughout the country could be connected through a central clearing house. Registries would thus be able to assist each other through the sharing of pertinent information on cancer-prone families, which would then be coordinated at the Central Clearing House level by computerization for rapid retrieval. It is well known that highly mobile families are often scattered widely throughout the United States. Nevertheless, individual registries established on the basis of geographic considerations, with appropriate computer terminals at each registry and the main interconnecting data channel at the Central Clearing House, could distribute pertinent information and pedigrees rapidly to any qualified physician in the United States.

In addition to rapid identification of patients at risk for cancer, it would be possible in certain familial and/or cancer genetic disorders to provide a relatively precise estimate of cancer risk for specific target organs. When reliable diagnostic markers exist, such as calcitonin assay in Sipple's syndrome (MEN II) or the multiple mucosal neuroma syndrome (MEN III), this information would also be provided to the interested family physician with detailed explanation. The System would thus be more than a registry, since direct service is provided the patients and their physicians.

The development and implementation of a National Familial Cancer Registry System is feasible, particularly when one considers the success of similar endeavors elsewhere. A registry containing more than 200 families with familial polyposis coli at St. Mark's Hospital in London, the long experience with functionally useful cancer registries in the Netherlands and Scandinavian countries, and the many noncancer registries for genetic diseases serve well to emphasize our point. With respect to the latter, i.e., noncancerous genetic diseases, Huntington's chorea serves as an excellent example. A concerted effort by the Committee to Combat Huntington's Disease (New York, N.Y.) to register individuals has provided an outstanding service to patients and physicians alike. The Committee, with its vested interest in contributing to the welfare of patients with the disease, has been able to ascertain more than 2,000 individuals in the United States who were members of a number of families with this exceedingly rare disease. In turn, they were able to provide investigators with useful information about more than 66% of the family membership (46). This serves to show how a properly organized group can succeed in such an educational venture. There are other similar organizations devoted to specific genetic diseases, for example: juvenile diabetic clinics; cystic fibrosis organizations; parents of mentally retarded; osteogenesis imperfecta registries; and many others. Thus we see clearly that given sufficient impetus and a well organized plan for the common good, interested individuals will participate in such organizations.

For such a program to work at maximum efficiency, it requires the backing of the medical community, including the medical societies, practicing physicians, hospitals, pathology laboratories, and most important, it would also require the cooperation of individual patients.

Perhaps the first step toward the initiation of such a large scale program would be to secure consultation from individuals in those areas of the world who currently work with registries of cancer-prone families that have been compiled and that have been utilized effectively by practicing physicians. Assistance might also be given by members of the Latter-Day Saints Church who have assumed scientific as well as administrative roles in their very elaborate Genealogy Center. Cancer geneticists could also provide consultation through the sharing of their own techniques and expertise in eliciting cooperation from families and the medical community, so that detailed family studies can be performed expeditiously. They can also show clearly how this information can be disseminated to family physicians and utilized for maximum gain by the patients.

At first glance this might seem to be a formidable operation. Furthermore when one considers the obstacles posed by security and confidentiality requirements of personal data, one might wonder how such a program could ever get off the ground. The fact of the matter is the offering of a rather unique cancer control program with the recognition of patients who may be at inordinately high cancer risk for specific target organs should speak for itself. The success of the entire program might rest upon the very first phases of development in terms of smoothness of operation and objectively measurable patient and physician benefit. Of course, uniform establishment of cancer as a reportable disease would greatly expedite the operation of the registry system.

GENETIC COUNSELING IMPLICATIONS

There has accumulated little experience in genetic counseling for cancer problems. Those problems most noteworthy for genetic counseling implications are retinoblastoma (autosomal dominant), familial polyposis coli (autosomal dominant), and XP (autosomal recessive). The limited experience in genetic counseling in cancer is undoubtedly due to the fact that until recently a paucity of knowledge has existed in the field of cancer genetics. We now know that there are more than 50 Mendelian inherited precancerous and cancerous disorders (14). A threefold increased risk (empiric risk) for site-specific cancer to first degree relatives of an affected patient has been shown for several of the commonly occurring cancers including carcinoma of the breast, stomach, colon, endometrium, prostate gland, lung, leukemia, lymphoma, and others.

Extensive experience in genetic counseling exists for numerous noncancerous disorders, much of which can be readily applied to cancer genetic problems. One of the most striking features about genetic counseling is the fact that the overwhelming majority of patients are much more concerned about the medical aspects of their particular disease, including diagnosis, prognosis, and treatment, than they are about the actual genetic or familial transmission (15). This has been well documented recently in the case of Huntington's chorea by Stern and Eldridge (46) who showed that the least concern among patients and close relatives pertains to genetic risk for the disease. The overwhelming majority of patients were more disturbed about the physical and mental aspects of Huntington's disease than social or genetic factors. Those affected or at high risk were most concerned about physical symptoms such as chorea, ataxia, mental and physical deterioration, and overall prognosis. In our own experience in genetic counseling of several hundred cancer-prone families, we have observed similar findings. Concern about etiology, including genetic risk, has been secondary. It therefore becomes important in counseling cancer-prone families that the counselor meet the needs of the patient and provide him with as detailed an account as possible about diagnosis and natural history of the particular cancer problem (15,21).

SUMMARY

Cancer control can be maximized when the physician is aware of his patient's cancer risk for specific anatomic target organs. Such risk factors can be assessed with precision based on Mendelian inheritance patterns. Such inherited disorders as retinoblastoma, von Recklinghausen's neurofibromatosis, familial polyposis coli, Gardner's syndrome, Sipple's syndrome, and several others contribute to a minority of the familial cancer load. A significantly larger number of syndromes are comprised of some of the more common tumors such as carcinoma of the breast, colon (in the absence of familial polyposis coli), stomach, endometrium, Hodgkin's disease, and leukemia. In these syndromes, so-called empiric risk figures, which in general indicate a threefold increased cancer risk to first degree relatives of the cancer proband, are often observed. The finding of physical markers such as the cutaneous signs of sebaceous cysts, lipomas and fibromas in Gardner's syndrome, or biochemical markers such as elevated calcitonin levels in Sipple's syndrome, provide additional aids to the physician's cancer control program. These physical or biochemical markers enable him to use these indicators as adjuncts to pedigree methods, thereby indicating more specifically those individuals at extremely high risk for development of cancer. Unfortunately, physical signs and laboratory markers are few when all familial and/or hereditary cancer is considered. Thus, in many cases such as the cancer family syndrome, the physician must laboriously gather family data and develop a pedigree from the data so that greater precision about cancer risk for specific anatomic sites can be obtained. It is here that the patient can be of great help in assisting the physician by gathering these data so that management of familial cancer can be improved through recognition of cancer risk. Once such family pedigrees are compiled, it would seem a pity not to make this painstakingly assembled information available to all interested physicians who may be managing these families. Indeed some of the families such as Family G (32) and Family N (16), under study by us, may contain as many as 2,000 or 3,000 relatives once the pedigrees are significantly extended. These relatives may be scattered across the United States with as many as 100 or more physicians involved in the total management. These facts are raised because this problem of dissemination of familial risk information could be significantly simplified through development of a National Registry of Cancer-Prone Families patterned to some extent after the ongoing tumor registry systems of the Third National Cancer Survey. This would provide a central clearing house for collection and dissemination of familial cancer risk information. A plan for development of such a registry system is given.

REFERENCES

1. Anderson, D. E. (1972): A genetic study of human breast cancer. *J. Natl. Cancer Inst.,* 48:1029–1034.
2. Anderson, D. E. (1971): Clinical characteristics of the genetic variety of cutaneous melanoma in man. *Cancer,* 28:721–725.
3. Bailar, J. C., III (1976): Mammography—a contrary view. *Ann. Intern. Med.,* 84:77–84.
4. Cawley, E. P. (1952): Genetic aspects of malignant melanoma. *AMA Arch. Dermatol. Syph.,* 65:440–450.
5. Cleaver, J. E. (1970): DNA repair and radiation sensitivity in human (xeroderma pigmentosum) cells. *Int. J. Radiat. Biol.,* 18:557–565.
6. Cleaver, J. E. (1969): Xeroderma pigmentosum: A human disease in which an initial state of DNA repairs is defective. *Proc. Natl. Acad. Sci. USA,* 63:428–435.
7. Cleaver, J. E., and Bootsma, D. (1975): Xeroderma pigmentosum: Biochemical and genetic characteristics. *Ann. Rev. Genet.,* 9:19–38.
8. Dukes, C. F. (1958): Cancer control in familial polyposis of the colon. *Dis. Colon Rectum,* 1:413–423.
9. Fraumeni, J. F., Jr., Grundy, G. W., Creagan, E. T., and Everson, R. B. (1975): Six families prone to ovarian cancer. *Cancer,* 36:364–369.
10. Keiser, H. R., Beaven, M. A., Doppman, J., Wells, S., Jr., and Buja, L. M. (1973): Sipple's syndrome: Medullary thyroid carcinoma, pheochromocytoma, and parathyroid disease. Studies in a large family. *Ann. Intern. Med.,* 78:561–579.
11. Kopf, A. W., Mintzis, M., and Bart, R. S. (1975): Diagnostic accuracy in malignant melanoma. *Arch. Dermatol.,* 111:1291–1292.
12. Li, F. P., and Fraumeni, J. F., Jr. (1969): Soft-tissue sarcomas, breast cancer, and other neoplasms: A familial syndrome? *Ann. Intern. Med.,* 71:747–752.
13. Krush, A. J., Lynch, H. T., and Magnuson, C. (1965): Attitudes toward cancer in a "cancer family": Implications for cancer detection. *Am. J. Med. Sci.,* 249:432–438.
14. Lynch, H. T. (ed.) (1976): *Cancer Genetics.* Charles C. Thomas, Springfield, Ill.
15. Lynch, H. T. (1969): *Dynamic Genetic Counseling for Clinicians.* Charles C. Thomas, Springfield, Ill.
16. Lynch, H. T. (1974): Familial cancer prevalence spanning eight years. *Arch. Intern. Med.,* 134:931–938.
17. Lynch, H. T. (1967): Hereditary factors in carcinoma. *Recent Results Cancer Res.,* 12:1–184.
18. Lynch, H. T. (1969): Skin, heredity, and cancer. *Cancer,* 24:277–287.
19. Lynch, H. T. (1972): *Skin, Heredity, and Malignant Neoplasms.* Medical Examination Publ., Flushing, N.Y.
20. Lynch, H. T. (1976): Studies of familial melanoma *(in progress).*
21. Lynch, H. T., Anderson, D. E., Krush, A. J., and Mukerjee, D. (1967): Cancer, heredity, and genetic counseling: Xeroderma pigmentosum. *Cancer,* 20:1796–1801.
22. Lynch, H. T., Anderson, D. E., Smith, J. L., Jr., Howell, J. B., and Krush, A. J. (1967): Xeroderma pigmentosum, malignant melanoma, and congenital ichthyosis. *Arch. Dermatol.,* 96:625–635.

23. Lynch, H. T., Brodkey, F. D., Lynch, P., Lynch, J., Maloney, K., Rankin, L., Kraft, C., Swartz, M., Westercamp, T., and Guirgis, H. A. (1976): Familial risk and cancer control. *JAMA,* 236:582–584.
24. Lynch, H. T., Frichot, B. C. III, and Lynch, J. F. (1976): Xeroderma pigmentosum and cancer control *(in press).*
25. Lynch, H. T., Frichot, B. C., Lynch, P., Lynch, J., and Guirgis, H. A. (1975): Family studies of malignant melanoma and associated cancer. *Surg. Gynecol. Obstet.,* 141:517–522.
26. Lynch, H. T., Guirgis, H., Albert, S., and Brennan, M. (1974): Familial breast cancer in a normal population. *Cancer,* 34:2080–2086.
27. Lynch, H. T., Guirgis, H. A., Brodkey, F. D., Maloney, K., Lynch, P. M., Rankin, L., and Lynch, J. (1976): Early age of onset in familial breast cancer. Genetic and cancer control implications. *Arch. Surg.,* 111:126–131.
28. Lynch, H. T., Guirgis, H. A., Brodkey, F. D., Lynch, J., Maloney, K., Rankin, L., and Mulcahy, G. M. (1976): Genetic heterogeneity and familial carcinoma of the breast. *Surg. Gynecol. Obstet.,* 142:693–699.
29. Lynch, H. T., Harlan, W., Swartz, M., Marley, J., Becker, W., Lynch, J. F., Kraft, C. A., and Krush, A. J. (1972): Multiphasic mobile cancer screening: A positive approach to early cancer detection and control. *Cancer,* 30:774–781.
30. Lynch, H. T., Kaplan, A. R., and Lynch, J. F. (1974): Klinefelter syndrome and cancer: A family study. *JAMA,* 229:809–811.
31. Lynch, H. T., and Krush, A. J. (1969): Breast carcinoma and delay in treatment. *Surg. Gynecol. Obstet.,* 128:1027–1032.
32. Lynch, H. T., and Krush, A. J. (1971): Cancer family "G" revisited: 1895–1970. *Cancer,* 27:1505–1511.
33. Lynch, H. T., and Krush, A. J. (1971): Carcinoma of the breast and ovary in three families. *Surg. Gynecol. Obstet.,* 133:644–648.
34. Lynch, H. T., and Krush, A. J. (1967): Heredity and adenocarcinoma of the colon. *Gastroenterology,* 53:517–527.
35. Lynch, H. T., and Krush, A. J. (1968): Heredity and malignant melanoma: Implications for early cancer detection. *Can. Med. Assoc. J.,* 99:17–21.
36. Lynch, H. T., and Krush, A. J. (1971): The cancer family syndrome and cancer control. *Surg. Gynecol. Obstet.,* 132:247–250.
37. Lynch, H. T., Krush, A. J., and Guirgis, H. A. (1973): Genetic factors in families with combined gastrointestinal and breast cancer. *Am. J. Gastroenterol.,* 59:31–40.
38. Lynch, H. T., Krush, A. J., Harlan, W. L., and Sharp, E. A. (1973): Association of soft tissue sarcoma, leukemia, and brain tumors in families affected with breast cancer. *Am. Surg.,* 39:199–206.
39. Lynch, H. T., Krush, A. J., Lemon, H., Kaplan, A. R., Condit, P. T., and Bottomley, R. H. (1972): Tumor variation in families with breast cancer. *JAMA,* 222:1631–1635.
40. Lynch, H. T., Lynch, J., and Kraft, C. (1973): A new approach to cancer screening and education. *Geriatrics,* 28:152–157.
41. Lynch, H. T., Lynch, J., and Lynch, P. (1975): Breast cancer genetics and cancer control: Tumor association. *Arch. Surg.,* 110:1227–1229.
42. Lynch, H. T., Shaw, M. W., Magnuson, C. W., Larsen, A. L., and Krush, A. J. (1966): Hereditary factors in cancer: Study of two large midwestern kindreds. *Arch. Intern. Med.,* 117:206–212.
43. Pathak, M. A., and Epstein, J. H. (1971): Normal and abnormal reactions of man to light. In: *Dermatology in General Medicine,* edited by T. B. Fitzgerald, K. A. Arndt, W. H. Clark, Jr., A. Z, Eisen, E. J. VanScott, and J. H. Vaughn, pp. 977–1036. McGraw-Hill, New York.
44. Pearse, A. G. E. (1973): Cell migration and the alimentary system: Endocrine contributions of the neural crest to the gut and its derivatives. *Digestion,* 8:372–385.
45. Sipple, J. H. (1961): The association of pheochromocytoma with carcinoma of the thyroid gland. *Am. J. Med.,* 31:163–166.
46. Stern, R., and Eldridge, R. (1975): Attitudes of patients and their relatives to Huntington's disease. *J. Med. Genet.,* 12:217–223.
47. Williams, E. D. (1965): A review of 17 cases of carcinoma of the thyroid and pheochromocytoma. *J. Clin. Pathol.,* 18:288–292.

Discussion

Murphy: I agree with Dr. Lynch about the need for accurate empirical information. We have been acutely sensitive to the problem of ascertainment bias. In our study of polyposis of the colon, we very carefully selected our cases for analysis in such a way that we eliminated bias from this source. We have been fitting age-at-involvement curves for the relatives of cases of Gardner's syndrome who should be at 50% risk; and our best data so far suggest that the lifetime risk among these people is not one-half, but one-third. I think this raises a very interesting and fundamental question. Do we really understand the mechanism of inheritance of this trait? There may be some influence from, let us say, a partially or totally epistatic gene located elsewhere. I am no longer certain that Gardner's syndrome is inherited as a simple classic autosomal dominant.

Lipkin: Dr. Lynch mentioned thymidine labeling of intestinal cells and correctly indicated its potential for predicting neoplasia. The presence of abnormally proliferating cells on the mucosal surface is not in itself a malignant sign, but rather appears to be an early step in the sequence that leads to polyp formation and then to cancer (Chapter 34). This information can be combined with other studies, including cytologic measurements of colonic washings, to develop indicators of actual malignancy as well as early premalignant changes.

Sanford: As a geneticist I have great enthusiasm for looking at the genetic background in cancer, but Dr. Lynch's proposal is a little bit frightening if I understand it correctly. The idea of having centers all over the country keeping track of cancer-prone families, given our current state of knowledge, really concerns me. Dr. Lynch, do you actually have in mind centers that would keep track of people with familial predisposition to breast cancer, to lung cancer, to colon cancer, and so forth?

H. T. Lynch: I find the lack of such a registry system frightening, particularly when you realize the work that goes into family studies and the good that can be accomplished through early cancer detection. We do not need to include all family aggregations, such as those of lung cancer in which the role of a genetic factor is unclear. However, as a point of embarkation we should identify families in which the elevated risk is quite firm and highly significant. At the moment virtually nothing along these lines is available. The present cancer registries throughout the country have a paucity of information that is functionally useful to the clinical oncologist.

Gatti: I have related questions. What psychological problems have been encountered in contacting family members who think they are healthy and are then told that they may be cancer-prone? What is being done in these studies to minimize this trauma?

H. T. Lynch: Certainly in these families, there exists psychological trauma that has a deleterious effect on cancer control. That is why I think we, as clinicians, must be more aggressive in our approach. To those of you who have not worked with cancer-prone families, this may sound a little unusual, but we are obviously dealing with a life-threatening disease. In these families many of the members are extremely fatalistic, particularly the older people who have been saddened by the loss of so many relatives. In some families, such as the one I discussed with polyposis coli, the fatality rate has been virtually 100% among affected persons. Death from this disease should be preventable, and in this family much effort is being directed toward early diagnosis by proctoscopy. Discussions with family members are instrumental in working through the psychological problems. The family registry would help to promote medical counseling, surveillance, and other services that would involve and inform the family physician as well. Finally, more research should be directed towards understanding the psychological factors in cancer in general, but particularly in familial cancer.

Gatti: Dr. Lynch, my concern is that you may proctoscope these people, and tell them that you see no evidence of cancer; but this is like telling someone "We see no evidence of heart attack.'' This does not exclude the possibility of an attack. I am concerned that you may be sending people away with almost as much fear as when they came, as you can say only that they do not have cancer at the moment. Perhaps we should follow Dr. Sanford's advice and postpone some of these family studies until a test is available, for example, that can pick up the heterozygotes; then at least we can send people away with peace of mind. One of the roles of the physician, besides diagnosis and treatment, is to comfort patients who are concerned about a medical problem. In this instance, we may be creating a problem, although I think we all understand the benefits of the registry.

H. T. Lynch: The medical and psychological problems are there long before we ever encounter a family and before the physician intervenes either as a researcher or family practitioner. We cannot turn away from people who have familial polyposis or other high-risk states. More affirmative measures must be taken to allow early diagnosis and treatment and to advise and support these individuals.

I want to congratulate you, Dr. Utsunomiya, for having the wisdom to establish a registry for familial cancer in Japan. Is cancer a reportable disease in Japan and, if your registry proves successful, would you include various forms of familial cancer eventually?

Utsunomiya: Cancer is not a reportable disease in Japan. My registry includes familial polyposis coli, Gardner's syndrome, Peutz-Jeghers' syndrome and familial cancer without multiple polyposis. I would like to extend the registry to other forms of familial cancer eventually.

Gerald: The only caution I would urge, Dr. Lynch, is that what is acceptable in Nebraska may not be acceptable in other parts of the country.

Lipkin: Dr. Gatti's question concerning the psychological effect of these types of examinations on families is extremely important. A prime example of the successful development of projects of this type is in the field of cardiology. Broad screening and prevention programs for cardiovascular disease, based on the identification of high-risk factors determined in the Framingham and other studies, have been successfully applied to individuals. Evidently, the participants are able to accept the blood testing and general physical examinations that prevention entails.

Hirschhorn: The rising trend of cardiovascular disease may be partly related to increasing awareness and detection of disease. We may be reaching a time when the true incidence is known, and not really be preventing any additional rise. So I am not sure that we can call that program successful as yet.

Dr. Lynch suggested in his presentation that the genetic risk factors are of somewhat secondary importance to the cancer-prone family in terms of counseling, but I think this depends on how one approaches genetic counseling. We have found that when one spends enough time and starts digging a bit the concern of many family members (particularly younger women) is actually much greater for potential offspring than for themselves. One should not neglect trying to reach that concern even though it is not expressed at the time of initial counseling.

Cleaver: One of my concerns over the years has been that, even with the amount of interest in and work being done on xeroderma pigmentosum (XP), therapy and treatment are really no better than they were in 1870 when the disease was first described. It is very gratifying to see some contribution to the health of the family being made through prophylactic care. XP can now be added to the list of diseases that can be successfully diagnosed prenatally [*Science,* 174:147–150 (1974)]. The moment a child with XP is born, obviously there is a family at risk. There is no technical obstacle to the prenatal diagnosis of subsequent pregnancies. The only time required is that needed to establish cultures, followed by about a week of measurements to establish the DNA repair capacity of cultured amniotic cells. This has been done successfully in recent years.

Gorlin: In practically all lists of genetic conditions, one sees Turcot's (gliomatosis-polyposis) syndrome. Am I being apostate when I question the existence of this syndrome?

H. T. Lynch: I think the syndrome is rather convincing from the cases reported to date, but I would like to hear Dr. Fraumeni's ideas.

Fraumeni: There is no doubt that there have been a series of families reported in which intestinal polyps are associated with the occurrence of brain tumors [*Dis. Colon Rectum,* 18:514–515 (1975)]. However, I question whether the condition represents a genetic variant of intestinal polyposis, like Gardner's syndrome, as many have suggested. I would favor putting it in the category of a family cancer syndrome.

Genetics of Human Cancer, edited by J. J.
Mulvihill, R. W. Miller, and J. F. Fraumeni, Jr.
Raven Press, New York, 1977.

21

Family History: A Criterion for Selective Screening

David E. Anderson and Marvin M. Romsdahl

*The University of Texas System Cancer Center M.D. Anderson Hospital and Tumor
Institute, Houston, Texas 77030*

As emphasized by Lynch (Chapter 20), eliciting a family history of cancer is important to the identification of high-risk groups and to early cancer detection, prevention, and treatment. This is particularly true for various Mendelian inherited neoplasms whereby high-risk individuals may be readily identified by pedigree analysis and/or by specific diagnostic procedures, as in polyposis, nevoid basal cell carcinoma syndrome, neurofibromatosis, retinoblastoma, neuroblastoma, and more recently, multiple endocrine neoplasia types I and II (8–10). But, what of the more common types of familial-occurring neoplasms, such as those of the stomach, uterus, breast, or colon, where the tumor distribution does not behave as a Mendelian trait or no specific diagnostic means are available for identifying relatives at high risk?

Some preliminary evidence is available suggesting that early detection and treatment are possible in patients with at least two such neoplasms—colorectal cancer or breast cancer. This evidence derives from examinations of three groups of relatives: relatives of patients with colorectal cancer developing independently of polyposis, relatives of patients with colorectal cancer developing in association with some form of polyposis, and relatives of breast cancer patients. The only criterion for examination of a relative was that he or she have at least two relatives with colorectal cancer or breast cancer. In the majority of cases, the examination involved a first-degree relative, usually a sib or child, of one or more of the affected family members.

COLORECTAL CANCER

The colonic examinations were initiated in 1968 and were conducted in the Surgery Clinic, and the breast examinations the latter part of 1969 in the Surgical Breast Clinic. The colonic evaluation included a history and physical examination, proctosigmoidoscopy, air-contrast barium enema study, and for women, pelvic and breast examinations as well. The results of these examinations are summarized in Table 1. Significantly, among the 188 examinations in 76 men and 112 women, five colonic cancers were detected, two in men and three in women. In addition, one woman was found to have an ovarian mass by pelvic examination. This mass was subsequently diagnosed as an adenocarcinoma. Another woman was found to have a breast tumor which proved to be carcinoma. The average age at examination was 42.5 years and at colonic cancer detection, 52.4 years. The detection rates of 2.7/100 examinations at all ages and 3.7/100 examinations at ages 35 and over exceed those reported for detection programs of the general population, where the rates approach 1/1000 and the age range is older (5,6).

The detection rate was much higher among the examinations of relatives known to belong to polyposis families. Ten of 16 relatives were found to have polyps and three also had carcinoma, for a cancer detection rate of 18.8%. The average age of the examined group was 26.4 years and 30.0 years for those with carcinoma.

An important point regarding the colonic examinations was that only two of the five cancers detected in the colonic cancer families were within the range of the proctosigmoidoscope. Colonic cancer in general develops most often in the cecal and rectosigmoid areas, the latter area having about two-thirds of the neoplasms (7). In the hereditary polypoid diseases the distribution is similar but with approximately three-quarters of the carcinomas developing in the rectosigmoid area (1), although in Gardner's syndrome, they may extend into the small intestine. As shown in Table 2, the tumor distribution is different in familial and nonfamilial patients with colorectal cancer occurring independently of polyposis (4). Neoplasms in nonfamilial patients, as also noted in other surveys (7), most frequently occurred in the cecal and rectosigmoid areas, whereas in familial patients they were more uniformly distributed throughout the colon. In fact, 52%

TABLE 1. *Colonic cancer detection in families with a history of colonic cancer or polyposis*

Age at exam	Colonic cancer			Polyposis		
	No. exams	Ca.[a] colon	Other cancer	No. exams	Polyps	Ca colon
15–24	21			8	5	1
25–34	32			5	4	1
35–44	50	1		3	1	1
45–54	41		2			
55–64	26	4				
65–74	16					
75–84	2					
Total	188	5	2	16	10	3
Ca detection rate		2.7%	1.1%		62.5%	18.8%
Ca detection rate ≥ 35		3.7%	1.5%		—	—

[a] Ca = cancer.

TABLE 2. *Percent distribution of colonic cancer in patients with and without a family history of colonic cancer (M. D. Anderson Hospital, September 1964 to August 1974)*

Colonic site	Non-familial	Familial
Cecum	10.5	15.0
Ascending	5.1	18.7
Hepatic flexure	0.9	3.7
Transverse	5.4	14.0
Splenic flexure	1.6	5.6
Descending	5.7	5.6
Sigmoid	27.8	19.6
Rectosigmoid	6.6	3.7
Rectum	36.2	14.0
Total patients	1799	107

of the carcinomas in familial patients involved the transverse and right side as compared to only 22% in these sites in the nonfamilial group. Further analysis of 11 families with hereditary colonic cancer occurring independently of polyposis suggested that the tumor distribution was a familial characteristic, some families having clustering of lesions in the transverse colon and other families having clustering of lesions in either the right or left colon (4). It is important, therefore, that examinations for familial-occurring colorectal cancer utilize methods that encompass the entire colon and not merely the distal portion.

BREAST CANCER

The detection program for breast cancer included a physical breast examination, thermography, and xeromammography. A total of 107 examinations have now been conducted on 102 asymptomatic women ranging in age from 15 to 79 years (Table 3). The average age at examination was 42.4 years. At initial examination, suspicious masses were detected in ten women, six of whom underwent biopsy. Three of these were histologically diagnosed as duct cell carcinoma, adenocarcinoma, and lobular carcinoma *in situ* at ages 45, 48, and 68 years, respectively. The present detection rates of 2.8/100 examinations at all ages and 4.2/100 examinations at ages 35 and over are in excess of those observed in screening programs of the general population. Strax (11), using similar examination procedures, reported a detection rate of 9.4/1000 among 40,341 initial examinations and a rate of 5.9/1000 among 80,442 initial and subsequent examinations of a slightly older group of women from the New York area. In a survey conducted at M. D. Anderson Hospital by the Department of Radiology, four proven breast cancers were detected among 630 nonhospitalized women by thermography and xeromammography, a detection rate of 6/1000.

Breast examinations were also conducted on women belonging to the colonic cancer families. A total of 114 breast examinations were performed on 86 women averaging 42.7 years of age. Five were found to have benign masses and one a carcinoma at age 46. Interestingly, the one woman with breast cancer had a family history of the disease in two paternal aunts and a cousin. The breast cancer detection rate for this group was thus 0.88/100 examinations at all ages and 1.2/100 examinations at ages 35 and over. These rates are similar to those reported for women from the general population. It would appear, therefore, that a family history of breast cancer can serve to identify a risk group in which breast cancer can be detected at a higher frequency and at a slightly earlier age than in women from the general population or women with a family history of colorectal cancer.

Additionally, Table 3 provides a unique demonstration by a prospective approach that women with a family history of the disease have a threefold to fourfold higher risk for the disease than women not having a family history of this neoplasm.

The women in the present survey, as previously stated, belonged to families having at least two members with breast cancer. These affected members were related as sisters in 36% of the families, mother and daughter in 41%, and as second degree relatives in 23%. The lifetime probability of breast cancer development in these families, using retrospective data, was calculated to be 13%, about twofold higher than the 6% generally cited for women in general. However, the risks for breast cancer development in relatives were previously shown to be significantly influenced by the age at which it was first diagnosed in the patient, whether the disease was bilateral or unilateral, and who in the family, in addition to the patient, had the disease (2). Three groups of patients were identified by these criteria. One group was characterized by early and bilateral disease and disease occurrence in the mother of the patient. The lifetime risk of breast cancer development in the sisters of such patients was about 30%. Another group was

TABLE 3. *Breast cancer detection in families with a history of breast cancer or colonic cancer*

Age at exam	Breast cancer families			Colonic cancer families		
	No. breast exams	No. masses	Ca [a] breast	No. breast exams	No. masses	Ca breast
15–24	16			13		
25–34	19			20		
35–44	21	3		32	2	
45–54	28	5	2	28	2	1
55–64	19	1		13		
65–74	3	1	1	6		
75–84	1			2	1	
	107	10	3	114	5	1
Ca detection rate			2.8%			0.88%
Ca detection rate ⩾ 35			4.2%			1.2%

[a] Ca = cancer.

characterized by a later-occurring disease and in one breast, and where the mothers were unaffected but a sister of the patient had breast cancer prior to ascertainment of the patient. The lifetime risk to the remaining sisters of such patients was 11%. Another group of patients was identified in which the lifetime risk was little different from controls (3). The women in the present survey, based on the breast cancer occurrence in the affected relatives, were classified into these three groupings in an attempt to provide evidence of detection differences that might relate to the differences in empiric risks. Of the 107 examinations, 45 pertained to women belonging to the highest risk group. Four women were found to have suspicious masses, three of which were biopsied, disclosing one carcinoma. In the moderate-risk group, there were 38 examinations. Four masses were detected, three of which were biopsied, and two were carcinoma. In the low-risk group, two suspicious masses were detected among 24 examinations, neither of which has as yet been biopsied. Consequently, these numbers are still too small to provide evidence of detection differences among pedigree groups at varying risk for the disease.

CONCLUSION

The results from these groups of relatives indicate the feasibility of using a family history of a common cancer as a criterion for defining a risk group, and that appropriate examination of individuals belonging to such groups will lead to the detection of tumors at a higher than expected frequency, and apparently, the higher the empiric risks, i.e., a family history vs no family history or polyposis vs colonic cancer per se, the higher will be the detection rate. The present numbers are still much too small and the follow-up period too short to determine whether these early detections will lead to increased survival rates. Clearly, however, the detections were at an earlier age, and treatment was instituted earlier than had the tumors been detected after the onset of symptoms.

These detection programs will continue with emphasis on follow-up examinations. Effort will also be directed toward identifying families with early onset and multiplicity of tumors, and perhaps in the case of colonic cancer, a more proximal than distal tumor distribution. Such families might lead to the isolation of a homogeneous group of patients and families in which a Mendelian inheritance mechanism might be demonstrated. The identification of homogeneous groupings of a familial neoplasm has applicability not only to defining risk groups for detection purposes, but also in serving as a source of experimental material for evaluating the biochemical and physiological events underlying the development of a specific neoplasm. Insight into the disease processes ultimately relates to improved treatment and management practices. But until such insight comes into being, and in the absence of specific diagnostic tests by which high-risk relatives may be identified, the minimum requirement for control of familial-occurring cancer should be to at least examine family members for early diagnosis and treatment.

ACKNOWLEDGMENT

Supported in part by Medical Genetics Center Grant GM-19513, C1 from the National Institute of General Medical Sciences.

REFERENCES

1. Alm, T., and Licznerski, G. (1973): Intestinal polyposes. *Clin. Gastroenterol.*, 2:577–602.
2. Anderson, D. E. (1974): Genetic study of breast cancer: Identification of a high risk group. *Cancer*, 34:1090–1097.
3. Anderson, D. E. (1976): Genetic predisposition to breast cancer. *Recent Results Cancer Res.*, 57:10–20.
4. Anderson, D. E., and Strong, L. C. (1974): Genetics of gastrointestinal tumors. *Proc. XIth Int. Cancer Cong., Florence, Italy*. p. 267. Excerpta Medica Series No. 351.
5. Editorial (1969): Cancer of the large intestine. *Br. Med. J.*, 1:589–590.
6. Ellis, H. (1968): Carcinoma of the caecum and colon. *Br. Med. J.*, 3:37–39.
7. Falterman, K. W., Hill, C. B., Markey, J. C., Fox, J. W., and Cohn, I., Jr. (1974): Cancer of the colon, rectum, and anus: A review of 2313 cases. *Cancer*, 34:951–959.
8. Gerson, J., Chatten, J., and Eisman, S. (1974): Familial neuroblastoma — a follow-up. *N. Engl. J. Med.*, 290:1487.
9. Li, F. P., Melvin, K. E. W., Tashjian, A. H., Levine, P. H., and Fraumeni, J. F., Jr. (1974): Familial medullary thyroid carcinoma and pheochromocytoma: Epidemiologic investigations. *J. Natl. Cancer Inst.*, 52:285–287.
10. Mallette, L. E., Bilezikian, J. P., Ketcham, A. S., and Aurbach, G. D. (1974): Parathyroid carcinoma in familial hyperparathyroidism. *Am. J. Med.*, 57:642–648.
11. Strax, P. (1975): Utilization of diagnostic technique for cancer of the breast — early diagnosis. *Proc. Natl. Breast Cancer Conf., Montreal, Canada, Oct. 31-Nov. 1, 1975*.

Genetics of Human Cancer, edited by J. J.
Mulvihill, R. W. Miller, and J. F. Fraumeni, Jr.
Raven Press, New York, 1977.

22

Investigative Approach to Familial Cancer: Clinical Studies

Frederick Pei Li

*Clinical Studies Section, Clinical Epidemiology Branch, National Cancer Institute, and
Sidney Farber Cancer Center, Boston, Massachusetts 02115*

Familial aggregation of cancer can provide clues to causes of neoplasia in man. I wish to highlight some methods of identifying etiologic factors through clinical *bedside* studies of cancer families. Since the following chapter considers the role of *laboratory* investigations of affected kindreds, it should be emphasized at the outset that the clinical and laboratory approaches are complementary, often synergistic in effect, and together, provide a powerful investigative tool for etiologic studies.

Because cancer develops during the lifetime of one in four persons in the United States, a history of tumors in close relatives is not extraordinary. Thus, even striking familial aggregations of malignancies can occur solely on a chance basis. Clinically, several techniques can help distinguish familial tendency from chance association of neoplasms. To illustrate these approaches, I shall briefly recount our investigations in recent years of a series of families with sarcomas and other tumors (4, 5).

The first study began when a clinician told us of a child with rhabdomyosarcoma, history of acute leukemia in his father, and unknown types of cancers in other relatives (Family A). Interviews with the parents and grandparents indicated a high frequency of cancers in paternal relatives in California and Arizona (Fig. 1). Other relatives, descendents of the sisters of patient II-1, resided elsewhere and had been lost to contact for many years. However, a search of old family records (made at our request) uncovered a letter written in 1937 to report the death of patient II-3 in a small Ohio town (Fig. 2). The law office which handled her estate was identified and contacted for the names of her heirs, but these files were destroyed in a fire in 1953. Finally, the relatives residing in Ohio were located through court records of a sale of family property. In this part of the kindred (II-2, II-3, and her progeny), five of ten persons had died with cancer. The types of cancer in members of the entire family were then established through hospital,

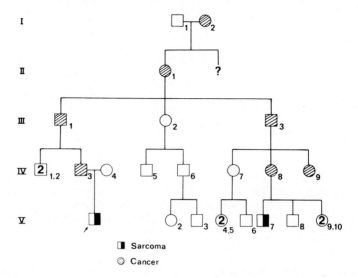

FIG. 1. Pedigree of Family A, as initially reported by the father and paternal grandfather of the proband.

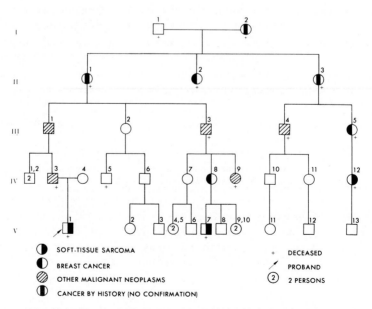

FIG. 2. Pedigree of Family A showing all descendents of patients I-1 and I-2. The types of cancer in family members were documented with appropriate medical records. Among the 10 relatives in Ohio (II-2, II-3, and her progeny), five had died with cancer before 1969.

pathology, and mortality records, and review of histologic materials. A high proportion of the neoplasms developed in children and young adults; 8 of 14 tumors, including three soft-tissue sarcomas were diagnosed before age 35 years. The findings suggested a tendency for familial aggregation of soft-tissue sarcomas in association with other neoplasms, particularly breast cancer. The investigation also showed that the pursuit of family studies may involve the type of detective work in epidemiology described in Berton Roueché's fascinating book, *Eleven Blue Men* (10).

This experience prompted a search for other family aggregates of soft-tissue sarcomas, which developed in three members of family A. The investigation involved review of the history recorded on medical records of children treated for rhabdomyosarcoma (5). Because of the rarity of the neoplasm (approximately five cases per million U.S. children per year) (12), 17 hospital centers had to be visited to abstract the records of 280 affected children. In addition, examination was made of death certificates for U.S. children under age 15 years who died of the neoplasm, 1960 to 1964. The records were from our Branch's registry of recent cancer deaths in U.S. children which, in other studies, identified excessive sib-aggregation of soft-tissue sarcomas with brain tumor and adrenocortical carcinoma (9). In our study, the hospital and mortality data yielded three new sets of young sibs with soft-tissue sarcomas (Fig. 3). Among their close relatives in Families B, C, and D, a high proportion of persons had cancer, including sarcoma and breast cancer.

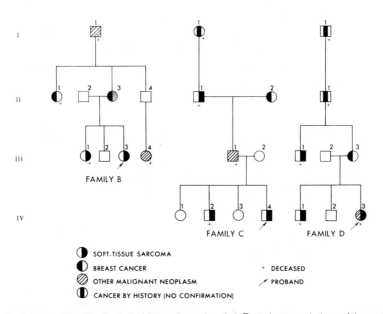

SOFT-TISSUE SARCOMA
BREAST CANCER
OTHER MALIGNANT NEOPLASM
CANCER BY HISTORY (NO CONFIRMATION)

+ DECEASED
/ PROBAND

FIG. 3. Pedigrees of Families B, C, and D, as shown in ref. 4. First-degree relatives of the proband and selected portions of the extended family are depicted.

The four families (A-D) were then studied, when feasible, in the following manner: (1) complete history and physical examination of family members for the influences of host and environmental factors; (2) a battery of laboratory studies tailored to the types of cancers in the kindreds, described elsewhere in this volume; (3) medical follow-up. After these families were reported in 1969, eight members of Families A, B, and C, including children and young adults, were diagnosed with new cancers (Table 1) (6). Six of the eight were among the 31 living members of these families who were identified in the 1969 report (the two other patients with cancer were omitted from that study) (4); 0.6 cases of cancer were expected in these 31 persons over the period, 1969 to 1975, on the basis of age-, sex-specific cancer incidence data from the Connecticut Tumor Registry (11). In each of two families (B and C), two additional patients developed breast cancer. In family C, medical examinations in 1969, prompted in part by our investigation of the family history, revealed breast cancer in a 30-year-old sister (IV-1) of the index patient with sarcoma, and a benign breast nodule in another sister (IV-3) in whom breast cancer developed five years later (at age 32). Four new patients in family A had five, possibly six, primary lesions of diverse sites: Wilms' tumor (V-6); glioma (V-11); carcinoma of the larynx followed by probable primary lung carcinoma (IV-10); and prostatic adenocarcinoma and ileal leiomyosarcoma in a patient with previously reported skin cancers (III-1). Thus, the prediction of high risk of sarcomas, breast cancer, and other neoplasms, including multiple primaries, has been realized in these families.

Familial cancers can sometimes be identified, as in Families B, C, and D, through retrospective studies of hospital and death records. However, death certificates contain only the names of the patient and the parents, including the mother's maiden name, which represent fragmentary family data. Similarly, hospital records seldom provide a complete pedigree or full identification of relatives with cancer. Thus, the recorded information is at best a starting point for later studies. To increase the number of potential families for study, we have developed

TABLE 1. *Cancers diagnosed in 8 members of Families A, B, and C, 1969–1975*

Family	Case no.	Sex	Age at diagnosis (yr)	Tumor type
C	IV-1	F	30	Breast cancer
	IV-3	F	32	Breast cancer
B	—	F	43	Breast cancer
	—	F	68	Breast cancer
A	V-6	M	3	Wilms' tumor
	V-11	F	18	Glioma
	IV-10	M	35	Carcinoma of larynx
			38	Carcinoma of lung
	III-1[a]	M	63	Carcinoma of prostate
			66	Leiomyosarcoma of ileum

[a] Patient previously diagnosed with skin cancers.

and administered to cancer patients a questionnaire to collect more complete family history and other etiologic data. Investigators at other centers may wish to use the forms, particularly in patients with findings that show a strong familial tendency (2): e.g., cancers diagnosed at an unusually early age, including adult-type cancers that develop in a child; neoplasms with a large hereditary component such as certain tumors of neural crest origin; bilateral or multicentric cancers, and multiple primary neoplasms (e.g., retinoblastomas, and pheochromocytoma with medullary thyroid carcinoma).

On occasion, detection of a familial condition requires astute observation at the bedside, as well as knowledge of clinical and etiologic features of cancer in man. Let us consider two examples. In the first, Wilms' tumor developed in three siblings who attended clinic during a period of years; another sib had duplication of one ureter. Dr. Anna Meadows (7) noticed that the mother's left shoe was unusually large. Examination revealed hemihypertrophy. The finding indicates that association of the constitutional disorder with Wilms' tumor may occur not only in the same patient, as reported by others (8), but also individually in close relatives. In the second example (3), a child's tumor was classified under the rubric of malignant lymphoma, and there was no history of cancer in close relatives. The patient actually had Burkitt's lymphoma of the jaw, and several years later the father developed a "cancer of the throat" which, on further inquiry, was nasopharyngeal carcinoma. Epstein-Barr virus is implicated as an etiologic agent in both of these rare cancers (1), and an unusual opportunity was discovered for study of the viral etiology of neoplasia in this family. Serologic examination revealed an absence of antibodies to Epstein-Barr virus in the child, thus effectively eliminating the virus as the cause of the Burkitt's tumor and the familial aggregation of cancers. The point of these examples is that the findings were based on bedside observations which are nonstatistical. In fact, a statistical approach would likely have failed to detect the unusual features in these families which led to more detailed investigation.

Etiologic studies can effectively be made by a clinician-etiologist who is experienced with management of cancer patients and their families. Studies of familial cancer by the bedside clinician are then part of the thorough work-up at a university center for purposes of patient care, research, and teaching. The clinical approach should also lead younger physicians to obtain more detailed family histories, and to participate in etiologic studies. Because many oncogenic factors in man were first identified by astute physicians at the bedside, the skill in making etiologic observations needs to be fostered in clinical training programs. For members of cancer-prone families, the studies provide opportunities for counseling, prevention, and early tumor detection and treatment.

REFERENCES

1. Epstein, M. A., and Achong, B. G. (1973): Various forms of Epstein-Barr virus infection in man: established facts and a general concept. *Lancet*, 2:836–839.
2. Fraumeni, J. F., Jr. (1973): Genetic determinants of cancer. In: *Host-Environment Interactions*

in the Etiology of Cancer in Man, edited by R. Doll, and I. Vodopija, pp. 49–55. International Agency for Research on Cancer, Lyon.

3. Li, F. P. (1976): Familial Burkitt lymphoma and nasopharyngeal carcinoma. *Lancet,* 1:687–688.

4. Li, F. P., and Fraumeni, J. F., Jr. (1969): Soft-tissue sarcomas, breast cancer, and other neoplasms: a familial syndrome? *Ann. Intern. Med.,* 71:747–751.

5. Li, F. P., and Fraumeni, J. F., Jr. (1969): Rhabdomyosarcoma in children: epidemiologic study and identification of a familial cancer syndrome. *J. Nat. Cancer Inst.,* 43:1365–1373.

6. Li, F. P., and Fraumeni, J. F., Jr. (1975): Familial breast cancer, soft-tissue sarcomas, and other neoplasms, *Ann. Intern. Med.,* 83:833–834.

7. Meadows, A. T., Lichtenfeld, J. L., and Koop, C. E. (1974): Wilms's tumor in three children of a woman with congenital hemihypertrophy. *N. Engl. J. Med.,* 291:23–24.

8. Miller, R. W., Fraumeni, J. F., Jr., and Manning, M. D. (1964): Association of Wilms's tumor with aniridia, hemihypertrophy and other congenital malformations. *N. Engl. J. Med.,* 270:922–927.

9. Miller, R. W. (1971): Deaths from childhood leukemia and solid tumors among twins and other sibs in the United States, 1960-1967. *J. Nat. Cancer Inst.,* 46:203–209.

10. Roueché, B. (1956): *Eleven Blue Men, and Other Narratives of Medical Detection,* pp. 1–156. Berkley Publishing, New York.

11. *Cancer in Connecticut: Incidence Characteristics, 1935–1962* (1967): Hartford, State of Connecticut Department of Health, p. 34.

12. Young, J. L., Jr., and Miller, R. W. (1975): Incidence of malignant tumors in U.S. children. *J. Pediatr.,* 86:254–258.

Genetics of Human Cancer, edited by J. J.
Mulvihill, R. W. Miller, and J. F. Fraumeni, Jr.
Raven Press, New York, 1977.

23

Family Studies: The Interdisciplinary Approach

William A. Blattner

*Environmental Epidemiology Branch, National Cancer Institute, Bethesda, Maryland
20014*

Laboratory investigation of familial cancer aggregations provides an opportunity for evaluating hypotheses and delineating mechanisms of cancer risk especially as they relate to host factors.

THE INTERDISCIPLINARY APPROACH

The interdisciplinary approach entails studies of human cancer and high-risk groups with laboratory techniques that measure environmental exposures, genetic susceptibility, or other risk factors identifiable on a subclinical level (9). This approach to familial cancer depends on the cooperation of the laboratory investigator with the bedside etiologist. Such collaboration was initiated in the Epidemiology Branch of the National Cancer Institute in 1966 when Joseph F. Fraumeni, Jr. investigated the occurrence of urinary bladder cancer in a father and three sons (10). At the time abnormal tryptophan metabolism had been incriminated in the genesis of bladder cancer. An interested biochemist tested specimens, and although no abnormality was detected, the interdisciplinary approach to "cancer families" was established. [Subsequently, abnormalities of tryptophan metabolism have been found in another kinship prone to bladder cancer (27).]

Role of the Bedside Etiologist

Since this first effort, the basic approach to cancer families has remained the same (Fig. 1). The bedside etiologist plays a central role in collecting and synthesizing clinical information, formulating protocols, implementing and coordinating laboratory studies, and analyzing results. Families are referred by interested colleagues, professionals, and lay individuals, including family members themselves. For successful interaction and study, the first contact is crucial especially for identifying a key family member who will act as liason and provide essential detailed information on the genealogy.

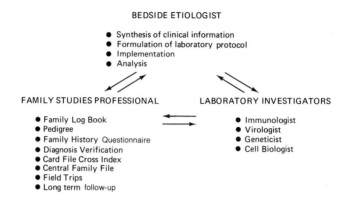

Role of the Family Studies Professional

Sometimes the first contact raises the need for an emergency field trip, when fresh biopsy or pretreatment blood may be obtained from a patient with a newly diagnosed neoplasm. A more systematic approach to the family is usually undertaken in conjunction with the family studies professional. This person provides continuity to the interdisciplinary approach and to long-term follow-up, as the permanent contact between the Epidemiology Branch and the cohort under study. When a family is ascertained, he records the key information (unique pedigree number, name, date, method of ascertainment or referral source, and major tumor type) in the family studies log book and draws the first of a series of progressively more complete pedigrees. The history is expanded by phone or field interviews and a medical questionnaire (see Appendix) that elicits detailed information about the dates and places of hospitalization and death, so that verification can be sought through vital records, hospital charts, and genealogy searches. This detailed clinical information is cross-indexed by disease and by names of all contacted individuals.

Role of the Laboratory Investigator

The clinical evaluation of families is one cornerstone of the interdisciplinary approach; laboratory investigation is the other. Most families are evaluated for etiologic clues suggested by the clinical information. The questions are asked: what is already known about the etiology of the tumor and any associated medical condition and what are the demographic and medical antecedents? The answers identify certain kinships to be studied in greater depth by laboratory tests. If enough potentially informative members are available and cooperative, a laboratory protocol is developed in conjunction with a team of laboratory specialists.

In a typical laboratory protocol, for example, for familial chronic lymphocytic leukemia (CLL) (Table 1), some assays are used as a screen for abnormalities because they require small samples and are easy to perform, whereas other more sophisticated tests are directed to a specific etiologic hypothesis. In the sample

TABLE 1. *Laboratory Protocol—Familial chronic lymphocytic leukemia*

I.   Immunologic studies
   A.   Skin tests
         1.   Recall antigens (PPD, SK-SD, mumps)
         2.   Induction with DNCB, KLH
   B.   Humoral immunity
         1.   Serum protein electrophoresis
         2.   Quantitative immunoglobulins (IgM, IgG, IgA, IgD, IgE)
         3.   Immunoelectrophoresis
         4.   Isoantibodies
         5.   Direct and indirect Coombs' test
         6.   Antinuclear antibody
         7.   Rheumatoid factor
         8.   Antithyroid antibodies
         9.   Antiparietal cell antibodies
        10.   Syphilis serology
   C.   Cell populations
         1.   Rosette-forming cells
             a. Sheep red cells
             b. Sheep red cells coated with IgM
             c. Sheep red cells coated with antibody and complement
         2.   Surface-bound immunoglobulin (fluorescent-labeled
             IgM, IgG, IgA, IgD)
   D.   Cellular immune function
         1.   Lymphocyte stimulation *in vitro*
             a. Nonspecific mitogens (PHA, PWM, Con A)
             b. Specific antigens (as used above for skin tests)
         2.   Mixed leukocyte culture
         3.   Cellular cytotoxicity
             a. PHA and antibody-dependent cytotoxicity
             b. Cr^{51} cellular cytotoxicity
II. Genetic markers
   A.   HL-A
   B.   Red blood cell phenotype
   C.   Red blood cell enzymes
   D.   Chromosome analysis
III. Hematologic studies
   A.   Complete blood count and differential
   B.   Erythrocytic sedimentation rate
   C.   Bone marrow for cytogenetics
IV. Viral studies
   A.   Epstein-Barr virus titers (early antigen, viral capsid antigen)
   B.   Oncornavirus markers in leukemic cells
         1. Reverse transcriptase
         2. DNA hybridization
         3. Cellular enzymes (terminal transferase)
V.   Nonspecific markers
   A.   Leukemia associated antigen
   B.   *In vitro* induction of SV-40 T antigen in skin fibroblasts
VI. General studies
   A.   Chest radiographs
   B.   Chemistry profile

SK-SD, streptokinase-streptodornase; DNCB, dinitrochlorobenzene; KLH, keyhole limpet hemocyanin, PHA, phytohemagglutinin, PMN, pokeweed mitogen; Con A, concanavalin A.

protocol, hypothesis-specific probes, such as assays of immune function applied to diseased as well as clinically normal family members, allow a test of the hypothesis that subclinical immunodeficiency predisposes to CLL. Additional tests, such as for oncornavirus markers, are so complex and the sample requirements so large that clinically normal relatives are evaluated only if tumor patients have abnormalities.

In short, a pragmatic approach is taken. Many general tests and some hypothesis-specific probes with small specimen requirements are offered to all available family members. If abnormalities are identified, then selected individuals may be studied in depth with more sophisticated assays.

Overall, the success of the interdisciplinary approach depends upon the cooperation of suitable families with an appropriate constellation of tumors, the availability of hypothesis-specific probes, and the active participation of interested laboratory researchers.

THE STATE OF THE ART

The interdisciplinary approach has evolved as more families are studied. Refinements include (a) closer search for host and environmental antecedents to explain familial aggregation, (b) rapid incorporation of recent laboratory advances into protocols, especially for lymphoproliferative neoplasms, and (c) the use of long-term follow-up.

Host and Environmental Antecedents

Chromosomal Abnormalities

Because of trisomy 18 in cousins, other family members were karyotyped and several were identified as carriers of a balanced translocation between chromosome 13 and chromosome 18 (1a).

One translocation carrier developed acute myelogenous leukemia (AML) during the course of evaluation. The association may not be coincidental since karyotypic abnormalities are frequent in AML (43) and in persons at high risk for leukemia (32). To investigate this possibility, fibroblasts of family members were exposed to SV-40 *in vitro,* and elevated T antigen expression was observed in translocation carriers but not in a karyotypically normal brother. One translocation carrier had normal SV-40 T antigen expression. The translocation carriers with increased SV-40 T antigen expression, although hematologically normal now, may be at increased risk for leukemia (35,44), possibly through defects in cellular growth imposed by the abnormal position of chromosomes (5,23).

Metabolic Abnormalities

Numerous hormonal abnormalities have been seen in women with breast cancer and in their relatives at high risk, especially abnormalities involving estrogen metabolites (19). Elevated urinary estrogens were found in three men from two families at increased risk for male breast cancer (8); two men with increased estrogen excretion had prophylactic mastectomies, and histopathologic analysis revealed mild dysplasia suggestive of a premalignant state. Thus, an abnormality in estrogen metabolism may predispose to breast cancer in men as it seems to in women.

Searching for Environmental Factors

When gastric carcinoma occurred in four generations ot an inbred kindred from rural Virginia, environmental factors were suspected because the county had significantly higher mortality from stomach cancer than the surrounding area (31). No common environmental factors were identified, and soil samples from the homestead had no unusual concentrations of trace metals. However, the laboratory protocol revealed a high frequency of antibody to gastric parietal cells and defects in cell-mediated immunity in clinically normal relatives (6). The observations suggest that mechanisms of autoimmunity and immunodeficiency, consistent with a genetic defect of T lymphocytes, are involved in this familial susceptibility to stomach cancer (13,20,45,46). The findings concur with the observation that persons with common variable immunodeficiency appear at high risk for carcinoma of the stomach (Chapter 30, *this volume*) and recall a family prone to ataxia-telangiectasia and gastric carcinoma (15).

Adding Recent Laboratory Advances

Putative Immune Response Locus

Immune defects are much more likely in lymphoproliferative disorders. Adolescent brothers separated by 11 months in age developed acute lymphatic leukemia (ALL) within 3 weeks of each other (51), a pattern of onset resembling that observed for monozygous twins in whom leukemia develops (33,34,36). A familial autoimmune disorder was suggested by the finding of clinical seropositive rheumatoid arthritis in both parents and subclinical elevations of rheumatoid factor in three clinically healthy sibs (26). The immune defects observed in the leukemic sibs could result from the leukemia or its therapy and probably are not an etiologic factor. A leukemia-associated antigen was identified in the leukemic sibs but not in their clinically normal sibs or parents (16,41).

The leukemic sibs were found to be HL-A and MLC identical, and their combination of parental haplotypes was not shared with any other sib. Because a human immune response gene may lie within the HL-A gene complex (48), the leukemic sibs could be homozygous for an HL-A-linked defect in the immune response to leukemia (tumor) transplantation, analogous to that underlying certain forms of murine leukemia (29). The unusual presentation in this family raises the question of whether a similar defect in immune surveillance allows for the emergence of leukemia derived from placental exchange of cells in monozygous twins (4).

Immune Function

Another family was studied for evidence of immunodeficiency because of the striking occurrence of lymphoproliferative neoplasms in seven members, including five siblings (12). Lymphocytic and histiocytic lymphomas, Waldenström's macroglobulinemia, Hodgkin's disease, and acute lymphocytic leukemia were distributed over three generations. A subclinical lymphoproliferative disorder was suggested in three healthy relatives by the finding of polyclonal elevations of IgM, the same immunoglobulin with a monoclonal increase in the proband with Waldenström's macroglobulinemia. Since many of the malignancies in this family may be of B cell origin (2), the array of lymphoproliferative disorders may be based in part on the anomalous genetic control of IgM-bearing lymphocytes at various stages of differentiation. As in a similar kinship (42), the finding of impaired *in vitro* response to PHA in the same individuals with IgM elevations supports the hypothesis that subclinical immunodeficiency, analogous to the heritable immunodeficiency syndromes that occasionally underlie lymphoma, predisposed members of this family to malignancy (22, 47). The occurrence of lung adenocarcinoma in two members of this family recalls the excess risk of adenocarcinoma of the lung observed in immunosuppressed renal transplant recipients (9), supporting the hypothesis that immunodeficiency plays a role in the pathogenesis of this tumor.

Immunoglobulin Markers on Cells

The sample protocol (Table 1) was applied to a family in which CLL developed in a father and four offspring (1). No evidence of immune deficiency was detected in any of the clinically normal members of the family, and no linkage to HL-A was found. The immunologic abnormalities of the diseased siblings resembled those observed in sporadic cases of CLL (17).

Sophisticated cell surface immunoglobulin techniques shed light on the mechanism of risk in this family. An unusual heavy-chain type (IgD) and a shared light chain (kappa) were the only surface immunoglobulin markers found on the leukemic cells in three of the four sibs (50). The fourth and youngest sib to be affected, with the mildest clinical disease, had no immunoglobulin detectable on the surface of her cells, suggesting that she may be in an early stage of the disease (40). Since the surface immunoglobulin on B lymphocytes appears to be genetically determined, the finding of the same heavy- and light-chain immunoglobulin on cells of the leukemic sibs suggests an inherited defect, possibly a germinal mutation, in the pool of cells destined to express IgD and kappa on their surface (24).

Longitudinal Studies

In 1969, a consanguineous family was studied because of the occurrence of CLL in three sibs. Selective immunoglobulin deficiency and impaired *in vitro* lymphocyte transformation were discovered in the proband (a patient at the National Institutes of Health being treated for CLL) and several of his clinically healthy sibs (11).

In 1973, the family was recontacted. The proband's brother, previously abnormal by immunologic testing, had subsequently died from bronchogenic carcinoma. The proband's daughter had developed well differentiated lymphocytic lymphoma, the solid tumor equivalent of CLL. As a child, she had been unusually susceptible to infections, and attempted vaccinations had failed, suggesting an immunodeficiency syndrome similar to those known to predispose to lymphoproliferative disorders (21). The son, daughter, and grandchildren of the proband were investigated and had immunologic abnormalities like those originally found in other relatives. All individuals with subclinical immunodeficiency had HL-A2,12, but so did two siblings without abnormalities; hence, the significance of this association is unclear. In another kinship, this haplotype has recently been reported to be associated with diverse tumors (30).

Whereas the initial report postulated a recessively inherited immunodeficiency disorder, because of sib aggregation of leukemia and parental consanguinity, longitudinal follow-up suggested a dominantly inherited defect underlying the lymphoproliferative disorder in this family.

PITFALLS OF THE INTERDISCIPLINARY APPROACH

The role of host susceptibility in the etiology of most cancer is probably subtle. Conventional epidemiologic techniques have defined genetic mechanisms poorly. The interdisciplinary approach explores the role of host factors in a setting where mechanisms of risk may be clearer. Despite this potential, certain limitations of the approach arise from study design and from the laboratory techniques themselves.

Weaknesses in Design

Studies start with the "cancer family," but what is an excessive frequency of a disease as common as cancer? The number of tumors in a family is less important than the pattern of tumors, temporal relationships at diagnosis, and association with other medical conditions. The objective of the interdisciplinary approach is to define processes and mechanisms rather than to enumerate cases.

Interpreting the biologic significance of an association between cancer in a family and a laboratory result is even more difficult. One major pitfall is the tendency to ascribe significance to an observation because it occurs in the family setting. The occasional laboratory abnormality found in a spouse of a family member emphasizes this point. For example, the husband of a family member with CLL (1) was discovered to have a monoclonal IgA spike. Had this abnormality been found in a blood relative, a defect in B cells might have been evoked to explain the observation. (As it was, longstanding chronic osteomyelitis offered a more suitable explanation.) In addition, when an abnormality is identified, the relationship of the observation to the type of tumor must be considered. For example, because persons with immunodeficiency are prone to stomach cancer (Chapter 30, *this volume*), the suggestion is more tenable that immunologic abnormalities found in a gastric cancer family play an etiologic role. The results of a family study cannot be interpreted in a vacuum and must be related to what is already known about a tumor and its antecedents.

Although spouses are usually studied, they are only partially adequate as controls. The logistics of studying numerous people sometimes prohibit repetitive sample collection to control for daily laboratory variations especially in bioassays. The rarity and lethality of certain familial cancer aggregations make confirmatory study nearly impossible. The small size of most families limits the opportunity to do linkage studies and to quantitate the significance of observed abnormalities. Longitudinal studies for clinical correlation are arduous but essential if subclinical abnormalities are to become useful in counseling for cancer control.

Weaknesses in Laboratory Techniques

Interpretation of a laboratory result depends on (a) a statistically valid normal range, (b) confirmatory studies to insure that observed abnormalities did not result from day-to-day laboratory variation, and (c) clinical correlation as defined by a long-term follow-up. The latter is essential if useful information about the importance of subclinical abnormalities in families is to have application to genetic counseling. Many collaborating investigators with research goals different from those of the family studies investigator have little statistically normative data. For example, information about the frequencies of abnormalities in cancer-free families or in those with only one case of a particular malignancy is generally unavailable. Further, problems in interpretation arise from the premature application of new laboratory assays, developed primarily for purposes other than family studies. Assays originally billed as having tumor specificity may turn out to be nonspecific and consequently less useful in the definition of an etiologic hypothesis. The multifaceted protocols addressing many hypotheses sometimes call for an excessive amount of blood or an otherwise unobtainable specimen.

DEVELOPING HYPOTHESIS—SPECIFIC PROBES

The paucity of hypothesis-specific probes is an important barrier to the development of protocols for the evaluation of cancer families, but there are many promising areas of laboratory research that may find application.

New concepts of immunologic regulation are being defined: tests for helper lymphocytes, suppressor T cells, and regulator macrophages may offer new precision in the delineation of mechanisms underlying immunologic disorders (3,49). The development of tumor-specific immune response assays, such as migration inhibition, may provide opportunities for better definition of the role of host immune response (38). Understanding of the hormonal determinants of malignancy may come from study of hormonal markers on tumors (39) and measurements of serum and urinary metabolities (19). The recent isolation of C type virus from human leukemia cells has led to the development of new assays that may help clarify the role of viruses in leukemia (14). DNA hybridization techniques and characterization of molecular enzymes, such as terminal transferase, may lead to identifying specific clones of cells (37). The SV-40 T antigen assay may help define the role of host regulatory genes in the pathogenesis of tumors (Chapter 35, *this volume*). Tests of DNA repair and sister chromatid exchange may permit precise characterization of the inherited molecular defects that may underlie certain familial cancer syndromes (18). Techniques of somatic cell hybridization may be utilized for localizing inherited abnormalities to specific chromosomes (7). Lipkin's assay of cellular kinetics may identify the premalignant phenotype (Chapter 34, *this volume*). Improved chromosomal analysis by computer (25) and new staining techniques (28,52) may offer opportunities for delineating chromosomal defects predisposing families to cancer. As the technology becomes more precise, the genetics of familial malignancy should come into better focus.

CONCLUSION

Studies of familial malignancy are in their infancy because the tools available to define the genetic factors underlying familial susceptibility are primitive. Today we speak of "associations" between laboratory observations and the clinical pattern, but as the tools for investigation are improved, the interdisciplinary approach to familial cancer offers promise for defining genetically determined mechanisms that predispose to malignancy. In this respect, the approach could be considered a pilot for studying in man the role of host factors in carcinogenesis with broader application to cancer etiology and environmental carcinogenesis.

REFERENCES

1. Blattner, W. A., Strober, W., Muchmore, A. V., Blaese, R. M., Broder, S., and Fraumeni, J. F., Jr. (1976): Familial chronic lymphocytic leukemia: Immunologic and cellular characterization. *Ann. Intern. Med.,* 84:554–557.
1a. Blattner, W. A., Whang-Peng, J., and Kistenmacher, M. (1976): Familial translocation and leukemia *(unpublished data).*
2. Braylan, R. C., Jaffe, E. S., and Berard, C. W. (1975): Malignant lymphomas: Current classification and new observations. *Pathol. Annu.,* 213–270.
3. Broder, S., Humphrey, R., Durm, M., Blackman, M., Meade, B., Goldman, C., Strober, W., and Waldman, T. (1975): Impaired synthesis of polyclonal (non-paraprotein) immunoglobulins by circulating lymphocytes from patients with multiple myeloma, role of suppressor cells. *N. Engl. J. Med.,* 293:887–892.
4. Clarkson, B. D., and Boyse, E. A. (1971): Possible explanation of the high concordance for acute leukemia in monozygotic twins. *Lancet,* 1:699–701.
5. Comings, D. E. (1973): A general theory of carcinogenesis. *Proc. Natl. Acad. Sci. USA,* 70:3324–3328.
6. Creagan, E. T., and Fraumeni, J. F. Jr. (1973): Familial gastric cancer and immunologic abnormalities. *Cancer,* 32:1325–1331.
7. Croce, C. M., Aden, D., and Koprowski, H. (1975): Somatic cell hybrids between mouse peritoneal macrophages and Simian-Virus-40 transformed human cells: II. Presence of human

chromosome 7 carrying Simian Virus 40 Genome in cells of tumors induced by hybrid cells. *Proc. Natl. Acad. Sci. USA,* 72:1397–1400.

8. Everson, R. B., Li, F. P., Fraumeni, J. F. Jr., Fishman, J., Wilson, R. E., Stout, D., and Norris, H. J. (1976): Familial male breast cancer. *Lancet,* 1:9–12.

9. Fraumeni, J. F. Jr. (1975): Respiratory carcinogenesis: An epidemiologic appraisal *J. Natl. Cancer Inst.,* 55:1039–1046.

10. Fraumeni, J. F. Jr., and Thomas, L. B. (1967): Malignant bladder tumors in a man and his three sons. *JAMA,* 201:507–509.

11. Fraumeni, J. F. Jr., Vogel, C. L., and DeVita, V. T. (1969): Familial chronic lymphocytic leukemia. *Ann. Intern. Med.,* 71:279–284.

12. Fraumeni, J. F. Jr., Wertelecki, W., Blattner, W. A., Jensen, R. D., and Leventhal, B. G. (1975): Varied manifestations of a familial lymphoproliferative disorder. *Am. J. Med.,* 59:145–151.

13. Fudenberg, H. H. (1971): Genetically determined immune deficiency as the predisposing cause of ''autoimmunity'' and lymphoid neoplasia. *Am. J. Med.,* 51:295–298.

14. Gallager, R. E., and Gallo, R. C. (1975): Type C RNA tumor virus isolated from cultured human acute myelogenous leukemia cells. *Science,* 187:350–353.

15. Haerer, A. F., Jackson, J. F., and Evers, C. G. (1969): Ataxia-telangiectasia with gastric adenocarcinoma. *JAMA,* 210:1884–1897.

16. Halterman, R. H., Leventhal, B. G., and Mann, D. L. (1972): An acute-leukemia antigen: Correlation with clinical status. *N. Engl. J. Med.,* 287:1272–1274.

17. Han, T. (1973): Studies of correlation of lymphocyte response to phytohemagglutinin with the clinical and immunologic status in chronic lymphocytic leukemia. *Cancer,* 31:280–285.

18. Hayashi, K., and Schmid, W. (1975): The rate of sister chromatid exchanges parallel to spontaneous chromosome breakage in Fanconi's anemia and to trenimon-induced aberrations in human lymphocytes and fibroblasts. *Humangenetik,* 29:201–206.

19. Henderson, B. E., Gerkins, V., Rosario, I., Casagrande, J., and Pike, M. C. (1975): Elevated serum levels of estrogen and prolactin in daughters of patients with breast cancer. *N. Engl. J. Med.,* 293:790–795.

20. Hermans, P. E., and Huizenga, K. A. (1972): Association of gastric carcinoma with idiopathic late-onset immunoglobulin deficiency. *Ann. Intern. Med.,* 76:605–609.

21. Kersey, J. H., and Spector, B. D. (1975): Immune deficiency diseases. In: *Persons at High Risk of Cancer: An Approach to Cancer Etiology and Control,* edited by J. F. Fraumeni, Jr., pp. 55–67. Academic Press, New York.

22. Kersey, J. H., Spector, B. D., and Good, R. A. (1973): Primary immunodeficiency diseases and cancer: The immunodeficiency-cancer registry. *Int. J. Cancer,* 12:333–347.

23. Klein, G. (1975): The Epstein–Barr virus and neoplasia. *N. Engl. J. Med.,* 293:1353–1357.

24. Knudson, A. G. Jr., Strong, L. C., and Anderson, P. E. (1973): Heredity and cancer in man. *Prog. Med. Genet.,* 9:113–152.

25. Ladda, R., Atkins, L., Littlefield, J., Neurath, P., and Marimuthu, K. M. (1974): Computer assisted analysis of chromosomal abnormalities: Detection of deletion in aniridia/Wilms' tumor syndrome. *Science* 185:784–787.

26. Lawrence, J. S. (1973): Rheumatoid factors in families. *Semin. Arthritis Rheum.,* 3:177–188.

27. Leklem, J. E., and Brown, R. R. (1976): Abnormal tryptophan metabolism in a family with a history of bladder cancer. *J. Natl. Cancer Inst.,* 56:1101–1104.

28. Lewandowski, R. C., and Yunis, J. J. (1975): New chromosomal syndromes. *Am. J. Dis. Child* 129:515–529.

29. Lilly, F., and Pincus, T. (1973): Genetic control of murine viral leukemogenesis. *Adv. Cancer Res.,* 17:231–277.

30. Lynch, H. T., Thomas, R. J., Terasaki, P. I., Ting, A., Guirgis, H. A., Kaplan, A. R., Chaperon, E., Magee, H., Lynch, J., and Kraft, C. (1975): HL-A in cancer ''Family N.'' *Cancer,* 36:1315–1320.

31. Mason, T. J., and McKay, F. W. (1974): *U.S. Cancer Mortality by County: 1950–1969.* DHEW Publication No. (NIH) 74–615.

32. Miller, R. W. (1967): Persons with exceptionally high risk of leukemia. *Cancer Res.,* 27:2420–2423.

33. Miller, R. W. (1968): Deaths from childhood cancer in sibs. *N. Engl. J. Med.,* 279:122–126.

34. Miller, R. W. (1971): Deaths from childhood leukemia and solid tumors among twins and other sibs in the United States, 1960–67. *J. Natl. Cancer Inst.,* 46:203–209.

35. Mulvihill, J. J. (1975): Congenital and genetic disease. In: *Persons at High Risk of Cancer: An*

Approach to Cancer Etiology and Control, edited by J. F. Fraumeni, Jr., pp. 3–37. Academic Press, New York.

36. MacMahon, B., and Levy, M. A. (1964): Prenatal origin of childhood leukemia. *N. Engl. J. Med.,* 270:1082–1085.

37. McCaffrey, R., Harrison, T. A., Parkman, R., and Baltimore, D. (1975): Terminal deoxynucleotidy 1 transferase activity in human leukemic cells and in normal human thymocytes. *N. Engl. J. Med.,* 292:775–780.

38. McCoy, J. L., Jerome, L. F., Dean, J. H., Cannon, G. B., Alford, T. C., Doering, T., and Herberman, R. B. (1974): Inhibition of leukocyte migration by tumor associated antigens in soluble extracts of human breast carcinoma. *J. Natl. Cancer Inst.,* 53:11 17.

39. McGuire, W. L. (1975): Current status of estrogen receptors in human breast cancer. *Cancer,* 36:638–644.

40. McLaughlin, H., Wetherly-Mein, G., Pitcher, C., and Hobbs, J. R. (1973): Non-immuno-globulin-bearing 'B' lymphocytes in chronic lymphocytic leukaemia? *Br. J. Hematol.,* 25:7–14

41. Pendergrass, T. W., Stoller, R. G., Mann, D. L., Halterman, R. H., and Fraumeni, J. F. Jr. (1975): Acute myelocytic leukaemia and leukaemia-associated antigens in sisters. *Lancet,* 1:429–431.

42. Potolsky, A. I., Heath, C. W. Jr., Buckley, C. E. III, and Rowlands, D. T. Jr. (1971): Lymphoreticular malignancies and immunologic abnormalities in a sibship. *Am. J. Med.,* 50:42–48.

43. Sakurai, M., and Sandberg, A. A. (1976): Chromosomes and causation of human cancer and leukemia, XI. Correlation of karyotypes with clinical features of acute myeloblastic leukemia. *Cancer,* 37:285–299.

44. Snyder, A. L., Li, F. P., Henderson, E. S., and Todaro, G. J. (1970): Possible inherited leukaemogenic factors in familial acute myelogenous leukaemia. *Lancet,* 1:586–589.

45. Twomey, J. J., Jordan, P. H., Jarrold, T., Trubowitz, S., Ritz, N. D., and Conn, H. O. (1969): The syndrome of immunoglobulin deficiency and pernicious anemia. *Am. J. Med.,* 47:340–350.

46. Twomey, J. J., Jordan, P. H., Laughter, A. H., Meuwissen, M. D., and Good, R. A. (1970): The gastric disorder in immunoglobulins deficient patient. *Ann. Intern. Med.,* 72:499–504.

47. Twomey, J. J., Levin, W. C., Melmik, M. B., Trobaugh, F. E., and Allgood, J. W. (1967): Laboratory studies on a family with father and son affected by acute leukemia. *Blood,* 29:920–930.

48. Vladistin, A. O., and Rose, N. R. (1974): HL-A antigens: Association with disease. *Immunogenetics,* 1:305–328.

49. Waldman, T. A., Ourm, M., Broder, S., Blackman, M., Blaese, M., and Strober, W. (1974): Role of suppressor T-cells in pathogenesis of common variable hypogammaglobulinaemia. *Lancet,* 2:609–613.

50. Warner, N. L. (1975): Membrane immunoglobulins and antigen receptors on B and T lymphocytes. *Adv. Immunol.,* 19:67–216.

51. Wimmer, R. S., Blattner, W. A., Naiman, J. L., Fraumeni, J. F. Jr., and Dean, J. H. (1975): Familial ALL: Genetic and immunologic determinants. *Proc. Am. Soc. Hematol.,* 48 (Abstr.).

52. Yunis, J. J. (1976): High resolution of human chromosomes. *Science,* 191:1268–1270.

Discussion

Lynch: Dr. Blattner, in the family in which you reported an immunologic deficiency and HLA2,12 haplotype, what were the predominant tumors? Have you seen type 2,12 in other family aggregates, including the cancer family syndrome?

Blattner: Chronic lymphocytic leukemia and well differentiated lymphocytic lymphomas, which are derived from the same cells essentially, were the major tumors in our family, although one member had bronchogenic carcinoma. We have not had the opportunity to carry out detailed studies in other family syndromes.

Gatti: You mentioned that the two children with leukemia shared perhaps the same histocompatibility locus. This may be true, but the bone marrow transplant program for leukemia is based on finding such siblings that are HLA matched and they are all free of leukemia.

Blattner: You have a good point. However cofactors in the family may suggest an autoimmune disorder, just as in the murine system where there are multiple factors. The situation may be analogous to the H-2 factor associating leukemia with tumor transplantation antigens, although I doubt this mechanism explains all familial leukemia.

Hirschhorn: In the various pedigrees that we have seen from you, Dr. Li and Dr. Fraumeni, I am struck by the peculiar form of segregation; there are simply too many affected individuals. I wonder if this has ever been analyzed as to the possibility of chance; it suggests that familial aggregations of cancer cannot always be explained in a straightforward Mendelian fashion. They may involve vertical transmission of various agents or cytoplasmic inheritance—which incidentally does not have to be maternal, at least in mammals, because mitochondria are plentiful in sperm. The word dominant has been tossed about a good bit, perhaps too loosely, in relation to these families.

Li: Your point is well taken, and you may be right. On the other hand, we identified these families for study because there were so many affected cases, indicating a selection factor. But we really do not know what the mode of inheritance is, or whether, in fact, inheritance is a factor.

Blattner: In addition to having biased families, we have biased data in the sense that not all family studies show abnormalities by the experimental techniques used. We are successful only when the laboratory investigators are able to develop hypothesis-specific probes to uncover mechanisms of familial susceptibility.

German: I thought I might mention a family we had in New York Hospital in the 1960s. It was a ''sarcoma family'' in which one child had rhabdomyosarcoma of the face, a second child had a sarcoma of the brain, and many relatives were affected by various other types of cancer.

Li: Dr. German's comments are a good illustration of how we accumulate information on cancer families. However, since he did not report the family earlier, his observation might well have become lost. We really should report cancer-prone families one by one, if necessary, when new observations are made.

Nance: I would like to ask about the titers of fetal antigens from patients in cancer families compared to patients with nonfamilial cancer.

Li: We have studied a multiple-case family with colon cancer, and did not find elevations of carcinoembryonic antigen in clinically normal family members [*Cancer*, 37:946–948 (1976)].

Lynch: We have several carcinoma-prone families with increased carcinoembryonic antigen titers apparently in normal members [*JAMA*, 224:1042 (1973)]. We are also working with investigators at the Mayo Clinic and have seen two melanoma-prone families with elevation of alphafetoprotein.

Genetics of Human Cancer, edited by J. J.
Mulvihill, R. W. Miller, and J. F. Fraumeni, Jr.
Raven Press, New York, 1977.

24

Genetic Markers and Cancer

Mary-Claire King and Nicholas L. Petrakis

*G. W. Hooper Foundation and the Department of International Health, University of
California School of Medicine, San Francisco, California 94143*

Customarily the epidemiologic characteristics of populations have been described in terms of age, sex, ethnic or racial origin, marital, occupational, and
socioeconomic status, and so on. In recent years, polymorphic genetic markers
have provided an additional tool for epidemiologic studies of disease frequency in
various populations. We will discuss the use of genetic markers in the definition
of groups at high risk for cancer. By *genetic marker,* we refer to a protein or other
phenotype determined by a single locus with two or more alleles present at
significant frequencies in the population of epidemiologic interest. We exclude
from our consideration chromosomal markers associated with certain cancers,
especially leukemias (25), as well as proteins which undergo quantitative change
(for physiological rather than genetic reasons) in tissues associated with tumor
development.

Genetic markers can contribute to two genetic-epidemiologic approaches to the
study of human cancer. First, allelic frequencies at the marker locus may differ in
cancer subjects compared with a healthy control population. Such studies of
associations between genetic markers and disease have been by far the most
common use of genetic markers in cancer epidemiology to date. A significant,
reproducible statistical association between a genetic marker and cancer indicates
either (1) an etiological relationship (quite possibly indirect) between marker and
disease, or (2) a more susceptible subpopulation, defined in part by the frequency
of particular alleles at the marker locus, although the genetic marker has no
clinical significance itself. An example of (1) is the possible causal relationship
between breast cancer and the cerumen marker. An example of (2) might be the
use of the Duffy blood group (whose allelic frequencies differ markedly in
African and Caucasian populations) to help determine whether black cancer
patients have genotypes derived in greater measure from Caucasian, rather than
African, ancestry more frequently than healthy black persons.

A second approach to cancer epidemiology using genetic markers is *linkage analysis,* which, unlike the study of associations, investigates whether loci are closely linked physically on the same chromosome so that they are inherited together in families. The relevance of linkage analysis to cancer epidemiology lies in finding a genetic marker (quite probably with no clinical significance itself) which is inherited with a neoplastic phenotype in cancer-prone families. If a marker gene is located on its chromosome very close to a (possibly undetectable) cancer-related gene or gene complex so that crossing over during meiosis seldom occurs, the presence of the genetic marker would serve as a warning that the closely linked cancer-related gene complex is also present. The presence of the genetic marker could, of course, be detected long before the process of carcinogenesis is clinically apparent. If, in addition, the chromosomal site of the genetic marker is known, the location of closely linked cancer-related genes could also be estimated. Recently, particularly with the application of somatic cell hybridization techniques, almost 100 genes have been mapped on specific chromosomes (26). Therefore, considerable material is available for linkage analysis.

To be useful for either association or linkage analysis, potential "marker" genes should produce traits that are clearly defined manifestations of single loci. The protein or phenotypic characteristic determined by the marker gene should be easy to detect, with (ideally) the heterozygote and homozygote genotypes clearly distinguishable, and should be highly polymorphic in the population of epidemiologic interest. The characteristic coded by the marker gene should be unaffected by physiological or environmental factors. Meeting these specifications are more than 60 polymorphic blood groups, red cell and serum proteins, and physical traits now in use as genetic markers.

ASSOCIATIONS OF SINGLE GENETIC MARKERS AND SPECIFIC CANCERS

The modern history of the possible association of genetic markers and cancer began in 1951 when Aird and Bentall (1) reported a slight but significant association between blood group A and cancer of the stomach. Since that time an extensive and controversial literature has developed. A simple statistical technique for measuring the relative incidence of disease in individuals with or without any specific characteristic, and for determining the statistical significance of the association between the presence of disease and the marker (43), permits comparisons of results from various research centers with differing gene frequencies in their populations. Blood group A appears to be associated with a higher risk for several major cancers (Table 1). The literature on the possible associations between blood groups and cancer has been reviewed by Vogel (38) and by Vogel and Helmbold (39), and has been severely criticized by others (22,42). Critics correctly point out that spurious associations may arise from inappropriately lumping together different diagnostic conditions, from selection of control groups from populations that differ genetically from populations to which affected subjects belong, and/or from the failure to publish negative results so that occasional positive associations result simply by chance from large numbers of tests. In

TABLE 1. *Some reported associations between polymorphic blood group markers and cancer*

Polymorphism	Ref.	Cancer	Phenotypes compared	Relative risk [a]
ABO	38	Stomach	A:O	1.22
		Colon and rectum	A:O	1.10
		Salivary gland	A:O	1.64
		Pancreas	A:O	1.23
		Mouth and pharynx	A:O	1.25
		Cervix	A:O	1.13
		Corpus uteri	A:O	1.15
		Ovary	A:O	1.27
		Breast	A:O	1.08
	33	Acute leukemia	A:O	1.12
		Chronic leukemia	A:O	1.08
Secretor	38	Lung cancer	se:Se	0.41
Rh	38	Stomach	D(+):D(−)	0.77
		Esophagus	D(+):D(−)	0.64
		Pancreas	D(+):D(−)	0.72
		Breast	D(+):D(−)	1.25
S	6	Breast	ss:S−	1.82
	24	Breast	ss:S−	N.S.
	2	Breast	ss:s−	N.S.

[a] Calculated from published data; all numbers are statistically significant at $P \leq 0.05$. N.S., not significant.

contrast to the abundance of literature on possible associations of cancer and blood groups, relatively few studies have been made of the possible association of other polymorphic biochemical markers and cancer. Tables 1 to 3 list some of the reported associations and lack of associations between genetic markers and neoplasia. Terasaki et al. discuss the HL-A data in detail elsewhere in this volume.

A different experimental approach has revealed possible etiological associations between several other markers and specific cancers. In each of these cases, quantitative variation in protein levels was observed in healthy populations. A trimodal distribution of protein levels led in each instance to the hypothesis that two alleles at a single locus controlled enzyme production. When protein levels of cancer patients appeared to be clustered disproportionately in one or two modes of the distribution, the possible role of the protein in the etiology of the disease became the subject of intense scrutiny. The advantage of this approach is that a biological hypothesis underlies investigation of the marker; the limitations of these studies lie in poor reproducibility of quantitative results, the physiological variability in activity level for any individual, and the uncertainty surrounding a single-locus Mendelian model suggested only by quantitative information. The development of direct detection methods (such as specific staining procedures) for alternative alleles in these systems would greatly increase their value as genetic markers.

Individuals heterozygous or homozygous for the Z allele at the *Pi* locus produce α_1-antitrypsin which is not completely released from the liver where it is synthe-

TABLE 2. *Reported associations between HL-A antigens and neoplasia*

Cancer	Ref.	Association
Acute lymphocytic leukemia	40	HL-A2 increased
	31	HL-A2 increased
	17	HL-A9 more favorable prognosis
Breast	27	HL-A7 increased
	8	No association
Hodgkin's disease	5	HL-A5, W5, W15,W18 increased
Nasopharynx	35	HL-A2 increased
Multiple myeloma	4	W18 increased
"Cancer family syndrome"	21	HL-A2-HL-A12 increased

sized, and individuals homozygous for the much rarer 0 allele apparently do not produce α_1-antitrypsin at all (13). Deficiency of serum α_1-antitrypsin is associated with emphysema in adults and hepatitis in infants. It now appears that $Pi^M Pi^Z$ and $Pi^Z Pi^Z$ individuals may also be highly susceptible to liver cancer (3,7,9,20,30). The Z allele in hepatoma patients in these studies was detected indirectly by the presence of cytoplasmic globules in liver samples, rather than by direct determination of the *Pi* genotype in serum. Since most enzyme-deficient individuals do not develop infantile hepatitis, emphysema, or liver cancer, and since most patients with these diseases are not α_1-antitrypsin deficient, this system presents interesting questions of environmental influences on potentially susceptible individuals.

The use of 16α-hydroxylase activity as a genetic marker related to breast cancer risk has been suggested by Lemon (18,19). He postulates a two-allele, single-locus genetic basis for reduced 17β-estradiol and estrone hydroxylation to estriol by 16α-hydroxylase, based on variation in Caucasian women of urinary excretion of estriol compared to estrone and 17β-estradiol, plasma clearance rates of estrone and estradiol, and leukocyte 16-hydroxylase activity. At least three clusters of activity appear in healthy Caucasian populations, and breast cancer cases repeatedly aggregate in the lowest activity groups. The demonstration of the Mendelian inheritance of 16α-hydroxylase levels, by study of the enzyme in families and by development of a direct detection technique for the low-activity allele, would be a major contribution to the clinical usefulness of this marker.

Aryl hydrocarbon hydroxylase may prove a valuable genetic marker in the study of lung cancer. Kellerman et al. (15) reported that inducibility of this enzyme appears to be controlled by a single locus with two alleles, and that persons heterozygous or homozygous for the allele determining high inducibility have a much increased risk of lung cancer. However, this work is fraught with technical problems in development of a reproducible assay and in confirmation of Kellerman's original results. Nebert reviews current research on the possible association of aryl hydrocarbon hydroxylase and lung cancer elsewhere in this volume.

Preliminary results indicate that adenosine deaminase (ADA) levels in lymphocytes from untreated chronic lymphocytic leukemia patients are significantly lower

TABLE 3. *Some reported associations between polymorphic serum proteins and cancer*

Polymorphism	Ref.	Cancer	Phenotypes compared	Relative risk [a]
Haptoglobin	28	"Leukemias"	1-1:2-1 + 2-2	1.8
		.	2-1:1-1 + 2-2	2.0
			2-2:1-1 + 2-1	N.S.
	41	"Leukemias"	1-1:2-2	3.2
	32	Breast cancer	All combinations	N.S.
	16	Breast cancer	All combinations	N.S.
		Uterus, ovary, and cervix	2-2:1-1 + 2-1	2.96
		Melanoma	All combinations	N.S.
		Bronchogenic cancer	All combinations	N.S.
		Reticulosis	All combinations	N.S.
		Colon	All combinations	N.S.
	23	Cervix	All combinations	N.S.
GC component	14	Stomach	All combinations	N.S.
		Colon	2-1:2-2 + 1-1	0.59
		Breast	All combinations	N.S.
		Ectodermal cancers	All combinations	N.S.
		Endodermal cancers	2-2:2-1 + 1-1	2.36
			2-1:2-2 + 1-1	0.65
		Mesodermal cancers	1-1:2-1 + 2-2	0.68
			2-2:2-1 + 1-1	3.55
	12	Acute myeloid leukemia	2-2:2-1 + 1-1	2.41
		Chronic myeloid leukemia	All combinations	N.S.
		Chronic lymphatic leukemia	All combinations	N.S.

[a] Calculated from published data; all numbers are statistically significant at $p \leqslant 0.05$; N.S., not significant.

than ADA levels in normal lymphocytes (37). ADA genotypes were directly determined, using electrophoresis, for 16 chronic lymphocytic leukemia patients in the study. Unexpectedly, the 2-1 genotype was more frequent (38%) than in normal populations (10%). This preliminary sample is far too small to indicate ADAs usefulness as a genetic marker, but further study of this system is certainly worthwhile.

Investigation of possible associations of single genetic markers and specific cancers continues, but results are still contradictory and not clinically useful. Little is known about possible physiological mechanisms underlying most of the observed associations. Recent studies suggest that carcinoembryonic antigens are closely related to blood group precursor substances (34), and that HL-A antigens have chemical structures very similar to the immunoglobulins (36). Many bacteria and viruses have been reported to contain blood group specific antigens, and differences in immunoglobulin levels have been found to be associated with blood group and secretor status (11). It is likely that future studies will clarify interrelationships of these factors and their associations with malignant disease. Meanwhile, from the clinical standpoint, it is evident that, although statistically significant associations between individual genetic markers and cancer do exist, they are

TABLE 4. *Percentage of individuals heterozygous for blood polymorphisms at selected loci–Caucasian U.S. population*

Erythrocyte enzymes	%	Serum proteins	%	Blood group systems	%
Acid phosphatase	54	Group-specific component	42	ABO	44
Adenosine deaminase	10	Haptoglobin α chain	48	Duffy A and B	49
Adenylate kinase	9	Third component of complement	36	Lewis A and B	36
Glutamate-pyruvate transaminase (soluble)	50	Immunoglobulins: G1m (z, a, x, and f); G3m (b0, b1, b3, b5,		MN	50
Peptidase A	41	c3, c5, g, s, t, and v);		Rh (CcDEe)	49
Phosphoglucomutase 1	35	A_2m (1 and 2); Km^a(1)	50	Secretor	50
Esterase D	18			Ss	40
				Kell	9

[a] Km was formerly referred to as Inv.
Data from refs. 10, 13, and 29.

for the most part relatively slight. They are not yet useful for the detection of individuals at high risk for cancer nor in the differential diagnosis of cancer.

LINKAGE ANALYSIS

In cooperation with Drs. Henry Lynch, Paul Terasaki, Robert Elston, and Mel Schanfield, our laboratory has begun the investigation of genetic linkage between segregating genetic markers and putative cancer-susceptibility loci in families at high risk for breast cancer. Segregation analysis in conjunction with linkage analysis will enable us to suggest possible modes of inheritance of cancer phenotypes in families. Using breast cancer as a model, we are studying 18 extended families, characterized by at least one mother-daughter or sister-sister pair with histologically verified breast cancer. Twenty enzyme and blood group systems polymorphic in Caucasian populations, as well as 23 leukocyte (HL-A) antigens, have been analyzed in blood samples from more than 300 members of these families (Table 4). Preliminary results indicate that at least several of these markers are segregating in each family. We plan to test two alternative models by segregation and linkage analysis. First, we will investigate the pattern of inheritance of breast cancer in the families and the possible linkage of the breast cancer phenotype with marker loci; second, the analysis will be repeated with breast, cervical, ovarian, and/or endometrial cancer classified positive for the cancer characteristic.

DISCRIMINANT ANALYSIS USING GENETIC MARKERS

Another approach to the study of possible associations of genetic markers and cancer involves combining multiple genetic markers and more traditional epidemiologic (environmental) parameters in order to determine a constellation of factors defining a high-risk group. The goal of this approach is to accurately assign asymptomatic persons in a given age, sex, ethnic, and socioeconomic group to a high or low cancer-risk group. Again, starting with breast cancer, we are using 23 genetically and environmentally influenced factors measured for each of approximately 200 breast cancer patients, 200 patients with cancer at a site other than the breast, and 200 healthy women matched in case-control triplets. The values of the 23 factors for each woman will be used to produce a function that most effectively distinguishes the three groups.

In a preliminary test of this approach, 81 breast cancer patients from the University of California hospitals and the Hooper Foundation breast screening clinic were matched with 81 healthy women from the breast screening clinic. Cases and controls were matched by age (within 5 years), ethnicity (white, black, Chinese, Japanese, Filipino, or Mexican-American), years of education (grade school, high school, college, postgraduate, or professional school) and hospital status (clinic or private patient). Age and ethnicity are, of course, known to affect breast cancer risk, so these variables were controlled in order to obtain a preliminary index independent of these factors. We matched education and hospital status in a rough attempt to control for socioeconomic status in our sample.

Three types of variables were measured for each of the women in our sample: personal history (age at menarche, first pregnancy, and menopause; marital history; number of livebirths, miscarriages, or stillbirths, and children breastfed; use of contraceptive pills and hormones; and history of hysterectomy prior to breast cancer diagnosis), family history of breast cancer (mother, sister, grandmother, or aunt), and genotypic information (11 of the systems from Table 4). Linear discriminant analysis was used to distinguish between the breast cancer patients and their healthy controls by finding the linear function of the measured variables that best characterized the two groups by maximizing the genetic and environmental distance between them.

Individually, none of the genetic markers in Table 4 differed significantly in gene frequency in the cancer and control groups. Nevertheless, this collection of markers did add significantly to our ability to distinguish the two samples. When clinical data were removed from each record, and subjects classified into "high-risk" or "low-risk" groups on the basis of this preliminary analysis alone, more than 60% of the breast cancer patients were correctly assigned to the "high-risk" group and over 75% of the healthy controls to the "low-risk" group.

Although the genetic markers in this analysis may not be physiologically involved in breast cancer etiology, they may be demographically associated as a group with loci of clinical interest. Since cases and controls in the study were matched for ethnicity, these genetic markers do reflect more than simple differences in gene frequencies among ethnic groups.

Several lines of investigation are possible now using the multivariate statistical approach with multiple genetic markers. First, we will determine how effectively the preliminary function correctly assigns new cases to breast cancer or healthy groups. Second, additional genetic, demographic, biochemical, and clinical data that we have collected on the larger sample of patients and controls will be integrated into the analysis in order to increase the discriminating power. Third, we will determine the constellation of genetic and other factors contributing to risk for a number of separate subpopulations: blacks, whites, premenopausal, and postmenopausal samples are now large enough to allow separate analyses.

ACKNOWLEDGMENTS

Supported by Public Health Service Grant CA 13556 and Contract CB 44003 from the National Cancer Institute and by a gift from Mrs. Viola K. Schroeder.

REFERENCES

1. Aird, I., and Bentall, H. H. (1951): A relationship between cancer of the stomach and the ABO blood groups. *Br. Med. J.*, 1:799–801.
2. Anderson, D. E. (1971): Some characteristics of familial breast cancer. *Cancer*, 28:1500–1504.
3. Berg, N. O., and Eriksson, S. (1972): Liver disease in adults with alpha$_1$-antitrypsin deficiency. *N. Engl. J. Med.*, 287:1264–1267.
4. Bertrams, J., Kuwert, E., Böhme, U., Reis, H. E., Gallmeier, W. M., Wetter, O., and Schmidt, C. G. (1972): HL-A antigens in Hodgkin's disease and multiple myeloma: Increased frequency of W18 in both diseases. *Tissue Antigens*, 2:41–46.
5. Bodmer, W. F. (1973): Genetic factors in Hodgkin's disease: Association with a disease—susceptibility locus (DSA) in the HL-A region. *Natl. Cancer Inst. Monogr.* 36:127–134.
6. Boston Collaborative Drug Surveillance Program (1971): Relation between breast cancer and S blood-antigen system. *Lancet*, 1:301–304.
7. Brunt, P. W. (1974): Progress report: Antitrypsin and the liver. *Gut*, 15:573–580.
8. Cordon, A. L., and James, D. C. O. (1973): HL-A and carcinoma of the breast. *Lancet*, 2:565.
9. Eriksson, S., and Hagerstrand, I. (1974): Cirrhosis and malignant hepatoma in alpha$_1$-antitrypsin deficiency. *Acta Med. Scand.*, 195:451–458.
10. Giblett, E. R. (1969): *Genetic Markers in Human Blood.* Blackwell, Oxford.
11. Grundbacher, F. J., and Shreffler, D. C. (1970): Effect of secretor, blood, and serum groups on isoantibody and immunoglobulin levels. *Am. J. Hum. Genet.* 22:194–202.
12. Gurda, M. (1969): Die Korrelation zwischen dem Gc-Typ und den verschiedenen Leukämie formen. *Folia Haematol*, 91:452–456.
13. Harris, H. (1975): *Principles of Human Biochemical Genetics,* pp. 360–362. Elsevier. New York.
14. Hughes, N. R. (1968): Gc group distributions in patients with cancer. *J. Natl. Cancer Inst.*, 41:303–313.
15. Kellerman, G., Shaw, C. R., and Luyten-Kellerman, M. (1973): Aryl hydrocarbon hydroxylase inducibility and bronchogenic carcinoma. *N. Engl. J. Med.*, 289:934–936.
16. Larkin, M. F. (1967): Serum haptoglobin type and cancer. *J. Nat. Cancer. Inst.*, 39:633–638.
17. Lawler, S. D., Klouda, P. T., Smith, P. G., Till, M. M., and Hardisty, R. M. (1974): Survival and the HL-A system in acute lymphoblastic leukaemia. *Br. Med. J.*, 1:547–548.
18. Lemon, H. M. (1972): Genetic predisposition to carcinoma of the breast: Multiple human genotypes for estrogen 16 alpha hydroxylase activity in Caucasians. *J. Surg. Oncol.*, 4:255–273.
19. Lemon, H. M., and Reilly, D. (1974): Genotypic variations in Caucasian leukocyte estradiol 16 hydroxylase activity: A measurable deterrent of breast cancer risk? *Nebr. State. Med. J.*, 59:151–155.
20. Lieberman, J. (1974): Emphysema, cirrhosis, and hepatoma with alpha$_1$-antitrypsin deficiency. *Ann. Intern. Med.*, 81:850–852.
21. Lynch, H. T., Thomas, R. J., Terasaki, P., Ting, A. Guirgis, H. A., Kaplan, A. R., Magee,

H., Lynch, J., Kraft, C., and Chaperon, E. (1975): HL-A in cancer family "N". *Cancer*, 36:1315–1320.

22. Manuilia, A. (1958): Blood groups and disease—hard facts and delusions. *JAMA*, 167:2047–2053.

23. Milunicôva, A., Jandovà, A., and Skoda, V. (1969): Serum haptoglobin type in females with genital cancer. *J. Natl. Cancer Inst.*, 42:749–752.

24. Morosini, P., Lee, E. G., Jones, M. N., and Vessey, M. P. (1972): Breast cancer and the S blood-group system. *Lancet*, 1:411–412.

25. Mulvihill, J. J. (1975): Congenital and genetic diseases. In: *Persons at High Risk of Cancer. An Approach to Cancer Etiology and Control,* edited by J. F. Fraumeni, Jr., pp. 3–37. Academic Press, New York.

26. New Haven Conference (1974): Human gene mapping. *Birth Defects*, 10(3):1–216.

27. Patel, R., Habal, M. B., Wilson, R. E. Birtch, A. G., and Moore, F. D. (1972): Histocompatibility (HL-A) antigens and cancer of the breast: Association with HL-A7. *Am. J. Surg.*, 124:31–34.

28. Peacock, A. C. (1966): Serum haptoglobin type and leukemia: An association with possible etiological significance. *J. Natl. Cancer Inst.*, 36:631–639.

29. Race, R. R. and Sanger, R. (1968): *Blood Groups in Man, 5th edition.* Blackwell, Oxford.

30. Rawlings, W., Jr., Moss, Jr., Cooper, H. S., and Hamilton S. R. (1974): Hepatocellular carcinoma and partial deficiency of alpha₁-antitrypsin (MZ). *Ann. Intern. Med.*, 81:771–773.

31. Rogentine, G. N., Yankee, R. A., Gart, J. J., Nam, J., and Trapani, R. J. (1972): HL-A antigens and disease: Acute lymphocytic leukemia. *J. Clin. Invest.*, 51:2420–2428.

32. Scholz, W., Gilly, L., and Gilly, G. (1968): Bestimmung von Blutgruppen und Serumgruppen bei Karzinompatienten. *Strahlentherapie,* 136:448–453.

33. Shirley, R., and Desai, R. G. (1965): Association of leukemia and blood groups. *J. Med. Genet.,* 2:189–191.

34. Simmons, D. A. R., and Perlmann, P. (1973): Carcinoembryonic antigen and blood group substances. *Cancer Res.,* 33:313–322.

35. Simons, M. J., Wee, G. B., Day, N. E., Morris, P. J., Shanmugaratnam, K., and De-Thé, G. B. (1974): Immunogenetic aspects of nasopharyngeal carcinoma: 1. Differences in HL-A antigen profiles between patients and control groups. *Int. J. Cancer,* 13:122–134.

36. Strominger, J. L., Cresswell, P., Grey, H., Humphreys, R. H., Mann, D., McCune, J., Parkam, P., Robb, R., Sanderson, A. R. Springer, T. A., Terhorst, C., and Turner, M. J. (1974): The immunoglobulin-like structure of human histocompatibility antigens. *Transpl. Rev.,* 21:126–143.

37. Tung, R., Conklyn, M., Selber, R., and Hirschhorn, R. (1974): Adenosine deaminase in lymphocytes from normal subjects and patients with chronic lymphocytic leukemia. *Blood,* 44:923.

38. Vogel, F. (1970) : ABO blood groups and disease. *Am. J. Hum. Genet.,* 22:464–475.

39. Vogel, F., and Helmbold, W. (1972): Blutgruppen-Populationsgenetik und Statistik. In: *Humangenetik: Ein kurzes Handbuch, Vol. 1/4,* edited by P. E. Becker, pp. 129–557. Georg Thieme Verlag, Stuttgart.

40. Walford, R. L., Smith, G. S., and Waters, H. (1971): Histocompatibility systems and disease states with particular reference to cancer. *Transpl. Rev.,* 7:78–111.

41. Wendt, G. G., Krüger, J., and Kindermann, I. (1968): Serumgruppen und Krankheit. *Humangenetik,* 6:281–299.

42. Wiener, A. S. (1970): Blood groups and disease. *Am. J. Hum. Genet.,* 22:476–483.

43. Woolf, B. (1955): On estimating the relation between blood group and disease. *Ann. Hum. Genet.,* 19:251–253.

Discussion

Rashad: Linkage of the Hawaii Household Registration file (1942–1943) and the death record file (1950–1973) was carried out. Of 87,016 death records, 20,409 were linked and provided information on cancer patients who lived in Hawaii in 1942. Additional information from the Hawaii Household Registration file was extracted including age in 1942, sex, race, blood group, and dermatoglyphic traits. Each cancer death was matched with another individual of the same sex, age, and race, and a study of the distribution of dermatoglyphic traits and the ABO blood groups in the cancer deaths and their controls was carried out.

An excess of group A subjects in cancer patients when compared with the controls was significant for cancer of the stomach and ovary. A similar trend was also demonstrated for other cancer types, but the differences were not statistically significant.

Significant differences in dermatoglyphic traits occurred between cancer cases and controls. A consistent reduction of the frequency of ulnar loops in cancer cases was associated with an excess of unusual patterns: an excess of arches for cancer of the rectum and cervix and in leukemia; an excess of double loops for cancer of the stomach, lung, breast, prostate, and thyroid; and an excess of true whorls in cancer of the pancreas.

Genetics of Human Cancer, edited by J. J.
Mulvihill, R. W. Miller, and J. F. Fraumeni, Jr.
Raven Press, New York, 1977.

25

Endocrine Function and Breast Cancer

B. E. Henderson, V. R. Gerkins, M. C. Pike, and J. T. Casagrande

University of Southern California School of Medicine, Los Angeles, California 90033

The familial risk of breast cancer has been well-documented (28). Overall, a two- to threefold increased risk for the disease has been demonstrated in first-degree relatives. Among premenopausal women with bilateral breast cancer the increased risk for first-degree relatives is at least ninefold (1,2). The interpretation of this remarkable familial risk is complicated as it is difficult to separate the genetic from the environmental components.

In mice, there is also a familial risk of breast cancer. Type B virus can be transmitted through the milk producing very high incidence strains (5). Such a mechanism of virus transmission via milk does not seem important in humans (16). Genetic transmission (germ cell) of type B virus occurs in practically all strains of mice and variations in tumor incidence also can be associated with variations in genetic expression of type B virus (4). Information on genetic inheritance of this type in humans is still inconclusive (16). Perhaps of more relevance to humans, is the knowledge that hormones are also a key factor in the development of breast cancer in mice and that there may be hereditary factors determining hormone production or metabolism (20). In humans, there is considerable evidence that alterations in female hormones underlie the risk to breast cancer (28).

The risk factors associated with breast cancer, such as age at menarche (19,34), first delivery (19,28,30), and menopause, natural or artificial (19,26,28,37), have focused attention on ovarian activity and the interrelationship of gonadal and pituitary secretion. Several workers have studied the relative amounts of the three estrogen fractions (estradiol, estrone and estriol) (10,23,24,28). A relative excess of estriol, a metabolite of estrone and the least estrogenic of the three fractions, was hypothesized to protect against breast cancer (10). Case-control studies of women with breast cancer have produced conflicting results concerning this hypothesis (3,15,24). Indirect support for the role of estrogen fractions has come from comparative international studies (29). American women have a lower urinary estriol ratio (estriol/estradiol plus estrone) than their Asian counterparts. Asian women in Hawaii, whose breast cancer rates are intermediate between their homeland rates and those of Caucasian Americans, have a similarly intermediate estriol ratio (11).

The role of pituitary hormones, particularly prolactin, has been the object of study because this hormone is an important regulator of susceptibility to breast cancer in rodents (28,33,35,38). Human studies have yielded conflicting results concerning the basal levels of serum prolactin in breast cancer cases and controls (32,38). At least some of these discrepancies may be due to persistent difficulties in achieving a standardized, repeatable assay for prolactin. In a recent study, however, increased prolactin levels were found in nonaffected members of nine families with a high frequency of breast cancer (22).

Patients with benign and malignant breast disease have been reported to have decreased levels of plasma androgens and urinary androgen metabolites; these changes can be detected several years before onset of disease (6,8,9). The decreased androgen excretion may not be of direct etiological significance but may reflect a fundamental alteration in endocrine status of women at risk of breast cancer (28). Finally, relative thyroid deficiency has been suggested as a characteristic of breast cancer patients, although whether this precedes the onset of disease and how it relates to pathogenesis remain unclear (31).

In a series of studies we have attempted to amalgamate the familial risk of breast cancer with the variety of hormone interactions referred to above (17–19). Initially we observed that mothers of women with breast cancer have the increased ages at first delivery and menopause characteristic of the patients themselves (19). Subsequent studies suggested that the sisters of patients also had an earlier age at menarche and later age at first delivery than did the sisters of matched controls (17). Thus, the familial risk seemed at least in part to be associated with risk factors common to the patient and her first degree relatives, suggesting that the underlying endocrinopathy associated with breast cancer could at least partially be inherited.

In order to further define this familial endocrinopathy, we studied the secretion of certain hormones in the teenage daughters of breast cancer patients and matched controls (17). By study of girls at this age, the confounding effects of pregnancy and exogenous estrogens on the underlying hormone pattern could be avoided. Elevated levels of plasma estrone, estradiol, progesterone, and prolactin were observed in the daughters of breast cancer patients. There was a distinct pattern of high estrogen and prolactin in 14 of the 24 case daughters. The dehydroepiandrosterone (DHEA) sulfate levels were similar in both groups of daughters.

It seemed likely that these elevated hormone levels are what determines risk of breast cancer. Estradiol, progesterone, and prolactin are apparently all implicated in the genesis of breast cancer in the rat (7). These findings also agree with the international studies of MacMahon and coworkers (11,29), as the lower estriol ratio in American Caucasians and Asian immigrants to Hawaii was due to increased estrone and estradiol levels in the face of unchanging estriol levels. Serum concentrations of estradiol have been found elevated in women with malignant and benign breast disease by England et al. (12).

The mechanism producing these elevated hormone levels may, in part, be related to the same factors influencing age at menarche. Menarche is determined by the attainment of a critical weight (14,36). The net effect of alterations in those dietary habits that are associated with increases in total calories and fat consumed is to lower the age at menarche and to lead to hypersecretion of several pituitary and gonadal steroids after menarche (14,21). However, alterations in hormone levels can presumably be the result of genetic factors as well. Lemon (24) has proposed that there is a genetically determined variation·in estrogen 16α-hydroxylase activity in Caucasians. This enzyme is necessary for the conversion of estrone to estriol (Fig. 1). At least three population clusters were identified based on clearance rates of estrone and estradiol. Individuals with reduced 16α-hydroxylase activity were suggested to be at increased risk for breast cancer (25).

Recently Everson et al. (13) described two families in each of which three men developed breast cancer. In one of the families, there was also an aggregation of breast cancer in female relatives. Increased urinary estrogen excretion was reported in the one case tested and three nonaffected male family members. These observations further strengthen the possibility that there are genetically determined variations in hormonal excretion and metabolism. As suggested above by the work of Lemon (24), genetically determined variations in any of the several individual enzymes necessary for the synthesis of steroids could produce altered levels of circulatory estrogens and other hormones (Fig. 1). Similarly, biological variation in excretion of certain pituitary hormones could be influenced by genetic differences in the biosynthesis of the hormone itself, or, as in the case of prolactin, in

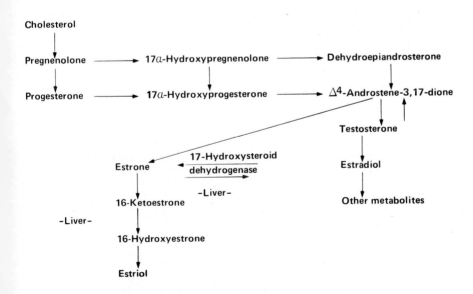

FIG. 1. Biosynthesis and metabolism of estrogens.

the hypothalamic inhibitory factor controlling the release of prolactin. It is likewise feasible that certain of these (hypothetical) genetically determined hormone patterns, particularly those affecting the hypothalamic-pituitary axis, could lead to hormone levels that predispose not only to breast cancer but to other related cancers, producing familial clusters such as those reported for the breast and ovary (27).

In the hope of moving from the realm of speculation to a more solid understanding of the molecular basis of hormone produced neoplasms, we have started an in-depth study of family members of women with bilateral breast cancer diagnosed prior to age 50. As expected, compared to patients with unilateral breast cancer and to controls, first degree relatives of women with bilateral breast cancer have a markedly increased risk as others have reported (1,2). Women with bilateral breast cancer share with women with unilateral breast cancer a reduced mean age at menarche and a delayed age at first delivery. Hormone levels (prolactin, FSH, LH, TSH, estradiol, estrone, progesterone, and DHEA-sulfate) are being determined on the cases and their sisters and offspring.

ACKNOWLEDGMENTS

This study was conducted under Contract NO. N01-CP-53500 within the Virus Cancer Program and Grant No. PO ICA 17054-01 of the National Cancer Institute, National Institutes of Health, U.S. Public Health Service.

REFERENCES

1. Anderson, D. E. (1972): A genetic study of human breast cancer. *J. Natl. Cancer Inst.,* 48:1029–1034.
2. Anderson, D. E. (1974): Genetic study of breast cancer: Identification of a high risk group. *Cancer,* 34:1090–1097.
3. Arguellas, A. E., Hoffman, C., Poggi, U. L., Chekherdenian, M., Saborida, C., and Blanchard, D. (1973): Endocrine profiles and breast cancer. *Lancet,* 1:165–167.
4. Bentvelzen, P., Daams, J. H., Hogeman, P., and Calafat, J. (1970): Genetic transmission of viruses that incite mammary tumors in mice. *Proc. Natl. Acad. Sci. USA,* 67:377–384.
5. Bittner, J. J. (1936): Some possible effects of nursing on the mammary gland tumor incidence in mice. *Science,* 84:162.
6. Brennan, M. J., Bulbrook, R. D., Deshpande, N., Wang, Y., and Hayward, J. L. (1973): Urinary and plasma androgens in benign breast disease. *Lancet,* 1:1076–1079.
7. Brown, C. E., Chute, R. N., and Porter, M. W. (1975): The effect of nephrectomy on the incidence of breast carcinoma in irradiated parabiased rats. *Cancer Res.,* 35:37–44.
8. Bulbrook, R. D. and Hayward, J. L. (1967): Abnormal urinary steroid excretion and subsequent breast cancer. A prospective study in the Island of Guernsey. *Lancet,* 1:519–522.
9. Bulbrook, R. D., Hayward, J. L., and Spicer, C. C. (1971): Relation between urinary androgen and corticoid excretion and subsequent breast cancer. *Lancet,* 2:395–398.
10. Cole, P., and MacMahon, B. (1969): Estrogen fractions during early reproductive life in the etiology of breast cancer. *Lancet,* 1:604–606.
11. Dickinson, L. E., MacMahon, B., Cole, P., and Brown, J. B. (1974): Estrogen profiles of Oriental and Caucasian women in Hawaii. *N. Engl. J. Med.,* 291:1211–1213.
12. England, P. C., Skinner, L. G., Cottrell, K. M., and Sellwood, R. A. (1974): Serum estradiol-17 in women with benign and malignant breast disease. *Br. J. Cancer.,* 30:571–576.
13. Everson, R. B., Li, F. P., Fraumeni, J. F., Jr., Fishman, J., Wilson, R. E., Stout, D., and Norris, H. J. (1976): Familial male breast cancer. *Lancet,* 1:9–12.

14. Frisch, R. E., Revelle, R., and Cook, S. (1973): Components of weight at menarche and the initiation of the adolescent growth spurt in girls: Estimated total water, lean body weight and fat. *Hum. Biol.*, 45:469–483.
15. Gronos, M., and Aho, A. J. (1968): Estrogen metabolism in postmenopausal women with primary and recurrent breast cancer. *Eur. J. Cancer*, 4:523–527.
16. Henderson, B. E. (1974): Type B virus and human breast cancer. *Cancer*, 34:1386–1389.
17. Henderson, B. E., Gerkins, V. R., Rosario, I., Casagrande, J., and Pike, M. C. (1975): Elevated serum levels of estrogen and prolactin. *N. Engl. J. Med.*, 293:790–795.
18. Henderson, B. E., Gerkins, V. R., and Pike, M. C. (1975): Sexual factors and pregnancy. In *Persons at High Risk of Cancer. An Approach to Cancer Etiology and Control,* edited by J. F. Fraumeni, Jr., pp. 267–283. Academic Press, New York.
19. Henderson, B. E., Powell, D., Rosario, I., Keys, C., Hanisch, R., Young, M., Casagrande, J., Gerkins, V. R., and Pike, M. C. (1974): An epidemiologic study of breast cancer. *J. Natl. Cancer Inst.*, 53:609–614.
20. Heston, W. E., and Andervont, H. B. (1944): Importance of genetic influence on the occurrence of mammary tumors in virgin female mice. *J. Natl. Cancer Inst.*, 4:403–407.
21. Kulin, H. E., Grumbach, M. M., and Kaplan, S. L. (1969): Changing sensitivity of the pubertal gonadal hypothalamic feedback mechanism in man. *Science*, 166:1012–1013.
22. Kwa, H. G., De-Jong Bakker, M., and Engelsman, E. (1974): Plasma-prolactin in breast cancer. *Lancet*, 1:433–435.
23. Lemon, H. M. (1969): Endocrine influences on human mammary cancer formation. A critique. *Cancer*, 23:781–790.
24. Lemon, H. M. (1972): Review—Genetic predisposition to carcinomas of the breast: Multiple human genotypes for estrogen 16 alpha hydroxylase activity in Caucasians. *J. Surg. Oncology*, 4:255–273.
25. Lemon, H. M., and Reilly, D. (1974): Genotypic variations in Caucasian leukocyte estradiol 16 hydroxylase activity: A measurable deterrent of breast cancer risk? *Nebr. State Med. J.*, 59:151–155.
26. Lilienfeld, A. M. (1956): Relationship of cancer of the female breast to artificial menopause and marital status. *Cancer*, 9:927–934.
27. Lynch, H. T., and Krush, A. J. (1971): Carcinoma of the breast and ovary in three families. *Surg. Gynecol. Obstet.*, 133:644–648.
28. MacMahon, B., Cole, P., and Brown, J. (1973): Etiology of human breast cancer: A review. *J. Natl. Cancer Inst.*, 50:21–42.
29. MacMahon, B., Cole, P., Brown, J. B., Aoki, K., Lin, T. M., Morgan, R. W., and Wood, N. C. (1974): Urine estrogen profiles of Asian and North American women. *Int. J. Cancer*, 14:161–167.
30. MacMahon, B., Cole, P., Lin, T. M., Lowe, C. R., Mirra, A. P., Ravnihar, B., Salber, E. J., Valaoras, V. G., and Yuasa, S. (1970): Age at first birth and breast cancer risk. *Bull. WHO*, 43:209–221.
31. Mittra, I., Hayward, J. L., and McNeilly, A. S. (1974): Hypothalamic-pituitary-thyroid axis in breast cancer. *Lancet*, 1:885–889.
32. Rolandi, E., Barreca, T., Masturzo, P., Polleri, A., Indiveri, F., and Barabino, A. (1974): Plasma prolactin in breast cancer. *Lancet*, 2:845–846.
33. Smith, O. W., and Smith, G. V. (1970): Urinary estrogen profiles and etiology of breast cancer. *Lancet*, 1:1152–1155.
34. Staszewski, J. (1971): Age at menarche and breast cancer. *J. Natl. Cancer Inst.*, 47:935–940.
35. Talwalker, P. K., Meites, J., and Mizienan, H. (1962): Mammary tumor induction by estrogen on anterior pituitary hormones in ovariectomized rats given 7, 12-dimethyl-1,2-benzanthracene. *Proc. Soc. Exp. Biol. Med.*, 116:531–534.
36 Tanner, J. M. (1962): *Growth at Adolescence*, p. 37. Blackwell, Oxford.
37. Trichopoulos, D., MacMahon, B., and Cole, P. (1972): The menopause and breast cancer risk. *J. Natl. Cancer Inst.*, 48:605–613.
38. Wilson, R. G., Buchan, R., Roberts, M. M., Forrest, A. P. M., Boyns, A. R., Cole, E. N., and Griffiths, K. (1974): Plasma prolactin and breast cancer. *Cancer,* 33:1325–1327.

Genetics of Human Cancer, edited by J. J.
Mulvihill, R. W. Miller, and J. F. Fraumeni, Jr.
Raven Press, New York, 1977.

26

Genetic Cerumen Type, Breast Secretory Activity, and Breast Cancer Epidemiology

Nicholas L. Petrakis

*G. W. Hooper Foundation and the Department of International Health, University of
California School of Medicine, San Francisco, California 94143*

A genetic marker that we have studied from an anthropological, biochemical, and epidemiologic viewpoint provides some clues to the possible interaction between genetic, endocrine, and environmental factors in breast cancer epidemiology. Several years ago we reported an association between the frequency of wet-type cerumen and increased breast cancer mortality (9). This association is based on the apocrine nature of the ceruminous glands, axillary apocrine sweat glands, and the breast. Cerumen types are inherited in a simple Mendelian fashion, in which the allele for wet type is dominant over that for dry. The recessive dry type is markedly prevalent in Oriental and American Indian populations, in contrast with the wet type that predominates in European and African populations (6,9). In a study of Japanese-American women, wet cerumen was found to be twice as frequent in patients with breast cancer as in control subjects (9). However, in a larger case-control study in Hong Kong, these findings were not substantiated (4).

For the past several years we have investigated the secretion of breast fluid by the nonlactating adult human breast. These studies have confirmed the previously known fact that the adult nonlactating breast secretes and resorbs fluid within the alveolar-ductal system (1–3). Recently, we reported an association between breast fluid secretion with race, age, menopausal status, and cerumen type [a known genetic indicator of apocrine system activity (11)]. The highest proportion of breast fluid secretors was found among Caucasian women and the lowest among Oriental and American Indian women having dry-type cerumen. In all groups studied, the proportion of secretors declined after menopause, but was lowest among Chinese and Japanese women, in whom only a small proportion yielded fluid after the menopause. In contrast, over half of postmenopausal Caucasians gave fluid, suggesting that a persistent hormonal stimulus present in this group, probably estrogen, maintained breast secretory activity into older age.

That the fluid secreted is a true secretory product of the breast is indicated by the presence of lactose, α-lactalbumin, immunoglobulins, cholesterol, fatty acids, and other substances that are in breast milk and colostrum (8). Because many drugs and other chemicals are secreted by the lactating breast (5), we have begun to investigate the secretion of exogenous substances into fluids of the *nonlactating* breast, employing techniques of gas liquid chromatography-mass spectrometry and radioisotopes. It has been found that, as in lactating mothers, such diverse substances as radioactive technetium, barbiturates, fatty acids, and products of cigarette smoke are rapidly secreted into breast fluid of the nonlactating breast (10; Petrakis et al., *in preparation*; Petrakis, *unpublished observations*).

These findings, when combined with previous information on secretory activity, indicate that the adult human breast, through its biological role in reproduction, appears to provide a mechanism for preferentially secreting and concentrating substances from the blood. It is hypothesized that endocrine factors, through their influence on breast epithelial maintenance and secretion, may interact with exogenous environmental and genetic factors to determine breast cancer risk.

Evidence that a genetic factor may affect breast secretion is suggested by our findings in Oriental women who are dimorphic for cerumen type. A significantly lower frequency of secretors was found among those women with dry cerumen compared with women with wet cerumen, suggesting that the alleles which determine cerumen type also affect breast secretory activity. A similar association has been reported between cerumen type and the quantity of axillary apocrine secretion (15).

Based upon these considerations, we have developed a working model that relates the known epidemiologic evidence associating reproductive experience and the risk of breast cancer to our findings of breast secretory activity, evidence of secretion of exogenous substances, and genetic variation in quantity of secretions. These factors may be related as in the following diagram:

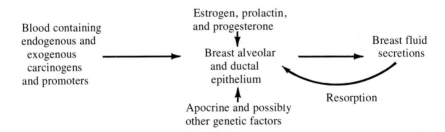

In this hypothesis, the turnover rate of secreted substances and their rates of resorption are primary determinants of the extent and duration of exposure of the breast epithelium to environmental and endogenous carcinogens. The estrogen-dependent secretory activity of the nonlactating breast can provide a mechanism permitting initiating mutagens and cocarcinogenic factors to reach the breast epithelium. These cocarcinogenic factors can lead, with advancing age, to the accumulation of mutant cells. Many histological studies of the human breast have demonstrated striking increases in the frequency of alveolar atypia and metaplasia in breasts of women over 30 years of age (13–16).

This model may help to explain the significant excess of breast cancer in Caucasian compared to Oriental women. The lower risk in Orientals may be due to their overall decrease in breast secretory activity, especially marked in those with genetically dry-type apocrine systems. A low or absent epithelial secretory activity may minimize the contact of the breast with exogenous carcinogens.

Many avenues for clinical, genetic, and epidemiologic research are suggested by these studies. The model presented emphasizes the interaction of genetic, physiological, endocrine, and environmental factors in the pathogenesis of breast cancer.

ACKNOWLEDGMENT

This work was supported by Public Health Service Grant CA 13556 and Contract CB 33882 from the National Cancer Institute and by a gift from Mrs. Viola K. Schroeder

REFERENCES

1. Besser, G. M., and Edwards, C. R. (1972): Galactorrhoea. *Br. Med. J.,* 2:280–282.
2. Bonser, G. M., Dossett, J. A., and Jull, J. W. (1961): *Human and Experimental Breast Cancer.* Charles C. Thomas, Springfield, Illinois.
3. Keynes, G. (1923): Chronic mastitis. *Br. J. Surg.,* 11:89–121.
4. Ing, R., Petrakis, N. L., and Ho, H. C. (1973): Evidence against association between wet cerumen and breast cancer. *Lancet,* 1:41.
5. Knowles, J. A. (1965): Excretion of drugs in milk—a review. *J. Pediatr.,* 66:1068–1082.
6. Matsunaga, E. (1962): The dimorphism in human normal cerumen. *Ann. Hum. Genet. (London),* 25:273–286.
7. McFarland, J. (1922): Residual lactation acini in the female breast. *Arch. Surg.,* 5:1–64.
8. Petrakis, N. L. (1973): Analysis of breast secretions. *First Breast Cancer Task Force Working Conference,* National Cancer Institute. Williamsburg, Virginia.
9. Petrakis, N. L. (1971): Cerumen genetics and human breast cancer. *Science,* 173:347–349.
10. Petrakis, N. L., Kaufman, L., Swann, S., Price, D., and Mason, L. (1975): Studies of the secretory activity of the nonlactating breast as determined by the secretion rate of ^{99m}Tc into breast duct fluid. *Proc. Am. Soc. Clin. Oncology,* (Abstr.) 16:256.
11. Petrakis, N. L., Mason, L., Lee, R., Sugimoto, B., Pawson, S., and Catchpool, F. (1975): Association of race, age, menopausal status, and cerumen type with breast fluid secretion in nonlactating women, as determined by nipple aspiration. *J. Natl. Cancer Inst.,* 54:829–834.
12. Petrakis, N. L., Pingle, U., Petrakis, S. J., and Petrakis, S. L. (1971): Evidence for a genetic cline in earwax types in the Middle East and Southeast Asia. *Am. J. Phys. Anthropol.,* 35:141–144.
13. Sandison, A. T. (1962): An Autopsy Study of the Adult Human Breast. *Natl. Cancer Inst. Monogr. 8.*
14. Symington, T., and Currie, A. R. (1958): Pathology: discussion and summary. In: *Endocrine Aspects of Breast Cancer,* edited by A. R. Currie, pp. 135–137. E & S Livingstone, Ltd., Edinburgh and London.
15. Yamashita, S. (1939): On the offensive odor of the armpit and the soft earwax among the Formosans in Canton. *Jap. J. Anthropol.,* 54:444–446.
16. Wellings, S. R., Jensen, H. M., and Marcum, R. G. (1975): An atlas of subgross pathology of the human breast with special reference to possible precancerous lesions. *J. Natl. Cancer Inst.,* 55:231–273.

Discussion

Rowley: If breast fluid is continually being secreted, I assume there is some mechanism for resorption?

Petrakis: Yes, secretion and resorption go on all the time beginning at puberty. In many Caucasian women, the turnover continues to old age; whereas in most Oriental women, it appears to practically cease soon after menopause.

Bolande: What effect does oophorectomy have on breast secretory activity? And, conversely, what is the effect of estrogen use in artificially and therapeutically menopausal and postmenopausal women?

Petrakis: Applying the breast pump technique, we could find no effect of oophorectomy on breast secretion in Caucasian women. However, this is a crude measure of secretion and we need to develop more sophisticated techniques to measure breast secretory activity. I assume that the postmenopausal women who still secrctc have some source of estrogen, probably the adrenals or fat depots, that helps maintain the secretory epithelium. Another problem is that we cannot examine the epithelium of the living patient. We have found much cytologic atypia in fluids aspirated from the remaining breast following mastectomy for breast cancer and from women with fibrocystic disease. These observations support the notion that secretory functions may be altered in women with cancer and benign breast disease.

Hirayama: Have you tested breast fluid for mutagenicity in a microbial system?

Petrakis: No; but, we are preparing to collect fluid for testing by Bruce Ames.

Genetics of Human Cancer, edited by J. J.
Mulvihill, R. W. Miller, and J. F. Fraumeni, Jr.
Raven Press, New York, 1977.

27

Aryl Hydrocarbon Hydroxylase Induction (*Ah* Locus) as a Possible Genetic Marker for Cancer

Daniel W. Nebert and Steven A. Atlas

Developmental Pharmacology Branch, National Institute of Child Health and Human Development, National Institutes of Health, Bethesda, Maryland 20014

Analysis of hereditary and nonhereditary human cancers suggests a model for carcinogenesis implicating two or more events in the initiation of cancer. At least one of these events is stochastic, a term used broadly to include all random somatic mutational events (8,33). Such events can presumably be caused by radiation, viruses, or chemicals. Environmental agents have been implicated as the cause of 80% or more of all human cancers (25a). There are counties throughout the United States that have abnormally high rates for a number of tumor types (43); studies on migrant populations also suggest that the location of residence for approximately the first 20 years of life may inordinately influence predisposition to certain types of cancers (6,23,64,68).

The purpose of this report is to provide a current view of the enzyme systems which metabolize most environmental carcinogens, to review the genetic regulation of these enzymes in the mouse, to demonstrate an association of the mouse *Ah* locus with increased susceptibility to chemical carcinogenesis, and to evaluate the current status of attempts at defining and ascertaining the *Ah* locus in man.

THE MONOOXYGENASES

Environmental contaminants are, in general, hydrophobic chemicals that are metabolized by a group of enzymes known collectively as the cytochrome P-450-mediated monooxygenases (9,24,28,51,66). These membrane-bound enzyme systems are known to metabolize: Polycyclic aromatic hydrocarbons such as benzo[a]pyrene, 3-methylcholanthrene (MC), methylated benz[a]anthracenes, dibenzanthracenes, biphenyl, and other benzene derivatives; strong mutagens such as N-methyl-N′-nitro-N-nitrosoguanidine and nitrosamines; aminoazo dyes and diazo compounds; N-acetylaryl-amines and nitrofurans; numerous aromatic amines, nitroaromatics, and heterocyclics; epoxides; carbamates; alkyl halides; safrole derivatives; certain fungal toxins and antibiotics; many of the chemotherapeutic agents used to treat human cancer; and endogenous and synthetic steroids. These enzyme systems may metabolically potentiate the detrimental effects of an inert parent compound by converting it to a reactive or toxic intermediate [e.g., benzo(a)pyrene (50,67)] or may detoxify a reactive parent compound to an inactive product [e.g., N-methyl-N'-nitro-N-nitrosoguanidine (12)]. By "reactive" intermediate or parent compound, we mean an alkylating or arylating agent or electrophile capable of random damage to nucleic acids or proteins, thereby producing the one or more stochastic "hits" predisposing to cancer.

Figure 1 illustrates the possible pathways during the metabolism of a polycyclic hydrocarbon such as benzo[a]pyrene. Monooxygenation of the parent compound by the P-450-mediated enzyme systems produces the reactive epoxide (also called arene oxide), which can (1) rearrange spontaneously to phenols, (2) be converted to *trans*-dihydrodiols by microsomal epoxide hydrases, (3) conjugate with glutathione, or (4) combine covalently with cellular macromolecules (24,28,50, 51,66,67). Ample evidence in intact animals (28,50,51,66,67), the *in vitro* *Salmonella*/microsomal mutagenesis test system (14,15), and cultured cells undergoing malignant transformation (24) indicates that a reactive epoxide(s) is most likely the proximal carcinogen.

What factors, then, will influence the steady-state level of the proximal chemical carcinogen in the cell? Increases in monooxygenase activity or decreases in the formation of phenols, dihydrodiols, and glutathione-conjugated products will increase the steady-state level of reactive intermediate. Studies using compounds which stimulate or induce the monooxygenase systems or which inhibit the epoxide hydrase or glutathione S-epoxide transferase indicate that covalent binding of the reactive chemical to cellular macromolecules increases and that hepatic necrosis, mutagenesis, or chemical carcinogenesis often increase concomitantly (24,28,50,51,66,67). A primary factor is the genetically mediated response of

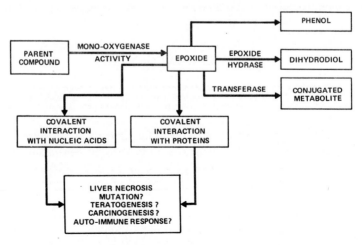

FIG. 1. Possible subcellular pathways for reactive epoxide intermediates of carcinogenic polycyclic hydrocarbons (48).

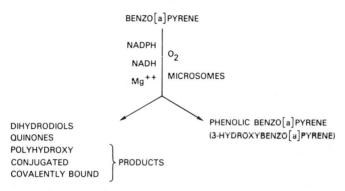

FIG. 2. Current concept of the aryl hydrocarbon (benzo[a]pyrene) hydroxylase (AHH) "activity." The substrate benzo[a]pyrene is oxygenated to an arene oxide which rearranges nonenzymically to the phenol. Oxygenation via direct oxygen insertion to form phenolic derivatives (28) is a second possible mechanism. Other oxygenated derivatives of benzo[a]pyrene, including dihydrodiols and quinones, are not measured by this assay (27,51).

the monooxygenases to enzyme inducers. In addition, the reactivity of the intermediate(s) produced may depend upon inherent differences in the enzyme-active sites of various forms of cytochromes P-450. These latter two factors will be examined in greater detail with data from the laboratory animal.

ARYL HYDROCARBON HYDROXYLASE "ACTIVITY"

Evidence has been presented (49) for a single gene difference between C57BL/6N and DBA/2N inbred mouse strains in the induction of a monooxygenase activity, hepatic aryl hydrocarbon hydroxylase (AHH), and newly formed cytochrome P_1-450 by MC. Figure 2 outlines the AHH assay *in vitro*. The autosomal dominant trait for AHH induction by polycyclic hydrocarbons was found to be expressed in nonhepatic tissues as well (18,51). Careful dose-response curves of AHH inducers (53) indicate, however, that the amount of induced AHH activity in liver, kidney, bowel, or lung in the C57BL/6N mouse is always slightly greater than that in the (C57BL/6N) (DBA/2N)F_1 heterozygote and is always considerably greater than that in the DBA/2N mouse. Similar results exist in skin (5,18), lymph nodes (5), bone marrow (41), and the retinal pigmented epithelium of the eye (65)—although differences in inducible AHH activity in these tissues between C57BL/6N and DBA/2N mice are often not as striking as those in bowel, kidney, and liver. The fact that the magnitude of AHH and cytochrome P_1-450 induction by polycyclic hydrocarbons appears to be genetically regulated in most tissues of the mouse (38,51) is of importance for the remainder of this report.

GENETICS OF AHH INDUCTION

The induction of a certain group of monooxygenase activities, including AHH, by polycyclic aromatic compounds is regulated at or near the same genetic locus

[*Ah* locus (20,51] controlling the formation of cytochrome P_1-450 (also called P-448). Certain inbred strains of mice are "responsive" (Ah^b) to such induction whereas others are "nonresponsive" (Ah^d) (20,51). The original hypothesis (18,49,72) that aromatic hydrocarbon "responsiveness" is expressed as a single autosomal dominant trait was complicated by the dose-response data (53) and by experiments involving crosses between 12 responsive and nonresponsive strains (61,70).

In the mouse the simplest model which accommodates all of the information involves a minimum of six alleles at two loci (61) (Fig. 3). In all this scheme we suggest a structural gene P_1-450, by means of which induction-specific RNA and protein are necessary for new cytochrome P_1-450 synthesis and the associated induced monooxygenase activities. Whether one cytochrome or a family of different cytochromes P_1-450 exists remains to be determined. Aromatic hydrocarbon responsiveness involves two or more regulatory genes (shown here as *Ah-1* and *Ah-2*) which activate or control in some manner the structural gene P_1-450. At least one of the gene products is a soluble receptor (21) which binds with high affinity specific polycyclic aromatic compound inducers. Inactive analogs cannot displace active inducer molecules, whereas active analogs can (21, 57a). In primary liver cell cultures (19), aromatic hydrocarbon inducers can also direct at some posttranslational level, a further rise in AHH activity in which the normal rate of decay of induced AHH activity is slowed. Lastly (Fig. 3, right), we suggest that other P-450 structural loci exist and that each of these other loci may respond to a single stimulus, or multiple stimuli, thereby forming other induction-specific RNA species and proteins and ultimately leading to the expression of other basal and inducible

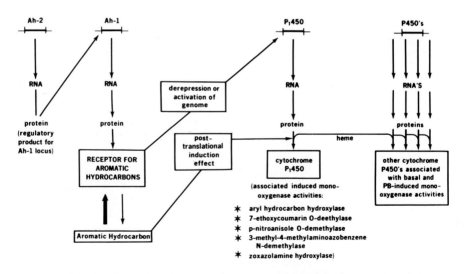

FIG. 3. Hypothetical scheme for the overall genetic control of cytochrome P_1-450 formation and the associated induction of certain monooxygenase "activities" by aromatic hydrocarbons in mice (51). Only the first five of 11 associated monooxygenase activities are included.

monooxygenase activities. The metabolism of benzo[a]pyrene by both basal and MC-induced AHH activities is associated quite specifically with the P_1-450 enzyme-active site (1,51). But major contributions are also made to the basal activity by metabolism at enzyme-active sites associated with at least one of these other P-450 cytochromes which is inducible by phenobarbital (1,51). The coumarin 7-hydroxylase activity, inducible by phenobarbital but not by aromatic hydrocarbons (76), is a recent example of rather simple genetic control of a monooxygenase activity probably associated with one or more P-450 structural loci other than the P_1-450 locus.

DIFFERENCES IN METABOLITES PRODUCED BY DIFFERENT FORMS OF CYTOCHROMES P-450

As suggested above and recently reviewed in detail (51), several lines of evidence indicate that at least two different AHH activities exist and are associated with different cytochromes P-450: The enzyme from MC-treated responsive mice associated with cytochrome P_1-450 and the enzyme from control or phenobarbital-treated responsive and nonresponsive mice and from MC-treated nonresponsive mice associated principally with some form other than P_1-450. This finding becomes increasingly important because it is apparent that different forms of cytochromes P-450 may generate different ratios of metabolites from the same substrate. Comparing MC versus phenobarbital as the inducer in rat liver, for example (Fig. 4), various groups have shown that hydroxylations may occur predominantly in different chemical positions on the molecule for such substrates as biphenyl (10), testosterone (40), 2-acetylaminofluorene (44,74), bromobenzene (77), n-hexane (16), and benzo[a]pyrene (26,59). Such differences in the metabolite profile of a polycyclic hydrocarbon or other foreign chemical reflect presumed differences in the nature of the intermediates formed; differences in the reactivity of these intermediates might result in marked dissimilarities in the carcinogenicity or toxicity of a given compound. One of the best examples to date is the metabolism of bromobenzene in the rat. The p-phenolic derivative of bromobenzene, presumably arising from the 3,4-oxide, is associated in some manner with hepatic necrosis, whereas the o-phenolic derivative, presumably arising from the 2,3-oxide, is not (77). Incidentally, this finding is an example in rats in which higher amounts of cytochrome P_1-450 are beneficial to the animal.

With a similar goal in mind, members of our laboratory for the past several years have searched for differences in drug metabolism, toxicity, and susceptibility to cancer which can be shown to be associated with differences in a single gene (or small number of genes). Although tumorigenesis initiated by 7,12-dimethylbenz[a]anthracene was shown (47) *not* to be associated with the *Ah* locus, subcutaneous sarcomas initiated by MC were associated with inducible AHH activity among 14 inbred strains of mice (36,39,48) (Fig. 5). With the use of offspring from the F_1 to parent backcrosses and $F \times F_1$ intercross, MC-initiated tumorigenesis was shown recently to be highly correlated with the Ah^b allele (37). Table

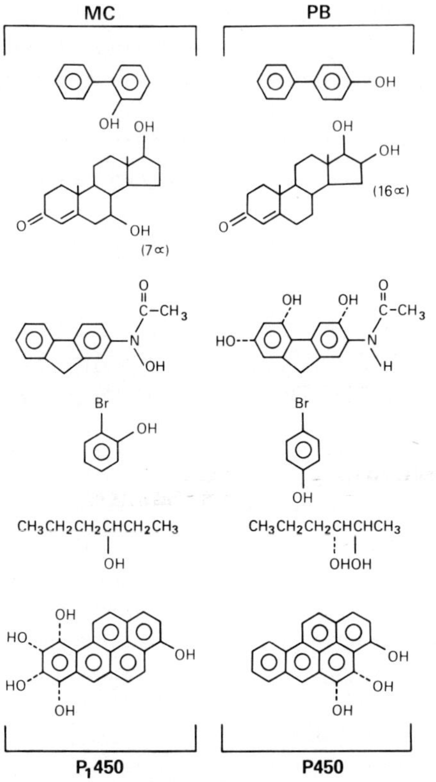

FIG. 4. Chemical structures of known differences in metabolite formation when each of these six substrates is oxygenated *in vitro* with liver microsomes from rats treated with MC or phenobarbital (PB) (50). Similar differences in metabolite profile exist in mice for biphenyl (1), 2-acetylaminofluorene (73), and benzo[a]pyrene (27), but not for testosterone (2) or bromobenzene (62); to our knowledge *n*-hexane has not been examined in MC- and phenobarbital-treated mice.

1 summarizes the various effects caused by differences in xenobiotic metabolism due to the *Ah* locus, which have been reported by us as well as by Kouri, Hutton and coworkers. 7,12-Dimethylbenz[a]anthracene-produced skin inflammation, MC- or 7,12-dimethylbenz[a]anthracene-caused birth defects, benzo[a]pyrene-initiated tumors, and acetaminophen-produced cataracts have been studied to date only as differences among inbred strains. All other effects listed in Table 1 have been demonstrated to be correlated specifically with the *Ah*[b] or *Ah*[d] allele by means of studies using siblings from the (C57BL/6N) (DBA/2N) F_1 × DBA/2N backcross. *In vitro* effects shown to be correlated with the *Ah* locus include MC, 6-aminochrysene, and 2-acetylaminofluorene mutagenesis (14,15) (as determined by the *Salmonella*/microsomal system developed by Ames), and differences in the profile of benzo[a]pyrene metabolites that bind to DNA nucleosides (50).

SEARCH FOR THE *Ah* LOCUS IN MAN

In 1973, two reports (31,32) gave initial hope to clinical geneticists and on-cologists. The extent of AHH induction in cultured mitogen-activated lympho-cytes by MC was examined in 353 healthy subjects, ranging in age from 2 to 89 years and including 67 families with 165 children (31). Cultured leukocytes from each individual were treated with phytohemagglutinin M and pokeweed mitogen for 3 days, at which time they were divided into an MC-treated sample and a control sample receiving the vehicle (acetone) alone. The cells were harvested 24 hr later and AHH activity was assayed at pH 7.5 (31). Thus each person served as his own control, and emphasis was placed on *fold induction*—which ranged between 1.3 and 4.5 times the basal level (31). The distribution of inducibilities in the patients tested in the Houston area was allegedly trimodal, the groups being designated low, intermediate, and high inducible. The data were consistent with a

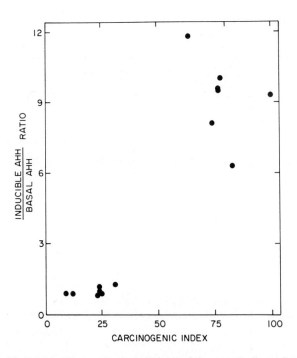

FIG. 5. Relationship between the carcinogenic index and the genetically mediated induction of AHH activity by MC for each of 14 inbred mouse strains (48). The correlation coefficient *r* is 0.90 (p<0.001). Each *dot* represents a group of 30 mice of a particular inbred strain. The carcinogenic index was evaluated 4 to 8 months later after a subcutaneous dose of 150 μg of MC had been given to weanling mice (39). The "inducible AHH/basal AHH ratio" reflects the mean of hepatic hydroxylase activity in MC-treated mice of a given strain divided by the mean hepatic enzyme activity in control mice (N$\geq$5 for each of the two groups). Whether the MC-inducible AHH activity in the nonhepatic tissues is expressed in a manner similar to that in the liver has not been tested in all 14 of these strains.

TABLE 1. *Conditions in the mouse associated with the Ah^b allele or with aromatic hydro-carbon responsiveness*

	Condition	Ref.
1.	Increased susceptibility to MC-initiated subcutaneous sarcomas	36,37,39,48
2.	Increased susceptibility to 7,12-dimethylbenz[a]-anthracene-produced skin inflammation	71
3.	Shorter zoxazolamine paralysis time	63
4.	Increased susceptibility to acetaminophen-caused hepatic necrosis	73
5.	Shorter survival time when given large doses of polycyclic aromatic compounds or polychlorinated biphenyls intraperitoneally	62
6.	Increased resistance to lindane given intraperitoneally	62
7.	Increased resistance to polycyclic hydrocarbons or lindane given orally	62
8.	Increased resistance to aplastic anemia caused by oral benzo[a]pyrene	41,62
9.	Shorter survival time when given polychlorinated biphenyls orally	62
10.	Increased susceptibility to stillborns, fetal resorptions, and malformations caused by MC or 7,12-dimethylbenz[a]anthracene given to pregnant mother	52
11.	Increased susceptibility to benzo[a]pyrene-initiated subcutaneous sarcomas	34,50
12.	Increased susceptibility to squamous cell carcinomas of the lung initiated by intratracheal instillation of MC	34
13.	Increased susceptibility to cataract formation caused by acetaminophen given intraperitoneally	a

[a]G. H. Lambert, D. W. Nebert, and H. Shichi, manuscript in preparation

hypothesis of two alleles at a single locus, and gave an excellent fit to the Hardy-Weinberg equilibrium, with a frequency of 0.717 for the low-inducibility allele and 0.283 for the high-inducibility allele (although the sample was biased by the inclusion of parents and siblings). Family studies also conformed to a monogenic codominant model, not a single individual of unexpected phenotype (e.g., an illegitimate child) being uncovered among 130 children. The deviation in extent of induction for each individual tested several times ranged between 5 and 10%, indicating a coefficient of variation of 0.01 to 0.04.

In the second report (32), 50 patients with bronchogenic carcinoma were compared with 46 patients having other types of tumors and 85 healthy controls; no attempt was mentioned to match the latter two control groups to the bronchogenic carcinoma group with respect to age or smoking history. Whereas the gene frequencies for the low- and high-inducibility alleles, respectively, were 0.676 and 0.324 for the healthy controls and 0.663 and 0.337 for the tumor controls, the gene frequencies were reversed—0.370 for the low-inducibility allele and 0.630 for the high-inducibility allele—among patients with bronchogenic carcinoma (32). The authors concluded that a person having the "intermediate" phenotype has a 16-fold increased risk, and a person having the "high" phenotype has a 36-fold increased risk, of developing bronchogenic carcinoma, compared with persons having the "low" inducibility phenotype (32).

In 1974, our laboratory emphasized the day-to-day experimental variability, the variations within each assay, and the fact that no patient having the "high" inducibility phenotype was found among 42 individuals tested (35). The AHH assay was performed at pH 7.8. Gurtoo and co-workers (22) used Ficoll-Hypaque purified lymphocytes, different culture medium, a larger surface area during culture, a shorter time of lymphocyte exposure to the mitogens, and an assay pH of 8.5, thereby enhancing the sensitivity of the AHH determination an average of 17-fold. They also showed that the AHH activity at pH 7.5 was only one-fourth to one-half that at the pH optimum of 8.5.

Because of the variability of the lymphocyte system, even after incorporating some of Gurtoo's modifications, and because several laboratories besides ours were unable to confirm readily the monogenic hypothesis, we undertook a study of twins in order to assess the extent to which lymphocyte AHH reflected genetic differences, irrespective of the mode of heritability. We found that the intratwin variance between identical twin pairs is statistically significantly less than that between fraternal twin pairs, with regard to the fold induction of AHH activity in cultured mitogen-activated lymphocytes (3) (Fig. 6). A heritable trait is measurable if monozygotic twins show a common response more frequently than fraternal twins, and this heritability index (h^2) can be quantitated by the equation:

$$h^2 = \frac{V_d - V_m}{V_d} \tag{1}$$

in which V_d and V_m denote, respectively, intratwin variance between dizygotic and monozygotic twin pairs (57). Hence, if V_d and V_m are the same, h^2 is zero and variations in the trait are said to be due to environment. Conversely, if variation is smaller between monozygotic twins than between dizygotic twins, h^2 approaches unity and the observed variations are said to be principally due to heredity. The h^2 for our study with 16 twin pairs tested two to five times (always together in the same experiment) is 0.80, indicating a detectable heritable component for AHH inducibility in cultured mitogen-activated lymphocytes (3). It previously had been shown (45,46) that genetic differences in the extent of AHH induction in fetal mouse cell cultures correlated quite well with the expression of the *Ah* locus in the intact mouse. However, the h^2 for either the absolute basal or the absolute MC-induced AHH activity in our lymphocyte study (3) is near zero,

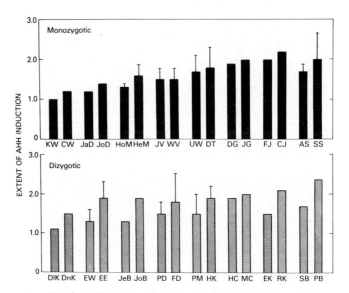

FIG. 6. Variance in the extent of AHH induction in cultured mitogen-activated lymphocytes from identical and fraternal twins (3). *Brackets:* standard deviation in those pairs whose lymphocytes were tested in at least three separate experiments. A single experiment originated from a single drawing of blood, and two to five determinations of AHH activity were each carried out on MC-treated and control cultures. Each twin pair was studied simultaneously under identical conditions. The AHH assay was performed at pH 8.5. The heritability index for these data is 0.80. If, however, these 16 twin pairs are compared using a single lot of fetal calf serum in culture, a value of 0.77 is obtained.

indicating that variations in the basal and inducible AHH activities exist because of environmental factors (in this case, most likely day-to-day variations in the cell culture experimental conditions).

A significant, inverse correlation was recently reported between the level of inducibility, measured by induction of AHH in cultured mitogen-activated lymphocytes by MC, and plasma half-lives of antipyrine and phenylbutazone (29), and vice versa. In this same study, the basal AHH level was highly correlated with both the MC-induced AHH level and "fold inducibility," suggesting that an individual could be classified as having a "low," "intermediate," or "high" phenotype on the basis of the basal AHH activity alone. An attempt (3) in this laboratory was made to confirm these data, and no such relationship was found between AHH inducibility in lymphocyte cultures and the plasma clearance rates of phenylbutazone or dicumarol; there was a significant ($0.03 < p < 0.05$) correlation between AHH induction in culture and the plasma antipyrine clearance rate.

Ah LOCUS IN MAN: UNANSWERED QUESTIONS

Is AHH induction in man controlled by two alleles at a single locus? This was thought to be the case in 1972 for the mouse (18,49,72) but now is clearly not so (51,61). Whereas one can easily envision a monogenic model for an all-or-none phenomenon such as that obtained in mouse liver, it is difficult to fit such a simple genetic model to the *gradations* in induction response observed in human lymphocytes (31). Interestingly, except for the claim that the basal activity correlates with the extent of induction (29), which is certainly not the case in the mouse (18,34,51,61), the lymphocyte data are in fact similar to the graded response observed in certain nonhepatic mouse tissues, such as the lung (34), in which MC treatment results in small increases in AHH of "nonresponsive" strains and much larger increases in responsive strains.

Is the "high" inducibility phenotype more susceptible to bronchogenic carcinoma? Evidence in the mouse with MC (34,36,37,39,48) and with benzo[a]pyrene (34,50) indicates that highly inducible AHH activity is associated with an increased incidence of fibrosarcomas and rhabdomyosarcomas as well as squamous cell carcinoma of the lung. In all probability, these associations are due to polycyclic hydrocarbon metabolism by local tissues rather than the liver. It is thus conceivable that the lymphocyte may be a reasonable indicator for AHH inducibility among nonhepatic tissues. The peripheral blood monocyte, for instance, is generally believed to be the precursor for pulmonary macrophages (4,58).

Can AHH induction in cultured mitogen-activated lymphocytes be an indicator of plasma clearance of commonly used classes of drugs? The plasma clearance of every drug tested in humans during the past 20 years has been shown to be Gaussian (75) and therefore presumably under multifactorial polygenic control,[1] whereas the extent of AHH induction in cultured lymphocytes is claimed (31) to be regulated by two alleles of unequal frequency at a single locus. If this is the case, it is not surprising that we find (3) no correlation between AHH induction in culture and the plasma half-lives of two drugs known to be metabolized principally by cytochrome P-450-mediated monooxygenases. However, several laboratories, including our own (35), currently find that distribution of the lymphocyte AHH inducibilities in the general population falls into a skewed unimodal (rather than a trimodal) distribution. Thus, provided that the appropriate drugs are studied, the possibility remains that the lymphocytes can reflect the activity of the liver (the major site of drug metabolism).

Is there promise for the use of AHH inducibility in cultured lymphocytes as a biochemical marker of susceptibility to cancers, such as bronchogenic carcinoma? One consideration concerns the fact that mitogen stimulation of the lymphocytes is necessary in order to detect the basal and inducible AHH activity. The responsiveness of the B or T lymphocytes to the mitogens might therefore be what one is measuring, rather than the responsiveness of the lymphocytes to MC. Variation in responsiveness to mitogens between B and T cells are known to exist between

---

[1]However, we cannot state categorically that any statistical methodology will enable us to predict the range of phenotypic possibilities which are inherent in any genotype, nor that any technique of statistical estimation can provide a convincing argument for a genetic mechanism more complicated than one or two Mendelian loci with low and constant penetrance.

individuals; and, in the same individual, the percentage of circulating B or T cells varies daily and at different times of day (42). The response of lymphocytes from lung cancer patients to mitogens is known to be poor (13,17,69). In fact, even therapeutic doses of aspirin suppress the cultured lymphocytes' response to mitogens (11). Studies using cultured peripheral blood monocytes (4,58), in which inducibility of AHH activity ranges from about 7- to 35-fold without the need for mitogens, might be one promising approach to determine whether "mitogen responsiveness" is an important factor. Studies using pulmonary alveolar macrophages obtained by tracheal lavage (7) show that AHH activity is measurable in fresh (i.e., uncultured) cells, that the activity is higher in smokers than in nonsmokers, and that one can measure a rise and fall in activity in sequential samples from an individual who begins and stops smoking. These cells (and perhaps the antecedent monocytes) are thus subject to environmental influences *in vivo*. Ironically, then, the requirement for mitogen stimulation may be, in one sense, advantageous in assessing a genetic trait, since the mature lymphocyte *in vivo*, which cannot express AHH, is presumably resistant to such environmental influences. Such a dilemma arises principally because we are seeking to measure in cell culture—an inherently variable system—quantitative variations among individuals rather than the qualitative all-or-none phenomena found in many recessive inborn errors of metabolism.

Cell growth or lymphoblast formation may influence AHH activity. A correlation is claimed between the basal and MC-induced AHH activity in lymphocyte cultures (31); this is not the case in tissues of the intact mouse (18,51,61). A correlation between MC-induced AHH activity and MC-induced epoxide hydrase activity has been reported (30); no such correlation exists in mouse liver (54). The basal AHH activity, MC-induced AHH activity, and fold inducibility are higher by a factor of about two in the late summer and autumn than in the late winter and spring (Beverly Paigen, *personal communication*). The skewed-to-the-left distribution of AHH inducibility for 588 different individuals was very similar to that for the same individual tested 33 different times (C. R. Shaw, *personal communication*).

On the other hand, variables unrelated to cell growth also influence the expression of AHH activity. Unknown factors in the serum (19), numerous hydrophobic chemicals (55), and even superoxides generated from riboflavin in the presence of light (56) have been shown to stimulate AHH activity in cell culture; the presence of vitamin A in the growth medium (60) can, under certain circumstances, enhance the effects of AHH inducers. The particular lot of fetal calf serum (which is required for cell growth) used in lymphocyte cultures has been found by all laboratories involved to be one of the principal variables affecting levels of AHH. This variation is not accounted for by differences in rates of DNA synthesis as measured by incorporation of radioactive thymidine (S. A. Atlas and D. W. Nebert, *unpublished observations*). If other classes of AHH inducers[2] are present

---

[2] At least three classes of AHH inducers exist in mammalian cell culture, represented by polycyclic aromatic compounds, phenobarbital, and catecholamines (19). Induction by each class is additive with

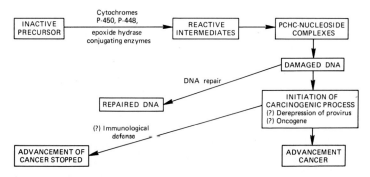

FIG. 7. Hypothetical scheme by which polycyclic hydrocarbons (PCHC) may initiate tumorigenesis. Following metabolic activation by the various drug-metabolizing enzymes (24,28,51, 66), interaction of reactive intermediates with base pairs may damage DNA. The advancement of cancer, however, can still be prevented or modified by the host's mechanisms of DNA repair and immunological competence.

to variable degrees in different lots of serum, their effects may be additive with those of MC, thereby obscuring the true extent of induction due to MC alone. If, on the other hand, trace amounts of potent aromatic hydrocarbon inducers variably contaminate the water supply used to make up media, their concentration, which determines the extent of submaximal AHH induction, becomes a critical factor in determining the extent of induction by added MC. For all these reasons, the coefficient of variation ranges between 0.10 and 0.50 in most laboratories, compared with 0.01 to 0.04 in the study of Kellermann et al. (31). One promising modification, currently being examined in the laboratory of Kouri and co-workers, is the use of markers for endoplasmic reticulum proliferation which are not induced by MC.

CONCLUDING COMMENTS

When tumors are initiated by polycyclic hydrocarbons (Fig. 7), factors other than metabolic activation with resultant cellular macromolecular damage, such as DNA repair and immunological competence, are also presumably important. The susceptibility or resistance to chemically induced pulmonary tumors in the mouse is associated with specific genes on six different linkage groups (25), and it has been suggested (48) that the *Ah* locus is one of these loci. The relationship between chemically induced cancers and loci controlling DNA repair and immunological competence in the mouse remains to be determined.

With respect to benzo[a]pyrene-initiated tumorigenesis, the rates of monooxygenation, phenol, quinone, dihydrodiol, and conjugate formation (pathways of Fig. 1), DNA repair, and immune surveillance quite likely differ among different

induction by either or both of the others, thus indicating three distinct mechanisms of induction. Only induction by the polycyclic aromatics such as MC is responsible for significant cytochrome P_1-450 formation *in vivo* (18,51).

tissues, strains, and species; age, nutritional status, hormonal balance, diurnal and pH variations, as well as saturating versus nonsaturating substrate concentrations, may be important factors in affecting these various metabolic rates, DNA repair, and immunological competence. It remains possible that the monooxygenation of benzo[a]pyrene is under relatively simple genetic control in man and that this step is of such overwhelming importance, compared with subsequent metabolic steps or with DNA repair or immunological competence, that this singular response (i.e., AHH induction in cultured lymphocytes) can be shown to be correlated with increased risk of bronchogenic carcinoma. Such an association with the *Ah* locus has been demonstrated for MC-initiated (36,37,39,48) and benzo[a]pyrene-initiated (34,50) sarcomas and MC-initiated lung cancer (34) in two prototype strains of mice. Until one can increase the range of fold inducibility of AHH and/or decrease the amount of experimental "noise" (i.e., nonspecific factors inducing AHH activity in culture to varying degrees), however, AHH inducibility in cultured mitogen-activated lymphocytes cannot be used as a biochemical marker for determining who is at risk for bronchogenic carcinoma or other cancers. Consistent differences between two individuals can be found if the samples are always carried together through the same experiment, and this presumably accounts for the success of our data (ref. 3; Fig. 6) on identical and fraternal twin pairs.

ACKNOWLEDGMENTS

We greatly appreciate valuable conversations with Drs. Richard E. Kouri, Charles R. Shaw, Beverly Paigen, Harry V. Gelboin, and Gottfried Kellermann, with regard to recent studies with AHH inducibility in man.

REFERENCES

1. Atlas, S. A., and Nebert, D. W. (1976): Genetic association of increases in naphthalene, acetanilide, and biphenyl hydroxylations with inducible aryl hydrocarbon hydroxylase in mice. *Arch. Biochem. Biophys.*, 175:495–506.
2. Atlas, S. A., Taylor, B. A., Diwan, B. A., and Nebert, D. W. (1976): Inducible monooxygenase activities and 3-methylcholanthrene-initiated tumorigenesis in mouse recombinant inbred sublines. *Genetics*, 83:537-550.
3. Atlas, S. A., Vesell, E. S., and Nebert, D. W. (1976): Genetic control of interindividual variations in the inducibility of aryl hydrocarbon hydroxylase in cultured human lymphocytes. *Cancer Res.*, 36:4619–4630.
4. Bast, R. C. Jr., Whitlock, J. P. Jr., Miller, H., Rapp, H. J., and Gelboin, H. V. (1974): Aryl hydrocarbon (benzo[a]pyrene) hydroxylase in human peripheral blood monocytes. *Nature*, 250:664–665.
5. Benedict, W. F., Considine, N., and Nebert, D. W. (1973): Genetic differences in aryl hydrocarbon hydroxylase induction and benzo[a]pyrene-produced tumorigenesis in the mouse. *Mol. Pharmacol.* 9:266–277.
6. Buell, P., and Dunn, J. E. (1965): Cancer mortality among Japanese Issei and Nisei of California. *Cancer*, 18:656–664.
7. Cantrell, E. T., Warr, G. A., Busbee, D. L., and Martin, R. R. (1973): Induction of aryl hydrocarbon hydroxylase in human pulmonary alveolar macrophages by cigarette smoking. *J. Clin. Invest.*, 52:1881–1884.

8. Comings, D. E. (1973): A general theory of carcinogenesis. *Proc. Natl. Acad. Sci. USA,* 70:3324–3328.
9. Conney, A. H. (1967): Pharmacological implications of microsomal enzyme induction. *Pharmacol. Rev.,* 19:317–366.
10. Creaven, P. J., and Parke, D. V. (1966): The stimulation of hydroxylation by carcinogenic and non-carcinogenic compounds. *Biochem. Pharmacol.,* 15:7–16.
11. Crout, J. E., Hepburn, B., and Ritts, R. E. Jr. (1975): Suppression of lymphocyte transformation after aspirin ingestion. *N. Engl. J. Med.,* 292:221–223.
12. Czygan, P., Greim, H., Garro, A., Schaffner, F., and Popper, H. (1974): The effect of dietary protein deficiency on the ability of isolated hepatic microsomes to alter the mutagenicity of a primary and a secondary carcinogen. *Cancer Res,,* 34:119–123,
13. Ducos, J., Migueres, J., Colombies, P., Kessous, A., and Poujoulet, N. (1970): Lymphocyte response to P.H.A. in patients with lung cancer. *Lancet,* 1:1111–1112.
14. Felton, J. S., and Nebert, D. W. (1975): Mutagenesis of certain activated carcinogens *in vitro* associated with genetically mediated increases in monooxygenase activity and cytochrome $P_1 450$. *J. Biol. Chem.,* 250:6769–6778.
15. Felton, J. S., Nebert, D. W., and Thorgeirsson, S. S. (1976): Genetic differences in 2-acetyl-aminofluorene mutagenicity *in vitro* associated with mouse hepatic aryl hydrocarbon hydroxylase activity induced by polycyclic aromatic compounds. *Mol. Pharmacol.,* 12:225–233.
16. Frommer, U., Ullrich, V., and Orrenius, S. (1974): Influence of inducers and inhibitors on the hydroxylation pattern of *n*-hexane in rat liver microsomes. *FEBS Lett.,* 41:14–16.
17. Garrioch, D. B., Good, R. A., and Gatti, R. A. (1970): Lymphocyte response to P.H.A. in patients with non-lymphoid tumours. *Lancet,* 1:618.
18. Gielen, J. E., Goujon, F. M., and Nebert, D. W. (1972): Genetic regulation of aryl hydrocarbon hydroxylase induction. II. Simple Mendelian expression in mouse tissues *in vivo. J. Biol. Chem.,* 247:1125–1137.
19. Gielen, J. E., and Nebert, D. W. (1972): Aryl hydrocarbon hydroxylase induction in mammalian liver cell culture. III. Effects of various sera, hormones, biogenic amines, and other endogenous compounds on the enzyme activity. *J. Biol. Chem.,* 247:7591–7602.
20. Green, M. C. (Chairman, Committee on Standardized Genetic Nomenclature for Mice): Guidelines for nomenclature of genetically determined biochemical variants in the house mouse, *Mus musculus. Biochem. Genet.,* 9:369–374.
21. Guenthner, T. M., Poland, A. P., and Nebert, D. W. (1976): Evidence for possible receptors active in aryl hydrocarbon hydroxylase induction in established cell lines by 2,3,7,8-tetra-chlorodibenzo-*p*-dioxin. *Fed. Proc. (in press).*
22. Gurtoo, H. L., Bejba, N., and Minowada, J. (1975): Properties, inducibility, and an improved method of analysis of aryl hydrocarbon hydroxylase in cultured human lymphocytes. *Cancer Res.,* 35:1235–1243.
23. Haenszel, W., and Kurihara, M. (1968): Studies of Japanese migrants. I. Mortality from cancer and other diseases among Japanese in the United States. *J. Natl. Cancer Inst.,* 40:43–68.
24. Heidelberger, C. (1975): Chemical carcinogenesis. *Annu. Rev. Biochem.,* 44:79–121.
25. Heston, W. E. (1963): Genetics of neoplasia. In: *Methodology in Mammalian Genetics,* edited by W. J. Burdett, p. 247. Holden-Day Inc., San Francisco.
25a. Higginson, J., and Muir, C. S. (1973): Epidemiology. In: *Cancer Medicine,* edited by J. F. Holland and E. Frei, pp. 241–306. Lea & Febiger, Philadelphia.
26. Holder, G., Yagi, H., Dansette, P., Jerina, D. M., Levin, W., Lu, A. Y. H., and Conney, A. H. (1974): Effects of inducers and epoxide hydrase on the metabolism of benzo[a]pyrene by liver microsomes and a reconstituted system: Analysis by high pressure liquid chromatography. *Proc. Natl. Acad. Sci. USA,* 71:4356–4360.
27. Holder, G. M., Yagi, H., Jerina, D. M., Levin, W., Lu, A. Y. H., and Conney, A. H. (1975): Metabolism of benzo[a]pyrene: Effect of substrate concentration and 3-methylcholanthrene pretreatment on hepatic metabolism by microsomes from rats and mice. *Arch. Biochem. Biophys.,* 170:557–566.
28. Jerina, D. M., and Daly, J. W. (1974): Arene oxides: A new aspect of drug metabolism. *Science,* 185:573–582.
29. Kellermann, G., Luyten-Kellermann, M., Horning, M. G., and Stafford, M. (1975): Correlation of aryl hydrocarbon hydroxylase activity of human lymphocyte cultures and plasma elimination rates for antipyrine and phenylbutazone. *Drug Metab. Dispos.,* 3:47–50.

30. Kellermann, G., Luyten-Kellermann, M., and Shaw, C. R. (1973): Presence and induction of epoxide hydrase in cultured human leukocytes. *Biochem. Biophys. Res. Commun.*, 52:712–716.
31. Kellermann, G., Luyten-Kellermann, M., and Shaw, C. R. (1973): Genetic variation of aryl hydrocarbon hydroxylase in human lymphocytes. *Am. J. Hum. Genet.*, 25:327–331.
32. Kellermann, G., Shaw, C. R., and Luyten-Kellermann, M. (1973): Aryl hydrocarbon hydroxylase inducibility and bronchogenic carcinoma. *N. Engl. J. Med.*, 289:934–937.
33. Knudson, A. G. Jr. (1975): Genetics of human cancer. *Genetics*, 79 (Supplement):305–316.
34. Kouri, R. E. (1976): Relationship between levels of aryl hydrocarbon hydroxylase activity and susceptibility to 3-methylcholanthrene- and benzo[a]pyrene-induced cancers in inbred strains of mice. In: *Polynuclear Aromatic Hydrocarbons,* edited by R. I. Freudenthal and P. Jones, pp. 139–151. Raven Press, New York.
35. Kouri, R. E., Ratrie, H., Atlas, S. A., Niwa, A., and Nebert, D. W. (1974): Aryl hydrocarbon hydroxylase induction in human lymphocyte cultures by 2,3,7,8-tetrachlorodibenzo-*p*-dioxin. *Life Sci.*, 15:1585–1595.
36. Kouri, R. E., Ratrie, H., and Whitmire, C. E. (1973): Evidence of a genetic relationship between susceptibility to 3-methylcholanthrene-induced subcutaneous tumors and inducibility of aryl hydrocarbon hydroxylase. *J. Natl. Cancer Inst.*, 51:197–200.
37. Kouri, R. E., Ratrie, H., and Whitmire, C. E. (1974): Genetic control of susceptibility to 3-methylcholanthrene-induced subcutaneous tumors. *Int. J. Cancer*, 13:714–720.
38. Kouri, R. E., Rude, T., Thomas, P. E., and Whitmire, C. E. (1976): Studies on pulmonary aryl hydrocarbon hydroxylase activity in inbred strains of mice. *Chem. Biol. Interact.* 13:317–331.
39. Kouri, R. E., Salerno, R. A., and Whitmire, C. E. (1973): Relationships between aryl hydrocarbon hydroxylase inducibility and sensitivity to chemically induced subcutaneous sarcomas in various strains of mice. *J. Natl. Cancer Inst.*, 50:363–368.
40. Kuntzman, R., Levin, W., Jacobson, M., and Conney, A. H. (1968): Studies on microsomal hydroxylation and the demonstration of a new carbon monoxide binding pigment in liver microsomes. *Life Sci.*, 7:215–224.
41. Levitt, R. C., Felton, J. S., Robinson, J. R., and Nebert, D. W. (1975): A single-gene difference in early death caused by hypoplastic anemia in mice receiving oral benzo[a]pyrene daily. *Pharmacologist*, 17:213.
42. Ling, N. R., and Kay, J. E. (1975): *Lymphocyte Stimulation,* 2nd ed., 398 pp. North-Holland, Amsterdam.
43. Mason, T. J., McKay, F. W., Hoover, R., Blot, W. J., and Fraumeni, J. F. Jr. (1975): *Atlas of Cancer Mortality for U.S. Counties: 1950–1969.,* 103 pp. U.S. Dept HEW Publication, (NIH) 75–780. U. S. Govt. Print. Off., Washington, D.C.
44. Matsushima, T., Grantham, P. H., Weisburger, E. K., and Weisburger, J. H. (1972): Phenobarbital-mediated increase in ring- and *N*-hydroxylation of the carcinogen *N*-2-fluorenylacetamide, and decrease in amounts bound to liver deoxyribonucleic acid. *Biochem. Pharmacol.*, 21:2043–2051.
45. Nebert, D. W. (1973): Use of fetal cell culture as an experimental system for predicting drug metabolism in the intact animal. *Clin. Pharmacol. Therap.*, 14:693–699.
46. Nebert, D. W., and Bausserman, L. L. (1970): Genetic differences in the extent of aryl hydrocarbon hydroxylase induction in mouse fetal cell cultures. *J. Biol. Chem.*, 245:6373–6382.
47. Nebert, D. W., Benedict, W. F., Gielen, J. E., Oesch, F., and Daly, J. W. (1972): Aryl hydrocarbon hydroxylase, epoxide hydrase, and 7,12-dimethylbenz[a]anthracene-produced skin tumorigenesis in the mouse. *Mol. Pharmacol.*, 8:374–379.
48. Nebert, D. W., Benedict, W. F., and Kouri, R. E. (1974): Aromatic hydrocarbon-produced tumorigenesis and the genetic differences in aryl hydrocarbon hydroxylase induction. In: *Chemical Carcinogenesis,* edited by P.O.P. Ts'o and J. A. Dipaolo, pp. 271–288. Dekker, New York.
49. Nebert, D. W., and Gielen, J. E. (1972): Genetic regulation of aryl hydrocarbon hydroxylase induction in the mouse. *Fed. Proc.*, 31:1315–1325.
50. Nebert, D. W., Boobis, A. R., Yagi, H., Jerina, D. M., and Kouri, R. E. (1976): Genetic differences in mouse cytochrome P_1-450-mediated metabolism of benzo[a]pyrene *in vitro* and carcinogenic index *in vivo*. In: *Biological Reactive Intermediates,* edited by D. J. Jollow, J. J. Kocsis, R. Snyder, and H. Vainio, pp. 125–145. Plenum Press, New York *(in press)*.
51. Nebert, D. W., Robinson, J. R., Niwa, A., Kumaki, K., and Poland, A. P. (1975): Genetic expression of aryl hydrocarbon hydroxylase activity in the mouse, *J. Cell Physiol.*, 85:393–414.

52. Nebert, D. W., Thorgeirsson, S. S., and Lambert, G. H. (1976): Genetic aspects of toxicity during development. *Environ. Health Perspect. (in press)*.

53. Niwa, A., Kumaki, K., Nebert, D. W., and Poland, A. P. (1975): Genetic expression of aryl hydrocarbon hydroxylase activity in the mouse. Distinction between the "responsive" homozygote and heterozygote at the *Ah* locus. *Arch. Biochem. Biophys.* 166:559–564.

54. Oesch, F., Morris, N., Daly, J. W., Gielen, J. E., and Nebert, D. W. (1973): Genetic expression of the induction of epoxide hydrase and aryl hydrocarbon hydroxylase activities in the mouse by phenobarbital or 3-methylcholanthrene. *Mol. Pharmacol.*, 9:692–696.

55. Owens, I. S., and Nebert, D. W. (1975): Aryl hydrocarbon hydroxylase induction in mammalian-liver-derived cell cultures. Stimulation of "cytochrome P_1-450-associated" enzyme activity by many inducing compounds. *Mol. Pharmacol.*, 11:94–104.

56. Paine, A. J., and McLean, A. E. M. (1974): Induction of aryl hydrocarbon hydroxylase by a light-driven superoxide generating system in liver cell culture. *Biochem. Biophys. Res. Commun.*, 58:482–486.

57. Penrose, L. S. (1963): *The Biology of Mental Defect*, 3rd ed., pp. 92–95. Sidgwick and Jackson, London.

57a. Poland, A. P., Glover, E., and Kende, A. S. (1976): *J. Biol. Chem.*, 251:4936–4946.

58. Ptashne, K., Brothers, L., Axline, S. G., and Cohen, S. N. (1974): Aryl hydrocarbon hydroxylase induction in mouse peritoneal macrophages and blood-derived human macrophages. *Proc. Soc. Exp. Biol. Med.*, 146:585–589.

59. Rasmussen, R. E., and Wang, I. Y. (1974): Dependence of specific metabolism of benzo[a]pyrene on inducer of hydroxylase activity. *Cancer Res.*, 34:2290–2295.

60. Rasmussen, R. E., Wang, I. Y., and Crocker, T. T. (1972): Modification of aryl hydrocarbon metabolism in Syrian hamster cell cultures by vitamin A. *Proc. Am. Assoc. Cancer Res.*, 13:53.

61. Robinson, J. R., Considine, N., and Nebert, D. W. (1974): Genetic expression of aryl hydrocarbon hydroxylase induction. Evidence for the involvement of other genetic loci. *J. Biol. Chem.*, 249:5851–5859.

62. Robinson, J. R., Felton, J. S., Levitt, R. C., Thorgeirsson, S. S., and Nebert, D. W. (1975): Relationship between "aromatic hydrocarbon responsiveness" and the survival times in mice treated with various drugs and environmental compounds. *Mol. Pharmacol.*, 11:850–865.

63. Robinson, J. R., and Nebert, D. W. (1974): Genetic expression of aryl hydrocarbon hydroxylase induction presence or absence of association with zoxazolamine, diphenylhydantoin, and hexobarbital metabolism. *Mol. Pharmacol.*, 10:484–493.

64. Schenker, J. G., Polishuk, W. Z., and Steinity, R. (1968): An epidemiologic study of carcinoma of the ovary in Israel. *Isr. J. Med. Sci.*, 4:820–826.

65. Shichi, H., Atlas, S. A., and Nebert, D. W. (1975): Genetically regulated aryl hydrocarbon hydroxylase induction in the eye: Possible significance of the drug-metabolizing enzyme system for the retinal pigmented epithelium-choroid. *Exp. Eye Res.*, 21:557–567.

66. Sims, P., and Grover, P. L. (1974): Epoxides in polycyclic aromatic hydrocarbon metabolism and carcinogenesis. *Adv. Cancer Res.*, 20:165–274.

67. Sims, P., Grover, P. L., Swaisland, A., Pal, K., and Hewer, A. (1975): Metabolic activation of benzo[a]pyrene proceeds *via* a diol-epoxide. *Nature*, 252:326–328.

68. Staszewski, J., and Haenszel, W. (1965): Cancer mortality among the Polish-born in the United States. *J. Natl. Cancer Inst.*, 35:291–297.

69. Suciu-Foca, N., Buda, J., McManus, J., Thiem, T., and Reemtsa, K. (1973): Impaired responsiveness of lymphocytes and serum-inhibitory factors in patients with cancer. *Cancer Res.*, 33:2373–2377.

70. Thomas, P. E., and Hutton, J. J. (1973): Genetics of aryl hydrocarbon hydroxylase induction in mice: Additive inheritance in crosses between C3H/HeJ and DBA/2J. *Biochem. Genet.*, 8:249–257.

71. Thomas, P. E., Hutton, J. J., and Taylor, B. A. (1973): Genetic relationship between aryl hydrocarbon hydroxylase inducibility and chemical carcinogen induced skin ulceration in mice. *Genetics*, 74:655–659.

72. Thomas, P. E., Kouri, R. E., and Hutton, J. J. (1972): The genetics of aryl hydrocarbon hydroxylase induction in mice: A single gene difference between C57BL/6J and DBA/2J. *Biochem. Genet.*, 6:157–168.

73. Thorgeirsson, S. S., Felton, J. S., and Nebert, D. W. (1975): Genetic differences in the aromatic hydrocarbon-inducible *N*-hydroxylation of 2-acetylaminofluorene and acetaminophen-produced hepatotoxicity in mice. *Mol. Pharmacol.*, 11:159–165.
74. Thorgeirsson, S. S., Jollow, D. J., Sasame, H. A., Green, I., and Mitchell, J. R. (1973): The role of cytochrome P-450 in *N*-hydroxylation of 2-acetylaminofluorene. *Mol. Pharmacol.*, 9:398–404.
75. Vesell, E. S. (1972): Pharmacogenetics. *N. Engl. J. Med.*, 287:904–909.
76. Wood, A. W., and Conney, A. H. (1974): Genetic variation in coumarin hydroxylase activity in the mouse *(Mus musculus)*. *Science*, 185:612–614.
77. Zampaglione, N., Jollow, D. J., Mitchell, J. R., Stripp, B., Hamrick, M., and Gillette, J. R. (1973): Role of detoxifying enzymes in bromobenzene-induced liver necrosis. *J. Pharmacol. Exp. Ther.*, 187:218–227.

Discussion

Blattner: I understand the AHH assay using monocytes is being applied to Dr. Minna's lung cancer service at the Veterans Administration Hospital of Washington, D.C. Dr. Minna, would you give a progress report?

Minna: The source is easily acquired and gives levels of AHH for our hybrid cell work even in bone marrow samples, which do not need culture or stimulation.

Nebert: The ideal clinical test for a biochemical marker of those at high risk for cancer must be simple, reproducible, and reliable with few falsely positive or falsely negative results. Therefore, drawing 10 or 20 cc of blood and culturing lymphocytes is simple; aspiration of bone marrow or a skin or liver biopsy is unreasonable. Dr. Minna, you are correct that bone marrow samples or monocytes would alleviate the problem of mitogen stimulation. The monocyte assay under development by Bast, Miller, Gelboin, and others at the National Cancer Institute [*Nature*, 250:664–665 (1974)] requires 50 to 100 cc of blood—a prohibitive amount for a simple clinical test.

Comings: Do fibroblasts give a clearer picture than lymphocytes?

Nebert: Using fibroblasts introduces all the problems of tissue culture techniques—differences in cell density, cell growths, particularly lots of fetal calf serum and powdered prepared media, etc. But, again, the need for skin biopsy prohibits wide clinical use.

Gatti: What about using lymphoblastoid lines?

Nebert: Gurtoo and co-workers [*Cancer Res.*, 35:1235–1243 (1975)] tested AHH induction in 10 stable lymphocyte cell lines and found significant activity in at least three; however, it is not known whether the level of AHH induction in the established cell lines reflects a genetic trait of the patient from which the cells were derived.

Hirschhorn: It is not surprising that lymphoblast lines do not work. Preliminary results from Dr. Popper's laboratory and ours suggest that the whole P-450 system is low or absent in these lines.

Nebert: With regard to established lymphocyte cell lines, I am reminded of the report by Kowal and co-workers [*J. Biol. Chem.*, 245:2438–2443 (1970)]. Whereas long-term culture—for periods of up to 2 years—does not change the levels of the mitochondrial respiratory chain cytochromes in monolayer cultures of mouse adrenal cortex tumors, cytochrome P-450 essentially falls to undetectable levels. But the P-450 content can be restored to normal by passage of the tumor cells into the abdominal cavity of recipient mice and then returning the cells to culture. This study indicates that a genetic measurement in freshly cultured cells is certainly subject to possible changes during subsequent passaging of the cells. Treatment with trypsin and growing logarithmically a sparse cell density to confluency, week after week, will therefore undoubtedly alter numerous enzymes and other macromolecules in established cell lines.

Swift: To avoid the variability seen in tumor patients possibly related to their primary disease, one might study the *offspring* of patients instead of the patients themselves.

Nebert: Yes, this is a good point. Lymphocytes from cancer patients receiving chemotherapy might not respond normally to mitogens in culture. I understand such a project is currently underway at Roswell Park Memorial Institute in Buffalo.

Hirschhorn: Calling this trait a dominant one presents a couple of obvious curiosities: first, supposedly inbred mice are now segregating a dominant trait; and, secondly, if you consider the trait an enzyme deficiency, most such deficiencies are recessives.

Nebert: The first studies indicated that AHH induction by methylcholanthrene (MC) was inherited as a single autosomal dominant trait [*J. Biol. Chem.*, 247:1125–1137 (1972); *Nature* [*New Biol.*], 236:107–110 (1972); *Biochem. Genet.*, 6:157–168 (1972)]. The present feeling is that a minimum of two loci and six alleles is required to explain all of the data in the mouse [*J. Cell. Physiol.*, 85:393–414 (1975)]. It is interesting, if Kellermann is correct, that AHH induction in a species as outbred as man is expressed simply as two alleles at a single locus, whereas AHH induction among about 12 inbred strains of mice is under a more complex genetic control.

Mulvihill: The fact that "AHH" is a shorthand word for a series of enzymes would argue against a single locus.

Nebert: Yes. "AHH activity" represents one of several dozen well defined cytochrome P-450-mediated drug metabolizing monooxygenases. But even with benzo[a]pyrene as the substrate, aryl hydrocarbon (benzo[a]pyrene) hydroxylase "activity" is different between control animals and MC-treated genetically responsive animals [*J. Cell Physiol.*, 85:393–414 (1975)]. The MC-inducible AHH is associated with cytochrome P_1-450 (P-448), and the basal AHH activity is associated with one or more forms of P-450 other than P_1-450. This is true in the mouse, rat, hamster, and guinea pig. The two forms are under different genetic control in mice [*J. Biol. Chem.*, 249:5851–5859 (1974)]. There is now evidence (O. Pelkonen, *personal communication*) that at least three different forms of AHH activity exist in human placenta, fetal liver, and fetal adrenal gland. I suppose that it is conceivable, although unlikely, that AHH induction in man might be expressed as simply as two alleles at a single locus.

Petrakis: The Paigens described a seasonal variation of AHH inducibility in the people of Buffalo who drink the water of Lake Erie. Could fluctuations in the concentration of carcinogens in the drinking water account for the seasonal variation in the assay?

Nebert: This variability could not be caused by carcinogens in the water drunk by the lymphocyte donors, just as there is no influence on the lymphocyte culture system by cigarette smoking. Any AHH activity induced by outside factors, such as benzo[a]pyrene in cigarette smoke, will disappear during the first 12 to 24 hr that the lymphocytes are in culture. The inducer is then not added until after 48 or 72 hr of culture of the lymphocytes with pokeweed mitogen and phytohemagglutinin M. Although the seasonal variation might be caused by something inherent in the human lymphocytes, more likely there are factors in the fetal calf serum, or in the water used to prepare the medium, that differ between summer and winter.

Genetics of Human Cancer, edited by J. J.
Mulvihill, R. W. Miller, and J. F. Fraumeni, Jr.
Raven Press, New York, 1977.

28

HLA Frequencies in Cancer: A Second Study

Paul I. Terasaki, Sondra T. Perdue, and Max R. Mickey

*Departments of Surgery and Biomathematics, University of California, Los Angeles,
California 90024*

Earlier we reported that, unlike diseases such as ankylosing spondylitis, which has a high association with an HLA antigen (4), most cancers have a weak association, if any, with HLA (6). The recent finding of a high degree of linkage of cancer with a single HLA haplotype in a large cancer family (2) suggests that a cancer susceptibility gene could be linked to HLA, but that this linkage may not be apparent in random population studies. Although it is often stated that linked genes are not *associated* in a random population, as witnessed by ABO and the nail patella syndrome, this generalization is obviously not applicable to many HLA-associated diseases. Strong linkage disequilibrium exists between the A,B,C, and D loci of HLA and corresponding high associations among specificities of the four loci are seen in the random population. As we pointed out earlier (7), there is no reason to expect that the disease susceptibility gene might not have the same type of linkage with HLA specificities.

There is a possibility that cancer is an ancient disease, and that the susceptibility gene has crossed over extensively, reaching equilibrium with at least the first two loci of HLA. If there is any residual disequilibrium, a large study of possible association can be expected to reveal a linkage relationship. The most difficult complication of this approach is the problem of sampling variations. Some indications of association would be expected to occur by chance alone.

In the present study, we have attempted to deal with the sampling problem by studying a second independent sample and by increasing the number of patients in each group studied.

METHODS

For the present study (1973–1975), 2,005 cancer patients and 1,536 healthy controls who were typed between January, 1973, and August, 1975, were selected. Because of racial variations in frequencies of HLA antigens among various ethnic populations, only Caucasian patients and controls were used; family members and persons with Mexican surnames were eliminated.

A second group of 4,017 patients and 3,896 controls was selected from persons typed between January, 1970, and October, 1975. These were selected independently of the study from 1973 to 1975, although many patients and some controls appear in both groups. Disease categories that did not have cases occurring throughout the years 1970 to 1975 were not analyzed in the overall study, as these categories were not comparable to the controls from that period. For example, recording of the specific diagnoses acute lymphocytic leukemia (ALL), acute myelocytic leukemia (AML), and chronic myelocytic leukemia (CML) began in 1973; cases before that time were classified by the broader category of leukemia.

The microcytotoxicity test was used to test for 25 HLA specificities using at least four selected antisera per specificity in Tables 1 and 2. Analysis was done using chi-square computations performed at the UCLA Health Sciences Computing Facility.

Patients were divided into broad categories by tumor site based on the diagnosis reported by the physician submitting the specimen.

RESULTS

Among the 17 cancers tested from 1973 to 1975, there were 14 deviations from the normal control frequencies which were significant at the $p \leq 0.05$ level (Table 1). In no instance was the association sufficiently high to reach $p \leq 0.05$ when corrected by multiplying by the number of comparisons, i.e., 25. The relatively consistent frequency of each of the antigens for the different cancers can be noted. Within this 1973–1975 series of patients, the HLA associations with cancers are quite comparable to the general findings of the 1970–1972 series for solid tumors reported earlier (6).

During a longer time period, larger numbers of cancer patients were typed in each category (Table 2). With these larger numbers, the frequencies are more stable for each disease, even though detection of certain low frequency antigens has changed from 1970 to 1975. There are 22 comparisons which are significant at the $p \leq 0.05$ level. Again, none of the alterations is significant when corrected for the number of comparisons.

Some variation in frequencies among series separated in time can be expected because of technical variations in definition of antigens over a long time period.

The associations which have shown a statistical significance level of $p \leq 0.05$ in at least one of our studies are listed in Table 3. ALL had a high frequency of HLA-A2 in the 1973–1975 series. HLA-B27 was also high in ALL. Cancer of the prostate appears the most likely of the cancers tested to have valid HLA associations. In the first (1970–1972) and second (1973–1975) patient series, A1 and B8 were low. A28 and BW22 were both high, particularly in the second series.

The association of kidney, liver, and lung cancer with AW29 may be of some importance. The low B12 frequency in both series of ovarian cancers may not be

TABLE 1. *Frequencies of HLA specificities in various types of cancers in Caucasians (1973–1975)*

Cancer[b]	N	A 1	A 2	A 3	A 9	A 10	A 11	A 28	A 29	AW 30	AW 32	B 5	B 7	B 8	B 12	B 13	B 14	B 18	B 27	BW 15	BW 16	B 17	BW 21	BW 22	BW 35	BW 40
Normal controls	1536	31	47	26	21	14	12	9	6	10	7	11	23	21	24	5	10	7	7	10	10	10	6	4	21	12
A.L.L.	215	26	56[a]	30	20	13	11	11	6	12	8	12	21	20	28	7	6	10	11[a]	13	7	7	3	3	20	14
A.M.L.	151	25	47	30	20	13	11	11	9	7	12[a]	11	22	22	23	4	11	9	7	12	5	6	4	9[a]	24	12
Bladder	148	28	47	32	19	13	9	9	7	7	10	10	30	17	28	3	7	6	11	7	11	11	7	3	14	17
Breast	327	26	53	22	22	13	11	9	8	9	8	10	24	17	21	6	8	6	7	11	8	8	7	5	25	11
Cervix	107	34	44	28	24	12	6	6	6	13	7	7	28	24	34[a]	3	8	0	6	8	6	14	4	5	14	10
C.M.L.	37	16	49	35	19	11	19	11	5	16	7	16	40[a]	8	16	3	5	8	8	14	14	8	11	8	27	16
Colon	82	29	45	24	19	23	15	6	4	4	11	8	23	15	32	2	8	8	8	15	6	6	4	2	27	13
Endometrium	41	24	54	29	19	19	17	7	12	2	7	15	24	22	20	2	7	7	7	15	7	5	7	10	17	10
Hodgkin's disease	101	37	41	22	24	17	8	7	7	10	8	11	25	19	17	6	9	12	5	16	8	9	6	7	20	9
Kidney	45	33	47	27	19	11	8	7	7	7	0	7	27	29	22	4	18	11	0	4	9	11	2	6	18	13
Larynx	38	29	39	32	21	21	8	3	16[a]	13	10	10	29	16	29	0	13	10	5	16	8	8	10	8	10	16
Leukemia, unspecified	104	28	48	23	22	12	7	11	8	7	13[a]	10	23	16	26	9	10	12	5	9	9	12	6	5	18	16
Lung	180	29	44	32	13	14	14	8	10	7	7	10	27	20	28	4	11	7	5	12	7	9	6	6	17	10
Lymphoma	100	29	44	18	24	12	14	9	14[a]	12	7	9	21	15	24	2	12	6	7	12	12	9	5	9	23	9
Melanoma	159	35	49	25	20	13	11	8	6	9	10	8	24	23	22	2	11	10	7	12	6	12	6	3	20	14
Ovary	74	26	50	31	26	14	11	7	4	12	5	18	26	18	14[a]	0	9	5	12	5	9	9	7	8	23	18
Prostate	96	19[a]	50	24	24	14	5	16[a]	6	14	7	8	20	14	31	5	11	7	9	10	6	9	6	10[a]	12	14

[a] $p \leq 0.05$ without correction for number of comparisons.

[b] Abbreviations: A.L.L., acute lymphoblastic leukemia; A.M.L., acute myelogenous leukemia; C.M.L., chronic myelogenous leukemia.

TABLE 2. Frequencies of HLA specificities in various cancers in Caucasian population (1970–1975)

Cancer	N	A 1	A 2	A 3	A 9	A 10	A 11	A 28	A 29	AW 30	AW 32	7	B 5	B 7	B 8	B 12	B 13	B 14	B 18	B 27	BW 15	BW 17	BW 21	BW 22	BW 35	BW 40
Normal controls	3896	31	47	27	20	13	12	8	6	10	7	10	25	21	26	4	9	8	7	10	9	5	4	4	19	12
Bladder	264	25	45	30	22	14	11	9	8	7	8	9	28	17	26	6	9	9	6	9	8	10	7	4	14	13
Brain	35	14	60	34	23	9	9	6	3	6	3	9	34	9	29	11	9	11	11	11	11	9	0	3	11	9
Breast	705	28	48	23[a]	23	15	12	8	7	9	7	10	22	20	23	4	9	10	10	8	9	8	5	5	22	12
Cervix	253	35	42	28	20	10	8[a]	11	10	13	6	9	28	24	30	5	6	7	7	7	4	9	4	6	19	13
Colon	189	28	47	24	21	16	11	8	4	10	8	10	25	16	25	4	7	6	6	8	13	9	3	6	22	13
Endometrium	102	25	46	28	25	12	14	8	10	7	8	13	24	20	21	6	5	5	9	7	10	8	7	6	20	11
Esophagus	47	28	51	36	13	14	4	13	4	4	13	14[a]	45[a]	8	40[a]	8	13	5	8	6	8	6	0	6	13	8
Hodgkin's disease	411	32	44	26	24	14	11	8	7	10	3	11	21	24	24	8	6	13	9	6	8	6	5	6	13	10
Kidney	79	28	38	30	23	14	10	8	11	11	3	10	22	20	19	5	15	10	10	3	11	11	4	1	23	8
Larynx	109	30	45	34	18	14	7	12	11	8	6	11	25	15	31	4	7	8	8	4	13	14	10[a]	4	16	13
Leukemia, unspecified	140	27	49	24	24	10	8	11	8	12	12[a]	11	24	16	25	1	9	9	12	6	10	14	4	4	19	16
Leukemia, granulocytic	24	33	46	29	25	17	12	0	4	12	0	8	29	25	12	8	4	4	8	21[a]	21	17	8	0	8	8
Liver	56	20	50	27	11	12	12	12	16[a]	11	5	11	16	21	36	4	10	4	7	12	5	11	4	0	20	9
Lung	405	28	47	25	19	11	8	8	10[a]	10	5	10	23	25	25	5	10	9	8	5	11	9	4	5	19	11
Lymphoma	150	30	51	18[a]	25	13	11	11	11	9	5	11	21	17	23	4	12	12	9	7	11	9	5	7	25	10
Lymphosarcoma	63	30	46	24	22	8	10	16[a]	11	5	10	13	16	24	27	5	11	11	6	2	6	13	2	3	21	16
Melanoma	226	33	50	26	19	11	13	6	6	11	9	9	23	20	24	4	8	8	9	7	11	12	7	4	19	13
Mouth	61	31	46	28	23	10	16	7	3	15	3	11	18	18	18	8	8	11	8	7	7	13	2	8	16	13
Ovary	138	26	44	27	26	14	10	9	6	12	6	14	24	18	18	2	8	10	7	12	6	13	5	8	16	13
Pancreas	40	32	60	25	12	15	2	10	12	8	10	8	32	12	33	8	2	10	8	12	12	18	5	8	23	13
Prostate	299	22[a]	51	22	20	12	11	13	5	12	4[a]	11	25	13	24	6	10	10	7	10	11	8	2	8[a]	15	10
Rectum	88	31	47	26	25	9	11	3	6	10	5	16	25	20	26	2	11	11	2	4	12	10	2	6	24	8
Stomach	58	28	43	22	24	24[a]	2[a]	3	9	9	10	19	21	12	26	2	12	14	14	7	5	10	3	3	17	10
Uterus, not specified	39	28	51	13	26	18	8	13	8	21	0	21	15	18	26	8	3	11	11	13	15	10	3	5	10	8

[a] $p \leq 0.05$ without correction for the number of comparisons.

TABLE 3. *Significant trends in HLA specificities for various cancers (p ≤ 0.05 in at least one study)*

		Antigen frequencies								
		1970-1975			1973-1975			1970-1972 [f]		
		Disease			Disease			Disease		
Cancer	Ag	Total	With anti-gen	Normal[a] with antigen	Total	With anti-gen	Normal[b] with antigen	Total	With anti-gen	Normal[c] with antigen
Acute lymphoblastic leukemia	A2	ND[d]			215	56*	47	NR[e]		
	B27					11*	7			
Acute myelogenous leukemia	AW32	ND			151	12*	7	NR		
	BW22					9*	4			
Bladder	BW35	264	14	19	148	14	21	139	13*	22
Breast	A1	705	28	31	327	26	31	384	32*	27
	A3		23*	27		22	26		24	24
Cervix	A1	253	35	31	107	34	31	142	35*	27
	A9		20	20		24	21		15	21
	A11		8	12		6	12		11	12
	B12		30	26		34	24		32	24
Chronic myelogenous leukemia	B7	ND			37	40*	23	NR		
Colon	A10	189	16	13	82	23*	14	121	11	11
	BW35		22	19		27	21		14	22
Esophagus	B7	47	45*	25	ND			NR		
	B12		40*	26						
Hodgkin's disease	B5	411	14*	10	101	11	11	321	17*	11
	B7		21	25		25	23		19*	25
Kidney	A29	79	11	6	45	16*	6	NR		
Larynx	BW21	109	10*	5	38	10	6	NR		
Liver	A29	56	16*	6	ND			NR		
Lung	A29	405	10*	6	180	10	6	250	9	7
Lymphoma	A3	150	18*	27	100	18	26	51	27	24
	A29		11	6		14*	6		12*	7
	BW35		25	19		23	21		35*	22
Lymphosarcoma	A28	63	16*	8	ND			39	26*	12
Ovary	B12	138	16*	26	74	14*	24	69	14	24
Prostate	A1	299	22*	31	96	19*	31	214	21	27
	A28		13*	8		16*	9		14	12
	AW32		4*	7		7	7		5	8
	B8		13*	21		14	21		14	21
	BW22		8*	4		10*	4		6	5
Rectum	A9	88	25	20	ND			55	36	21
Stomach	A10	58	24*	13	ND			63	19	11
	A11		2*	12					6	12

[a]N = 3896
[b]N = 1536
[c]N = 906
[d]ND = Not done
[e]NR = Not reported
[f]Frequencies reported earlier (Takasugi et al., Ref. 2).
*p ≤ 0.05 without correction for the number of comparisons.

attributable to chance alone. The higher A10 frequency in stomach cancer appeared in the earlier study and the overall study along with a parallel lower ALL frequency.

It is of some interest that ALL is associated with B27, AML with BW22, and CML with B7, since these three B locus antigens are strongly crossreacting. The significant first locus antigens in leukemias may be A2 in ALL and AW32 in AML.

DISCUSSION

The general conclusion of our earlier report (6) that HLA is not strongly associated with cancers has been confirmed. Lack of genetic linkage, however, has not been proven. From the data given here, it appears that a linkage may well exist. In the study of a second set of patients and an overall larger group of patients, ALL and prostate cancer appear to show some degree of association with certain antigens which cannot be attributed entirely to chance. Other cancers may have a similar difference, such as the lower HLA-B12 incidence in ovarian cancer.

ALL has been reported previously to be associated with HLA-A2 by Walford, et al. (9), Rogentine et al. (3), and Thorsby et al. (8). There have also been some studies in which this association was not found (1). The finding of the same antigen association in separate studies suggests that the relationship is not a spurious one. However, factors such as the resistance to a disease once it is contracted may be an explanation for these associations (3).

Nasopharynx cancer (NPC) has been reported by Simons to have a high association in Chinese patients with a second locus antigen named Sin 2 (5). This association is the highest reported for a cancer and HLA. It will be important to see if Caucasian NPC patients have this or any other association with HLA. Our studies on the question will be reported elsewhere.

As larger numbers of cancer patients are tested, haplotype analysis will become feasible (7). It is possible that certain haplotypes may be linked to a cancer susceptibility gene. Simple comparisons of single specificities may fail to detect such an underlying difference in haplotypes.

SUMMARY

Frequencies of 25 HLA antigens in 2,005 cancer patients were compared to 1,536 healthy controls who were HLA-typed from 1973 to 1975 and also in a total group of 4,017 cancer patients and 3,896 healthy controls typed from 1970 to 1975. Some specificities were altered from control levels in cancers of the cervix, colon, esophagus, kidney, larynx, liver, lung, ovary, prostate, rectum, stomach, Hodgkin's disease, leukemia, lymphoma, and lymphosarcoma, but none of the differences was statistically significant when corrected for the number of comparisons. The most significant associations, when compared with those obtained in an earlier series, were an increase in HLA-A2 in acute lymphocytic leukemia and lower HLA-A1 and HLA-B8 along with elevated HLA-A28 and HLA-BW22 in prostate cancer.

ACKNOWLEDGMENT

This work was supported in part by contract number N01 CP 43211 within the Virus Cancer Program of the National Cancer Institute.

REFERENCES

1. Lawler, S. D., and Klouda, P. T. (1971): The HL-A system in lymphoblastic leukemia. *Br. J. Haematol.,* 21:595–605.
2. Lynch, H. T., Thomas, R. J., Terasaki, P. I., Ting, A., Guirgis, H. A., Kaplan, A. R., Chaperon, E., Magee, H., Lynch, J., and Kraft, C. (1975): HL-A in cancer "Family N". *Cancer,* 36:1315–1320.
3. Rogentine, G. N., Trapani, R. J., Yankee, R. A., and Henderson, E. S. (1973): HL-A antigens and acute lymphocytic leukemia: The nature of the HL-A2 association. *Tissue Antigens,* 3:470–476.
4. Schlosstein, L., Terasaki, P. I., Bluestone, R., and Pearson, C. M. (1973): High association of an HL-A antigen W27, with ankylosing spondylitis, *N. Engl. J. Med.,* 288:704–705.
5. Simons, M. J., Wee, G. B., Day, N. E., Morris, P. J., Shanmugaratnam, K., and De-The, G. B. (1974): Immunogenetic aspects of nasopharyngeal carcinoma: I. Differences in HL-A antigen profiles between patients and control groups. *Int. J. Cancer,* 13:122–134.
6. Takasugi, M., Terasaki, P. I., Henderson, G., Mickey, M. R., Menk, H., and Thompson, R. W. (1973): HL-A antigens in solid tumors. *Cancer Res.,* 33:648–650.
7. Terasaki, P. I., and Mickey, M. R. (1975): HL-A haplotypes of 32 diseases. *Transplant. Rev.,* 22:105–119.
8. Thorsby, E., Engeset, A., and Lie, S. O. (1971): HL-A antigens and susceptibility to diseases. A study of patients with acute lymphoblastic leukemia, Hodgkin's disease, and childhood asthma. *Tissue Antigens,* 1:147–152.
9. Walford, R. L., Finkelstein, S., Neerhout, R., Konrad, P., and Shanbrom, E. (1970): Acute childhood leukemia in relation to the HL-A human transplantation genes. *Nature,* 225:461–462.

Discussion

Gerald: Have you looked at Wilms' tumor?

Terasaki: No, we have not.

Gerald: The reason for asking is rather tortuous logic: in man, Wilms' tumor is associated with malformations. In mice, teratologic lesions are associated with mutations of the *T* locus, which normally regulates the expression of fetal antigens and is next to the *H2* locus.

Terasaki: We would be interested in pursuing that.

Hirschhorn: Regarding the cancer family in which you found an association to HLA 2,12, I think another explanation besides ascertainment bias is needed. As I remember, Dr. Lynch ascertained the family because of a *few* cancer patients. Then, when the extended pedigree was collected, a massive number of cancers was found.

Terasaki: Not all branches of that family were cancer prone. The branch we looked at had the most 2,12s and the most cancers. Incidentally, it is by chance, I think, that the two families of Lynch and Blattner both have 2,12. In Caucasians, 1,8 is the most common haplotype; 2,12 and 2,7 are next. So, one might expect them to often be linked to cancer.

Blattner: What mechanisms might explain the association you found?

Terasaki: Two speculations come to mind. First, we and others seek a possible homologue to the mouse *IR* and *HLA* loci. The weak association of cancer with HLA, in contrast to, for example, the strong association between W27 and ankylosing spondylitis, might suggest that cancer is a more ancient disease and, through the centuries, more crossovers have occurred, or that a cancer gene locus is farther from the *HLA* loci than the ankylosing spondylitis gene.

Gatti: Since neither parent in the family was homozygous 2,12, I wonder if you checked the mother for antibodies against other paternal antigens, for example, something that might destroy sperm?

Terasaki: No, we have not.

Nebert: Have you looked at healthy, cancer-free 80- to 100-year-old persons to determine what types are *not* associated with cancer.

Terasaki: Yes, we found the same distribution of types among 80- to 90-year-olds as in 20-year-olds, suggesting no special longevity associated with HLA.

Genetics of Human Cancer, edited by J. J.
Mulvihill, R. W. Miller, and J. F. Fraumeni, Jr.
Raven Press, New York, 1977.

29

Role of Immunological Factors in Cancer Susceptibility

Richard A. Gatti

*Division of Pediatric Oncology and Immunology, Cedars-Sinai Medical Center,
Los Angeles, California 90048*

Of the many immunologic aspects of cancer susceptibility, three will be discussed: (1) the association of cancer and oncogenesis with immunodeficiency; (2) the association of cancer with the major histocompatibility locus, H-2, in the mouse; and, (3) new technology that may permit close study of the HLA-D locus in man which is part of the human histocompatibility locus and homologous to H-2 in mouse.

CANCER AND IMMUNODEFICIENCY

My initial introduction to cancer biology came from Dr. Robert A. Good who taught me that many children with primary immunodeficiency disorders were developing cancer. We set out to document this fact and were able to show that there was an incidence of malignancy among the patients with primary immunodeficiency which exceeded that of the general pediatric population by several logs (2). Despite much interpretation on whether or not immunosurveillance relates to tumor formation, these incontrovertible data remain: Immune function bears on oncogenesis.

Our survey (2) initiated the formation of a registry of cancer with primary immunodeficiency which has accumulated many more cases over the past years. In general, if one compares the types of malignancies seen among children with and without primary immunodeficiency (Figs. 1 and 2), one finds that the distribution is quite different. Unlike in the general pediatric population, in children with primary immunodeficiency disease, three quarters of the cancers are lymphoid (Fig. 2). Neuroblastoma, Wilms' tumor, and bone tumors are not seen in the immunodeficient population. If faulty immunosurveillance were the whole story here, one would expect to see the same spectrum of tumors in both groups. Therefore, other pathogenetic mechanisms must exist as well. (It is important to point out that both lymphoma *and* leukemia are seen in the same groups of

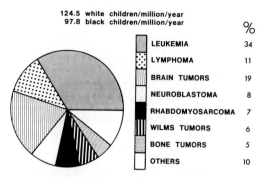

124.5 white children/million/year
97.8 black children/million/year

	%
LEUKEMIA	34
LYMPHOMA	11
BRAIN TUMORS	19
NEUROBLASTOMA	8
RHABDOMYOSARCOMA	7
WILMS TUMORS	6
BONE TUMORS	5
OTHERS	10

FIG. 1. Incidence and distribution of various forms of malignancy in the general pediatric (under 15 years) population of the United States. [Based on Young and Miller, *J. Pediatr.*, 86:254 (1975).]

patients, such as in ataxia telangiectasia (AT) and Wiskott-Aldrich syndrome.)

Among the patients with AT and tumors, there are five families in which more than one sibling with AT has developed cancer (2). In every case, the second sibling has developed the identical type of cancer. In one family, three children developed lymphoma over a 2 year period. In these families, siblings unaffected by AT did not develop cancer.

There are several ways to interpret the above findings. The two most obvious are: (1) a faulty immunosurveillance secondary to the underlying immunodeficiency, and (2) a genetic propensity to cancer and AT via some related genetic defect since, after all, AT is an inherited disorder. Parenthetically, Dr. Good still periodically suggests that the clinical pattern in AT resembles a slow-virus infection.

With regard to the first alternative, we are still far from isolating and identifying the immunological mechanisms responsible for faulty immunosurveillance. For instance, what little is understood about the immunological deficiency in AT is summarized in Fig. 3. In about 60% of the cases, serum IgA is low; there is a variable deficiency of their cell-mediated immunity. At post-mortem examination, the histology of the thymus is characteristically very abnormal. The cell-mediated

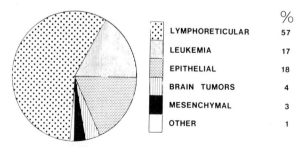

	%
LYMPHORETICULAR	57
LEUKEMIA	17
EPITHELIAL	18
BRAIN TUMORS	4
MESENCHYMAL	3
OTHER	1

FIG. 2. Distribution of various forms of malignancy among patients with primary immunodeficiency disease. [Modified from Kersey, Spector, and Good, *Int. J. Cancer*, 12:333 (1973).]

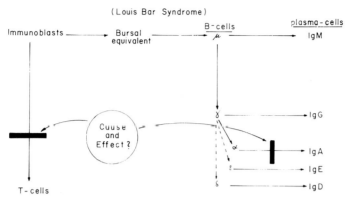

FIG. 3. Immunological defects in AT patients.

disturbance may mediate the humoral deficiencies in this disease, but this is not proven. In short, much more must be learned about the immunodeficiency disorders before they can be meaningfully related to oncogenesis. In particular, many more patients must be studied before and after they develop tumors.

In the late 1960's Todaro and others reported an association of SV-40 transformation of cultured fibroblasts with cancer susceptibility (13). In collaboration with Todaro's laboratory, Kersey and I studied 15 patients with primary immunodeficiency disease and found that all but one were within normal ranges for transformation; the other result was borderline (5). We concluded that by this one parameter, at least, we failed to demonstrate a genetic propensity in patients with immunodeficiency disease.

Any working hypothesis of how oncogenesis occurs must take into account many factors. For example, in some laboratory models leukemia is induced with 100% success by injection of virus-containing preparations while the same viral preparation does not induce leukemia in other mouse strains. Figure 4 is a working model of oncogenesis which, I think, assimilates most of these influences. Briefly, certain genetic backgrounds may predispose the host to certain viruses or other carcinogens; the two, however, must be paired appropriately since certain carcinogens have little or no effect on certain hosts. A target cell is transformed and begins to multiply during which time it may be influenced by hormones, poietins, microenvironments, and other mechanisms of development and differentiation. For example, in AKR mice with lymphoma and leukemia, the thymus apparently plays a major role in the expansion of the malignant population; for, when this organ is removed, the mice do not develop their spontaneous leukemia (8). Similarly, it may be that the pediatric age distribution of acute lymphoid leukemia is related to the stage of development of the thymus so that even the same host, infected with the same virus, but after pubescent involution of the thymus, may no longer be capable of developing the same form of leukemia. At some point in the development of the malignant clone, immunosurveillance most likely plays a role, for when an immunodeficiency exists or a patient is on long-term immunosuppression, certain tumors are manifested with a far greater incidence (2,11).

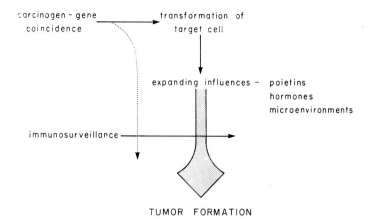

FIG. 4. The multifactorial etiology of tumor formation.

The specific role of immunosurveillance in tumor formation is difficult to analyze further because most carcinogens, including viruses, also act as immuno-suppressants, making it almost impossible to separate the carcinogenic effects of an agent from its possible effects on immunosurveillance. For this reason, the dashed line in Fig. 4 extends from the carcinogen-gene interaction to the line representing the influence of immunosurveillance on tumor formation. I feel that this is a somewhat more comprehensive view of oncogenesis than mentioned elsewhere in this volume.

HISTOCOMPATIBILITY LOCUS AND CANCER IN MICE

Over the past 10 years, the H-2 area (on chromosome 17) of mice has been strongly associated with susceptibility to a number of leukemias and other malig-nancies, including Gross virus-induced leukemia, Friend virus-induced erythroid leukemia, radiation-induced (viral) leukemia, Balb/Tennant virus-induced leu-kemia, Moloney virus-induced leukemia, Bittner virus-induced mammary tumor and vaccinia virus-related neoplasms (6). In each of these situations, however, the susceptibility gene located in the H-2 area is clearly not the only gene affecting oncogenesis. There are other cancer susceptibility genes which are not located in the H-2 area.

The association of leukemogenesis by Gross virus with the H-2 complex has been studied extensively by Lilly and co-workers (7) and was reviewed recently by Klein (6). Figure 5 somewhat oversimplifies this work, but is meant to demonstrate the high incidence of Gross virus-induced leukemia among those mouse strains with H-2^k or H-2^d haplotypes as compared with the low incidence among strains with H-2^b or H-2^j haplotypes. Further, the time onset of symptoms after viral infection is much longer in the resistant strains and correlates inversely and very dramatically with genetic susceptibility; for instance, in C57 B1/6 mice symptoms do not appear until 200 days after infection. Such observations suggest

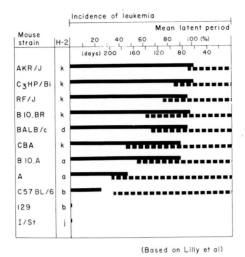

FIG. 5. Association of leukemogenesis by Gross virus with H-2 complex.

that even the Gross leukemia virus is capable of acting as a slow virus in the appropriate host. Other observations in patients with multiple sclerosis (4) and subacute progressive panencephalitis (10) also suggest that the "slow" property of certain viruses is more a property of the host being infected than of the infecting virus. Perhaps some leukemia viruses are also capable of behaving as slow virus under appropriate circumstances.

Exactly where in the H-2 complex the gene for resistance to Gross virus leukemia (Rgv-1) is located is still not completely clear, but it appears to lie near the *k* end of the region as demonstrated below:

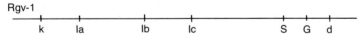

This very same area includes the Ia and immune response (Ir) genes as well as those genes that control responsiveness of lymphocytes in mixed leukocyte culture (MLC) reactions and cell-mediated immune responses (3). In fact, these genes may be so closely related in function that their products may be expressed on the same molecule and that molecule may be one of the many cell surface receptors involved in recognition and response to antigenic stimuli. Thus, it is possible that the Rgv-1 gene for resistance to one form of virally induced leukemia may dictate the formation (or lack thereof) of cell surface receptors which are essential to oncogenesis induced by the Gross virus.

HISTOCOMPATIBILITY AND CANCER IN MAN

The clinical implications of this branch of immunogenetics are most provocative. Balner et al. (1) have demonstrated that Ir genes similar to those of mice and guinea pigs exist in the analogous area in rhesus monkeys. Further, they have shown that monkeys may produce little or much antibody to (TG)AL, a synthetic copolymer of polyalanine and polylysine, and that this trait segregates with the gene controlling responsiveness of the lymphocytes of those animals in MLC. In man, genes controlling immune responsiveness may also be clustered around the major locus which controls lymphocyte responsiveness in MLC. This locus, formerly called MLR, is known as HLA-D by the new nomenclature (14).

Although typing for allelic determinants at HLA-A (LA) and HLA-B (FOUR) loci is relatively easy today and well standardized throughout the world, thanks to periodic histocompatibility workshops, typing at the HLA-D locus has been problematic. The antigenic determinants expressed by HLA-D have not been easily identified by serological means; they must be defined by MLC responsiveness. The classical test that is performed is to use the lymphocytes from individuals known as "typing donors" and known to be homozygous at this locus (each for a different allele) to stimulate the cells of the person being typed. When the responder shares at least one allele with the stimulating (typing) cell, there is little or no response (9). Until recently, the logistics of providing enough stimulator cells for such typing experiments have been difficult.

In 1974, we observed that the lymphoblastoid cell lines (LCL) derived from two typing donors stimulated very much in the same way as did their peripheral lymphocytes (Table 1) (12). Leibold and I have continued to establish such lines from other HLA-D homozygous typing donors from various laboratories world-wide in hopes of creating a panel of stimulating LCL cells that will be useful for HLA-D typing. We now have 35 such cell lines established and growing in our laboratories in Los Angeles and in Hannover, West Germany. All are Epstein-Barr virus transformed lines with cell surface markers characteristic of B lympho-cytes.

The single most important problem with this approach has been dealing with the autologous stimulation observed when using such lines as stimulators in MLC. When obligate heterozygotes of a typing donor were used as responders to the LCL cells of that donor, their response was only as high as the autologous responder. Unrelated responders showed much more vigorous responses (Fig. 6).[1] Thus, our current problem is to find an experimental system in which the level of the low responses is clear without the use of autologous responding cells for each typing line. Of course, as our panel grows, low and high responses to homozy-gous LCL cells with similar D alleles become cumulative.

At present, we are: (1) studying the stimulating and surface characteristics of each newly established typing line; (2) preparing frozen typing plates for family studies (low-volume plates) and for large population surveys (high-volume plates); and (3) defining the normal distribution of the various D alleles in the general population, thereby establishing a baseline for similar studies of cancer patients and their families. On the basis of the animal work outlined above, it is entirely possible that similar

---

[1]With cell line MS-LCL we have encountered occasional exceptions to this rule as can be noted in Table 1. These discordant responders, being analyzed further, might represent the influence of a second MLR locus.

TABLE 1. *Comparison of MLC responses to PBL versus LCL cells*

Responder	Stimulating cells			
	LV-PBLm	LV-LCLm	MS-PBLm	MS-LCLm
HP	−	−	+	+
BP	−	−	+	+
LV	−	−	+	+
KP	−	−		
CP	−	−		
MP	−	−		
BL	−	−	+	−
IE	−	−	+	−
HW	−	−	(−)	−
PG	−	−		
WL	−	−		
IL	+	+		
GP	(+)	(+)	−	−
GD	+	+	(−)	−
RG	+	+	+	+
SF	+	+	+	+
MH	+	+	−	−
RJ			−	−
AS	+	+	+	+
MS	+	+	−	−
ES	+	+	−	−
PS			−	−
BS			−	−
KS			−	−
JS			−	−

PBL = peripheral blood lymphocytes; + =positive MLC response; − = negative MLC response; ( ) = marginal MLC response. Brackets indicate families.

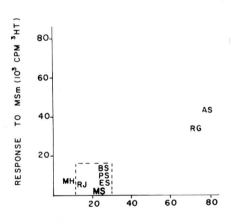

FIG. 6. Graph comparing MLC responses of obligate heterozygotes to responses of autologous donor and histoincompatible unrelateds. Stimulating cells (mitomycin-treated): Fresh lymphocytes from D-locus homozygote, MS; lymphoblastoid cells from same typing donor, MS-B.

cancer susceptibility genes exist in the HLA region of man and may be closely linked or in genetic disequilibrium with HLA-D.

SUMMARY

We have examined the relationship of immunosurveillance to oncogenesis. The available data suggest that immunosurveillance does play some role in oncogenesis of some tumors and that it may be difficult to separate, *in vivo,* the effects of most carcinogens on basic intercellular mechanisms leading to malignant transformation from those effects which produce immunosuppression of the host. Faulty immunosurveillance is probably *not* the sole or even the primary cause of oncogenesis; much more likely is a multifactorial hypothetical model of oncogenesis such as presented here.

Genetics factors leading to cancer susceptibility have been amply defined in many animal systems. One of the prime foci in the search for cancer susceptibility genes has been the major histocompatibility area. Leukemogenesis in mice has been irrefutably linked to the H-2 area. On the other hand, it is equally clear that other genes are also involved in this leukemogenesis which are not associated with the H-2 area. There is good reason to believe that the HLA area in man shares much homology with the major histocompatibility areas of other species. Whereas studies of the HLA-A and -B loci have thus far not revealed any strong association of particular alleles with cancer (see Terasaki, Chapter 28), this homology predicts that such cancer susceptibility genes are more likely to be located in the proximity of HLA-D than near either the HLA-A or -B loci.

A new methodology for defining the HLA-D locus has been initiated in our laboratories. It involves the use of established lymphoblastoid cell lines from D locus homozygous donors as stimulators in mixed leukocyte cultures. A panel of 35 such typing lines has been established and frozen in typing plates. Genetic studies of cancer patients and their families are underway.

ACKNOWLEDGMENT

Part of this work was supported by the Amie Karen Cancer Fund.

REFERENCES

1. Balner, H., Dorf, M. E., de Groot, M. L., and Benacerraf, B. (1973): The histocompatibility complex of Rhesus monkeys: III. Evidence for a major MLR locus and histocompatibility-linked Ir genes. *Transpl. Proc.,* 5:1555–1560.
2. Gatti, R. A., and Good, R. A. (1971): Occurrence of malignancy in immunodeficiency diseases. *Cancer,* 28:89–98.
3. Green, I. (1974): Genetic control of immune responses. *Immunogenetics,* 1:4–21.
4. Jersild, C., Dupont, B., Fog, T., Platz, P. J., and Svejgaard, A. (1975): Histocompatibility determinants in multiple sclerosis. *Transpl. Rev.,* 22:148.
5. Kersey, J. H., Gatti, R. A., Good, R. A., Aaronson, S. A., and Todaro, G. J. (1972): Susceptibility to SV 40 virus transformation of diploid fibroblast strains from immunodeficiency patients. *Proc. Natl. Acad. Sci. USA,* 69:980–982.
6. Klein, J. (1976): Genetic control of virus susceptibility. In: *Biology of the Mouse*

Histocompatibility-2 Complex, pp. 389–410. Springer-Verlag, New York.

7. Lilly, F., Boyse, E. A., and Old, L. J. (1964): Genetic basis of susceptibility to viral leukemogenesis. *Lancet,* 2:1207.

8. McEndy, D. P., Boon, M. C., and Furth, J. (1944): On the role of the thymus, spleen and gonads in the development of leukemia in a high-leukemia stock of mice. *Cancer Res.,* 4:377–383.

9. Mempel, W. L., Grosse-Wilde, H., Baumann, P., Netzel, B., Steinbauer-Rosenthal, I., Scholz, S., Bertrams, J., and Albert, E. D. (1973): Population genetics of the MLC responses: Typing for MLC determinants using homozygous and heterozygous reference cells. *Transpl. Proc.,* 5:1529–1534.

10. Norrby, E. (1973): Subacute sclerosing panencephalitis and measles virus. *Ann. Clin. Res.,* 5:288–292.

11. Penn., I., and Starzl, T. E. (1970): Malignant lymphomas in transplantation patients: A review of the world experience. *Int. J. Clin. Pharm. Therap. Toxicol.,* 3:49–54.

12. Svedmyr, E. A. J., Leibold, W., and Gatti, R. A. (1975): Possible use of established cell lines from MLR locus typing. *Tissue Antigens,* 5:186–195.

13. Todaro, G. J., Green, H., and Swift, M. R. (1966): Susceptibility of human diploid fibroblast strains to transformation by SV 40 virus. *Science* 153:1252–1253.

14. World Health Organization—IUIS Terminology Committee (1976): New nomenclature for the HLA system, 116-573–574, *J. Immunol.*

HLA system. *J. Immunol.,* 116:573–574.

Discussion

Heston: You used the term, "linkage," with reference to the histocompatibility complex. In some cases, what is observed may be the result of linkage but in other cases it is more likely simply an association. For instance, to test the effects of the mammary tumor virus, Mühlbock injected it into lines of C57 black mice that had different histocompatibility genotypes. He then determined whether any of the different histocompatibility types was associated with an increased frequency of tumors. Now what he could detect with this experiment would be an association between two events, but using other experimental designs one could examine the question of true gene linkage.

Gatti: You are more familiar with that literature that I am. You are absolutely right in saying that this type of study will not prove linkage. The primary method used to study linkage is to backcross the F_1 and the F_2 generations. One can use recombinants, but I doubt they were available when that work was done. I thought you were going to comment that in some cases histocompatibility type and tumor production may be the result of the same gene. Indeed, we may be looking directly at the gene, and calling it something else.

Koprowski. In multiple sclerosis, using the technique you have described, 60 to 70% of the patients have been shown to carry the DW-2 allele. It has also been determined that people who have optic neuritis and belong to the DW-2 group are much more likely than others to acquire multiple sclerosis. My questions to you and to people working on multiple sclerosis are: What do we do next? How has this approach advanced our knowledge of the mechanism leading to multiple sclerosis? What techniques and concepts can be developed using these approaches that will enhance our efforts to study the mechanisms leading to human cancer?

Gatti: Dr. Koprowski, as usual, your questions are never very simple. The studies on multiple sclerosis and related diseases indicate that a common viral infection of children (measles) may turn out to be the etiologic agent, but only in individuals who are type 7a. I do not know what we will do next. We may be advancing our knowledge into a cul-de-sac that may take us 100 years to get out of. What I have tried to do here is to bring a new dimension to Koch's postulates. It is well known that the mycobacterium infection leads to tuberculosis, but *only in a few people,* suggesting that host factors also influence the probability of developing an infectious disease. This is now a major issue in the field of arthritis. What do you tell an individual who has a brother with ankylosing spondylitis when you discover that the individual has the B27 antigen? The situation is illustrated by the recent experience which occurred on a destroyer off the coast of California. A banquet was held to celebrate the 10th anniversary of the boat. Two cooks had *Shigella* infection. Of 1,272 seamen in attendance, 605 become infected. It must have been a terrible place to be at that moment. The important point is that several weeks later Reiter's disease developed in nine of the exposed men. Six of the nine men were followed up and five were type B27 [*Ann. Intern. Med.*, 84:564–566, (1976)].

Genetics of Human Cancer, edited by J. J.
Mulvihill, R. W. Miller, and J. F. Fraumeni, Jr.
Raven Press, New York, 1977.

30

Immunodeficiency-Cancer Registry: 1975 Update

Beatrice D. Spector

Department of Laboratory Medicine and Pathology, University of Minnesota, Minneapolis, Minnesota 55455

The Immunodeficiency–Cancer Registry (ICR), established in 1971, has assembled data on over 200 case reports concerning children and adults who developed cancer subsequent to the diagnosis of a primary immunodeficiency disease. The original 80 case reports were collected and published by Gatti and Good in 1971 (1). The ICR has ascertained additional cases through a system of voluntary reporting from medical centers in the United States and abroad and from the literature. Earlier publications from ICR reported the numbers of *tumors,* whereas Table 1 presents a summary of *cases* assigning four patients with a total of eight primary tumors according to the first cancer diagnosed. Other variations from earlier reports arise from larger numbers, and there are continuing efforts to verify the accuracy of reported pathologic and immunologic diagnoses (2,3).

The 205 cases range from seven with IgM deficiency to 70 with ataxia telangiectasia (AT) and represent 26 years of experience; the years of cancer diagnosis range from 1949 to 1975. Grouping the 205 cases by immunodeficiency diagnosis and pathologic diagnosis of the tumor, in order of the proportion of lymphoid tumors seen, displays an unusual constellation of tumors.

In five immune disorders, lymphoreticular tumors (lymphosarcoma, reticulum cell sarcoma, Hodgkin's disease, etc.) predominated (117 cases, 57% of total), whereas the second most common malignancy was leukemia (all types) in some disorders and epithelial neoplasms in others. Leukemia was the most commonly reported tumor in X-linked (Bruton's) agammaglobulinemia, and carcinomas predominated in IgA deficiency. The remaining 13 cases had either nervous system tumors (9 cases, 4% of total) or mesenchymal cancers (4 cases, 2% of total).

Another unusual feature of cancer in these disorders is the distribution of tumors by age and sex (Table 2). The highest incidence of tumors for both sexes occurs in childhood and is composed mainly of lymphoreticular malignancies and

TABLE 1. *Immunodeficiency-Cancer Registry: Summary of cases*

| | Histologic type | | | | | | | | | | |
Primary immunodeficiency disease	Lymphoreticular %	No.	Leukemia %	No.	Epithelial %	No.	Mesenchymal %	No.	Nervous system %	No.	Total cases
IgA deficiency	31	4	—	—	54	7	7.5	1	7.5	1	13
X-linked (Bruton's) agammaglobulinemia	33	4	58	7	—	—	—	—	8	1	12
Variable immunodeficiency	48	28	6	4	41	24	2	1	2	1	58
Severe combined immunodeficiency	55	6	45	5	—	—	—	—	—	—	11
AT	60	42	23	16	13	9	1	1	3	2	70
IgM deficiency	71	5	—	—	14	1	—	—	14	1	7
Wiskott-Aldrich syndrome	82	28	6	2	—	—	3	1	9	3	34
Total	57	117	17	34	20	41	2	4	4	9	205

TABLE 2. Immunodeficiency-Cancer Registry: Distribution of cancers by age and sex (171 cases)

Age (yrs)	Males 0–9	10–14	15–19	20–29	30–39	40–49	50–59	60–74	Total	Females 0–9	10–14	15–19	20–29	30–39	40–49	50–59	60–74	Total
Lymphoreticular	34	14	6	5	3	—	3	1	66	13	6	2	—	1	6	1	3	32
Leukemia	12	5	—	1	—	—	2	—	20	5	1	—	—	—	—	—	1	7
Stomach	—	—	1	1	2	2	4	1	11	—	—	2	1	—	—	3	1	7
Other digestive organs	—	—	—	—	—	—	—	—	—	—	1	1	—	—	1	1	1	5
Lung	—	—	—	—	—	—	1	1	2	—	—	—	—	—	—	1	—	1
Breast	—	—	—	—	—	—	—	—	—	—	—	—	—	1	1	—	—	2
Genitourinary	—	—	—	—	—	—	—	—	—	—	—	2	—	—	1	—	—	3
Nervous system	2	1	—	—	—	—	—	—	3	1	2	—	—	—	—	—	—	3
Skin	—	—	—	1	1	1	—	1	4	1	—	—	—	—	—	—	—	1
Other sites	—	—	—	—	—	—	—	—	—	—	—	1	—	1	—	1	1	4
Totals	48	20	7	8	6	3	10	4	106	20	10	8	1	3	9	7	7	65

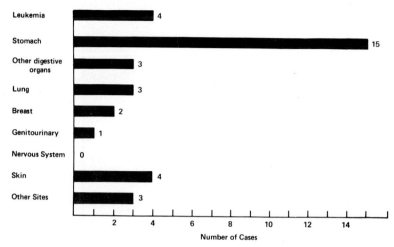

FIG. 1. Nonlymphoreticular tumors in 35 patients over 19 years of age at diagnosis.

leukemias which develop in individuals with immunodeficiencies that have very early ages of onset, e.g., X-linked (Bruton's) agammaglobulinemia, severe combined immunodeficiency, Wiskott–Aldrich syndrome and AT. The high male-to-female ratio, overall 2:1, can be attributed to the X-linked disorders of childhood. Sex becomes a less significant variable beyond childhood.

In adults, lymphoma is the major cancer developing with primary immunodeficiency, but other tumors, particularly stomach carcinomas, also seem excessive. Of 35 cases, 15 are stomach tumors (Fig. 1), occurring chiefly in common variable immunodeficiency and IgA deficiency.

REFERENCES

1. Gatti, R. A., and Good, R. A. (1971): Occurrence of malignancy in immunodeficiency diseases. *Cancer,* 28:89–98.
2. Kersey, J. H., and Spector, B. D. (1975): Immune deficiency diseases. In: *Persons at High Risk of Cancer: An Approach to Cancer Etiology and Control,* edited by J. F. Fraumeni, Jr., pp. 55–67. Academic Press, New York.
3. Kersey, J. H., Spector, B. D., and Good, R. A. (1973): Primary immunodeficiency diseases and cancer: The Immunodeficiency-Cancer Registry. *Int. J. Cancer,* 12:333–347.

Genetics of Human Cancer, edited by J. J. Mulvihill, R. W. Miller, and J. F. Fraumeni, Jr. Raven Press, New York, 1977.

31

Genetic Analysis of Malignancy Using Somatic Cell Hybrids

John D. Minna

NCI-VA Medical Oncology Branch, Veterans Administration Hospital and National Cancer Institute, Washington, D.C. 20422

In its conception and design, the experiment is elegant and appealing; in addition, it probably initiated the era of mammalian hybrid somatic cell genetics. A malignant cell is fused to a nonmalignant cell, and a replicating hybrid cell containing the genes of both parents in a common nucleus is isolated. This hybrid cell is tested for its neoplastic behavior and compared with the parental cells. The testing can be done when a full complement of chromosomes of each parent is present and after chromosomes from either the nonmalignant or malignant parent are preferentially lost. One can ask several questions: Are the neoplastic characteristics heritable, and if so, as dominant or recessive traits? Can they be reexpressed? Are they associated (syntenic) with the presence or absence of particular chromosomes?

CRITIQUE OF PAST WORK

Over the past decade, many people have used this format, and analysis of this literature is perplexing. The properties interpreted as manifestations of "neoplasia" include, of course, tumor formation, but also numerous measures of cell-contact inhibition, other histomorphologic features, and expression of antigens, enzymes, or hormones, among others (Table 1). The biologic meaning of some parameters of "neoplasia" can be questioned, but that is a separate debate. A tacit assumption of most authors is that neoplastic properties of one species will apply to other species including humans. In addition, it is obvious that the majority of the properties studied represent the effects of many structural genes and their regulation. In short, the systems are complex and pleiotropic effects and genetic complexities must be anticipated.

To summarize the results of more than 40 reports (Table 1): Many neoplastic

TABLE 1. *Expression of genes for properties related to neoplasia in hybrid cells formed by matings of the type: Neoplastic property (+) × neoplastic property (–)*

Property	Hybrid phenotype	Refs.
Tumor formation	Tumor	TABLE 4
	No tumor	TABLE 4
	Noncomplementing	41,82,84
	No ascites formation	41
	Strain-specific homotrans-plantability	31
	In vivo hybrid formation	22,46,80
DNA synthesis	Expressed	39,65
Senescence	Hybrids: replicate (? segregation)	MANY
	Heterokaryons: DNA synthesis inhibited with senescent cells	62
	Nuclear, noncytoplasmic	86
Contact inhibition		
Saturation density	High	18,64
	Low	61
Disordered, piled up	Overgrowth	17,18,54,64,77
	No overgrowth	51
Thymidine labeling	Uniform	64
colonies	Uniform and peripheral	51,53
Agar colonies	High cloning efficiency	18
	High and low efficiency	8,9,54
	Microcolonies or low	53,55
Serum dependence	Low	64
In vitro invasiveness	Invasive	10
Histology-morphology		
Lymphocytic	Sarcoma or lymphocytic	43,79
Neuroblastoma	Fibroblast or neuroblastoma	57
Teratocarcinoma	Fibrosarcoma	25,41
Surface morphology	Rough	31
Gap junctions, coupling	Expressed	1,2
Melanoma	Fibroblast	19
Concanavalin A		
Agglutinability	Low	31
	Low, High	56
	Intermediate	10
Sensitivity	Not sensitive	47
Histocompatability antigen		
Expression	Codominant	72
Level of expression	Low, high	40,43
Segregation	Asymmetric	49
Complement-dependent antibody lysis	Resistant, nonresistant	31,66
Tumor-specific antigens	Expressed	12,42,43
	Higher levels	43
Cyclic AMP metabolism		
Catecholamine response	Nonresponsive	35
Prostaglandin response	Responsive	58
Phosphodiesterase	Expressed	58,74
Basal levels	Correlated with tumorigenicity	74
Aryl hydrocarbon		
Hydroxylase: basal	Expressed	7,73,78
Benzo (a) pyrene treatment	Inducible	
LDH B (LDH 1)	Expressed	MANY
Ectopic hormone	?	75

properties studied *in vitro* or *in vivo* are inherited from one mitotic division to the next, in clonal fashion; although many of the neoplastic phenotypes are expressed (dominantly inherited), they are often expressed at low or intermediate levels in the hybrid cells; few of the properties have been related to chromosome segregation or have shown the phenomenon of reexpression.

In addition, most studies have been done with hybrids involving the same rather than different species, which makes chromosome assignment almost impossible. Consequently, few neoplastic properties have been assigned to particular chromosomes. Desirable goals for future work are to study simple properties (e.g., those related to specific enzymes or other molecules), and to use *interspecies* hybrids to facilitate chromosome identification and segregation and for the determination of which species contributes the property under study. The use of normal diploid tissue or primary tumors taken directly from the animal or patient without intervening culture is also to be highly recommended.

STANDARDS FOR CURRENT STUDIES

In reviewing the literature, certain weaknesses recur. To avoid these, minimal requirements for any major study should include:

1. Proof of the hybrid nature of the cells under study.

2. Demonstration, by cloning of parental lines and/or subcloning of hybrids, that heterogeneity of parental cells is not the mechanism responsible for generating hybrids of several phenotypes (e.g., a "malignant" parent strain composed of malignant and nonmalignant cells).

3. Evidence that the observed effects occur only in hybrids and not in mixtures of unfused cells.

4. Evidence that trivial physiologic mechanisms, such as the ability of both hybrid *and* parental cells to grow in selective medium or infection with bacteria or mycoplasma does not explain the results.

5. Documentation of the general chromosome composition of the hybrids (i.e., whether the hybrids represent fusions of genomes equivalent in ploidy or of 2N with 1N cells which are commonly seen in interspecies hybrids) to indicate if gene dosage plays a role.

6. Evidence that the phenomena are reproducible in several hybrids and in independently derived clones, which are reported as being primary or secondary.

7. Proof, by clonal analysis, that the phenomena breed true (i.e., are genetic in nature). In other words, demonstration by subcloning analysis that stable clones can be obtained that segregate the phenotype in a stable fashion and thus are likely to have a chromosomal or episomal basis.

8. Indication of whether or not the stage of the growth cycle can affect the expression of the property under question; if it can, testing of parental and hybrid cells in similar stages.

9. Indication of whether or not the phenotypic changes can be related to chromosome loss or changes in composition. This is necessary because a major

goal of these experiments is the localization to specific chromosome of traits under study.

10. Indication of whether or not the phenomena can be seen in inter- as well as intraspecies hybrids and when several different parental cells, including cells from normal tissue freshly derived from the whole animal, have been used.

11. An effort to assign the phenotype to one of the parental genomes, an opportunity almost exclusively reserved for interspecies hybrids where the homologous gene products can be distinguished by biochemical, electrophoretic or immunologic techniques.

These may seem overly strict requirements; however, the interpretation of many reported studies is in doubt because of deficiencies in these areas. Although these criteria apply largely to *in vitro* studies, most *in vivo* tumor work with hybrid cells suffers similar deficiencies.

RELATION TO VIRAL ONCOLOGY

The metabolism of oncogenic viruses and their effects on neoplastic behavior of cells have also been studied by these techniques (Tables 2 and 3). We have applied the above criteria in examining studies of regulation of RNA tumor virus components in human × rodent hybrid cells. To summarize these results: Human genes are capable of regulating the activity of the virion-associated DNA polymerase (reverse transcriptase); this is seen in many independent hybrids in-

TABLE 2. *Expression of genes for type C virus metabolism in hybrid cells*

RNA tumor virus metabolism		Refs.
Exogenous virus		
Ecotropic, murine	Replicates	32,33,68
Primate (woolly monkey)	Replicates	68
Xenotropic-1	No replication	32,33,68
Xenotropic-2	Replicates	33
Amphotropic	Replicates	33
Murine FV-1 locus	Expressed	32,68
Endogenous virus		
Induction (AKR)	Induces (high frequency)	61a
Induction (BALB)	Noninducible (low frequency)	61a
Focus formation with sarcoma virus rescue (SVR)	Expressed	33,60
Particles capable of SVR	Variable	52
p30 antigen	Expressed	60
Morphologic particles	High	61,87
	Low	61,87
Reverse transcriptase	Low levels	61
	High levels	61
Cell surface antigen	Expressed	28
A-particle antigen	Expressed	59
XC plaque formation	Variable	26
Viral tropism	Variable	27,29

TABLE 3. *Expression of oncogenic DNA virus properties in hybrid cells*

Matings with cells transformed with	Refs.
SV40	
Expressed	
Transformed morphology	17,18,64
Agar cloning (high and reduced)	18,64
Saturation density, high	17,65
Nondensity-dependent DNA synthesis	64
Tumor formation	13
Selective retention of integration site	13,14,15
SV40 T antigen	14,17
SV40 tumor-specific transplantation antigen	13
Low serum growth	64
Functions syntenic	16
Polyoma	
Expressed	
Transformed morphology	54
Agar cloning	54
Transplantation antigen	21,22,55
Complement fixing antigen	21,22,54,55
Tumor formation variable	21,22,34
Functions asyntenic	54
EBV	
Expressed	
EBV nuclear antigen	36,50
EBV superinfection	63
Not expressed	
Antigens: EA, VCA, MA (counter selective)	36,37,38,50
EBV surface receptors, immunoglobulin	50
Variable expression	
IUDR induction: Human X human-positive	38,63,88
Human X mouse-negative	50

volving many different parental human (normal and neoplastic) and rodent cells. Clonal analysis and study of segregation of human gene markers will allow the assignment to several chromosomes of genes which participate in this regulatory activity in mouse L cell × human hybrids and indicate that other chromosomes are involved with the regulation different type C viruses from other rodent cells. Thus, the genetic control of one tumor virus component seems amazingly complex. For this reason, one must be especially cautious in performing and interpreting hybrid cell genetic analysis of malignant behavior.

RELATIONSHIP TO *IN VIVO* TUMOR FORMATION

Considerable controversy arises in interpreting experiments in which hybrids between malignant × nonmalignant cells are used to determine whether malignancy (ability to form tumors) is a dominant or recessive trait. The answer may well be that both types of genes exist. The results of many studies are summarized

TABLE 4. *Tumor formation by somatic cell hybrids*

Mating	Tumors[a] in #clones	Tumors[a] in #animals	Loss of chromosomes in tumors	Refs.
Mouse X mouse	30/45	626/1125	7/8	—[b]
Rat X rat	0/3	0/3	?	2
CH[c] X CH	3/3 (7/13)	101/214	2/2	8,9,56,71
Mouse X CH	1/1	35/35	1/1	5
Mouse X human	5/5	36/45	?	10
Human (SV40) X mouse	?	20/20	Chrom. "7" retained	13
Mouse X rat	3/3	20/21	0/1	53

[a] Independent clones, and appropriate syngenic or immunosuppressed hosts.
[b] See refs: 3,4,6,11,23,24,25,34,39,40,44,45,48,67,70,81,83.
[c] CH: Chinese hamster.

in Table 4. Hybrids before any passage *in vivo* have been either as malignant as the malignant parent, as nontumorogenic as the nonmalignant or low-malignant parent, or have been of intermediate malignancy. These three different outcomes can be seen even in hybrids from the same mating. Of obvious importance in interpreting these tests are:

1. Inter- versus intraspecies matings.
2. The degree of chromosome segregation.
3. The immunologic capability of the host (e.g., adult, young irradiated-reconstituted, or athymic).
4. Expression of antigens by hybrid cells (old or new, and their density).
5. The metabolic state of the hybrid (e.g., whether it was grown in selective medium before transplantation such that substrates present *in vitro* are not present *in vivo*).
6. Microbial infection or expression by the hybrid cells of viruses or bacteria.
7. The normality of nonmalignant lines (e.g., the mouse L cells used in many studies are considered nonmalignant, yet they readily form tumors in nude mice and have many other neoplastic properties, such as cloning in agar and lack of contact inhibition).

Taking all these objections into account, a reasonable summary of results is that, in some cases and for unknown reasons, malignancy is suppressed in fusions of some tumor cells, and may be related in a general way to the chromosome content of the cells. In addition, complementation testing between suppressible tumor lines (malignant × malignant crosses) has given no evidence of complementation (suppression of malignancy). Thus, one would have to postulate that all the recessive defects have some common features. Most suppressions have been seen in intraspecies crosses; only recently has similar evidence been found in interspecies crosses and in these only in rodent × rodent crosses.

Malignancy in SV-40-transformed cells may be a dominant trait. When expression of the malignant phenotype is dominant, this property can be used to selectively retain chromosomes coding for these functions while selectively eliminating those that code for nonmalignant properties. The work of Croce and coworkers with SV-40-transformed cells typifies this approach and indicates that human cells transformed with SV40 and fused to nonmalignant mouse cells selectively retain *in vitro* and *in vivo* human chromosome 7 which presumably carries the SV-40 integration site. Drs. Stuart Brown and Richard Lemons in our laboratory have seen other examples of the selective retention and/or exclusion of certain human chromosomes in human × mouse hybrids. They compared hybrids made with tissue culture mouse RAG cells crossed to fresh human acute myeloblastic leukemia bone marrow with those made in crosses to normal marrow. They isolated hybrids under standard culture conditions which select for rapid, uncontrolled growth. In assays of 19 isozymes, those assigned to human chromosomes 10, 14, and 21 were selectively retained in over 50% of many independent primary clones in RAG × normal marrow and RAG × AML marrow hybrids; and, in addition, isozymes assigned to chromosomes 11, 12, 18, 19 were retained in the RAG × AML hybrids. Thus, in hybrid cells under standard conditions of growth which allow the culture to be taken over by noncontact-inhibited, rapidly growing cells of high plating efficiency, it may be possible to identify the human chromosomes coding for neoplastic properties.

POTENTIAL FOR THE FUTURE

What will hybrid cell methodology be used for in the coming years? Several major areas are:

1. Mapping of specific human genes whose products are dominantly expressed and can be assayed in hybrid cells.
2. Selecting for human chromosomes coding for malignant properties either by growth as tumors in immunosuppressed hosts (e.g., nude mice) or as noncontact-inhibited strains in cultures. The corollary is, of course, the selective elimination of chromosomes carrying genes that code for properties governing ordered, nonmalignant growth.
3. Conducting interspecies assays for the presence of human genes and their products capable of regulating nonhuman oncogenic viruses or tumor viral antigens, or malignant growth behavior.
4. Developing cell lines for immunologic and immunotherapeutic studies. Such hybrids can be used to generate large amounts of material for immunization from clinically accessible biopsy samples. It is likely that patients may be able to respond to human tumor antigens on a predominantly nonhuman background (e.g., in a human–mouse hybrid) where previously they were not able to respond to this antigen.
5. Studying the role of *in vivo* cell hybridization in tumorigenesis or in the development of metastatic and invasive behavior.
6. Complementation testing for malignancy and for characterizing drug resistance in patients.
7. Assaying for the expression of differentiated functions such as polypeptide

hormones that are produced ectopically by tumors when these tumors are used to form hybrids.

SUMMARY

I have tried to indicate the state of the art with respect to analysis of neoplastic properties through hybridization of cells. I have indicated both the potential uses and pitfalls of such techniques and possible direction for future studies. I apologize for any authors slighted or misrepresented and feel the complications of the field should be viewed as a challenge to find the simple, underlying threads in a complex tapestry.

ACKNOWLEDGMENTS

I thank my colleagues whose discussions and work stimulated this paper: Drs. A. Gazdar, R. Lemons, and S. Brown. I thank Dr. T. Shows and L. Lyons for allowing me to quote their unpublished work.

REFERENCES

1. Azarnia, R., Larsen, W. J., and Loewenstein, W. R. (1974): The membrane junctions in communicating and noncommunicating cells, their hybrids, and segregants. *Proc. Natl. Acad. Sci. USA*, 71:880–884.
2. Azarnia, R., and Loewenstein, W. R. (1973): Parallel correction of cancerous growth and of a genetic defect of cell-to-cell communication. *Nature*, 241:455–457.
3. Barski, G., and Cornefet, F. (1962): Characteristics of "Hybrid"-type clonal cell lines obtained from mixed culture *in vitro*. *J. Natl. Cancer Inst.*, 28:801–821.
4. Barski, G. (1970): Expression of malignancy in somatic cell hybrids. *Nature*, 227:67.
5. Barski, G., Blanchard, M. G., Youn, J. K., and Leon, B. (1973): Expression of malignancy in interspecies Chinese hamster × mouse cell hybrids. *J. Natl. Cancer Inst.*, 51:781–792.
6. Belehradek, J. Jr., and Barski, G. (1971): Karyological patterns and expression of malignancy in some homologous mouse somatic hybrid cells. *Int. J. Cancer*, 8:1–9.
7. Benedict, W. F., Nebert, D. W., and Thompson, E. B. (1972): Expression of aryl hydrocarbon hydroxylase induction and suppression of tyrosine aminotransferase induction in somatic-cell hybrids. *Proc. Natl. Acad. Sci. USA*, 69:2179–2183.
8. Berebbi, M., and Meyer, G. (1972): Transformation cellulaire maligne et modifications caryologiques: Apport de l'hybridation somatique de lignées de hamster chinois. *Int. J. Cancer*, 10:418–435.
9. Blanchard, M. G., Barski, G., Leon, B., and Hemon, D. (1973): Expression of tumorigenic potential in isologous hybrid clones of Chinese hamster cells. *Int. J. Cancer*, 11:178–185.
10. Bordelon, M. R., Shows, T. B., Chen, T. R., and Stubblefield. E. (1976): The correlation of *in vivo* malignancy with *in vitro* properties of human-mouse hybrid cells. *J. Natl. Cancer Inst.*, 56:499–507.
11. Bregula, U., Klein, G., and Harris, H. (1971): The analysis of malignancy by cell fusion. *J. Cell Sci.*, 8:673–680.
12. Chen, L., and Watkins, J. F. (1970): *Nature*, 225:734–735.
13. Croce, C. M., Aden, D., and Koprowski, H. (1975): Somatic cell hybrids between mouse peritoneal macrophages and simian-virus-40-transformed human cells: II. Presence of human chromosome 7 carrying simian virus 40 genome in cells of tumors induced by hybrid cells. *Proc. Natl. Acad. Sci. USA*, 72:1397–1400.
14. Croce, C. M., Girardi, A. J., and Koprowski, H. (1973): Assignment of the T-antigen gene of simian virus 40 to human chromosome C-7. *Proc. Natl. Acad. Sci. USA*, 70:3617–3620.

15. Croce, C. M., Huebner, K., Girardi, A. J., and Koprowski, H. (1974): Rescue of defective SV40 from mouse-human hybrid cells containing human chromosome 7. *Virology,* 69:276–281.

16. Croce, C. M., and Koprowski, H. (1974): Concordant segregation of the expression of SV40 T antigen and human chromosome 7 in mouse-human hybrid subclones. *J. Exp. Med.,* 139:1350–1353.

17. Croce, C. M., and Koprowski, H. (1974): Positive control of transformed phenotype in hybrids between SV40-transformed and normal human cells. *Science,* 184:1288–1289.

18. Croce, C. M., and Koprowski, H. (1974): Somatic cell hybrids between mouse peritoneal macrophages and SV40-transformed human cells. I. Positive control of the transformed phenotype by the human chromosome 7 carrying the SV40 genome. *J. Exp. Med.,* 140:1221–1229.

19. Davidson, R. L., Ephrussi, B., and Yamamoto, K. (1966): Regulation of pigment synthesis in mammalian cells, as studied by somatic hybridization. *Proc. Natl. Acad. Sci. USA,* 56:1437–1440.

20. Defendi, V., Ephrussi, B., Koprowski, H., and Yoshida, M. C. (1967): Properties of hybrids between polyoma-transformed and normal mouse cells. *Proc. Natl. Acad. Sci. USA,* 57:299–305.

21. Defendi, V., Ephrussi, B., and Koprowski, H. (1964): Expression of polyoma induced cellular antigen in hybrid cells. *Nature,* 203:495–496.

22. Defendi, V., Ephrussi, B., Koprowski, H., and Yoshida, M. C. (1967): Properties of hybrids between polyoma-transformed and normal mouse cells. *Proc. Natl. Acad. Sci. USA,* 57:299–305.

23. Ephrussi, B., Davidson, R. L., and Weiss, M. C. (1969): Malignancy of somatic cell hybrids. *Nature,* 224:1314–1315.

24. Ephrussi, B. (1972): *Hybridization of somatic cells.* Princeton University Press. Princeton, N.J.

25. Finch, B. W., and Ephrussi, B. (1967): Retention of multiple developmental potentialities by cells of mouse testicular teratocarcinoma during prolonged culture *in vitro* and their extinction upon hybridization with cells of permanent lines. *Proc. Natl. Acad. Sci. USA,* 57:615–621.

26. Fenyo, E. M., and Grundner, G. (1973): Characteristics of murine C-type viruses. I. Independent assortment of infectivity in one *in vivo* and four *in vitro* assays. *Int. J. Cancer,* 12:452–462.

27. Fenyo, E. M., Grundner, G., and Klein, E. (1974): Changes in the properties of the resident L virus in somatic cell hybrid lines. *Exp. Cell Res.,* 87:326–332.

28. Fenyo, E. M., Grundner, G., Wiener, F., Klein, E., Klein, G., and Harris, H. (1973): The influence of the partner cell on the production of L virus and the expression of viral surface antigen in hybrid cells. *J. Exp. Med.,* 137:1240–1255.

29. Fenyo, E. M., Nazerian, K., and Klein, E. (1974): Characteristics of murine C-type viruses. *Virology,* 59:574–579.

30. Fenyo, E. M., Wiener, F., Klein, G., and Harris, H. (1973): Selection of tumor-host cell hybrids from polyoma virus and methylcholanthrene-induced sarcomas. *J. Natl. Cancer Inst.,* 51:1865–1875.

31. Fribert, S. Jr., Klein, G., Wiener, F., and Harris, H. (1973): Hybrid cells derived from fusion of TA3-HA ascites carcinoma with normal fibroblasts. II. Characterization of isoantigenic variant sublines. *J. Natl. Cancer Inst.,* 50:1269–1286.

32. Gazdar, A. D., Russell, E. D., and Minna, J. D. (1974): Replication of mouse-tropic and xenotropic strains of murine leukemia virus in human × mouse hybrid cells. *Proc. Natl. Acad. Sci. USA,* 71:2642–2645.

33. Gazdar, A. F., Russell, E. K., Stull, B., Oie, H., and Minna, J. D. (1976): Cellular control of murine type C virus. *Bibl. Haematol.,* 43:154–157.

34. Gershon, P., and Sachs, L. (1963): Properties of a somatic hybrid between mouse cells with different genotypes. *Nature,* 198:912–913.

35. Gilman, A. G., and Minna, J. D. (1973): Expression of genes for metabolism of adenosine 3',5'-cyclic monophosphate in somatic cells. I. Responses to catecholamines in parental and hybrid cells. *J. Biol. Chem.,* 248:6610–6617.

36. Glaser, R., and Nonoyama, M. (1973): Epstein–Barr virus: Detection of genome in somatic cell hybrids of Burkitt lymphoblastoid cells. *Science,* 179:492.

37. Glaser, R., and O'Neill, F. J. (1972): Hybridization of Burkitt lymphoblastoid cells. *Science,* 176:1245.

38. Glaser, R., Rapp, F. (1972): Rescue of Epstein–Barr virus from somatic cell hybrids of Burkitt lymphoblastoid cells. *J. Virol.,* 10:288.

39. Harris, H. (1970): *Cell Fusion.* Harvard Univ. Press, Cambridge, Mass.

40. Harris, H., Miller, O. J., Klein, G., Worst, P., and Tachibana, T. (1969): Suppression of malignancy by cell fusion. *Nature,* 223:363–368.

41. Jami, J., Failly, C., and Ritz, E. (1973): Lack of expression of differentiation in mouse teratoma-fibroblast somatic cell hybrids. *Exp. Cell Res.*, 76:191–199.
42. Jami, J., and Ritz, E. (1973): Expression of tumor-specific antigens in mouse somatic cell hybrids. *Cancer Res.*, 33:2524–2528.
43. Jami, J., and Ritz, E. (1975): Tumor-associated transplantation antigens in immune rejection of mouse malignant cell hybrids. *Proc. Natl. Acad. Sci. USA*, 72:2130–2134.
44. Jami, J., and Ritz, E. (1973): Nonmalignancy of hybrids derived from two mouse malignant cells. I. Hybrids between L1210 leukemia cells and malignant L cells. *J. Natl. Cancer Inst.* 51:1647–1653.
45. Jami, J., and Ritz, E. (1975): Nonmalignancy of hybrids derived from two mouse malignant cells. II. Analysis of malignancy of LM (TK-) CL ID parental cells. *J. Natl. Cancer Inst.*, 54:117–122.
46. Janzen, H. W., Millman, P. A., and Thurston, O. G. (1971): Hybrid cells in solid tumors. *Cancer*, 27:455–459.
47. Kao, F. T., and Harris, H. (1975): Lack of correlation between malignancy and sensitivity to killing by concanavalin A. *J. Natl. Cancer Inst.*, 54:767–768.
48. Klein, G., Bregula, U., and Wiener, F. (1971): The analysis of malignancy by cell fusion. I. Hybrids between tumour cells and L cell derivatives. *J. Cell Sci.*, 8:659–672.
49. Klein, G., Friberg, S. Jr., Wiener, F., and Harris, H. (1973): Hybrid cells derived from fusion of TA3—HA ascites carcinoma with normal fibroblasts. I. Malignancy, karyotype, and formation of isoantigenic variants. *J. Natl. Cancer Inst.*, 50:1259–1268.
50. Klein, G., Wiener, F., Zech, L., Zur, H. H., and Reedman, B. (1974): Segregation of the EBV-determined nuclear antigen (EBNA) in somatic cell hybrids derived from the fusion of a mouse fibroblast and a human Burkitt lymphoma line. *Int. J. Cancer*, 14:54–64.
51. Levisohn, S. R., and Thompson, E. B. (1973): *J. Cell Physiol.*, 81:225–232.
52. Long, C., Kelloff, G., and Gilden, R. V. (1972): Variations in sarcoma and leukemia virus activity in somatic cell hybrids. *Int. J. Cancer*, 10:310–319.
53. Lyons, L. B., and Thompson, E. B. (1976): Reduced malignancy and altered growth properties of somatic cell hybrids between rat hepatoma and mouse L-cells *(in preparation)*.
54. Marin, G. (1971): Segregation of morphological revertants in polyoma-transformed hybrid clones of hamster fibroblasts. *J. Cell Sci.*, 9:61–69.
55. Meyer, G., Berebbi, M., and Klein, G. (1974): Expression of polyoma-induced antigens in low malignant hybrids derived from fusion of a polyoma-induced tumour with a fibroblast line. *Nature*, 249:47–49.
56. Micco, D., and Berebbi, M. (1972): Tumorigenicity and agglutination by concanavalin A of Chinese hamster cells and their hybrids. *Int. J. Cancer*, 10:249–253.
57. Minna, J. D., Glazer, D., and Nirenberg, M. (1972): Genetic dissection of neural properties using somatic cell hybrids. *Nature*, 235:225–231.
58. Minna, J. D., and Gilman, A. G. (1973): Expression of genes for metabolism of adenosine $3',5'$-cyclic monophosphate in somatic cells. II. Effects of prostaglandin E1 and theophylline of parental and hybrid cells. *J. Biol. Chem.*, 248:6618–6625.
59. Minna, J. D., Kueders, K. K., and Kuff, E. L. (1974): Expression of genes for intracisternal A-particle antigen in somatic cell hybrids. *J. Natl. Cancer Inst.*, 52:1211–1217.
60. Minna, J. D., Gazdar, A. F., Iverson, G. M., Marshall, T. H., Strombert, K., and Wilson, S. H. (1974): Oncornavirus expression in human × mouse hybrid cells segregating mouse chromosomes. *Proc. Natl. Acad. Sci. USA*, 71:1695–1700.
61. Minna, J. D., Marshall, T., Burk, R., Lemons, R., Brown, S., and Wilson, S. (1976): On the somatic cell genetics of type C virus: Regulation of viral DNA polymerase in human × rodent hybrid cells *(in preparation)*.
61a. Minna, J. D., and Gazdar, A. F. (1976): *In preparation*.
62. Norwjod, T. H., Pendergrass, W. R., Sprague, C. A., and Martin, G. M. (1974): Dominance of the senescent phenotype in heterokaryons between replicative and post-replicative human fibroblast-like cells. *Proc. Natl. Acad. Sci. USA*, 71:2231–2235.
63. Nyormoi, O., Klein, G., Adams, A., and Dombos, L. (1973): Sensitivity to EBV superinfection and IUDR inducibility of hybrid cells formed between a sensitive and a relatively resistant Burkitt lymphoma cell line. *Int. J. Cancer*, 12:398–418.
64. Ozer, H. (1975): Personal communication.
65. Rao, P. N., and Johnson, R. T. (1970): Mammalian cell fusion. I. Studies on the regulation of DNA synthesis and mitosis. *Nature*, 225:159–164.

66. Rubio, N. (1974): Surface H-2 antigen concentration requirement of somatic hybrid cells for IgM-mediated cytotoxicity. *Nature,* 249:461–463.
67. Scaletta, L. J., and Ephrussi, B. (1965): Hybridization of normal and neoplastic cells *in vitro. Nature,* 205:1169.
68. Scolnick, E. M., and Parks, W. P. (1974): Host range studies on xenotropic type C viruses in somatic cell hybrids. *Virology,* 59:168–178.
69. Schneider, J. R., and Weiss, M. C. (1971): Expression of differentiated functions in hepatoma cell hybrids. I. Tyrosine aminotransferase in hepatoma-fibroblast hybrids. *Proc. Natl. Acad. Sci. USA,* 68:127–131.
70. Silagi, S. (1967): Hybridization of a malignant melanoma cell line with L cells *in vitro. Cancer Res.,* 27:1953–1600.
71. Sobel, J. S., Albrecht, A. M., Riehm, H., and Biedler, J. L. (1971): Hybridization of actinomycin D- and amethopterin-resistant Chinese hamster cells *in vitro. Cancer Res.,* 31:297–307.
72. Spencer, R. A., Hauschka, T. S., Amos, D. B., and Ephrussi, B. (1964): Co-dominance of isoantigens in somatic cells grown *in vitro. J. Natl. Cancer Inst.,* 33:893–903.
73. Thompson, E. B., Benedict, W. F., Owens, I. S., and Nebert, D. W. (1974): Aryl hydrocarbon hydroxylase and tyrosine aminotransferase activities in somatic cell hybrids derived from hepatoma tissue culture HTC (Rat) cells and 3T3 (Mouse) benzo[a]pyrene-resistant cells. *Biochem. Biophys. Res. Commun.* 56:605–616.
74. Tisdale, M. J., and Phillips, B. J. (1974): Apparent correlation between adenosine 3':5' cyclic monophosphate levels and malignancy in somatic cell hybrids. *Exp. Cell Res.,* 88:111–120.
75. Warner, T. F. C. S. (1974): Cell hybridisation in the genesis of ectopic hormone-secreting tumours. *Lancet,* 1:1259–1260.
76. Watkins, J. F., and Chen, L. (1969): *Nature,* 223:1018–1022.
77. Weiss, M. C., Todaro, G. J., and Green, H. (1967): Properties of a hybrid between lines sensitive and insensitive to contact inhibition of cell division. *J. Cell Physiol.,* 71:105–107.
78. Wiebel, F. J., Gelboin, H. V., and Coon, H. G. (1972): *Proc. Natl. Acad. Sci. USA,* 69:3580–3584.
79. Wiener, F., Cochran, A., Klein, G., and Harris, H. (1972): Genetic determinants of morphological differentiation in hybrid tumors. *J. Natl. Cancer Inst.,* 48:465–468.
80. Wiener, F., Fenyo, E. M., and Klein, G. (1974): Tumor-host cell hybrids in radiochimeras. *Proc. Natl. Acad. Sci. USA,* 71:148–152.
81. Wiener, F., Klein, G., and Harris, H. (1971): The analysis of malignancy by cell fusion. *J. Cell Sci.,* 8:681–692.
82. Weiner, F., Klein, G., and Harris, H. (1973): The analysis of malignancy by cell fusion IV. Hybrid between tumour cells and a malignant L cell derivative. *J. Cell Sci.,* 12:253–261.
83. Wiener, F., Klein, G., and Harris, H. (1974): The analysis of malignancy by cell fusion. V. Further evidence of the ability of normal diploid cells to suppress malignancy. *J. Cell Sci.,* 15:177–183.
84. Weiner, F., Klein, G., and Harris, H. (1974): The analysis of malignancy by cell fusion. VI. Hybrids between different tumour cells. *J. Cell Sci.,* 16:189–198.
85. Wiblin, C. N., and McPherson, I. (1973): *Int. J. Cancer,* 12:148–161.
86. Wright, W. E., and Hayflick, L. (1975): Contributions of cytoplasmic factors to *in vitro* cellular senescence. *Fed. Proc.,* 34:76–79.
87. Yotsuyanagi, Y., and Ephrussi, B. (1974): Behavior of three types of ribovirus-like particles in segregating hamster × mouse somatic hybrids. *Proc. Natl. Acad. Sci. USA,* 71:4575–4587.
88. Zimmerman, J. E. Jr., Glaser, R., and Rapp, F. (1973): Effect of dibutyryl cyclic AMP on the induction of Epstein–Barr virus in hybrid cells. *J. Virol.,* 12:1442–1445.

Note added in proof:

The reader's attention is drawn to several recent articles of interest: Suppression of malignancy in human cells by E. Stanbridge (*Nature,* 260:17–20, 1976); *In vitro* derived mouse A9 cell clones differing in malignancy: Analysis by somatic cell hybridization with YACIR lymphoma cell clones by G. B. Clements, E. M. Fenyo, and G. Klein *(Proc. Natl. Acad. Sci. USA,* 73:2004–2007, 1976); Release by human chromosome 3 of the block at G1 of the cell cycle, in hybrids between ts AF8 hamster and human cells by P. L. Ming, H. L. Chang, and R. Baserga *(Proc. Natl. Acad. Sci. USA,* 73:2052–2055, 1976).

Genetics of Human Cancer, edited by J. J. Mulvihill, R. W. Miller, and J. F. Fraumeni, Jr. Raven Press, New York, 1977.

32

Human Diseases with *In Vitro* Manifestations of Altered Repair and Replication of DNA

J. E. Cleaver

Laboratory of Radiobiology, University of California, San Francisco, California 94143

A large number of human cancers are known to have a hereditary factor. Among these conditions, several have been reported as having defects associated with repair or replication of DNA. Although some reports are merely anecdotal and have not been generally confirmed, others appear to have identified defects of repair and replication that are genuinely associated with the disease. The best established example is xeroderma pigmentosum (XP), which is in most cases associated with defects of excision repair of damaged bases in DNA (3,4,7, 37,38). Information now available on XP and other diseases warrants consideration to ascertain the relevance of repair and replication defects to general theories of carcinogenesis.

DNA REPAIR MECHANISMS

Three main kinds of DNA repair processes are known: photoreactivation, excision repair, and postreplication repair (6).

Photoreactivation

This repair system is specific for ultraviolet (UV)-induced damage in DNA (pyrimidine dimers) and consists of a single enzyme (DNA photolyase) that binds to dimers and, in the presence of visible light, monomerizes them without removing any material from DNA (9,10). This repair system functions in embryonic birds and placental mammals; but in human cells, the question of the presence and function of DNA photolyase is controversial. An enzyme with properties of a DNA photolyase, active on purified dimer-containing DNA, has been identified in extracts of human cells (42,43). But DNA photolyase does not appear to function *in vivo* to any major or easily identifiable extent (2,8,9);

therefore, its presence in cell extracts may represent a vestigial function of an enzyme with a different role *in vivo*.

Excision Repair

This is a versatile repair system by which DNA damage is excised and a replacement patch synthesized (6). For base damage the repair system involves sequential operation of an endonuclease, or an *N*-glycosidase plus endonuclease, followed by an exonuclease, polymerase, and ligase. For broken strands of DNA the repair system involves excising or modifying enzymes to convert the breaks to 3′ and 5′ termini and the subsequent action of polymerase and ligase.

Repair of crosslinked DNA is more complex, but may involve two sequential excision-repair events, one on each strand. In eukaryotic cells where DNA is part of a compact nucleoprotein structure, repair of DNA may also involve numerous enzymes or cofactors that modify protein-DNA binding and render damaged bases accessible to the endonucleases, etc., of the excision-repair system (31).

Postreplication Repair

This is a complex modification of normal DNA replication in which newly synthesized strands of DNA have gaps opposite damaged sites on the parental strands when replication occurs within the first few hours after irradiation. Subsequently, the gaps are filled in by a process involving mainly *de novo* synthesis (21,22,29), and a small amount of strand exchange between parental and daughter strands (30). A number of induced enzymes may also be involved in this process. Postreplication repair is unique among repair processes in being strongly inhibited by high concentrations of caffeine or theophylline (22). Although the mechanism of this inhibition is unknown, many early models fail to take into account the rapid intracellular degradation of caffeine (16), and the mechanisms may involve complex feedback inhibition from degradation products on the purine pathway.

Association of these repair processes with some hereditary human diseases appears clearly established for XP, but several other promising examples have been recently reported which are worth critical evaluation.

REPAIR-DEFICIENT DISEASES

XP and the de Sanctis Cacchione Syndrome

The clinical features of this disease are an extreme sensitivity to sunlight exhibited in the form of erythema, abnormal pigmentation, and a high incidence of sunlight-induced skin cancers of all cell types. Two main clinical forms are recognized: The common form of XP in which there are only skin symptoms, and a neurological form in which there can be a wide range of additional neurological abnormalities. The extreme of the neurological form, the de Sanctis Cacchione syndrome (12,35,37), shows choreoathetosis, sensoneural deafness, sexual dysfunction, and mental retardation. The common and neurological forms are genetically distinct and both are autosomal recessive (7,28,37). The disease has now been successfully diagnosed *in utero* (34).

The cellular characteristics of XP have been more extensively studied than those of any other disease with defects in repair or radiation responses. When exposed to UV light, most XP cells are more sensitive than normal cells to killing (Table 1), chromosome aberration production and mutagenesis (7,24,25,39). The frequency of sister chromatid exchanges in undamaged XP cells is the same as in normal cells, but is higher than normal cells following exposure to monofunctional alkylating agents and 4-nitroquinoline-l-oxide (47).

Two broad classifications made on the basis of clinical symptoms can be further subdivided on the basis of biochemical observations. Among common XP patients a small group can be distinguished known as the XP variants which are biochemically quite different from any other XP cases. The variants have normal excision-repair of UV damage but an abnormally slow postreplication repair system. Variant cells are only slightly more sensitive to killing by UV light than normal cells (Table 1), but killing is enhanced greatly by incubation in caffeine after irradiation (1,26). All other common and neurological forms of XP are defective to various degrees in excision-repair of UV damage. Five mutually complementing groups can be classified on the basis of *in vitro* cell hybridization (Table 2) (37), but there is no certainty that this list is exhaustive or that the properties which thus far characterize each group will be found to apply universally.

The biochemical defect in excision-repair-defective XP cells has been inferred as the UV endonuclease which initiates excision of UV-induced pyrimidine dimers from DNA. The existence of five complementation groups defining one enzymatic step has not been satisfactorily interpreted, but may indicate (a) that there are multiple subunits for the human UV endonuclease, or (b) that a number of cofactors are required for repairing chromatin, or (c) that the process of cell hybridization alters gene expression such that complementation *in vitro* is not a simple indicator of the number of different gene loci involved.

TABLE 1. *Survival curve parameters for fibroblasts from various human diseases*

Disease	Extrapolation number	D_{37}(J/m^2 or rads)
Normal (1,6,7,25,26)	1.6	5.5 J/m^2
XP (excision-defective, group A) (1,6,7,25)	1	0.5 J/m^2
XP variant (1,6,25,26)	1–1.5	4.4–5.5 J/m^2
Cockayne's syndrome (41)	1	2.0 J/m^2
Normal (45)	1	120–170 rad
AT (45)	1	50–60 rad

TABLE 2. *Summary of properties of excision repair and postreplication repair defective XP cells*

Disease	Skin	CNS	Complemen-tation group	Excision repair (% of normal)
XP (de Sanctis Cacchione)	+	+	A	2-5
XP + Cockayne's syndrome [a]	+	+	B	3-7
XP	+	−	C	5-20
XP	+	+	D	25-50
XP	+	−	E	40-50
XP variant	+	−		100

[a] Patient shows symptoms of both diseases.
From refs. 7-37.

Recent experiments have been able to restore normal levels of dimer excision (11) and unscheduled synthesis (44) by adding the UV repair endonuclease from T4-infected *E. coli* (endo V) to XP cells. These results show that all repair steps subsequent to endonucleolytic cleavage near pyrimidine dimers are normal in all XP complementation groups; however, the converse is not necessarily true —namely, that a human UV endonuclease is absent from XP cells. Experiments based on the ability of XP cell extracts to excise pyrimidine dimers from pure DNA *in vitro* indicate that XP groups A and C do contain functional UV endonuclease (31), but lack some factor(s) that are required to excise dimers from chromatin. The initial steps of DNA repair in man may, therefore, be considerably complicated in contrast to microorganisms because of the structure of eukaryotic chromatin.

Ataxia Telangiectasia (AT)

The main features of this disease are progressive cerebellar ataxia, telangiectases of skin and conjunctiva, proneness to sinopulmonary infection, immunological deficiencies, and a tendency to develop lymphatic malignancy. Some patients are hypersensitive to conventional doses of radiation therapy. Inheritance is autosomal recessive (28).

Cellular characteristics include multiple chromosome aberrations in lymphocytes and fibroblasts, and increased sensitivity to cell killing by X rays (Table 1) (15,27,45). Fibroblasts can perform excision repair of UV damage to a normal extent (3,5) and rejoin single-strand breaks made by X rays normally (45), but excise X-ray-damaged bases slower than normal (32). The biochemical defect associated with the clinical features and X-ray sensitivity may therefore involve a defect in X-ray repair.

Bloom's Syndrome

The main features of this disease are low birth weight, sensitivity to sunlight, characteristic facial features including a prominent nose, hypoplastic malar areas and retruded mandible, and a high risk for acute leukemia. Inheritance is autosomal recessive (28).

Cellular characteristics include multiple chromosome aberrations in lymphocytes and fibroblasts, the most specific being quadriradials (15), and a very high incidence of sister chromatid exchanges (1). Fibroblasts perform excision repair of UV damage normally (5), and appear to have a slightly reduced DNA chain growth rate (17). The biochemical defect in this disease has yet to be clearly identified.

Cockayne's Syndrome

The main features of this disease are dwarfism, premature senility, retinal pigment degeneration, optic atrophy, deafness, mental retardation, and sensitivity to sunlight. Inheritance is autosomal recessive (28).

Cellular characteristics include normal sensitivity to X rays but increased sensitivity to ultraviolet light (Table 1). A suggestion has been made that these cases show a decrease in the ability of cells to perform excision repair of UV-damaged DNA (41) and symptoms of Cockayne's syndrome are found in the one XP patient that constitutes complementation group B (37) (Table 2).

Fanconi's Anemia

The main features of this disease are hypoplasia of all blood elements, pigmentary changes in the skin, malformation of the heart, kidney and extremities, and a tendency to develop acute leukemia and certain kinds of solid tumors. Inheritance is autosomal recessive, and heterozygotes may also show a higher than normal incidence of malignancy (28).

Cellular characteristics include a high frequency of spontaneous chromosome aberrations, and after exposure to DNA-crosslinking agents, the frequency of chromosome aberrations is high (39) while that of sister chromatid exchanges is low (20). There may also be a slight defect in excision repair of UV damage resulting in a failure of cells to rejoin excision-related breaks, but evidence supporting this is poor (33). A disease with similar clinical symptoms, dyskeratosis congenita, shows normal repair of UV damage (5).

Progeria (Hutchinson-Gilford's Syndrome)

The main features of this disease are a striking degree of premature senility and patients often die of coronary artery disease before the age of 10. Patients show facial features of extremely rapid senility, small stature, almost complete absence of subcutaneous fat, and arteriosclerotic blood vessels. The disease is too rare to allow its mode of inheritance to be established (28).

Cellular characteristics include a normal ability to perform excision repair of UV damage (5), and increased sensitivity to X rays (13). Under some culture conditions, cells have a reduced ability to rejoin X-ray-induced DNA breaks and show premature aging *in vitro* (13,14,36), but clear demonstration of repair defects has been controversial.

Chronic Lymphocytic Leukemia

This disease, although not clearly established as an inherited disorder, does have a tendency for familial clustering.

Cellular characteristics include refractoriness to mitogens, an increased ability to perform excision-repair of UV damage to DNA (18), and the presence of high levels of a DNA binding protein (19). Whether or not these cellular properties are a definite feature of the disease or merely adventitious has not been established.

Solar Actinic Keratosis

This disease occurs in middle life in fair-skinned people exposed to chronic sunlight. Multiple keratotic and malignant lesions develop on sun-exposed areas even after the patients are removed from the sun. There is a tendency for clustering of the disease due to hereditary factors, race, life-style, and perhaps other causes (28).

Cellular characteristics include one report that fibroblasts developed from the keratotic regions of a patient performed more excision repair of UV damage than fibroblasts from other parts of the skin (Pitts, University of Glasgow, *personal communication*). This and other diseases associated with familial susceptibility to UV-induced skin cancer are worth further investigation.

SOME IMPLICATIONS OF REPAIR DEFICIENCIES

Probably only for XP is there a ready interpretation of the relationships between biochemical and clinical observations. In most other diseases the involvement of repair defects is not clearly established by experiments done in different laboratories and XP is probably the only disease for which the involvement of repair defects can be regarded as confirmed. AT and Cockayne's syndrome do, however, appear to be the most promising diseases of current interest with putative association between repair defects and clinical symptoms. The immunological disorders in AT may point to some role of DNA repair in the immune response (15,27,28).

XP is a striking illustration of a mutational theory of carcinogenesis, in which malignancy is induced by defective repair of UV-induced damage in cells of the skin. As such, it can be used as a model of other kinds of cancers induced by environmental DNA-damaging agents. But it is interesting to note that XP does not lend any support to theories of aging involving DNA damage and repair because the clinical symptoms and cellular characteristics of XP represent normal rates of aging.

If XP and other recessive genes associated with DNA repair also have small effects in the heterozygous state, it is conceivable that many more examples of carcinogenesis in man than those described here may be influenced by repair genes. The evaluation of these possible contributiors in the induction of human cancer, and, in particular, the confirmation or refutation of the involvement of DNA repair defects in many cancer-associated diseases would seem to be especially important in this field of cancer research.

ACKNOWLEDGMENTS

This brief summary has drawn upon a large amount of unpublished material and I am grateful to all those who made their material available to me. Work was supported by the United States Energy Research and Development Administration.

REFERENCES

1. Arlett, C. F., Harcourt, S. A., and Broughton, B. C. (1975): *Mutat. Res.,* 33:341–346.
1a. Chaganti, R. S. K., Schonberg, S., and German, J. (1974): A manyfold increase in sister chromatid exchanges in Bloom's syndrome lymphocytes. *Proc. Natl. Acad. Sci. USA,* 71:4508–4512.
2. Cleaver, J. E. (1966): Photoreactivation: A radiation repair mechanism absent from mammalian cells. *Biochem. Biophys. Res. Commun.,* 24:569–576.
3. Cleaver, J. E. (1968): Defective repair replication of DNA in xeroderma pigmentosum. *Nature,* 218:652–656.
4. Cleaver, J. E. (1969): Xeroderma pigmentosum: A human disease in which an initial stage of DNA repair is defective. *Proc. Natl. Acad. Sci. USA,* 63:428–435.
5. Cleaver, J. E. (1970): DNA damage and repair in light-sensitive human skin disease. *J. Invest. Dermatol.,* 54:181–195.
6. Cleaver, J. E. (1974): Repair processes for photochemical damage in mammalian cells. In: *Advances in Radiation Biology,* Vol. 4, edited by J. T. Lett, H. Adler, and M. Zelle, pp. 1–75. Academic Press, New York.
7. Cleaver, J. E., and Bootsma, D. (1975): Xeroderma pigmentosum: Biochemical and genetic characteristics. *Ann. Rev. Genet.,* 9:19–38.
8. Cleaver, J. E., Paterson, M., and Friedberg, E. C. (1976): Absence of photoenzymatic monomerization of pyrimidine dimers in normal and xeroderma pigmentosum cells. *Biophys. J.,* 16:185a.
9. Cook, J. S. (1972): Photoenzymatic repair in animal cells. In: *Molecular and Cellular Repair Processes,* edited by R. F. Beers, Jr., R. M. Herriott, and R. C. Tilghman, pp. 79–103. The Johns Hopkins Univ. Press, Baltimore, Md.
10. Cook, J. S., and McGrath, J. R. (1967): Photoreactivating-enzyme activity in Metazoa. *Proc. Natl. Acad. Sci. USA,* 58:1359–1364.
11. Cook, K., Friedberg, E. C., and Cleaver, J. E. (1975): Excision of thymine dimers from specifically incised DNA by extracts of xeroderma pigmentosum cells. *Nature,* 256:235–236.
12. deSanctis, C., and Cacchione, A. (1932): L'idiozia xerodermica. *Riv. Sper. Freniat.,* 56:269–274.
13. Epstein, J., Williams, J. R., and Little, J. B. (1973): Deficient DNA repair in human progeroid cells. *Proc. Natl. Acad. Sci. USA,* 70:977–981.

14. Epstein, J., Williams, J. R., and Little, J. B. (1974): Rate of DNA repair in progeric and normal human fibroblasts. *Biochem. Biophys. Res. Commun.*, 59:850–857.
15. German, J. (1972): Genes which increase chromosomal instability in somatic cells and predispose to cancer. *Progr. Med. Genetics*, 8:61–101.
16. Goth, R., and Cleaver, J. E. (1976): Metabolism of caffeine to nucleic acid precursors in mammalian cells. *Mutat. Res.*, 36:105–114.
17. Hand, R., and German, J. (1975): A retarded rate of DNA chain growth in Bloom's syndrome. *Proc. Natl. Acad. Sci. USA*, 72:758–762.
18. Huang, A. T., Kremer, W. B., Laszlo, J., and Setlow, R. B. (1972): DNA repair in human leukaemic lymphocytes. *Nature [New Biol.]*, 240:114–116.
19. Huang, A. T., Riddle, M. M., and Koons, L. S. (1975): Some properties of a DNA-unwinding protein unique to lymphocytes from chronic lymphocytic leukemia. *Cancer Res.*, 35:981–986.
20. Latt, S. A., Stetten, G., Juergens, L. A., Buchanan, G. R., and Gerald, P. S. (1975): Induction by alkylating agents of sister chromatid exchanges and chromatid breaks in Fanconi's anemia. *Proc. Natl. Acad. Sci. USA*, 72:4066–4070.
21. Lehmann, A. R. (1972): Post-replication repair of DNA in ultraviolet-irradiated mammalian cells. *J. Mol. Biol.*, 66:319–337.
22. Lehmann, A. R., Kirk-Bell, S., Arlett, C. F., Paterson, M. C., Lohman, P. H. M., de Weerd-Kastelein, E. A., and Bootsma, D. (1975): Xeroderma pigmentosum cells with normal levels of excision repair have a defect in DNA synthesis after UV-irradiation. *Proc. Natl. Acad. Sci. USA*, 72:219–223.
23. Lehmann, A. R., and Arlett, C. (1976): Survival of UV-irradiated xeroderma pigmentosum cells grown in caffeine. *Proc. Natl. Acad. Sci. USA (in press)*.
24. Maher, V. M., Mischke, B. S., and McCormick, J. J. (1976): Effect of DNA repair on the frequency of mutations induced in normal human skin fibroblasts and in strains of xeroderma pigmentosum by ultraviolet irradiation. *Proc. Natl. Acad. Sci. USA (in press)*.
25. Maher, V. M., and McCormick, J. J. (1975): Effect of DNA repair on the cytotoxicity and on the frequency of mutations induced in normal human skin fibroblasts and in strains of xeroderma pigmentosum by ultraviolet irradiation and by chemical carcinogens. In: *International Symposium. Protein and Other Adducts to DNA: Their Significance to Aging, Carcinogenesis, and Radiation Biology*. (Abstr.) p. 83. Energy Research and Development Administration, National Cancer Institute, and National Science Foundation, Washington, D.C.
26. Maher, V., Ovellette, L. M., Mittlestat, M., and McCormick, J. (1975): Synergistic effect of caffeine on the cytotoxicity of ultraviolet irradiation and of hydrocarbon epoxides in strains of xeroderma pigmentosum. *Nature*, 258:760–763.
27. McCaw, B. K., Hecht, F., Harden, D. G., and Teplitz, R. L. (1975): Somatic rearrangement of chromosome 14 in human lymphocytes. *Proc. Natl. Acad. Sci. USA*, 72:2071–2075.
28. McKusick, V. A. (1971): *Mendelian Inheritance in Man; Catalogs of Autosomal Dominant, Autosomal Recessive, and X-Linked Phenotypes*. 3rd ed. The Johns Hopkins Univ. Press, Baltimore, Md.
29. Menighini, R. (1976): Gaps in DNA synthesized by ultraviolet light-irradiated WI38 human cells. *Biochem. Biophys. Acta*, 425:419–427.
30. Menighini, R., and Hanawalt, P. (1976): T4-endonuclease V-sensitive sites in DNA from ultraviolet irradiated human cells. *Biochem. Biophys. Acta*, 425:428–437.
31. Mortelmans, K., Friedberg, E. C., Slor, H., Thomas, G. H., and Cleaver, J. E. (1976): Excision of thymine dimers by cell-free extracts of xeroderma pigmentosum cells. *Proc. Natl. Acad. Sci. USA*, 73:2757–2801.
32. Paterson, M. C., Smith, B. P., Lohman, P. H. M., Anderson, A. K., and Fishman, L. (1976): Defective excision repair of gamma ray damaged DNA in human (ataxia telangiectasia) fibroblasts. *Nature*, 260:440–225.
33. Poon, P. K., O'Brien, R. L., and Parker, J. W. (1974): Defective DNA repair in Fanconi's anaemia. *Nature*, 250:223–225.
34. Ramsay, C. A., Coltart, T. M., Blunt, S., Pawsey, S. A., and Gianelli, F. (1975): Prenatal diagnosis of xeroderma pigmentosum. Report of first successful case. *Lancet*, 2:1109–1112.
35. Reed, W. B., May, S. B., and Nickel, W. R. (1965): Xeroderma pigmentosum with neurological complication. The de Sanctis—Cacchione syndrome. *Arch. Dermatol.*, 91:224–226.
36. Regan, J. D., and Setlow, R. B. (1974): DNA repair in human progeroid cells. *Biochem. Biophys. Res. Commun.*, 59:858–864.
37. Robbins, J. H., Kraemer, K. H., Lutzner, M. A., Festoff, B. W., and Coon, H. G. (1974):

Xeroderma pigmentosum. An inherited disease with sun sensitivity, multiple cutaneous neo-plasms, and abnormal DNA repair. *Ann. Intern. Med.*, 80:221–248.

38. Rook, A., Wilkinson, D. S., and Ebling, F. J. G. (eds.) (1968): *Textbook of Dermatology, Vol. 1.* Blackwell Scientific Publications, Oxford.
39. Sasaki, M. S. (1973): DNA repair capacity and susceptibility to chromosome breakage in xeroderma pigmentosum cells. *Mutat. Res.*, 20:291–293.
40. Sasaki, M. S. (1973): A high susceptibility of Fanconi's anemia to chromosome breakage by DNA cross-linking agents. *Cancer Res.*, 33:1829–1836.
41. Schmickel, R. D., Chu, E. H. Y., Trosko, J. E., and Chang, C. C. (1976): Cockayne's syndrome: Increased UV sensitivity due to defect in DNA repair *(in press)*.
42. Sutherland, B. M. (1974): Photoreactivating enzyme from human leukocytes. *Nature*, 248:109–112.
43. Sutherland, B. M., Rice, M., and Wagner, E. K. (1975): Xeroderma pigmentosum cells contain low levels of photoreactivating enzyme. *Proc. Natl. Acad. Sci. USA*, 72:103–107.
44. Tanaka, K., Sekiguchi, M., and Okada, Y. (1975): Restoration of ultraviolet-induced unsched-uled DNA synthesis of xeroderma pigmentosum cells by the concomitant treatment with T4 endonuclease V and HVJ (Sendai virus). *Proc. Natl. Acad. Sci. USA*, 72:4071–4075.
45. Taylor, A. M. R., Harnden, D. G., Arlett, C. F.. Harcourt, S. A., Lehmann, A. R., Stevens, S., and Bridges, B. A. (1975): Ataxia telangiectasia: A human mutation with abnormal sensitivity. *Nature*, 258:427–429.
46. Wolff, S., Bodycote, J., Thomas, G. H., and Cleaver, J. E. (1975): Sister chromatid exchange in xeroderma pigmentosum cells that are defective in DNA excision repair or post-replication repair. *Genetics*, 81:349–355.
47. Wolff, S., Rodin, B., and Cleaver, J. E. 1976) Sister chromatid exchanges induced by carcinogens and mutagens in normal and xeroderma pigmentosum cells. *Nature (in press)*.

Discussion

Agarwal: Is there any evidence to support the suggestion that a number of diseases, including chronic lymphocytic leukemia, might have defective DNA repair mechanisms similar to those found in xeroderma pigmentosum (XP)?

Cleaver: During the years since the identification of the biochemical defect in XP, a large number of other diseases have been suggested as candidates for studies of repair defects. However, very few of these diseases have actually become the province of interest of more than one group. For example, progeria has been intensively investigated, but the results to date have been negative. When other diseases begin to be examined, I would hope that a number of research groups would study each condition.

Nance: I wonder if you would comment on meiosis in XP, and on whether different forms of XP might have different effects. Do these mutations influence meiotic crossing over and pairing?

Cleaver: To my knowledge there have been no experimental investigations of the meiotic processes in XP.

Gerald: Are there any animal models for XP?

Cleaver: No, I wish there were. I have spent a lot of time wandering around in herds of Hereford cattle in Colorado looking at eye cancer and a few similar diseases. If anybody knows of such disease in animals, I would be very interested.

Genetics of Human Cancer, edited by J. J.
Mulvihill, R. W. Miller, and J. F. Fraumeni, Jr.
Raven Press, New York, 1977.

33

DNA Repair in Human Lymphocytes

S. S. Agarwal, D. Q. Brown, E. J. Katz, and L. A. Loeb

*The Institute for Cancer Research, The Fox Chase Cancer Center, Philadelphia,
Pennsylvania 19111*

In order to determine whether deficiency in the ability of cells to repair damaged
DNA is a predisposing factor for oncogenesis (1,2), an assay based on the effect of
X-irradiation on the stimulation of human lymphocytes with phytohemagglutinin
(PHA) is being developed. This assay may permit one to screen for defects in DNA
repair. Results of our studies on normal, healthy volunteers are presented in this
chapter.

METHODS

Lymphocytes from the peripheral blood of normal, healthy volunteers were separated on nylon fiber columns and cultured in Eagle's MEM supplemented with 20%
fetal calf serum. One-ml cultures, containing 10^6 cells in 16×125 mm Falcon tissue
culture plastic tubes, were irradiated at room temperature with 225-KVP X-rays from
a General Electric Maximar X-ray machine. The radiation dose rate was determined
with a Victoreen condenser R-meter and was kept at 120 to 135 rads/min. After
irradiation, the cultures were maintained in a humidified incubator at 37°C with 5%
CO_2 in air. Four hr following irradiation, 50 μl of PHA–M (Grand Island Biological
Company, New York) was added to each culture. The cells were harvested 96 hr after
the addition of PHA. The rate of [^{3}H]-thymidine uptake (NEN, 6 Ci/mmole; 2.5
μCi/culture for 2 hr) and the amount of DNA polymerase activity in each culture
were measured as previously described (3).

RESULTS

A typical experiment of the effect of different doses of X-irradiation on the rate of
[^{3}H]-thymidine uptake and DNA polymerase activity is shown in Fig. 1. In unirradiated PHA-stimulated cultures at 96 hr, the [^{3}H]-thymidine incorporation was
$32,500 \pm 2,750$ cpm/10^6 cells every 2 hr and the DNA polymerase activity was 138
± 3 pmoles dTMP incorporated/10^6 cells. Irradiation of lymphocytes with X-ray

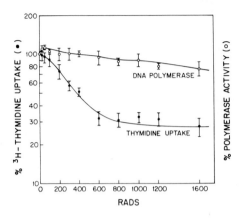

FIG. 1. Response of lymphocytes to PHA following X-irradiation.

doses up to 100 rads had no significant effect on the rate of thymidine uptake. However, above this dose and up to 600 rads, there was a linear decrease in the rate of [³H]-thymidine incorporation. Further increases in the X-ray dose had no additional effect. In contrast to the effect of X-irradiation on thymidine uptake, the DNA polymerase activity remained unaffected at all X-ray doses. Essentially similar results were obtained in five other individuals except that the response to the first 100 rads of irradiation was somewhat variable.

The decrease in thymidine uptake did not result from dilution of the radioactive thymidine by free thymidine in the cells. This was determined by measuring the thymidine incorporation in the presence of varying amounts of unlabeled thymidine in the medium.

On the basis of the above studies, three doses (200, 400, and 800 rads) were selected to quantitate the response to PHA following X-irradiation of lymphocytes from 12 normal, healthy individuals (Fig. 2). A repeat analysis after 1 week, on four of these individuals gave similar results. In one person out of the 12 persons studied, the decrease in [³H]-thymidine uptake in the X-irradiated lymphocytes was not so marked as in others, suggesting that the lymphocytes from this individual were uniquely resistant to X-irradiation. In the remaining 11, irradiation with 547 ± 180 rads resulted in 50% inhibition of thymidine uptake. The greatest variability in response was seen in cells irradiated with 800 rads.

We have also studied the response of lymphocytes from parents of two leukemic children and from age-sex matched normals (data not presented). There was no difference in the degree of inhibition of thymidine uptake for the corresponding X-ray doses in the two groups.

COMMENTS

In this study the response of lymphocytes to PHA following X-irradiation was measured at 96 hr after the addition of PHA. There was a marked inhibition of

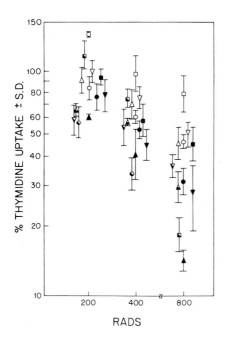

FIG. 2. Response of lymphocytes from 12 normal healthy volunteers to PHA after *in vitro* irradiation. The rate of [^{3}H]-thymidine uptake in unirradiated PHA-stimulated cultures was taken to be 100%. Each symbol identifies the response of lymphocytes from one individual.

[^{3}H]-thymidine uptake in irradiated cultures with essentially little effect on DNA polymerase activity when the lymphocytes were irradiated with doses between 100 and 800 rads. However, some residual DNA synthesis persisted even at very high doses of X-irradiation. This may be attributable to the presence of a subpopulation of cells that is highly radiation-resistant.

In order to interpret these results, a brief mention of the response of lymphocytes to PHA is pertinent. Other studies have shown that human lymphocytes obtained from the peripheral blood are in G$_0$ stage of the cell cycle. Addition of PHA stimulates them to undergo cell division. DNA synthesis in PHA-stimulated lymphocytes starts around 20 to 24 hr following the addition of PHA, and the first mitoses can be observed by 40 hr. Thereafter, the average cell cycle time is about 18 to 24 hr (4,5). Our earlier studies had shown that the initiation of DNA synthesis is correlated with the induction of DNA polymerase enzyme and that the latter is dependent on prior RNA and protein synthesis (6). The increase in the DNA polymerase activity has been shown to be the result of coordinate increase of all three (α, β, and γ) cellular polymerases (7).

In view of the normal DNA polymerase activity and the absence of significant alterations in the nucleotide pool in the PHA-stimulated irradiated lymphocytes, the impairment in the rate of thymidine uptake appears to be related to the inability of the cells to repair damage to DNA. The latter has been shown to be the primary target of biological damage in X-irradiated cells (8).

These results indicate that this test system can be used to screen for defects in DNA repair. Further studies in this direction are in progress.

ACKNOWLEDGMENTS

The study was supported by U. S. Public Health Service grants CA-11524, CA-06551, CA-15139, CA-06927, and RR-05539 from the National Institutes of Health, and by an appropriation from the Commonwealth of Pennsylvania. The technical help of Margaret Tuffner is acknowledged.

REFERENCES

1. Sneider, T. W. (1974): DNA replication, modification and repair. In: *The Molecular Biology of Cancer,* edited by H. Busch, pp. 107-186. Academic Press, New York.
2. Trosko, J. E., and Chu, H. Y. (1975): The role of DNA repair and somatic mutation in carcinogenesis. *Adv. Cancer Res.,* 21:391–424.
3. Leob, L. A., and Agarwal, S. S. (1971): DNA polymerase. Correlation with DNA replication during transformation of human lymphocytes. *Exp. Cell Res.,* 66:299–304.
4. Smith, M., Murray, D., and Gökcen, M. (1970): Life cycle of lymphoid cells *in vitro. Eur. J. Cancer,* 6:269–271.
5. Jhonson, L. I., LoBue, J., Chan, P., Monette, F. C., Rubin, A. D., Gordon, A. S., and Dameshek, W. (1969): Autoradiographic studies of human lymphocytes cultured *in vivo. Proc. Soc. Exp. Biol. Med.,* 130:675–679.
6. Agarwal, S. S., and Loeb, L. A. (1972): Studies on the induction of DNA polymerase during transformation of human lymphocytes. *Cancer Res.,* 32:107–113.
7. Mayer, R. J., Smith, R. G., and Gallo, R. C. (1975): DNA-metabolizing enzymes in normal human lymphoid cells. VI. Induction of DNA polymerase α, β and γ following stimulation with phytohemagglutinin. *Blood,* 46:509–518.
8. Okada, S. (1970): *Radiation Biochemistry, Vol. 1: Cells.* Academic Press, New York.

Genetics of Human Cancer, edited by J. J.
Mulvihill, R. W. Miller, and J. F. Fraumeni, Jr.
Raven Press, New York, 1977.

34

Gastrointestinal Neoplasia: An Investigative Approach

Martin Lipkin and Eleanor E. Deschner

Memorial Sloan-Kettering Cancer Center, New York, New York 10021

This paper discusses an approach to the analysis of individual susceptibility for gastrointestinal neoplasia, with particular emphasis on colon cancer and its premalignant antecedents. In the etiology of colorectal tumors and other neoplasms in the gastrointestinal tract, environmental factors that can modify the appearance of disease have been well-described (3,12,26). Additional evidence indicates that other factors, including genetic predisposition, are associated with increasing susceptibility of individuals to gastrointestinal tumors. Current findings suggest that interactions between inherited and environmental factors are involved in the evolution of cellular changes that lead to neoplastic transformation of gastrointestinal epithelial cells.

CLINICAL INDICES OF A HIGH RISK FOR COLORECTAL CANCER

A survey of clinical manifestations associated with the development of colorectal cancer indicates that certain factors play a significant role (Table 1). Especially noteworthy is the increased frequency with age. Individuals with dominantly inherited adenomatosis of the colon and rectum show an earlier age of onset of adenomas and cancer (1,19). The combined increase of colon and rectal cancer becomes greater in males than in females approaching the sixth decade of life (3).

The well-known variations of geographic distribution of incidence are interesting. Changing patterns of neoplasia are seen with shifts of populations, such as the migration of Japanese to Hawaii and California. The incidence of colonic cancer is high in North America, particularly the United States, and Northern and Western Europe, but low in parts of Africa, Asia, and South America (3,12,26). In addition to diet, factors such as exposure to stress and occupational and other environmental carcinogens may also be involved in modifying the expression of neoplastic transformation in gastrointestinal cells. Current studies have shown that similar proliferative abnormalities and morphologic changes develop in colonic epithelial cells of humans at high risk of inherited adenomatosis and colonic cancer, and rodents exposed to several chemical carcinogens (5,7,8,10,14,15,23,24).

TABLE 1. *Factors associated with increased susceptibility to colon cancer*

	Ref.
Autosomal dominant inheritance in adenomatosis of colon and rectum and "cancer families"	1,2,19
Increasing age	3,12
Geographic location (Western industrialized countries)	3,12
Multiple adenomas and increasing size	19
Family history of colon cancer	18
Early age of onset and multiple colonic malignancies	18
Inflammatory bowel disease	19

The development of multiple colonic tumors is an additional characteristic signaling a heightened susceptibility of some individuals to colorectal neoplasia. In man, individuals who have survived a previous cancer of the colon show a higher incidence of carcinoma than in the population at large (21). The subsequent lesions usually appear in the colon and rectum and occasionally in the stomach. Consideration of cellular, physiological, and environmental factors must be made in order to focus on the reasons for this observed susceptibility to tumor development.

Certain other groups appear to have an increased risk for the development of colonic neoplasms. In relatives of patients with colorectal cancer this appears to be three times greater than in the general population (4). Individuals under age 40 have been reported more likely to have a family history of colon cancer than those over age 40 (26). Patients with multiple primary colonic malignancies have a significantly earlier age of onset of colonic cancer than the population as a whole (18).

Associations also exist between the appearance of benign colonic neoplastic growths and the development of carcinomas. In man, several types of benign colonic growths appear to have premalignant potential (believed by some to be the major source of colorectal cancer). Only a minor fraction of all colonic excrescences of man are adenomatous; but these and villous adenomas are truly expanding neoplasms. Columnar epithelium lining the glands of these lesions show an increased number of nuclei. The probability of developing malignant cells increases as the size of the lesion expands (19).

Studies have also focused on cancer families because of the high frequency of primary malignancies in multiple anatomic sites (including colon and stomach), early age of onset, and apparent dominant inheritance (2). The most extensive studies, however, have been on the inherited disease, adenomatosis of the colon and rectum (ACR; familial polyposis). This is in part due to the well-defined expressions of neoplastic transformation occurring in cells of the colon and rectum. The changes in this disease lead to the early warning signal: the widespread formation of adenomatous polyps progressing to cancer. This disease can provide information related to the etiology and pathogenesis of colorectal cancer as some of the events occurring are detectable during the early stages of neoplastic transformation.

LABORATORY INDICES OF A HIGH RISK FOR COLORECTAL CANCER

Individuals with ACR, who are at high risk for colon cancer, best illustrate the progressive phases of abnormal cell growth. Normal colonic epithelial cells differentiate rapidly and more completely, and their DNA synthesis and proliferative activity are repressed as cells migrate to the mucosal surface (Fig. 1A). In contrast, colonic epithelial cells from persons with ACR have an increased ability to proliferate and accumulate in the mucosa before and during the formation of neoplastic lesions (8,14).

A further, early phenotypic expression of ACR, that has identified a genotypic propensity for cell transformation, has been a failure of colonic epithelial cells to repress DNA synthesis during migration to the surface of the mucosa, even before their accumulation as polyps (Fig. 1B). Failure of these cells to repress DNA synthesis does not itself indicate neoplasia, and additional changes in growth characteristics of the cells occur during their evolution.

A second observable phenotypic change is the accumulation of cells in the colonic mucosa and the initiation of adenomatous polyps which progress further to neoplasia (Fig. 2). Similar characteristics have been observed in other cells and species, including colonic epithelial cells of rodents after carcinogen exposure (6,13, 16,22,23,25) and in the development of nonhereditary gastrointestinal neoplasms in

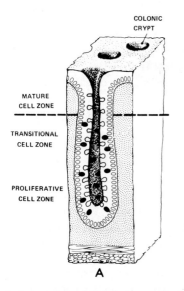
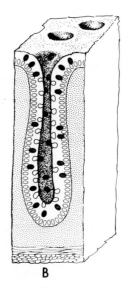

COLONIC CRYPT

MATURE CELL ZONE

TRANSITIONAL CELL ZONE

PROLIFERATIVE CELL ZONE

A   B

FIG. 1. A: Location of proliferating and differentiating cells in normal colonic crypt. Dark cells illustrate thymidine labeling in cells that are synthesizing DNA and preparing to undergo cell division. As cells pass from proliferative zone through the transitional zone, DNA synthesis and mitosis are repressed, and migrating epithelial cells leave the proliferative cell cycle to undergo normal maturation before they reach the surface of the mucosa. **B:** Colonic epithelial cells that fail to repress incorporation of thymidine ^{3}H into DNA during migration to the surface of flat colonic mucosa.

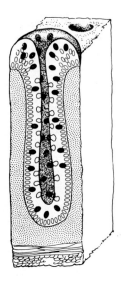

FIG. 2. Cells that incorporate thymidine ^{3}H into DNA develop additional properties that enable them to accumulate in the mucosa in increasing numbers, and to differentiate into pathologically defined neoplastic lesions including adenomatous polyps and villous adenomas.

the colon and stomach of man (10,11,15). Similar cellular mechanisms and somatic mutation could be involved in the development of abnormal proliferative characteristics in these cases.

Recent findings have suggested an additional expression of the inherited defect of adenomatosis of the colon and rectum. Normal-appearing skin fibroblasts of affected individuals demonstrate the ability, when plated at low density, to grow more actively in medium containing low serum than fibroblasts from normal persons. This low serum tolerance is a frequent characteristic of transformed cells (20). It may be associated with the basic genetic defect leading to ACR.

USING THE INDICES TO PREDICT INCREASED CANCER SUSCEPTIBILITY

In analyzing the significance of these expressions of abnormal cell growth, it is useful to study the degree of association that links the indices with each other and with the development of malignancy. We currently quantitate the cases in high-risk population groups that have significant simultaneous phenotypic attributes. The presence or absence of two phenotypic traits of interest are recorded, with a priori probabilities concerning their individual or simultaneous occurrence. The degree of association between phenotypic traits is quantitated in terms of ratios denoting fractions of cases with one trait occurring in subpopulations having another trait, which are then plotted in Venn diagrams (15).

The analysis can be used to estimate the probabilities with which the various phases of transformation and colon cancer will evolve in humans under specified conditions.

The utility of the analysis can be illustrated in relation to the development of colon cancer: s' denotes a failure of colonic epithelial cells to repress DNA synthesis, and n' represents an ability of s' cells to become adenomatous and accumulate in the mucosa initiating neoplastic lesions.

Our current data derived from affected individuals in the high-risk population group with inherited adenomatosis show the following comparison illustrated in Table 2: In the Venn analyses, the fraction of cases having s' in flat mucosa is 0.85, the fraction having n' is 0.64, and the fraction simultaneously having s' detected in flat mucosa and also developing n' is 0.49. All adenomatous polyps contain cells that fail to repress DNA synthesis. An individual with colonic cells in flat mucosa that fail to repress DNA synthesis at present has a 49% chance of developing polyposis. Accumulation of new cases will modify these values.

Quantitation of the early steps leading to neoplastic transformation in the cells of susceptible individuals and modification of the progression of transformation by known events is expected to improve both the surveillance and treatment of individuals and families at increased risk of cancer.

TABLE 2. *Cell phenotypes in inherited ACR*[a]

Tissue	Phenotype	Segment of Venn diagram	Fraction of cases
Adenomatous polyps	s'	S'	1.0
	n'	N'	1.0
Flat colonic mucosa	s'	S'	0.85
	n'	N'	0.64
	$s'n'$	S'N'	0.49

[a] Current data on inherited adenomatosis population showing observed relationship between the presence of adenomas (n'), and failure of colonic epithelial cells to repress DNA synthesis (s') in adenomas and flat colonic mucosa. The corresponding capital letters define the set of individuals with the given characteristic. The numerical values are continually modified as data of new cases are recorded.

ACKNOWLEDGMENTS

This research was supported by Contract and Grants CP 433661 and 08748, awarded by the National Cancer Institute, DHEW.

REFERENCES

1. Alm T., and Licznerski G. (1973): The intestinal polyposis. *Clin. Gastroenterol.*, 2:577–602.
2. Anderson D. E. (1970): Genetic varieties of neoplasia. In: *23rd Annual Symposium of Fundamental Cancer Research: Genetics Concepts of Neoplasia, Houston, Texas, 1969.* Williams & Wilkins, Baltimore, Maryland.
3. Berg, J. S., and Howell, M. A. (1974): Geographic pathology of bowel cancer. *Cancer*, 34:807–814.
4. Burdette, W. J. (1970): Heritable cancer of the colorectum. In: *Carcinoma of Colon and Antecedent Epithelium,* edited by W. J. Burdette. Charles C Thomas, Springfield, Illinois.

5. Cole, J. W., and McKalen, A. (1963): Studies on the morphogenesis of adenomatous polyps in the human colon. *Cancer,* 16:998–1002.
6. Deschner, E. E. (1974): Experimentally induced cancer of the colon. *Cancer,* 34:824–828.
7. Deschner, E. E., Lewis, C. M., and Lipkin, M. (1963): *In vitro* study of human epithelial cells. I. Atypical zone of H^3-thymidine incorporation in mucosa of multiple polyposis. *J. Clin. Invest.* 42:1922–1928.
8. Deschner, E. E., and Lipkin, M. (1975): Proliferative patterns in colonic mucosa in familial polyposis. *Cancer,* 35:413–418.
9. Deschner, E. E., Lipkin, M., Peterson, A., and Cooper, M. (1975): Cell proliferation kinetics in DMH induced neoplasms of mouse. *Proc. Am. Assoc. Cancer Res.* 16:139.
10. Deschner, E. E., Lipkin, M., and Solomon, C. (1966): *In vitro* study of human epithelial cells. II. H^3-thymidine incorporation into polyps and adjacent mucosa. *J. Natl. Cancer Inst.* 36:849–857.
11. Deschner, E. E., Winawer, S. J., and Lipkin, M. (1972): Patterns of nucleic acid and protein synthesis in normal human gastric mucosa and atrophic gastritis. *J. Natl. Cancer Inst.* 48:1567–1574.
12. Haenzel, W., and Correa, P. (1971): Cancer of the colon and rectum and adenomatous polyps. A review of eipdemiologic findings. *Cancer,* 28:14.
13. Kikkawa, N. (1974): Experimental studies on polypogenesis and carcinogenesis of the large intestine. *Med. J. Osaka Univ.* 24:293–314.
14. Lipkin, M. (1974): Phase 1 and phase 2 proliferative lesions of colonic epithelial cells in diseases leading to colonic cancer. *Cancer,* 34:878–888.
15. Lipkin, M. (1975): Biology of large bowel cancer: Present status and research frontiers. *Cancer,* 36:2319–2324.
16. Lohrs, U., Wiebecke, B., and Edgar, M. (1969): Morpholigische and autoradiographische untersuchung der darmschleim-hautveranderringen nach einmaliger injektion von 1,2-dimethylhydrazin. *Z. Ges. Exp. Med.,* 1.51:297–307.
17. Maskens, A. (1976): Histogenesis and growth pattern of 1,2-dimethylhydrazine-induced rat colon adenocarcinoma. *Cancer Res. (In press.)*
18. Moertel, C. G., Bargen, J. A., and Dockerty, M. B. (1958): Multiple carcinomas of the large intestine: A review of the literature and a study of 261 cases *Gastroenterol,* 34:285.
19. Morson, B. C., and Bussey, H., Jr. (1970): Predisposing causes of intestinal cancer. *Curr. Probl. Surg.,* pp. 1–50, February 1970.
20. Pfeffer, L., Kopelovich, L., and Lipkin, M. (1976): Phenotypic alterations in growth characteristics of human skin fibroblasts *in vitro:* A simple experimental approach for early detection of familial polyposis. *J. Cell Physiol., (In press).*
21. Schottenfeld, D., Berg, J. W., and Vitsky, B. (1969): Incidence of multiple primary cancers. *J. Natl. Cancer Inst.,* 43:77.
22. Springer, P., Springer, J., and Oehlert, W. (1970): Early stages of DMH induced carcinoma of the small and large intestine of rat. *Z. Krebsforsch* 74:236–240.
23. Thurnherr, N., Deschner, E., Stonehill, E., and Lipkin, M.(1973): Induction of adenocarcinomas of the colon in mice by weekly injections of 1,2-dimethylhydrazine. *Cancer Res.,* 33:940–945.
24. Weisburger, J. H., Reddy, B. S., Narisawa, T., and Wynder, E. L. (1975): Germ-free status and colon tumor induction by MNNG. *Proc. Soc. Exp. Biol. Med.,* 148:1119–1121.
25. Wiebecke, B., Krey, U., Löhrs, U., and Eder, M. (1973): Morphological and autoradiographical investigations on experimental carcinogenesis and polyp development in the intestinal tract of rats and mice. *Virchows Arch. Pathol. Anat.,* 360:179–193.
26. Wynder, E. L., and Shigematsu, T. (1967): Environmental factors of cancer of the colon and rectum. *Cancer,* 20:1520–1561.

Discussion

H. T. Lynch: Have you any evidence that different areas of the colon have different proliferative rates? Have you studied areas proximal to the sigmoid and rectum? I ask because of the predominance of right-sided tumors in one family I have seen with polyposis and in the kindred with juvenile polyposis coli reported by Stemper [*Ann. Intern. Med.,* 83:639–646 (1975)].

Lipkin: The instances you mentioned are unusual variations of what is usually seen. I would expect to see early proliferative changes in those areas.

Hirschhorn: Have chromosomes been analyzed from these atypical zones of proliferation?

Lipkin: Not yet, although this has been attempted in some laboratories.

Mulvhill: Can you distinguish Gardner's syndrome from typical famililial polyposis coli by the proliferative index or by the serum requirement of fibroblasts?

Lipkin: Gardner's syndrome, of course, can be distinguished by clinical findings. Separate classification cannot be made by using current subclinical *in vitro* tests.

Genetics of Human Cancer, edited by J. J.
Mulvihill, R. W. Miller, and J. F. Fraumeni, Jr.
Raven Press, New York, 1977.

35

SV-40 T Antigen Expression in Skin Fibroblasts from Normal Individuals, Patients with Fanconi's Anemia, and a Family at High Risk of Leukemia

A. S. Lubiniecki, *W. A. Blattner, and *J. F. Fraumeni, Jr.

*Life Sciences Division, Meloy Laboratories, Inc., Springfield, Virginia 22151, and
*Environmental Epidemiology Branch, National Cancer Institute, National Institutes of
Health, Bethesda, Maryland 20014*

In 1966, Todaro and co-workers (15) reported increased levels of colony formation or transformation in skin fibroblast cultures from certain individuals on *in vitro* exposure to SV-40, a monkey papovavirus oncogenic in hamsters. Soon thereafter, Miller and Todaro (8) suggested that such increased transformability was a marker of increased risk for cancer in conditions such as Down's syndrome and Fanconi's anemia.

While sporadic confirmatory cases were reported (4,9–13,16–18), the transformation assay had many drawbacks: the biological reagents were not standardized, laboratory variables were not explored, and the endpoint (colony or focus formation) was somewhat subjective and took 3 weeks to complete. We have established a more standardized and reproducible assay using the expression of SV-40 T antigen detected by immunofluorescence as the endpoint after only 3 days of infection.

MATERIALS AND METHODS

Cell Strains

Human skin fibroblast cell strains derived from punch biopsy materials were established and maintained as previously described (5).

Virus

The virus stocks employed for transformation and T antigen expression assays were plaque-purified and propogated as reported by Takemoto et al. (14).

Assays

Transformation (6) and T antigen (6,7) assays were performed as previously described. Briefly, replicate cultures of human fibroblast strains were seeded in Petri dishes ($1-2 \times 10^5$ cells/dish). One day later, cultures were infected with SV-40 at known input multiplicities (virus:cell ratio). After 3 days, replicate plates were fixed and stained by indirect immunofluorescent methods for SV-40 T antigen (6,7). The mean proportion of positive cells 70 hr after infection in quadruplicate fibroblast cultures, weighted to account for the differing cell numbers examined in each culture, was taken as the numerical value for T antigen expression. The inverse sin or arc sin of the square root of that average was calculated. This calculation did not change the biological results but is a mathematical device for reducing variance among values by changing scale.

RESULTS AND DISCUSSION

T Antigen Expression and Transformation

Following studies of variables affecting T antigen expression that resulted in numerous assay modifications, the relationship between the expression of T antigen and transformation in our modified system was evaluated. SV-40 T antigen and SV-40-induced transformation in seven cell lines were strongly correlated at two different virus concentrations. Among the types tested were cell lines from normal individuals, from cancer family members, and from actual human tumor cell lines. The correlation between expression of transformation and T antigen seemed independent of clinical history and virus concentration (6). Similar findings have been reported by several other laboratories (1,2,11,12).

T Antigen Expression in Normal Individuals

For 76 healthy individuals with no significant family history of cancer or genetic disease, the expression of T antigen followed a statistically normal distribution. The data for the normal population showed no significant differences by race, sex, age, or ethnic background. This information served to define a rational method for controlling future studies of various clinical groups and to delineate between normal and abnormal levels of T antigen expression on the basis of a simple parametric statistical test.

T Antigen Expression in Fanconi's Anemia Patients

Table 1 shows that all but one of 11 cases tested had significantly elevated expression of T antigen, with P-value less than 1%. The remaining case had a P-value less than 2%. Thus, skin fibroblasts from Fanconi's anemia patients express SV-40 T antigen more frequently than normal cells in our assay (7), confirming earlier observations using transformation assays (4,11,12,15,18).

TABLE 1. *Distribution of T antigen expression in skin fibroblasts from individuals and patients with Fanconi's anemia*

Source	N^a	Within 95%[b] confidence limit	Within 99%[b] confidence limit	Exceeded 99%[b] confidence limit
Normal controls	76	68	75	1
Fanconi's anemia	11	0	1	10

[a]Total number of individuals examined.
[b]Based on mean and standard deviation of healthy population.

T Antigen Expression in Family with Acute Myelogenous Leukemia

T antigen expression was investigated in a familial aggregation of acute myelogenous leukemia (AML) and malignant reticuloendotheliosis, described originally by Snyder et al. (13). The SV-40 transformation values reported (13) correlated with T antigen values obtained by us for the same cell strains (3). The kindred contains many individuals who showed an elevated expression of T antigen. All six women exhibited significantly elevated values of T antigen expression, whereas only one of the men did (Table 2). In both family branches studied, the offspring manifested SV-40 T antigen values that were intermediate between the values of the parents (3). It must be emphasized that the apparent hereditary nature of T antigen expression values and the sex effect are only preliminary findings obtained from a fairly small number of individuals. Further studies are in progress.

TABLE 2. *Distribution of T antigen expression in skin fibroblasts from members of a family at high risk of leukemia*

Source	N	Within 95% confidence limit	Exceeded 99% confidence limit
Kindred males	5	4	1
Kindred females	6	0	6
Spouses	2	2	0

REFERENCES

1. Aaronson, S. A. (1970): Susceptibility of human cell strains to transformation by simian virus 40 and simian virus 40 deoxyribonucleic acid. *J. Virol.*, 6:470–475.
2. Aaronson, S. A., and Todaro, G. (1968): SV-40 T antigen induction and transformation in human skin fibroblast cell strains. *Virology*, 36:254–261.

3. Blattner, W. A., Lubiniecki, A. S., and Fraumeni J. F., Jr. (1976): Increased levels of SV-40 T antigen expression in two families exhibiting multiple cases of acute myelogenous leukemia. *Lancet,* 1976 *(submitted for publication).*
4. Dosik, H., Hsu, L. Y., Todaro, G. H., Lee S. L., Hirschhorn, K., Selirio, E. S., and Alter, A. A. (1970): Leukemia in Fanconi's anemia: Cytogenetic and tumor virus susceptibility studies. *Blood,* 30:341–352.
5. Kaplan, M. M., Giard, D. J., Blattner, W. A., Lubiniecki, A. S., and Fraumeni, J. F., Jr. (1975): An improved method for immunofluorescent detection of SV-40 T antigen in infected human fibroblasts. *Proc. Soc. Exp. Biol. Med.,* 148:660–664.
6. Kaplan, M. M., Lubiniecki, A. S., Blattner, W. A., Mason, T., Giard, D. J., Gunnell, M., Triantafellu, N., and Fraumeni, J. F., Jr. (1976): Systematic variables affecting SV40-induced T antigen expression and transformation in human cells. *J. Clin. Microbiol.,* 3:593–598.
7. Lubiniecki, A. S., Blattner, W. A., Dosik, H., Sun, C., and Fraumeni, J. F., Jr. (1977): SV-40 T antigen expression in skin fibroblasts from clinically normal individuals and from ten cases of Fanconi's anemia. *Am. J. Hematol. (in press).*
8. Miller, R. W., and Todaro, G. J. (1970): Viral transformation of cells from persons at high risk of cancer. *Lancet,* 1:81–82.
9. Mukerjee D., Bowen, J., and Anderson, D. E. (1970): Simian papovavirus 40 transformation of cells from cancer patients with XY/XXY mosaic Klinefelter's syndrome. *Cancer Res.,* 30:1769–1771.
10. Mukerjee, D., Bowen, J., Trujillo, J. M., and Cork, A. (1972): Increased susceptibility of cells from cancer patients with XY-gonadal dysgenesis to simian papovavirus 40 transformation. *Cancer Res.,* 32:1518–1520.
11. Potter, A. M., and Potter C. W. (1970): Transformation of human cells by SV40 virus. *Br. J. Cancer,* 31:348–354.
12. Potter, C. W., Potter, A. M., and Oxford, J. S. (1970): Comparison of transformation and T antigen induction in human cell lines. *J. Virol.,* 5:293–298.
13. Snyder, A. L., Li, F. P., Henderson, E. S., and Todaro, G. J. (1970): Possible inherited leukemogenic factors in familial acute myelogenous leukemia. *Lancet,* 1:586–589.
14. Takemoto, K. K., Todaro, G. J., and Habel, K. (1968): Recovery of SV40 virus with genetic markers of original inducing virus from SV40-transformed mouse cells. *Virology,* 35:1–8.
15. Todaro, G. J., Green, H., and Swift, M. R. (1966): Susceptibility of human diploid fibroblasts to transformation by SV40 virus. *Science,* 153:1252–1254.
16. Todaro, G. J., and Martin, G. M. (1967): Increased susceptibility of Down's syndrome fibroblasts to transformation by SV40. *Proc. Soc. Exp. Biol. Med.,* 124:1232–1236.
17. Young, D. (1971): The susceptibility to SV40 virus transformation of fibroblasts obtained from patients with Down's syndrome. *Eur. J. Cancer,* 7:337–339.
18. Young, D., (1971): Transformation of cells from patients with Fanconi's anemia. *Lancet,* 1:294–295.

Discussion

Croce: How did you conduct the transformation tests?

Lubiniecki: We performed the assays in Petri plates approximately by the same method as Todaro.

Croce: You did not assay for colony formation?

Lubiniecki: No.

Croce: So you did not use very stringent criteria to determine whether cells were transformed or not. Also, your cells may be permissive to SV-40 due to superinfection with SV-40. Perhaps you are not looking at the difference in transformability but rather the differences in titer from the superinfectivity of cells with SV-40.

Lubiniecki: Our assays were performed in the presence of sufficient SV-40-neutralizing antiserum to neutralize in excess of 10^6 viruses, so I am not concerned about superinfection. Also, the multiplicities are sufficiently high so that, even with the low absorption rate of the virus, we feel confident that the vast majority of cells, certainly more than 90%, was infected the first time.

Blattner: The assay we are using is not measuring transformation. Perhaps the word should be banned from this discussion; it is a bag of worms that gets virologists discussing things that may not be relevant to what we are looking at. We may actually be assaying the ability of a host cell to regulate the expression of what is thought to be viral genome material.

Swift: Have you looked for trivial explanations of the differences between the susceptible and nonsusceptible cells? For example, Fanconi's anemia (FA) homozygous cells have a much reduced growth fraction. Perhaps nondividing cells are more likely to express the T antigen.

Lubiniecki: We have not examined this, but it sounds like a very good idea.

Auerbach: We have been doing some studies with an *in vitro* model that demonstrates genetic and environmental interactions; that is, we have exposed cells to chemical carcinogens and examined them for chromosome damage [*Nature,* 261:494–496 (1976)].

Fibroblasts from patients with FA, ataxia-telangiectasia (AT), xeroderma pigmentosum (XP), and various other fibroblast strains have been exposed to a carcinogen for 7 days at a nontoxic concentration that has no effect on growth rate, viability, or morphology of the cells tested. After 7 days the cells are replaced in carcinogen-free medium and 48 hr later are harvested for chromosome studies. This enables us to look at residual effects of the carcinogen on the surviving and dividing population of cells. In each experiment treated fibroblasts were compared to untreated cells from the same cell line, at the same passage number.

Using diepoxybutane we have demonstrated a highly significant increase ($p < 0.001$) in chromosome breakage in FA fibroblasts compared to untreated FA cells. In a representative experiment, we found 0.28 breaks per cell in 100 untreated FA cells examined, whereas the treated population of cells had 1.05 breaks per cell. These breaks were not concentrated in a few cells, but were distributed so that practically all cells examined had at least one break. The AT fibroblasts from a patient with chromosome breakage in the untreated cultured fibroblasts showed a slight increase in breakage after exposure to diepoxybutane, with a low level of significance; and an AT strain with no intrinsic breakage showed no further effect after exposure to the chemical. Fibroblasts from XP, trisomy 18, and normal individuals all showed no increased breakage after exposure to diepoxybutane. We are also looking at FA heterozygotes, but our data are incomplete.

Treatment of FA cells with ethylmethanesulfonate, a chemical mutagen, also resulted in a significant increase in chromosome aberrations compared with untreated FA cells. No aberrations were induced in normal cells using the same concentration of the chemical.

This system thus enables one to look at residual and possibly lasting effects of chemical carcinogens on cells of certain cancer-prone individuals.

Hirschhorn: By analogy, a few years ago we were able to demonstrate, by growth kinetic analysis, that benzo[a]pyrene treatment of FA cells caused what might be interpreted as contact inhibition of growth [M. D. Anderson Symposium: *Genetic Concepts and Neoplasia,* Williams & Wilkins, Baltimore, 1970, pp. 191–204.] This would certainly be compatible with the idea that these cells may very well be ideal, not only to test for lasting damage in the susceptible individual, but also to screen for environmental mutagens.

Swift: I understand that in a number of laboratories many experiments are being done using the same cell cultures. I would urge people to contribute their own cultures to the Genetic Mutant Cell Bank of the Institute for Medical Research (Camden, N.J.) or to other cell banks, because great heterogeneity may exist in some of these important syndromes. I would not like to see all results based on the same three patients.

Genetics of Human Cancer, edited by J. J.
Mulvihill, R. W. Miller, and J. F. Fraumeni, Jr.
Raven Press, New York, 1977.

36

Cellular Interaction as a Limiting Factor in the Expression of Oncogenic Mutations: A Hypothesis

Vincent M. Riccardi

Genetics Unit, Milwaukee Children's Hospital, Department of Pediatrics, Medical College of Wisconsin, Milwaukee, Wisconsin 53233

The expression of a mutation in a cell can depend on the influence of adjoining nonmutant cells. For example, normal cells are able to mask the mutant cells' phenotype in uncloned fibroblast cultures from Lesch–Nyhan syndrome heterozygotes (1). Recognition and characterization of the ability of nonmutant cells to nullify the expression of an oncogenic mutation could have important consequences. This nongenetic limitation would introduce another factor in elucidating genetic or mutational mechanisms in oncogenesis. It would also account for variable expression in many dominantly inherited disorders. The following hypothesis suggests a nongenetic determinant in the expression of certain somatic or germinal mutations. Such specific nongenetic modifiers of oncogenic mutations receive little notice, but particulars of the hypothesis may readily be tested in several experimental systems described elsewhere in this book.

The components of the hypothesis are: (a) von Recklinghausen's neurofibromatosis (NF) is a disorder of a particular cell type—the phenotypically abnormal (mutant) cells are derived from the neural crest; (b) although all other somatic cells contain the NF gene, it is not ordinarily expressed in them; (c) NF and certain other autosomal dominant disorders show a mosaicism or patchiness, not previously explained; (d) if the ratio of mutant to nonmutant cells in a given collection of cells does not exceed a critical value, the nonmutant cells circumvent or mask the mutant phenotype (*café-au-lait* spots, neurofibromas, etc.), accounting for the mosaicism; (e) malignant transformation is a time-dependent consequence of unmodified mutant gene expression in previously benign tumors (i.e., neurofibromas); (f) the ultimate NF gene-directed insult in premalignant tumor

383

cells is the abnormal intracellular accumulation of carcinogens or co-carcinogens such as 3-hydroxyanthranilic acid or phenoxazinones, or both, derived from the aberrant metabolism of tyrosine and tryptophan (2). An additional chemical, viral, or second mutational insult may also be necessary.

This schema takes into account the following considerations. Individuals with certain autosomal dominant malformations (e.g., brachydactyly, type E) show a mosaicism in the expression of the mutant gene, i.e., decreased or no expression in one or more limbs, with no constant pattern from one person to another (3). Similarly, individuals with NF have dark patches, but are *not* uniformly dark even though all melanocytes are derived from neural crest and there are no apparent physiologic or anatomic restrictions. Among the neural crest-derived elements, neurofibromas and other neural tumors also occur in an apparent random distribution. This apparently random, localized expression of the mutant gene (mosaicism) has not previously been explained. Because of their dominant nature, we would expect these mutations to be uniformly manifest unless there were some additional overriding mechanism. I suggest that this mechanism involves a correction of the intracellular defect by specific or nonspecific direct cellular interaction. That is, the mutation is dominant only in the permissive sense—as long as there is not cross-correction by nonmutant cells, the mutant cells would manifest the defect in the heterozygous state. This also allows for wide quantitative variation: below a critical ratio of mutant to nonmutant cells in any cell collection no mutant phenotype is seen, whereas, above that ratio, the severity or size of the lesion is a direct function of the proportion of mutant cells.

The basic clinical abnormalities in NF are *café-au-lait* spots and neurofibromas or other neural tumors. What these lesions have in common is the neural crest origin of their primary elements. Melanocytes, various peripheral and central neural elements, and certain structural elements of the face and head are derived from neural crest. In the course of embryologic migration they closely associate and even mix with cells of separate origin (4). Moreover, nonneural crest cells need not express the NF mutation, e.g., the expression of the achondroplasia mutation is essentially limited to cartilage cells, and the enzyme defect in phenylketonuria is not expressed in skin fibroblasts.

Thus, the NF *café-au-lait* spots would be expected only when, on the basis of random cell admixing, the NF melanocytes did not have their primary defect overridden in some way by the adjacent nonmutant cells. Likewise, neurofibromas would be expected to develop only when, on the basis of random cell admixing, the abnormal growth potential of NF neural crest elements was not overridden by adjacent nonmutant cells. This is consistent with the known multicellular origin of these tumors as described by P. Fialkow (Chapter 41). If, during growth, there were a differential mitotic rate so that the mutant cells grew slightly faster, then we would expect the progressive gradual increase in the number or aggressiveness of either type of lesion; such change is often seen clinically. Finally, it is in the larger or older neurofibromas, where the mutation has not been tempered by the interaction of nonmutant cells, that the development of malignant changes is anticipated. I suspect that the primary defect in this mutant cell type involves the abnormal metabolic packaging and handling of tyrosine and tryptophan metabolities, as suggested by investigations on the giant melanosomes of the NF *café-au-lait* spots (5,6). It is intriguing to consider that accumulations of tyrosine and tryptophan metabolites, such as 3-hydroxyanthranilic acid and phenoxazinones, known carcinogens or co-carcinogens, may be the metabolic mediators of malignant changes in the neurofibromas (2).

Studies are currently underway with cultured tumors (neurofibromas and an astrocytoma) from patients with NF to characterize growth properties, chromosome constitution, and SV-40 responsiveness. Whole cell autoradiography experiments are planned utilizing labeled tyrosine and tryptophan to provide a basis for testing the described hypothesis. The key is demonstration of the mutant intracellular phenotype which can then be assessed in terms of whether it can be ablated or modified by growth in the presence of cells from an unaffected person or cells from a separate source on the affected person. To date, general growth properties, chromosome analysis, electron microscopy, and SV-40 responsiveness (T antigen positiveness and colony formation) have been within normal limits.

REFERENCES

1. Friedmann, T., Seegmiller, J. E., and Subak-Sharpe, J. H. (1968): Metabolic cooperation between genetically marked human fibroblasts in tissue culture. *Nature,* 220:272–274.
2. Arcos, J. C., and Argus, M. F. (1974): *Chemical Induction of Cancer: Structural Bases and Biological Mechanisms,* Vol. II B, pp. 88–89. Academic Press, New York.
3. Riccardi, V. M., and Holmes, L. B. (1974): Brachydactyly, type E: Hereditary shortening of digits, metacarpals, metatarsals, and long bones. *J. Pediatr.,* 84:251–254.
4. Weston, J. A. (1970): The migration and differentiation of neural crest cells. *Adv. Morphog.,* 8:41–114.
5. Benedict, P. H., Szabó, G., Fitzpatrick, T. B., and Sinesi, S. J. (1968): Melanotic macules in Albright's syndrome and in neurofibromatosis. *JAMA,* 205:618–626.
6. Konrad, K., Wolff, K., and Hönigsmann, H. (1974): The giant melanosome: A model of deranged melanosome-morphogenesis. *J. Ultrastruct. Res.,* 48:102–123.

Discussion

Warkany: What you suggest is fine. Do you think you will find any common denominator in these cell studies, or do you just want to study them with regard to possible malignancies?

Riccardi: The reason for examining these cells is to identify the presumed defect that leads to neurofibroma or neurofibrosarcoma.

Genetics of Human Cancer, edited by J. J. Mulvihill, R. W. Miller, and J. F. Fraumeni, Jr. Raven Press, New York, 1977.

37

A General Theory of Carcinogenesis

David E. Comings

Department of Medical Genetics, City of Hope National Medical Center, Duarte, California 91010

A general framework for viewing several aspects of tumor cell biology has been suggested (1) and has the following features.

1. It is clear from studies of a number of temperature-sensitive mutants of polyoma and avian sarcoma viruses, and more recent studies of mapping with endonuclease fragments of various viruses, that a single gene in the virus is responsible for the induction of the transformed state of the host cell. These are called transforming (Tr) genes.

2. The observation that temperature-sensitive transformation of mammalian cells can also be induced by chemicals implies that the transforming genes may also exist as a normal part of the genome.

3. It is suggested that all cells possess multiple structural genes (Tr) capable of coding for transforming factors which can release the cell from its normal constraints on growth. It is reasonable to suggest that these structural genes are normally suppressed by a diploid pair of regulatory genes and that many of the transforming genes are tissue-specific.

4. On this basis it is possible to explain hereditary tumors by a slight modification of the Knudson hypothesis, suggesting that in disorders such as retinoblastoma there is one gene inherited in the germ line and a second somatic mutation then results in a tumor. On the basis of this hypothesis the germ line mutation would be for one of the regulatory loci, the somatic mutation for the other, and the double mutation would release the retinoblastoma tissue-specific transforming gene and result in retinoblastoma.

5. The literature on hybrid tumors in fish has already been explained on a similar genetic mechanism.

6. The Philadelphia chromosome can be visualized as inactivation of one regulatory locus for the myeloid cell Tr gene through a position effect involving translocation of 22p to any of several other chromosomes. The other allele could be inactivated by somatic mutation. By this proposal the approximate 10% of cases which are Philadelphia-negative would be double somatic mutants at the 22 locus. The Tr gene

for myeloid cells is presumably on chromosome 22. Results of aberrations of chromosome 14 in ataxia telangiectasia and Burkitt lymphoma suggest there may be a Tr gene for lymphocytes on chromosome 14. The association of some cases of retinoblastoma with aberrations of chromosome 13 suggest there may be a retinal Tr gene on this chromosome. The gene for Wilms' tumor may be on chromosome 8.

7. Such a proposal is also consistent with the cell hybridization studies suggesting that in many cases the malignancy behaves as a recessive trait. Diploid regulatory genes for the Tr locus would also be recessive.

8. Studies of the dinucleotide profile of tumor viruses show that they closely resemble mammalian DNA. It is not unlikely that many tumor viruses arose through the extraction of different genes from mammalian hosts, and presumably one of these genes was a host transforming gene. Reintroduction of these Tr genes into the host by an oncogenic virus could accomplish the same result as would a double somatic cell mutation of the regulatory loci controlling of the host Tr gene.

9. Such a framework is clearly consistent with the close relationship between carcinogenesis and mutagenesis.

ACKNOWLEDGMENT

This work was supported by National Institute of Health Grant GM 15886.

REFERENCE

1.   Comings, D. E. (1973): A general theory of carcinogenesis. *Proc. Natl. Acad. Sci. USA*, 70:3324–3328.

Discussion

Gerald: We appreciate your giving us one crystal clear point we can criticize, namely, the notion that one gene leading to cancer is the effect of translocation position. This is convenient, at least for debate, because it means that some individuals who are balanced carriers might then have this position effect.

Comings: That is correct.

Gerald: So, does anyone know of a balanced translocation carrier with cancer, hopefully of a familial nature, to determine whether such individuals are susceptible? They would be like hereditary retinoblastoma, that is, born with one mutant gene leading to malignancy.

Comings: I do not know of any.

Gerald: Nor do I.

Hirschhorn: Excuse me, but does it have to be a predisposition to malignancy? I think not, unless it is a very specific locus. Certainly parents who are balanced translocation carriers do not show related phenotypic abnormalities.

Gerald: I believe these are *not* familial but only sporadically occurring cases.

Hirschhorn: No, no, no. There are several reported cases of an abnormal child with the same balanced translocation as found in the phenotypically normal parent. Some people have interpreted these as possibly showing a position effect, although the French group sees them as some form of aneusomy arising by recombination.

Gerald: But, in such cases, the propositus is usually the reason for ascertainment and the first abnormal person in a family with perhaps many other normal translocation carriers. In short, I would say that at the moment there is no familial translocation associated with a predisposition to malignancy.

Riccardi: We have such a family [*Am. J. Hum. Genet.*, 27:76a (1975)]. The proband with acute myelogenous leukemia has the same reciprocal translocation found in his brother and sister and her son. The proband's mother died of visceral malignancy; but we believe she carried the translocation. Two of her sisters had cancer, one involving the breast. Their mother died of an unspecified type of leukemia. The proband had a cousin with breast cancer but normal chromosomes.

Comings: It is interesting that many acute leukemias have a double Philadelphia chromosome.

Gerald: The intriguing thing about this is the existence of two groups of individuals: those with both chromosome 22s replaced by the Ph^1 chromosome and others with three 22s of which two are Ph^1. That does not support your hypothesis.

Comings: I agree. It is probably a secondary phenomenon. It does point out, however, the value of looking for chromosomal abnormalities in hereditary tumors, and not just for the usual association with a tumor. Rather, there may be rare cases where a chromosomal abnormality results in a phenotypic mutation of a regulatory locus; such cases might help localize the position of some tumor-specific genes, like chromosome 22 in chronic myelogenous leukemia, chromosome 13 in retinoblastoma, and possibly chromosome 8 in Wilms' tumor.

Blattner: Dr. Comings, would you relate your hypothesis to the findings of Lipkin [*this volume*] concerning the relationship of these transformed phenotypes in colonic mucosa and skin fibroblasts?

Comings: It would be consistent; but, I am not certain ₁that that is a valid use of the hypothesis. There are so many ways to wiggle things that almost any observation could be made to fit.

Di Paolo: There are other ways to look at the same problem. Whereas most carcinogens can be mutagens, many mutagens are not carcinogens. Specifically, we have failed to transform human cells with the same compounds that cause few new mutations. Using ultraviolet light at certain wavelengths, Dr. Cleaver has reported a mutation rate of 10^{-5} in Chinese hamsters. The transformation frequency in Syrian hamsters was 10^{-1} [*Int. J. Radiat. Biol., in press* (1976)]. This 10^4-fold difference is hard to attribute to dominant structural genes. In sum, many data do not fit your unifying concept.

Comings: Are you sure that the high transformation rate is not explained by viral activation, for example?

Di Paolo: With Dr. Gallo, we have failed to demonstrate viral activation or the existence of virus by hybridization techniques. Now, we are left with a series of negative experiments that indicate that transformation in this system is direct and inductive, not indirect or selective [*Proc. Am. Assoc. Cancer Res.*, 17:702 (1976)].

Comings: If these high transformation rates are correct, it implies that epigenetic changes can also lead to transformation.

Genetics of Human Cancer, edited by J.J.
Mulvihill, R.W. Miller, and J.F. Fraumeni, Jr.
Raven Press, New York, 1977.

38

Genetic and Environmental Interactions in the Origin of Human Cancer

Alfred G. Knudson, Jr.

*Graduate School of Biomedical Sciences, University of Texas Health Science Center,
Houston, Texas 77030*

The most determining parameter operating in carcinogenesis is age. The great bulk of cancers occur in late adulthood and their incidences steadily increase with age. As has been noted by many investigators this increase in age-specific incidence (I) for most cancers follows a distinct pattern—it is a surprisingly simple power function of time. The age-specific prevalence *(P)*, i.e., the accumulated risk at a given age, or summed age-specific incidence, is therefore also a power function and may be formulated as $P = kt^r$, or $\ln P = r \ln t + \ln k$, i.e., the logarithm of the age-specific incidence is linearly related to the logarithm of age. On a log-log plot this curve is a straight line whose slope is r. Similarly, since $I = dP/dt = rkt^{r-1} = k't^{r-1}$, $\ln I = (r-1) \ln t + \ln k'$, and a similar plot of age-specific incidence yields a straight line of slope $(r-1)$. Any hypothesis, genetic or other, must take these patterns into account.

First of all, what happens in those instances in which a dominant gene strongly predisposes its host to cancer? For this purpose the best example is a gene that produces other phenotypic effects, thus permitting identification of its carrier, and that predisposes to a cancer known to display the aforementioned age-specific pattern. An excellent model is provided by polyposis of the colon, which inevitably gives rise to carcinoma of the colon. Mortality data for carcinoma of the colon in the white population in the United States may be compared with data on carcinoma of the colon arising in subjects with polyposis, as compiled by Ashley (3). As noted in Fig. 1 all polyposis subjects at risk developed this cancer, whereas only 3 to 4% of subjects in a general population would do so by the age of 100 years even without competing mortality (15). The ultimate risk for polyposis subjects is therefore approximately 30 times that of the general population.

In addition, carcinoma occurs much earlier in polyposis patients, so the age-specific incidence for cancer is increased more that 1,000 times for young adults. The probability of acquiring carcinoma of the colon is so high that most patients who do not undergo colectomy develop more than one carcinoma, while this is an uncommon

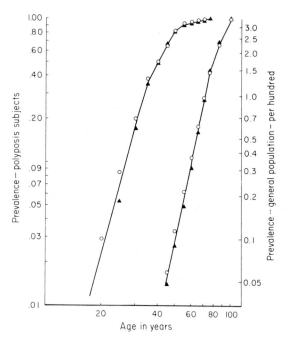

FIG. 1. Carcinoma of the colon. A comparison of the age-specific prevalences among poly-posis coli subjects *(left)* and all subjects *(right)*. (▲) Male; (○) female.

event (about 5%) in individuals who are not genetically predisposed. The curve for the general population therefore describes the rate of tumor production, but that for polyposis patients does not. The latter may be calculated if one assumes that tumor production in these individuals is a random event and that the mean number of tumors [$m(t)$] is small but continuously increasing. With these assumptions the Poisson distribution may be employed to relate age-specific prevalence, $P(t)$, and $m(t)$, as follows:

$$P(t) = P(\infty)[1 - e^{-m(t)}]$$

For each time for which $P(t)$ is known, a value of $m(t)$ may be calculated, since $P(\infty)$ may be set equal to 1.0. Now the time course of tumor development may be compared for the two populations, as shown in Fig. 2. We find that tumor production in a genetically predisposed subject is time-dependent, just as it is for nonpredisposed subjects. The slopes of the curves are not the same, however; those for the general population (male and female) are approximately 6 to 7, those for polyposis cases, approximately 4 to 5. These values differ by 2 to 3, as estimated also by Ashley (3) from the prevalence curves. We note that the mean number of tumors in polyposis exceeds 1.0 at an age when the mean number generally is 0.0005 (0.05 per 100 individuals).

   The combination of earlier onset and multiplicity is typical for dominantly inherited tumors. So also is time-dependence. From these facts two conclusions can be

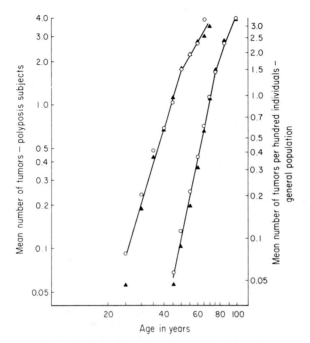

FIG. 2. Carcinoma of the colon. A comparison of tumor prevalence (mean number of tumors) among polyposis coli subjects *(left)* and all subjects *(right)*. (▲) Male; (○) female.

drawn. The first is that simple Mendelian genes can create a high probability for development of a tissue-specific tumor in the host. Secondly, at the level of the cell, tumor production is a rare event whose probability of occurrence increases with time. The inherited mutation does not itself "cause" cancer.

Earlier investigators, beginning with Muller (16) and Nordling (17), surmised that cancer may result from a sequence of mutations that occur in a single cell. If mutation is the only factor, if the population of target cells is constant with time, and if mutation rates in somatic cells are constant, then $P(t)$ should be proportional to the number of mutations required and therefore proportional to a power of time; thus if six mutations are required, $P(t)$ would be proportional to $(age)^6$. As suggested by Burch (7), this number would be smaller by one when tumor occurs in an individual who has inherited one of these mutations. But we have just noted for polyposis that the effect of inheriting a single dominant gene is to reduce the value of r by 2 to 3. This observation serves to notify us that the assumptions necessary for equivalence of r and number of mutations may not be correct.

One assumption that may never be correct is that the population of target cells is constant. This number may actually decrease at advanced age. On the other hand we have good reason to believe that for most adult tumors the susceptible cell population increases with age. This has to do with the possibility that cells that have sustained a first somatic mutation will grow into a clone of mutant cells, as suggested by Armitage and Doll (2) and by Fisher (9). This possibility then illuminates the finding noted above for polyposis that one mutation has the effect of two. In that case we know from the exuberance of polyps that mutant cells grow to a larger population than do normal colon cells. To the extent that any subsequent mutation might also exert a differential growth effect the true number of mutations would be somewhat less than the value of r, but, since one mutation is insufficient, at least two.

Another assumption that may not be correct is that somatic mutations are constant with time. If an environmental mutagen is introduced after birth then a significant increase in rate could occur. This is exemplified by lung cancer in smokers, as demonstrated by Doll (8). The slope of the age-specific incidence curve ($r - 1$) is steeper (7.5) for smokers than for nonsmokers (4.0), suggesting that more mutational steps are involved in smokers. However, when age at initiation of smoking is taken into account, the slopes are identical for the two groups ($r - 1 = 4$); smokers then differ in that the age-specific incidence curve is shifted more than 20 years.

If the dominantly inherited cancers provide evidence that at least one step in carcinogenesis is mutational, what evidence do we have to support the notion that somatic mutation plays a role in carcinogenesis? Originally this idea was developed because agents like X-rays and certain chemicals were known to be both mutagenic and carcinogenic in lower animals. Actually it has until recently been difficult to show that environmental agents exert their carcinogenic effect via mutation. We shall hear further in this session two lines of supportive evidence, which I shall only mention here. The first comes from the discovery by Dr. Cleaver that cells from patients with xeroderma pigmentosum are defective in their repair of ultraviolet-induced DNA damage. Here we have direct evidence that an environmental agent produces cancer by virtue of alteration of DNA, i.e., mutation. We note also the demonstration by Setlow and Regan (19) that N-acetoxy-2-acetylaminofluorene, a chemical carcinogen, produces damage which is not repaired by xeroderma pigmentosum cells. The second line of evidence comes from the breakthrough provided by Ames (1) with the development of a system to test for the mutagenicity of active forms of chemical carcinogens. The mass of evidence thus supports the idea that at least one somatic mutation is involved in carcinogenesis.

Although this activation of chemical carcinogens occurs in man, its efficiency is variable, due to a genetic polymorphism. Some individuals who smoke cigarettes are thought to be much more susceptible to lung cancer than others, due to a genetically enhanced activation of carcinogens by the enzyme, aryl hydrocarbon hydroxylase (11). As with xeroderma pigmentosum there is a genetic susceptibility to an environmental carcinogen. Other genetic conditions that predispose to cancer, such as Fanconi and Bloom syndromes, do so by mechanisms not yet understood at the molecular level, but known to cause chromosomal aberration. For them it is not known whether interaction with an environmental agent is involved in the carcinogenic process. It would also be of interest to know whether the excessive occurrence (5) of hepatic cancer in homozygotes, and even heterozygotes, for α_1-antitrypsin deficiency is mediated via an environmental carcinogen.

If there is evidence that at least one mutation, whether germinal or somatic, is necessary, what evidence is there that some further event on the carcinogenic pathway is mutational? Such evidence, although indirect, is available for at least two tumors (osteogenic sarcoma in hereditary retinoblastoma patients and basal cell carcinoma in the basal cell nevus syndrome) and is presented in this volume by Dr. Strong. This evidence leads us to the conclusion that a minimal requirement for any model of carcinogenesis is one which allows for two mutational events, one which can be either germinal or somatic, the other somatic. We must be cautious to note that the word "mutation" is used in its broadest context here and could include any genomic change, whether point mutation, deletion, insertion of viral genome, or other.

Environmental agents may increase these mutation rates and therefore the probability that cancer will occur. But the ability of these agents to increase mutation rates may in turn be influenced by the genetic constitution of the host. Finally, one of the mutational steps on the path to cancer can be acquired prezygotically and the rate of occurrence of that germinal mutation may be increased by environmental mutagens.

Now we must turn from the transformation of a normal cell into a tumor cell to the growth of a tumor cell into a clinical cancer, a process for which numerous factors have been implicated. Perhaps the best studied factors are hormones. Some cancers, notably breast cancer, are dependent upon one or more hormones for their growth. Such tumors may undergo somatic genetic change which relieves them of this dependence, however (12). There may also be genetic differences in endocrine metabolism that influence the elaboration of the sustaining hormone (10). And question has arisen whether environmental, perhaps dietary, factors may be influential in determining the level of such hormones (6).

This promotional phase of cancer was long ago shown to be influenced by certain chemicals (4). It is now very likely that some chemicals which increase the prospect of human cancer operate in this way. Thus asbestos workers are strongly predisposed to lung cancer. Careful analysis has shown, however, that the excessive incidence is attributable to that subset of workers who smoke cigarettes (18). Asbestos exposure alone does not seem to be predisposing but a synergism is noted for asbestos and smoking. The simplest explanation is that tobacco contains a mutagenic "initiator," and asbestos is a promoter of growth of transformed cells into clinically apparent tumors.

Other candidates for promoters include inflammatory processes such as cervicitis. But there is another kind of process which may influence cancer growth, viz., immunity. There is much argument regarding the possible role of immunity in protection against cancer, but I here only wish to note that it may be an important factor and to note further that the immune mechanisms may be modified by mutation (the immune deficiency diseases) and by environmental agents (immunosuppressive agents used in renal transplantation).

Any hypothesis on carcinogenesis must acknowledge a considerable array of interacting genetic and environmental factors. In Fig. 3 a scheme is presented which summarizes these interactions. Crucial elements are that more than one (mutational) event is necessary to transform a normal cell into a cancer cell. One of these events may be inherited and strongly predispose its host. Transformation will occur at some "background" or "spontaneous" rate in the absence of environmental carcinogens and some kinds of "carcinogenic" mutations. We should expect, therefore, to encounter a baseline incidence of cancer which is in essence an inherent biological

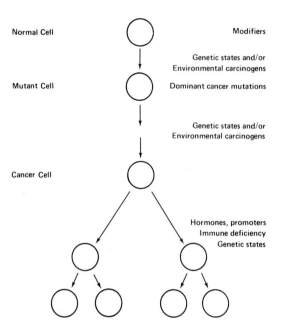

FIG. 3. The pathway to cancer. A schematic diagram relating steps in carcinogenesis to genetic, physiological, and environmental factors.

property. To the extent that increases in these rates can be avoided cancer is "preventable." The poorest prospects for prevention are therefore those tumors such as Wilms' tumor of the kidney and retinoblastoma that have a relatively constant incidence throughout the world, while the best prospects are those having large geographic variation in incidence.

Prevention must therefore be directed at identification of subjects who are genetically predisposed to cancer and of environmental agents which can increase the incidence of cancers. In addition to a group of individuals who develop cancer at a "spontaneous" or "background" rate there are three groups of predisposed individuals (14): (1) those who carry a highly penetrant cancer gene; (2) normal persons with exposure to environmental carcinogens; and (3) those persons who bear a relatively harmless mutation that renders them susceptible to environmental carcinogens. The first of these three will be relatively rare because it will be maintained in a population by the interaction of recurrent germinal mutation and natural selection. The second and third groups may both be large, especially in our contemporary chemical civilization. Since this civilization is of recent origin the third group may be rather large, but now subject to diminution by selection.

If we wish to identify genetic susceptibles and if we hope to treat the residual population of cancer subjects who are the end products of spontaneous mutation, we must learn more about the genes whose mutation leads to cancer. On both counts the study of genetically predisposed individuals and their cells should prove rewarding. Some encouragement may be taken from the possibility that the number of genetic changes on the carcinogenetic pathway may be very small. The simplest possibility is that the number is two and that cancer cells are homozygously defective for some tissue-specific developmental function (13); i.e., the multitude of cancers may be a set of single gene disorders resulting from a complex interaction of spontaneous mutation, physiological and genetic modulation, and environmental agents.

ACKNOWLEDGMENT

This work was supported in part by Medical Genetics Center Grant GM 19513 from the National Institute of General Medical Sciences.

REFERENCES

1. Ames, B. N., Durston, S. E., Yamasaki, E., and Lee, F. D. (1973): Carcinogens are mutagens: A simple test system combining liver homogenates for activation and bacteria for detection. *Proc. Natl. Acad. Sci. USA,* 70:2281–2285.
2. Armitage, P., and Doll, R. (1957): A two-stage theory of carcinogenesis in relation to the age distribution of human cancer. *Br. J. Cancer,* 11:161–169.
3. Ashley, D. J. B. (1969): Colonic cancer arising in polyposis coli. *J. Med. Genet.,* 6:376–378.
4. Berenblum, I., and Shubik, P. (1949): An experimental study of the initiating state of carcinogenesis, and a re-examination of the somatic cell mutation theory of cancer. *Br. J. Cancer,* 3: 109–118.
5. Berg, N. O., and Eriksson, S. (1972): Liver disease in adults with alpha₁—antitrypsin deficiency. *N. Engl. J. Med.,* 287:1264–1267.
6. Buell, P. (1973): Changing incidence of breast cancer in Japanese-American women. *J. Natl. Cancer Inst.,* 51:1479–1483.
7. Burch, P. R. J. (1962): A biological principle and its converse: Some implications for carcinogenesis. *Nature,* 195:241–243.
8. Doll, R. (1971): Cancer and aging: The epidemiologic evidence. In: *Oncology 1970,* Vol. 6, edited by R. L. Clark, R. W. Cumley, J. E. McCay, and M. M. Copeland, pp. 133–160. Year Book Medical, Chicago.
9. Fisher, J. C. (1958): Multiple-mutation theory of carcinogenesis. *Nature,* 181:651–652.
10. Henderson, B. E., Gerkins, V., Rosario. I., Casagrande, J., and Pike, M. C. (1975): Elevated serum levels of estrogen and prolactin in daughters of patients with breast cancer. *N. Engl. J. Med.,* 293:790–795.
11. Kellermann, G., Luyten-Kellermann, M., and Shaw, C. R. (1973): Aryl hydroxylase inducibility and bronchogenic carcinoma. *N. Engl. J. Med.,* 289:934–937.
12. Kim, U., and Depowski, M. J. (1975): Progression from hormone dependence to autonomy in mammary tumors as an in vivo manifestation of sequential clonal selection. *Cancer Res.,* 35:2068–2077.
13. Knudson, A. G. (1973): Mutation and human cancer. *Adv. Cancer Res.,* 17:317–352.
14. Knudson, A. G.: Mutation and cancer in man. *Cancer (in press).*
15. Mason, T. J., McKay, F. W., Hoover, R., Blot, W. J., and Fraumeni, J. F., Jr. (1975): *Atlas of Cancer Mortality for US Counties: 1950-1969. DHEW Publication No. (NIH) 75–780:75.*
16. Muller, H. J. (1951): Radiation damage to the genetic material. *Sci. Prog.,* 7:93–165, 481–493 [references].
17. Nordling, C. O. (1953): A new theory on the cancer-inducing mechanism. *Br. J. Cancer,* 7:68–72.
18. Selikoff, I. J., Hammond, E. C., and Churg, J. (1968): Asbestos exposure, smoking and neoplasia. *JAMA,* 204:106–112.
19. Setlow, R. B., and Regan, J. D. (1972): Defective repair of *N* acetoxy-2-acetylaminofluorene-induced lesions in the DNA of xeroderma pigmentosum cells. *Biochem. Biophys. Res. Commun.,* 46:1019–1024.

Discussion

Gerald: If homozygosity is the goal, then you should make comparisons with xeroderma pigmentosum (XP). Yet retinoblastoma does not seem to follow that kind of model, does it?

Knudson: At the cell level, retinoblastoma or polyposis of the colon may be the result of being homozygous; but, if a person inherits the pair of genes, he might just become a tumor *in utero*. XP is a different kind of problem because it does not represent one of the changes in the carcinogenic pathway, according to my hypothesis. Perhaps it is a gene that accelerates each of the steps that goes into making cancer cells.

Gerald: However, if homozygosity is essential, then you have literally one single locus to hit, and the probability of that is very small. If you have multiple other loci that could interact with the retinoblastoma locus, then you have many more loci that could be hit. The point becomes, at least numerically, quite important.

Knudson: We are talking about rare events, but there are lots of cells. The developing retina probably has millions of cells, so even though the mutation rate may be in the order of magnitude of 10^{-6}, if a person has inherited the first mutation, the chance that one or more cells will have the second mutation occur at the same locus becomes rather high. Our estimate is that for retinoblastoma the mean number of tumors of such carriers is three to four. So we are talking about a mutation rate of about 3 to 4×10^{-6} or 10^{-7}, which should not be unreasonable.

Nance: Dr. Knudson, I do not understand why you do not consider XP to be an example of your hypothesis. The only difference seems to be that in XP you know what the mechanism is. If you didn't know it, XP would simply be a condition in which two mutations inevitably caused cancer. Also, I wonder whether it is not a misnomer to talk about dominant cancer syndromes, if you really believe they require two mutations, possibly even homozygosity. The distinction between the so-called dominant cancer syndromes and the recessive ones like XP might be the number of loci at which the second mutation could occur. Perhaps in the dominantly inherited conditions the second mutation can occur at any of a large number of loci so that a person who has a first one inevitably develops the cancer. However, in the recessive conditions, the second mutation has to be locus-specific.

Knudson: In XP I am struck by the fact that one can protect against ultraviolet light and not get cancer. We know that the pathogenic mechanism influences rates of mutations, so I do not see any strong argument in favor of relating XP to the hypothesis. Not every cell becomes a cancer cell. It just seems to be a simpler hypothesis to assume that in XP each of the steps involved in changing a normal cell into a cancer cell is occurring at a much greater rate because the damage cannot be repaired.

Sanford: Your definition of mutation seems a little broader than usual if you include the presence of a virus in the genetic information. What do you mean by mutation?

Knudson: I use the original definition, that is, a change in the genome.

Sanford: Would your definition allow for an aberrant differentiation that gives rise to some cancers? Many workers are not convinced that cancer necessarily involves a specific mutation, but suggest that aberrant differentiation and epigenetic effects can also produce some forms of cancer.

Harnden: Could I follow on that point? Even if you suppose that in retinoblastoma you must have two mutational events, you must also have a third event: that is, differentiation along the correct pathway. If you require only two mutational events, you would have a prezygotic mutation in all cells of the body, and the second event could presumably occur in any other cell of the body. But you also must have differentiation into the appropriate cell type. So you have three events, even in retinoblastoma.

Knudson: You must have cell growth with multiplication.

Harnden: But you have to have more than that, namely, differentiation to the retinal cells, which sums to three events. Also, I think that it is wrong to make the assumption that, even supposing that two mutational events do occur, this necessarily leads to a neoplasm. There must be many occasions in which two mutational events occur plus differentiation, and then these cells are lost because of control mechanisms by the host. So to postulate only two mutational events seems a gross oversimplification.

Knudson: It may be. What I am trying to suggest is that if a small number of events occur, then it is worth thinking of cancer as a single gene process. For example, neuroblastoma or retinoblastoma may result when a person becomes homozygous for a mutant gene that in the normal state provides for differentiation of a blast cell into a normal cell. Homozygosity for the mutant gene, however, prevents the cell from differentiating in the normal way. The person then continues to have a primitive cell that grows into a tumor. On the other hand, leaky mutants might exist. You would then have some control, so that certain cells would develop tumors, such as neuroblastoma, which might then differentiate into ganglioneuroma or even disappear. So we would expect a wide spectrum of mutant phenotypes.

Harnden: I accept the importance of mutation, but to say that it is the only event of importance cannot be correct.

Jackson: In our patients with medullary thyroid carcinoma—the endocrine neoplasia type 2 syndrome—we have interpreted the C cell hyperplasia as resulting from the first mutational event, with the second mutational event producing medullary thyroid carcinoma. However, the ratio of affected to unaffected individuals so closely fits the 1:1 ratio expected for a dominant gene that the factors promoting the second event must be ubiquitous. Would you agree with that concept?

Knudson: I would like to have Dr. Fialkow find out whether the hyperplasia in medullary thyroid cancer is of single-cell origin. It seems to be a crucial question. Is it just once in a while that a cell or group of cells will become hyperplastic, without further events occurring by chance? We do not know, but there is some evidence that the carcinomas have a clonal origin [*Science*, 193:321–323 (1976)]. I believe that is the first demonstration that a person who has inherited a dominant gene has a tumor with single-cell origin.

Fialkow: That is correct.

Rowley: We have emphasized in the past the occurrence of chromosome abnormalities in leukemia. We should not lose sight of the fact that chromosome abnormalities occur also in potentially leukemic conditions. These defects can be quite stable over a period of time. They occur in roughly 10% of patients with unexplained hematologic disorders. In my own experience patients have gone from 1½ to 3 years with a majority of their bone marrow cells having chromosome abnormalities, frequently an extra chromosome 8 without exhibiting leukemic manifestations. All the patients who later develop acute leukemia show the same chromosome abnormalities at the time of the leukemic episode as they did prior to leukemia. If you look at a different group of hematologic disorders, particularly polycythemia vera, many patients live 10 years with chromosomal abnormalities and still have polycythemia and nothing else. So some of the events can take a long time to develop.

Genetics of Human Cancer, edited by J. J.
Mulvihill, R. W. Miller, and J. F. Fraumeni, Jr.
Raven Press, New York, 1977.

39

Theories of Pathogenesis: Mutation and Cancer

Louise C. Strong

Graduate School of Biomedical Sciences,
The University of Texas Health Science Center, Houston, Texas 77030,
and The University of Texas System Cancer Center,
M. D. Anderson Hospital and Tumor Institute, Houston, Texas 77030

CARCINOGENESIS: MUTATION AS A PRIMARY EVENT

There is a great deal of evidence that most known carcinogens, including chemicals, radiation, or viruses, are also mutagens in the broad sense of causing some genomic change (1,56,74). At least one disorder, xeroderma pigmentosum, predisposes to cancer through a defect in DNA repair (15,46, and *this volume*), greatly increasing the probability both of mutation and of cancer. Further, study of dominantly inherited tumors demonstrates that a single genetic change may vastly increase the probability of tumor development (42). Of course, a primary mutational model for carcinogenesis presupposes a single cell origin for cancer, as discussed by Dr. Fialkow *(this volume)*.

CARCINOGENESIS: A MULTISTAGE PROCESS WITH A MINIMUM OF TWO STEPS

Age-specific incidence studies have in general indicated that carcinogenesis is a multistage process, which might be explained by a minimum of two steps (4). Evidence from studies of chemical carcinogenesis (5), radiation carcinogenesis (53), and dominantly inherited tumors (42) have also suggested a two-step model for carcinogenesis. The second step apparently occurs with a frequency similar to that of a mutation (42). If one can assume from the vast evidence that one essential step is mutational, what is known about the subsequent step(s)?

One might examine that question by looking at the effect of mutagens on those individuals who have inherited the first mutation which predisposes to a specific tumor. One mutagen to which those individuals might be exposed, and the mutagenic effects observed, is radiation. Therefore, it is appropriate to review briefly some characteristics of radiation carcinogenesis.

RADIATION CARCINOGENESIS: GENERAL CONSIDERATIONS

While it is well known from *in vitro* studies that radiation can cause mutation (56), there is also *in vivo* evidence that the primary role of radiation in carcinogenesis is in the induction of mutation (70,71). Many studies involving laboratory animals (47,53) as well as human populations indicate that radiation does not cause new or unique diseases or mutations but increases the incidence of certain spontaneously occurring diseases (21,47,53). With carcinogenesis in particular, there is evidence from studies of experimental mice (53), from studies of those exposed to radiation *in utero* from obstetric X-rays (7), from those treated with radiation for benign conditions such as enlarged thymus gland in infancy (31) or ankylosing spondylitis at a later age (54), and from those survivors of the atomic bomb (36) that radiation does not cause unique malignancies but increases the incidence of those spontaneously occurring. Those "extra" radiogenic malignancies reflect the characteristics of the spontaneous malignancy with respect to demographic variables including age, sex, ethnic group, environmental exposure, and other known risk factors. Further, radiation-induced malignancies are similar in their histology and their biologic behavior to spontaneously occurring malignancies.

While it is well established that radiation increases the risk of spontaneously occurring tumors, there is debate over whether the increase is relative to the spontaneous incidence, or absolute (21). At present, although there are many variables outstanding, recent data appear to favor the relative increase model. Such data include:

1. Experimental studies by Mole (53) in radiation carcinogenesis in CBA mice revealed that the age-specific incidence of tumors increased in constant proportion for all ages.

2. Studies of the risk of cancer in those exposed *in utero* due to obstetric radiography revealed an increased risk of each childhood cancer in proportion to its spontaneous incidence (7).

3. Studies of the differences in the age-specific incidence of leukemia in Japanese atomic bomb survivors and English ankylosing spondylitics revealed that the age-specific incidence of radiogenic leukemia paralleled that of spontaneous leukemia in each population (18).

4. Study of thyroid cancer in those treated with radiation in infancy for thymic enlargement revealed an increased incidence of thyroid cancer in proportion to risk factors relevant to spontaneous thyroid cancer, including age, sex, and ethnic group (31).

5. Study of the interaction of radiation with other carcinogens through study of lung cancer in uranium miners and atomic bomb survivors revealed a multiplicative increase in the incidence of lung cancer in those who also smoked (65).

One apparent exception to the generalization that radiation acts to multiply the spontaneous incidence of cancer may be the absence of an excess of gastric carcinoma in Japanese survivors who were adults at the time of the atomic bomb (21,35). However, an excess of gastric carcinoma was observed in those exposed to the atomic bomb as children (37). The increased incidence of gastric carcinoma in those receiving radiation for ankylosing spondylitis in England suggests that the stomach is not insensitive to radiation, although that cancer might be attributed to the medication and high dosage of radiation to which that population was exposed (21).

If indeed radiation in general simply increases the spontaneous incidence of cancer, radiation carcinogenesis may reflect mechanisms or pathways operative in spontaneous carcinogenesis.

RADIATION CARCINOGENESIS AND A TWO-MUTATION MODEL

Studies in experimental radiation carcinogenesis as well as observations on radiogenic malignancy in man suggested to Mole (53) that more than a single mutation was necessary for carcinogenesis. Critical observations included:

1. The long latent period for most cancers independent of the dosage;
2. Saturation kinetics of the dose-response curve for radiation carcinogenesis;
3. An increased incidence of tumors in subjects receiving multiple exposures as compared to a single exposure of the same total radiation dose; and
4. The multiplicative effects of radiation in cancer induction in interaction with other carcinogens or risk factors.

The above observations led Mole to conclude that carcinogenesis was a two-step mutational process in which either step might occur spontaneously, might be induced by another carcinogen, or by radiation.

If radiation can increase the probability of either of two sequential mutagenic events critical to the development of cancer, then radiogenic tumors should occur in two distinct populations, one of which already has experienced the first mutational event.

Radiation and the First Mutational Step

Since the mutational events leading to cancer are rare at the cellular level, as described by Knudson in this volume, most of the exposed population will not have acquired the first step, and the role of radiation in carcinogenesis will be to induce the first mutation. The incidence of cancer in this population will depend on the likelihood of their acquiring the second mutation. This is another rare event, and thus one would anticipate a long latent period. The age-specific incidence curve for a radiogenic cancer should then parallel that of spontaneous cancer, each reflecting the probability of acquiring the second step, and thus maintaining the same demographic and age-specific characteristics. Exposure to other carcinogens would be expected to have a synergistic and multiplicative effect on cancer incidence.

Radiation and the Second Mutational Step

Occasionally one may encounter individuals who already have acquired or inherited the first mutational step in an exposed tissue. In this subpopulation one might anticipate the radiogenic tumor incidence to be high and the latent period relatively short. The incidence of radiogenic malignancy apparently depends on the total radiation dose, number of exposures, type of exposure, age at exposure, specific sensitivity of exposed tissues, and interaction with other carcinogens or risk factors related to spontaneous cancers. Thus, comparisons of the incidence of radiogenic tumors in populations not matched for the above variables is probably meaningless. However, the latent period for radiogenic malignancy in those exposed after birth is apparently independent of those variables with the exception of tissue specificity, and that primarily in differentiating between radiogenic leukemia with a relatively short latent period and other radiogenic tumors (21,31,36,58,63). Thus, the latent period might be comparable among populations receiving varying radiation exposures at varying ages, and may reflect sequential steps in carcinogenesis. Two disorders in which there is a tissue-specific hereditary predisposition to tumor and a frequent exposure to radiation are hereditary retinoblastoma and the nevoid basal cell carcinoma syndrome.

Hereditary Retinoblastoma

Retinoblastoma has been attributed by Knudson (42) to a two-step mutational model in which the first step may be inherited. The hereditary fraction includes all bilateral and a small fraction of unilateral retinoblastoma patients. Because most bilateral but only occasional unilateral patients receive radiation therapy, the subsequent discussion will be based on data from radiation exposure in patients with bilateral retinoblastoma.

The gene which predisposes to retinoblastoma increases the probability of retinoblastoma in a gene carrier by approximately 100,000 times. However, to a much lesser extent it also increases the probability of spontaneous osteogenic and other sarcomas (41). The mean number of retinoblastoma tumors for a gene carrier is three; the mean number of sarcomas may be less than 0.05.

Patients with bilateral retinoblastoma are frequently reported to develop radiogenic tumors. One might consider the characteristics of these radiogenic tumors with respect to the tumor type and the latent period as defined by the interval between initial radiation exposure and diagnosis of radiogenic malignancy. Of course there is no absolute control group matched with respect to age at treatment, type and number of treatments, treatment field, etc., in which all but the genetic background are comparable. However, as described above, the latent period may provide a valuable reference for differences in subsequent carcinogenic events following radiation.

To avoid reporting bias toward those radiogenic malignancies which occur soon after radiation exposure, one might consider radiogenic malignancy in patients ascertained through the primary disease and followed for an appropriate interval. Table 1 includes data on two such series of survivors of childhood cancer treated with radiation. Data were collected from a large series of survivors of bilateral retinoblastoma followed for up to 38 years (63) and from a series of long-term survivors of childhood malignancy followed for up to 24 years (48). In each series there were radiogenic malignancies observed during the interval (Tables 2 and 3). In general,

TABLE 1. *Radiogenic malignancy in survivors of childhood cancer[a]*

	Bilateral retinoblastoma[63]	Childhood malignancy[48]
Number of survivors[b]	243	288
Age at treatment (yrs)		
Range	<4	0–17
Median	Not stated	<4
Dose (rads)		
Range	3,500–18,000	200–8,000
Median	<6000	Not stated
Mean	Not stated	2,600
Follow-up (yrs)		
Range	4–38	4–24
Median	14	13
Radiogenic malignancy		
Number	21	14
Frequency	8.6%	4.9%
Latent period (yrs)[c]		
Median	11	14
Range	4–30	6–21
Peak	5–6	15–19

[a]Ascertained through primary malignancy.
[b]Five year survivors who received radiation.
[c]Interval between initial radiation exposure and diagnosis of radiogenic malignancy.

patients with retinoblastoma received a much higher total radiation dose, although those with other childhood malignancies had larger treatment fields. Although radiation factors are certainly not directly comparable, in each series more than 1,000 rads were given each patient who developed a radiogenic malignancy.

Although tumor type is influenced by total radiation dose and the numbers are very small, it may be noteworthy that radiogenic sarcomas were more common among survivors of bilateral retinoblastoma (67% of radiogenic malignancy) than among

TABLE 2. *Radiogenic malignancy in survivors of childhood cancer [a]: Primary and radiogenic tumor types*

Primary tumor	No. with radiogenic malignancy	No. with radiogenic sarcoma
Wilms' tumor	4	1
Neuroblastoma	2	0
Sarcoma, bone	3	1
Sarcoma, soft-tissue	3	2
Lymphoma	2	1
Total	14	5

[a]Ascertained through ref. 48.

TABLE 3. *Radiogenic malignancy in survivors of childhood cancer*[a]

Radiogenic malignancy	Bilateral retinoblastoma[(63)]		Childhood cancer[(48)]	
	No. cases	%	No. cases	%
Osteogenic sarcoma	9	43.0	0	
Soft-tissue sarcoma	5	24.0	5	35.7
Thyroid carcinoma	2	9.5	3	21.4
Acute leukemia	0		2	14.3
Skin carcinoma (basal and squamous cell carcinoma)	3	14.0	1	7.1
Adenocarcinoma of breast	0		2	14.3
Other	2[b]	9.5	1[c]	7.1
Total	21	100.0	14	100.0

[a] Ascertained through primary malignancy.
[b] Malignant mesenchymoma and malignant fibrous histiocytoma.
[c] Hepatoma.

survivors of other childhood malignancy (35.7% of radiogenic malignancy) (Table 3).

Of greater significance is comparison of the latent period for radiogenic malignancy following primary childhood cancer (Fig. 1). Although the period of follow-up was longer for patients with retinoblastoma, and no leukemia with the characteristic short latent period was observed, the latent period for radiogenic malignancy in patients with bilateral retinoblastoma was shorter with a unique peak incidence in the fifth and sixth posttreatment years. Radiogenic malignancies in survivors of other childhood cancers most often showed a latent period greater than 15 years despite their short follow-up period, an interval similar to that of children exposed to the atomic bomb (37) or thymic irradiation in infancy (31). The observed peak incidence of radiogenic malignancy 15 to 19 years after exposure in survivors of childhood malignancy may further increase or shift with longer follow-up.

Because different tissues may have characteristic latent periods, and the retinoblastoma predisposition may be specific for sarcoma, it is important to examine the latent period for radiogenic sarcoma in general.

To provide adequate numbers of cases for analysis requires a collection of cases from the literature ascertained largely by the radiogenic malignancy. Patients were included in the series only if sarcoma arose from normal bone or soft tissue following external radiation. The primary disease for which radiation was administered in 92 cases of subsequent radiogenic malignancies was benign in 29 cases and malignant in 63. Twenty-four cases were exposed during childhood. Most were exposed to greater than 1,000 rads (2,10,12,14,17,20,25,29,30,38,48,51,58,60,62,66,67,69,73). Although the series of radiogenic sarcomas is obviously heterogeneous with respect to age and radiation exposure, as discussed previously, the latent period may not be influenced by those variables.

To avoid referral and publication bias toward those who developed radiogenic tumors after a very short period, all radiogenic sarcomas following retinoblastoma

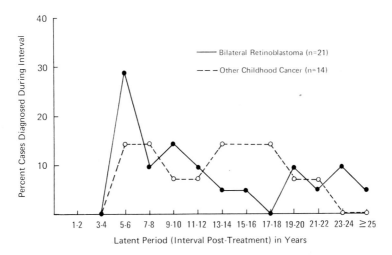

FIG 1. Latent period for radiogenic malignancy in survivors of childhood cancer ascertained through primary cancer. A comparison of the percentage of radiogenic malignancies diagnosed versus the interval in years from the time of initial radiation exposure to diagnosis of the radiogenic malignancy (latent period) for survivors of childhood cancers, bilateral retinoblastoma (63), or other childhood malignancy (48; Table 2).

were also collected from the literature (3,11,12,14,19,22-24,30,39,40,43-45,59,68,72,75,76) and the International Childhood Cancer Inventory [data collected by A. T. Meadows for the Late Effects Study Group, which includes one unpublished case from Philadelphia, three from Columbus, and seven from M. D. Anderson Hospital; A. T. Meadows et al., *in preparation*]. The latent period for radiogenic sarcomas in these two groups can be seen in Fig. 2. Again the rapid rate at which radiogenic sarcomas developed in children with retinoblastoma is evident. Radiogenic sarcomas were diagnosed in retinoblastoma patients at the most rapid rate from the fourth to sixth posttreatment years, and 50% were diagnosed by eight years posttreatment. Other patients developing radiogenic sarcomas did so at a more constant rate over the period of years observed following the fifth posttreatment year.

For no other solid radiogenic malignancy is there such a short interval (four to six years) between radiation exposure and peak incidence of radiogenic malignancy (18,26,54). The short interval is apparently not a biologic characteristic of radiation sarcomas, as they have not appeared early in survivors of the atomic bomb (37), patients treated for ankylosing spondylitis (20,53), or cases reported in the literature (Fig. 2). Further, it is not a consequence of childhood radiation exposure as solid tumors arising following thymic radiation (31), exposure to the atomic bomb (37), treatment for other childhood malignancy (48), or even obstetric X-ray (7) do not show this characteristic. One may conclude, therefore, that the patients with bilateral retinoblastoma represent that unique subgroup who have inherited the first mutational step predisposing to sarcoma and provide the opportunity to observe radiation effects on the subsequent events. Allowing for cell genera-

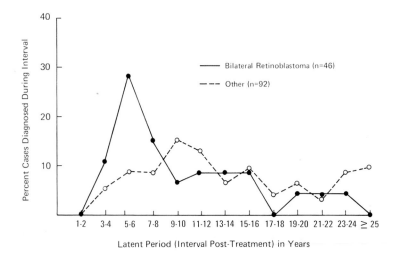

FIG. 2. Latent period in radiogenic sarcoma. A comparison of the percentage of radiogenic sarcomas diagnosed versus the interval in years from the time of initial radiation exposure to diagnosis of radiogenic sarcoma arising from normal bone treated with external radiation in 46 patients treated for retinoblastoma and 92 patients treated for various other malignant and benign disorders.

tion time from initiation to diagnosis of malignancy, the evidence is compatible with radiation providing the second mutation in the carcinogenic pathway.

Nevoid Basal Cell Carcinoma Syndrome

There is a second example of radiation carcinogenesis in a genetically predisposed population, that of the nevoid basal cell carcinoma syndrome. In this syndrome the gene predisposes to multiple systemic anomalies, the characteristic nevoid basal cell carcinomas, dentigerous cysts, and other less frequent neoplasms including medulloblastomas and ovarian fibromas. Due to genetic and environmental heterogeneity, as well as age-related factors among patients with the nevoid basal cell carcinoma syndrome, it is difficult to estimate the mean number of basal cell carcinomas which develop spontaneously in gene carriers; however, it may be in the range of 100. Although many may receive radiation following the onset of spontaneous tumors, the group in which radiation effects are most pronounced are those who develop medulloblastoma and are treated with radiation to the cranium and spinal axis in childhood.

There are now 11 such cases reported (27,28,32,33,52,55,57) and the following new case from the M. D. Anderson series.

Case Report.

L.M.B., a Caucasian female, was born June 26, 1967, after normal gestation, labor, and delivery. She reached normal developmental milestones during the first year of life, but thereafter showed some regression. At eighteen months of age she developed ataxia and signs of increased intracranial pressure which progressed until she was hospitalized

June 2, 1969. She was found to have obstruction of the fourth ventricle and underwent subtotal craniectomy with posterior fossa exploration and subtotal removal of a medulloblastoma of the vermis. At that time she was noted to have congenital rib anomalies. During the next two months she received radiation to the entire neural axis, including 2,350 roentgens in air to the calvarium and 3,000 roentgens in air to the cervical, thoracic, and lumbar spinal areas. Six months later, her parents noted eruptions of pigmented nevi on her neck, axillae, lumbosacral and intergluteal areas.

For the next several years, the patient did well although the skin lesions increased in size and number. She was referred to the M. D. Anderson Hospital in August, 1972, for consideration of prophylactic chemotherapy with respect to the medulloblastoma. There was no evidence of recurrence and further treatment was declined.

In July of 1973, biopsy of skin lesions from the occipital and temporal scalp areas and neck revealed basal cell carcinomas. Lesions on one side of her neck were removed with a plastic planing procedure.

The patient did not return to the M. D. Anderson Hospital from August, 1972, until July, 1974, when she required treatment for mandibular cysts. At that time, diagnosis of the nevoid basal cell carcinoma syndrome was made based on history and clinical findings which included a large head with hypertelorism and frontal bossing, palmar pits, multiple pigmented lesions of the occipital scalp, collar area about the neck, axillae, parallel fields down the vertebral axis, and intergluteal areas (Figs. 3-4). X-ray examinations in 1974 and 1975 revealed calcification of the falx cerebri and tentorium, bridging of the sella turcica, supernumerary teeth, multiple mandibular cysts, bilateral congenital anomalies of the ribs of fusion and bifurcation, and anomalous development of the midspine including hemivertebrae of T-2. There was no evidence of the nevoid basal cell carcinoma syndrome on clinical or X-ray examination of either parent, and no family history suggestive of the syndrome.

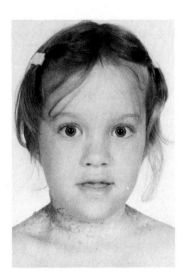
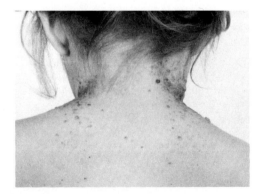

FIG. 3. Patient L. M. B. in July, 1974, age seven years. **Left:** The characteristic facies of the nevoid basal cell carcinoma syndrome, the concentration of skin lesions around the neck (except in the left anterior aspect previously treated by a plastic procedure), and the sparing of the facial areas most frequently spontaneously affected in patients with the nevoid basal cell carcinoma syndrome. **Right:** The distribution of skin lesions on neck and back.

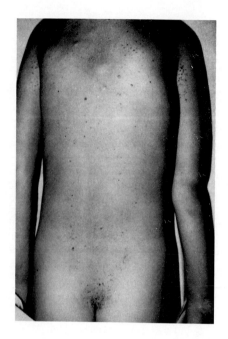

FIG. 4. Patient L. M. B. in December, 1975, showing distribution of skin lesions in the irradiated spinal and intergluteal areas.

The patient was followed at regular intervals for recurrent mandibular cysts and progression of the skin lesions. In April, 1975, she returned with a large, firm pelvic mass to the right of the midline. Exploratory laparotomy revealed a large right ovarian mass and a nodular left ovary. Right salpingo-oophorectomy with multiple biopsies of the left ovary were performed. The histologic report was multiple fibrosarcomas arising from ovarian fibromas. The patient is now six months postsurgery without evidence of recurrence.

Nevoid Basal Cell Carcinoma Syndrome and Radiation Carcinogenesis

·Among reported cases and those at the M. D. Anderson Hospital, all survivors of the nevoid basal cell carcinoma syndrome and medulloblastoma have developed a characteristic distribution of skin lesions (histologically basal cell carcinomas) from six months to three years posttreatment. These lesions are concentrated in the neck, shoulders, spinal areas, axillae, and scalp. This distribution of lesions is unlike that encountered in the syndrome in general, or in affected relatives of these patients (see case 1,57). The lesions have appeared at the very early ages of two to six years, and they demonstrate aggressive biologic behavior typical of the basal cell carcinomas encountered in the nevoid basal cell carcinoma syndrome.

Our case report is the only reported female survivor of the nevoid basal cell carcinoma syndrome and medulloblastoma known to the author. While ovarian fibromas are not uncommon in the syndrome (16), they have not been reported in prepubertal females. Fibrosarcoma of the jaw has been reported in a patient with the nevoid basal cell carcinoma syndrome following radiation (6).

TABLE 4. *Radiogenic malignancy in patients with medulloblastoma*[a]

No. cases	Tumor type	Latent period (yrs)
3	Thyroid adenocarcinoma	7–12
1	Fibrosarcoma of brain	8
1	Acute leukemia	1

[a] From ref. 50.

There is no large series of survivors with medulloblastoma in the absence of the nevoid basal cell carcinoma syndrome for comparison. Isolated case reports of patients with medulloblastoma and radiogenic malignancy have been encountered (Table 4) (50). However, there is nothing to suggest that, in general, patients with medulloblastoma are uniquely predisposed to radiogenic basal cell carcinomas or fibrosarcomas (Tables 4 and 5).

The latent period for radiogenic basal cell carcinoma in general is greater than 10 years, and is not related to age at exposure, total radiation dosage, or number of treatments (49,58). Although the radiogenic tumors are frequently multiple, a mean number of five has been reported (49), as contrasted to the hundreds developing in patients with the nevoid basal cell carcinoma syndrome (Figs. 3-4). Radiogenic basal cell carcinomas following other childhood malignancy, spinal radiation (ankylosing spondylitis), or benign disease in childhood do not demonstrate such multiplicity or early onset (Table 5). Instead, the evidence overwhelmingly suggests that those patients with the nevoid basal cell carcinoma syndrome represent a special subgroup with a hereditary predisposition to basal cell carcinoma in whom radiation may supply the subsequent mutation for tumor development and thus lead to a rapid onset of multiple radiogenic basal cell carcinomas.

TABLE 5. *Radiogenic basal cell carcinoma*

Series	No. of cases	Age at exposure (yrs)	Dose (rads)	Latent period (yrs)[d] Median	Range
Childhood malignancy (Table 2;[48])	1 in 288[a]	<1	3,100		21
Bilateral retinoblastoma[63]	1 in 243[a]	5	2,400		9
Medulloblastoma[b(8,9,13,34,50)]	1 in 95[a]	7	3,000–4,000		13
Ankylosing spondylitis [64]	5	17–37	2,000–8,875	23	11–28
X-ray epilation[61]	6	4–9	NS[c]	44	7–56
Benign disease of head and neck[49]	227	1–73 40%<21	NS[c]	23	1–64 94% > 10

[a] Five year survivors who received radiation.
[b] No evidence of the nevoid basal cell carcinoma syndrome.
[c] Not stated.
[d] Interval between initial radiation exposure and diagnosis of radiogenic malignancy.

CONCLUSION

If one assumes that radiation exerts its carcinogenic effect primarily through mutation, then the appearance of specific tumors to which one is genetically predisposed within a very short time following radiation may be considered evidence for two mutational steps in carcinogenesis. According to this model, the first mutation may be inherited or acquired; the second would always be acquired. Either step may occur spontaneously or be induced by environmental mutagens. Studies of those individuals who inherit the first mutation may reveal important characteristics of the sequential steps in carcinogenesis in general.

ACKNOWLEDGMENT

This research was supported in part by Medical Genetics Center Grant GM-19513 from The National Institute of General Medical Sciences.

REFERENCES

1. Ames, B. N., Durston, W. E., Yamasaki, E., and Lee, F. D. (1973): Carcinogens are mutagens: A simple test system combining liver homogenates for activation and bacteria for detection. *Proc. Natl. Acad. Sci. USA,* 70:2281–2285.
2. Arlen, M., Higinbotham, N. L., Huvos, A. G., Marcove, R. C., Miller, T., and Shah, I. C. (1971): Radiation-induced sarcoma of bone. *Cancer,* 28:1087–1099.
3. Arlen, M., Shah, I. C., Higinbotham, N., and Huvos, A. J. (1972): Osteogenic sarcoma of head and neck induced by radiation therapy. *NY State J. Med.,* 72:929–934.
4. Armitage, P., and Doll, R. (1957): A two-stage theory of carcinogenesis in relation to the age distribution of human cancer. *Br. J. Cancer,* 11:161–169.
5. Berenblum, I. (1941): The mechanism of carcinogenesis. A study of the significance of cocarcinogenic action and related phenomena. *Cancer Res.,* 1:807–814.
6. Binkley, G. W., and Johnson, H. H. (1951): Epithelioma adenoides cysticum: Basal cell nevi, agenesis of the corpus callosum and dental cysts. *A.M.A. Arch. Dermatol. Syph.,* 63:73–84.
7. Bithell, J. F., and Stewart, A. M. (1975): Pre-natal irradiation and childhood malignancy: A review of British data from the Oxford survey. *Br. J. Cancer,* 31:271–287.
8. Bloom, H. J. G., Wallace, E. N. K., and Henk, J. M. (1969) The treatment and prognosis of medulloblastoma in children. *Am. J. Roentgenol. Radium Ther. Nucl. Med.,* 105:43–62.
9. Bouchard, J., and Peirce, C. B. (1960): Radiation therapy in the management of neoplasms of the central nervous system, with a special note in regard to children: Twenty years' experience, 1939–1958. *Am. J. Roentgenol. Radium Ther. Nucl. Med.,* 84:610–628.
10. Cade, S. (1957): Radiation induced cancer in man. *Br. J. Radiol.,* 30:393–402.
11. Cahan, W. G., Woodard, H. Q., Higinbotham, N. L., Stewart, F. W., and Coley, B. L. (1948): Sarcoma arising in irradiated bone. *Cancer,* 1:3–29.
12. Castro, L., Choi, S.H., and Sheehan, F. R. (1967): Radiation induced bone sarcomas. *Am. J. Roentgenol. Radium Ther. Nucl. Med.,* 100:924–930.
13. Chatty, E. M., and Earle, K. M. (1971): Medulloblastoma. A report of 201 cases with emphasis on the relationship of histologic variants to survival. *Cancer,* 28:977–983.
14. Chavanne, G., Calle, R., and Gricouroff, G. (1970): Bone cancers induced by external irradiation: A few observations. In: *European Association of Radiology Symposium Ossium,* edited by A. M. Jelliffe and B. Strickland, pp. 204–207. E. and S. Livingstone, London.
15. Cleaver, J. E. (1968): Defective repair replication of DNA in xeroderma pigmentosum. *Nature,* 218:652–656.
16. Clendenning, W. E., Herdt, J. R., and Block, J. B. (1963): Ovarian fibromas and mesenteric cysts: Their association with hereditary basal cell cancer of the skin. *Am. J. Obstet. Gynecol.,* 87:1008–1012.
17. Cruz, M., Coley, B.L., and Stewart, F.W. (1957): Postradiation bone sarcoma. *Cancer,* 10:72–88.

18. Doll, R. (1971): Cancer and aging: The epidemiologic evidence. In: *Oncology 1970,* Vol. 6, edited by R. L. Clark, R. W. Cumley, J. E. McCoy, and M. M. Copeland, pp. 1–28. Year Book Medical, Chicago.

19. van Dongen, J.A., Montanari, G., and van Slooten, E. A. (1961): Oorspronkelijke stukken: Sarcomen van het skelet, onstaan na intensieve röntgenbestraling. *Ned. Tijdschr. Geneeskd.,* 105:1128–1134.

20. Edgar, M. A., and Robinson, M. P. (1973): Post-radiation sarcoma in ankylosing spondylitis. *J. Bone Joint Surg.,* 55B:183–188.

21. *Effects on Populations of Exposure to Low Levels of Ionizing Radiation. Report of the Advisory Committee on the Biological Effects of Ionizing Radiations* (1972): NAS-NRC, Washington, D.C. pp. 1–217.

22. Fabrikant, J. T., Dickson, R. J., and Fetter, B. F. (1964): Mechanisms of radiation carcinogenesis at the clinical level. *Br. J. Cancer,* 18:459–477.

23. Forrest, A. W. (1961): Tumors following radiation about the eye. *J. Am. Acad. Ophthal. Otolaryn.,* 65:694–717.

24. Frezzotti, F., and Guerra, R. (1963): Sarcoma following irradiated retinoblastoma. *Arch. Ophthalmol.,* 70:471–473.

25. Goldberg, M. B., Sheline, G. E., and Malamud, N. (1963): Malignant intracranial neoplasms following radiation therapy for acromegaly. *Radiology,* 80:465–470.

26. Goolden, A. W. G. (1972): Pharyngeal malignancy following irradiation of the neck. *Br. J. Radiol.,* 45:795.

27. Gorlin, R. J., Vickers, R. A., Kelln, E., and Williamson, J. J. (1965): The multiple basal-cell nevi syndrome. *Cancer,* 18:89–104.

28. Graham, J. K., McJimsey, B. A., and Hardin, J. C. (1968): Nevoid basal cell carcinoma syndrome. *Arch. Otolaryngol.,* 87:90–95.

29. Hatcher, C. H. (1945): The development of sarcoma in bone subjected to roentgen or radium irradiation. *J. Bone Joint Surg.,* 27:179–195.

30. Hatfield, P. M., and Schulz, M. D. (1970): Postirradiation sarcoma. *Radiology,* 96:593–602.

31. Hempelmann, L. H., Hall, W. J., Phillips, M. Cooper, R. A., and Ames, W. R. (1975): Neoplasms in persons treated with x-rays in infancy: Fourth survey in 20 years. *J. Natl. Cancer Inst.,* 55:519–530.

32. Hermans, E. H., Grosfeld, J. C. M., and Spaas, J. A. J. (1965): The fifth phacomatosis. *Dermatologica,* 130:446–476.

33. von Herzberg, J. J., and Wiskemann, A. (1963): Die fünfte phakomatose. *Dermatologica,* 126:106–123.

34. Hope-Stone, H. F., (1970): Results of treatment of medulloblastomas. *J. Neurosurg.,* 32:83–88.

35. Jablon, S. (1975): Radiation. In: *Persons at High Risk of Cancer: An Approach to Cancer Etiology and Control,* edited by J. F. Fraumeni, Jr., pp. 151–165. Academic Press, New York.

36. Jablon, S., and Kato, H. (1972): Studies of the mortality of A-bomb survivors. 5. Radiation dose and mortality, 1950–1970. *Radiat. Res.,* 50:649–698.

37. Jablon, S., Tachikawa, K., Belsky, J. L., and Steer, A. (1971): Cancer in Japanese exposed as children to atomic bombs. *Lancet,* 1:927–932.

38. Jones, A. (1953): Irradiation sarcoma. *Br. J. Radiol.,* 26:273–284.

39. Katzman, H., Waugh, T., and Berdon, W. (1969): Skeletal changes following irradiation of childhood tumors. *J. Bone Joint Surg.,* 51A:825–842.

40. Kaufman, S. L., and Stout, A. P. (1963): Extraskeletal osteogenic sarcomas and chondrosarcomas in children. *Cancer,* 16:432–439.

41. Kitchin, F. D., and Ellsworth, R. M. (1974): Pleiotropic effects of the gene for retinoblastoma. *J. Med. Genet.,* 11:244–246.

42. Knudson, A. G. (1971): Mutation and cancer. Statistical study of retinoblastoma. *Proc. Natl. Acad. Sci. USA,* 68:820–823.

43. Kolar, J., and Palecek, L. (1970): Radiation induced bone sarcoma. *Radiol. Diagn.,* 11:485–492.

44. Lathouwer, C. L. De, and Meulemans, G. (1972): Sarcomes ostéogéniques des maxillaires survenant en terrain irradié. *Rev. Stomatol. Chir. Maxillofac.,* 73:461–468.

45. Lee, W. R., Laurie, J., and Townsend, A. L. (1975): Fine structure of a radiation-induced osteogenic sarcoma. *Cancer,* 76:1414–1425.

46. Lehmann, A. R., Kirk-Bell, S., Arlett, C. F., Paterson, M. C., Lohman, P. H. M., de Weerd-Kastelein, E. A., and Bootsma, D. (1975): Xeroderma pigmentosum cells with normal levels of excision repair have a defect in DNA synthesis after UV-irradiation. *Proc. Natl. Acad. Sci. USA,* 72:219–223.

47. Lewis, E. B. (1975): Possible genetic consequences of irradiation of tumors in childhood. *Radiology,* 114:147–153.
48. Li, F. P., Cassady, J. R., and Jaffe, N. (1975): Risk of second tumors in survivors of childhood cancer. *Cancer,* 35:1230–1235.
49. Martin, H., Strong, E., and Spiro, R. H. (1970): Radiation-induced skin cancer of the head and neck. *Cancer,* 25:61–71.
50. McFarland, D. R., Horwitz, H., Saenger, E. L., and Bahr, G. K. (1969): Medulloblastoma—a review of prognosis and survival. *Br. J. Radiol.,* 42:198–214.
51. Meadows, A. T., D'Angio, G. J., Evans, A. E., Harris, C. C., Miller, R. W., and Mike, V. (1975): Oncogenesis and other late effects of cancer treatment in children. *Radiology,* 114:175–180.
52. Meerkotter, V. A., and Shear, M. (1964): Multiple primordial cysts associated with bifid rib and ocular defects. *Oral Surg.,* 18:498–503.
53. Mole, R. H. (1964): Cancer production by chronic exposure to penetrating gamma irradiation. *Natl. Cancer Inst. Monogr.,* 14:217–290.
54. Mole, R. H. (1973): Late effects of radiation: Carcinogenesis. *Br. Med. Bull.,* 29:78–83.
55. Moynahan, E. J. (1973): Multiple basal cell naevus syndrome—Successful treatment of basal cell tumours with 5-fluorouracil. *Proc. R. Soc. Med.,* 66:627–628.
56. Muller, H. J. (1954): The nature of the genetic effects produced by radiation. In: *Radiation Biology,* edited by A. Hollander, Vol. 1, pp. 351–474. McGraw-Hill, New York.
57. Neblett, C. R., Waltz, T. A., and Anderson, D. E. (1971): Neurological involvement in the nevoid basal cell carcinoma syndrome. *J. Neurosurg.,* 35:577–584.
58. Petersen, O. (1954): Radiation cancer: Report of 21 cases. *Acta Radiol. [Diagn.] (Stockh.),* 42:221–236.
59. Pettit, V. D., Chamness, J. T., and Ackerman, L. V. (1954): Fibromatosis and fibrosarcoma following irradiation therapy. *Cancer,* 7:149–158.
60. Phillips, T. L., and Sheline, G. E. (1963): Bone sarcomas following radiation therapy. *Radiology,* 81:992–996.
61. Ridley, C. M. (1962): Basal cell carcinoma following x-ray epilation of the scalp. *Br. J. Dermatol.,* 74:222–223.
62. Sabanas, A. O., Dahlin, D. C., Childs, D. S., and Ivins, J. C. (1956): Postradiation sarcoma of bone. *Cancer,* 9:528–542.
63. Sagerman, R. H., Cassady, J. R., Tretter, P., and Ellsworth, R. M. (1969): Radiation induced neoplasia following external beam therapy for children with retinoblastoma. *Am. J. Roentgenol. Radium Ther. Nucl. Med.,* 105:529–535.
64. Sarkany, I., Fountain, R. B., Evans, C. D., Morrison, R., and Szur, L. (1968): Multiple basal-cell epitheliomata following radiotherapy of the spine. *Br. J. Dermatol.,* 80:90–96.
65. Selikoff, I. J., and Hammond, E. C. (1975): Multiple risk factors in environmental cancer. In: *Persons at High Risk of Cancer: An Approach to Cancer Etiology and Control,* edited by J. F. Fraumeni, Jr., pp. 467–483. Academic Press, New York.
66. Senyszyn, J. J., Johnston, A. D., Jacox, H. W., and Chu, F. C. H. (1970): Radiation-induced sarcoma after treatment of breast cancer. *Cancer,* 26:394–403.
67. Sim, F. H., Cupps, R. E., Dahlin, D. C., and Ivins, J. C.: (1972): Postradiation sarcoma of bone. *J. Bone Joint Surg.,* 54A:1479–1489.
68. Skolnik, E. M., Fornatto, E. J., and Heydemann, J. (1956): Osteogenic sarcoma of the skull following irradiation. *Ann. Otol. Rhinol. Laryngol.,* 65:915–936.
69. Steiner, G. C. (1965): Postradiation sarcoma of bone. *Cancer,* 18:603–612.
70. Stewart, A. (1971): Low dose radiation cancers in man. *Adv. Cancer Res.,* 14:359–390.
71. Stewart, A. (1973): The carcinogenic effects of low level radiation. A re-appraisal of epidemiologists' methods and observations. *Health Phys.,* 24:223–240.
72. Tebbet, R. D., and Vickery, R. D. (1952): Osteogenic sarcoma following irradiation for retinoblastoma. *Am. J. Ophthalmol.,* 35:811–818.
73. Tefft, M., Vawter, G. F., and Mitus, A. (1968): Second primary neoplasms in children. *Am. J. Roentgenol. Radium Ther. Nucl. Med.,* 103:800–822.
74. Temin, H. M. (1974): On the origin of the genes for neoplasia: G. H. A. Clowes Memorial Lecture. *Cancer Res.,* 34:2835–2841.
75. Thompson, R. W., Small, R. C., and Stein, J. J. (1972): Treatment of retinoblastoma. *Am. J. Roentgenol. Radium Ther. Nucl. Med.,* 114:16–23.
76. Yoneyama, T., and Greenlaw, R. H. (1969): Osteogenic sarcoma following radiotherapy for retinoblastoma. *Radiology,* 93:1185–1186.

Discussion

Hirschhorn: In the ankylosing spondylitis patients and the Japanese survivors of the atomic bomb, there is a marked discrepancy reported between the latent periods for leukemia and solid tumors. Would you comment on this in relation to the model you presented?

Strong: An excess of myelogenous leukemia and, in some cases, acute lymphocytic leukemia is seen in a variety of population groups exposed to radiation. The relatively short latent period for radiogenic leukemia is, I think, simply a characteristic of growth pattern of bone marrow and of the probability of the cells acquiring a second mutational step. The solid tumors arise from tissues which proliferate less rapidly, and, as a consequence, display much longer latent periods in response to radiation exposure.

Hirschhorn: If the difference is based on cell turnover, how can you account for the long latency of tumors arising from the intestinal mucosal cells, which probably proliferate at least as rapidly as does the bone marrow; or of tumors arising from the skin, which also has quite a rapid cell turnover? In other words, this explanation is never completely satisfying.

Strong: I agree. In some manner the latent period may be a characteristic of each tumor cell line and may perhaps reflect the rate of repair mechanisms or other forces that affect the probability of developing the tumor. We know very little about the growth characteristics of the stem cell which presumably must undergo the specific mutations. The patterns are consistent for the various cell types in different populations exposed to radiation, but I really do not know the reason for this.

Skolnick: Have you tried to correct for an apparent bias, namely, that a person in whom a tumor develops in 2 years has a much greater probability of being ascertained than does someone in whom a tumor develops in 20 years?

Strong: I tried to avoid this bias by looking at two series of patients who were ascertained only through the first primary tumor and then followed: namely, the retinoblastoma patients traced for over 30 years, and the long-term survivors of childhood malignancy followed for up to 24 years. I am assuming that ascertainment of radiogenic tumors in retinoblastoma patients is similar to that of radiogenic tumors in any other patients.

Skolnick: But, with literature research, you are more likely to get a report of a case in which a second tumor developed soon rather than many years after the primary tumor.

Strong: The major findings are not based on case reports, but on two series with complete ascertainment and follow-up over a long period of time. Of the 243 bilateral retinoblastoma patients, we know how many developed any type of radiogenic malignancy, even the minor basal cell carcinomas. We know from Dr. Li's series how many survivors of other childhood cancers acquired any type of radiogenic malignancy over 24 years. The series of radiogenic sarcomas based on literature reports may be biased by reports of short latent periods, but no more so for retinoblastoma than for other primary disease.

Genetics of Human Cancer, edited by J. J.
Mulvihill, R. W. Miller, and J. F. Fraumeni, Jr.
Raven Press, New York, 1977.

40

Delayed Mutation Model: Carotid Body Tumors and Retinoblastoma

Jürgen Herrmann

Department of Pediatrics, University of Wisconsin, Madison, Wisconsin 53706

We use the term *oncogenesis* to designate the cause (etiology) of cancer and the term *oncoplasia* for the pathogenesis of cancer. The subject of delayed mutation relates to the genetic causes of cancer.

Charlotte Auerbach, in 1956, proposed a labile premutation as the cause of a new dominant mutation in several members of the same family (4). Auerbach postulated that the unaffected "connecting" relatives transmitted to the affected individuals a labile premutated gene which, by delayed mutation, gave rise to the (fully) mutant allele. Subsequent transmission of the gene was evident from the regularly dominant segregation pattern of the condition in the descendants of affected persons. As an illustration, Auerbach used a pedigree of ectrodactyly with six affected individuals: two sibs who had, combined, two out of five children affected and a first cousin of the sibs who had one affected child.

We have recently applied the delayed mutation model to further human conditions and have suggested that the change from the wild to the premutated allele be called *premutation* and the change from the premutated to the mutated allele be called *telomutation* (33). We noticed that the pattern of the pedigrees with multiple (unaffected) carriers was consistent for each condition but that significant differences exist between the pattern of different conditions (33,34). For instance, the rate of telomutation was equal and low in male and female carriers in achondroplasia while it was high in female carriers in the Wiedemann-Beckwith syndrome and apparently nonexistent in male carriers for this condition. The differences concerned the rate of telomutation, sex of carriers and affected individuals, the occurrence of delayed mutation in germinal and somatic cells, and the proportion of delayed and complete mutation at a particular locus.

These variables indicate (1) that several different mechanisms may be involved in delayed mutation and (2) that the model has broader implications than is generally assumed or was originally suggested by Auerbach. Not only the "tell-tale" pedigree with multiple unaffected relatives who "connect" the affected individuals may be indicative of delayed mutation but also the "pattern of pedigrees" of certain conditions, consisting of "dominant," "recessive," and "sporadic" pedigrees. In this paper we would like to illustrate these and further aspects of the delayed mutation model by applying it to data on carotid body tumors and retinoblastoma.

CAROTID BODY TUMORS (CHEMODECTOMAS)

Most cases of carotid body tumors (CBT) are sporadic and unilateral, but several instances of familial occurrence have been reported. In 1949 Kline et al. (45) summarized 291 unilateral sporadic cases and five bilateral cases, including two familial instances. In 1937 Phelps et al. (65) stated that 3% of cases are bilateral; after intensive follow-up studies Shamblin et al. (74) found bilateral occurrence in almost 8% of cases. Among familial cases the bilateral incidence is reported as 35% (16). Most authors report a higher incidence in males than in females (16), but Saldana et al. (71) observed CBT more often in females. The latter authors also observed it more often on the left than on the right.

In man, chemodectomas occur primarily in the carotid arteries, but concomitant occurrence of chemodectomas in other locations (16,19,60,62) and their embryologic, histologic, and physiologic similarities (53) suggest a close oncogenetic and/or oncoplastic relationship.

The prevalence of CBT is in part related to altitude. Saldana et al. (71) documented an approximate 10-fold increase of chemodectomas in Peruvian adults who had lived at altitudes over 2,000 m compared with Peruvians living at sea level; with one exception, these were all sporadic, unilateral cases. Chedid and Jao published a family with six affected individuals of which three had associated chronic obstructive pulmonary disease (16; pedigree 16 in Fig. 1). These authors suggested that chronic hypoxia per se may stimulate hyperplasia and perhaps tumor development of the carotid bodies. They pointed out the general correlation of carotid body hyperplasia with high altitude (3,23,71), emphysema (23), and cor pulmonale (31), but they also stated that in many individual instances of CBT no such associated findings were reported. Hayes and Fraumeni (30) investigated the epidemiology of chemodectomas in dogs, and they found an increased occurrence in two brachycephalic breeds (boxers and Boston terriers) and a positive correlation with male sex and advanced age. Chemodectomas in dogs were noticed more frequently in the aorta than in the carotid artery, and the concurrence of four other tumors was significant, namely seminomas, testicular interstitial cell tumors, thyroid adenomas, and hemangiomas.

The reported familial instances of CBT in man are summarized in Fig. 1, and the corresponding numerical data are in Table 1. Eight pedigrees showed affected members in one sibship, six showed members affected in consecutive generations, four pedigrees showed three or more carriers, and two pedigrees showed one carrier. For the purpose of tabulating the offspring of carriers in Table 1, we considered the sibs of pedigrees 1 to 8 to have a carrier parent. The pedigrees included an approximately equal number of male and female persons with unilateral and bilateral disease,

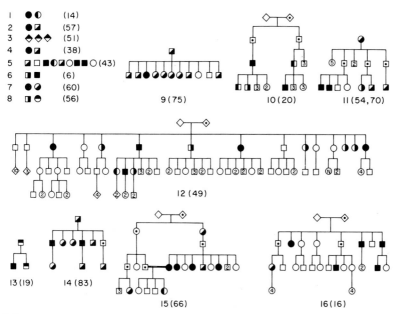

FIG. 1. Pedigrees of reported familial cases of carotid body tumors. Symbols: male □, female ○, unknown sex ◇; bilateral ■, left ◖, right ◆, unilateral ◈, undefined tumor ♦. Numbers in parentheses indicate reference. Pedigree 15 is subject to two alternate interpretations: ◖ is born to an affected mother as well as to a potential male carrier. That makes it a questionable case of female-to-female transmission. In Table 1 we treat the situation conservatively, i.e., as a case of male-to-female transmission.

but 11 male carriers and only one female carrier were identified; 41% of cases were bilateral. At least 25 instances of male-to-male transmission were seen in 8 pedigrees.

A most striking feature was the lack of affected persons among the offspring of affected females ($p < 0.001$). Nine of 12 affected males had affected offspring, and 3 had only normal children, while all children of 10 affected females were normal or, in 4 instances, carriers. The offspring of unilaterally affected males is not strikingly dissimilar from that of bilaterally affected males or of carriers. Unilaterally affected offspring are produced more often than bilaterally affected offspring. We recognize that reporting bias and ascertainment bias of these pedigrees demand caution in an analysis of the data, but it is noteworthy that carriers produced offspring in the ratio of 36% normal, 56% affected (half unilateral, half bilateral), and 8% carriers.

In the interpretation of these data several possible explanations come to mind. The investigation by Saldana et al. suggests either heterogeneity in the oncogenesis or a strong effect of hypoxia on the oncoplasia of carotid body tumors (16,71). The pedigrees in Fig. 1 are not compatible with decreased penetrance of an autosomal dominant gene since CBT occurred in sibs-only in eight instances and since pedigrees 10,15, and 16 show high penetrance in descendant, but low "penetrance" in ascendant relatives of affected persons. The familial instances of CBT are more compati-

TABLE 1. *Carotid body tumor: Familial cases*

Characteristics of affected persons and of carriers

	Bilateral	Unilateral	Unknown site	Carrier
Male	17	22	2	11
Female	13	22	1	1
Unknown sex	—	—	3	12
Total	30	44	6	24

Offspring of affected persons and of carriers

Parent	Affected					Carrier			Total
Sex	Male			Female		Male	Female	Unknown	
Site	U	B	Unk	U	B				
N	4	7	1	7	3	11	1	12	46
Offspring									
Normal	18	23	—	18	18	20	1	12	110
male	9	12	—	6	8	13	—	5	53
female	9	11	—	10	10	7	1	7	55
unknown	—	—	—	2	—	—	—	—	2
Affected	15	8	2	—	—	17	—	34	76
male U	5	3	—	—	—	5	—	8	21
male B	3	2	1	—	—	4	—	7	17
female U	6	3	—	—	—	4	—	7	20
female B	1	—	—	—	—	4	—	8	13
unknown	—	—	1	—	—	—	—	4	5
Carrier	1	—	—	4	—	—	2	5	12
male	1	—	—	4	—	—	2	4	11
female	—	—	—	—	—	—	—	1	1
Total	34	31	2	22	18	37	3	51	198

B, bilateral; U, unilateral; Unk, unknown.

ble with the Auerbach delayed mutation model involving a highly penetrant autosomal dominant mutant gene and transmission of a premutant allele through unaffected carriers. However, the offspring of affected females does not include any affected persons. If this were due to restriction of telomutation to somatic cells in females, one would expect to see affected offspring born to women who have an affected father. Figure 1 includes two such situations (pedigree 12), but these are not conclusive. From the number of affected females, it appears that the rate of somatic telomutation in females would have to be high.

Alternatively, one could speculate that affected females are unable to transmit the mutant gene to their offspring, or that expression of the mutant gene or development of the tumor is suppressed in their children. A mutant CBT allele which influences segregation would have different implications than a cytoplasmically transmitted suppressor episome or a placentally transmitted maternal antibody, but the existing pedigree data do not allow for a distinction between these possibilities. It is noted that the pedigrees do not contain a documented case of female-to-female transmission of the premutant or the mutant allele, but female-to-male transmission of a premutant allele (or a nonexpressed mutant allele) was observed in pedigrees 11 and 15.

In genetic counseling we suggest in familial cases to indicate a high risk for the offspring of affected males and carrier males and a low risk to affected females. Empiric recurrence risk figures for sporadic cases are not available and, therefore, it can not be estimated what proportion of sporadic cases is similar to the familial cases. Apparently, the risk is low for the offspring of most sporadic cases. The recurrence risk for affected sibs should be arrived at from similar considerations and not without an extensive family history.

RETINOBLASTOMA

Review of Genetic Data

The genetic data on retinoblastoma (RB) were recently reviewed by Warburg (80) and by François et al. (26). We have summarized the pertinent data in Table 2. Since

TABLE 2. *Retinoblastoma: Summary of genetic data*

Incidence: Slightly less than 1:20,000 (13,17,21,26,39,79)

Mutation rate: $3.7-6 \times 10^{-6}$ (13,17,78); 1.23×10^{-5} (72)

Paternal age increased for sporadic bilateral cases (17,26,64)

Possibly slightly higher incidence in males than in females (26,39,72)

Low rate of consanguinity: 3/48 cases (32); 9/360 cases (72); 2/114 cases (27)

Familial occurrence: In about 5-10% of cases (13,17,26,55,72); in 6.5% of unilateral and 17.7% of bilateral cases (13)

Bilateral occurrence: In over 30% of sporadic cases and over 60% of familial cases (10,13,26,39,72)

Age at diagnosis: Within 18 months in 73% of bilateral cases and 29% of unilateral cases (22); mean age: 14 months for bilateral cases and 30 months for unilateral cases (46); mean age: 10.5 months for bilateral cases and 31 months for unilateral cases (1)

Spontaneous regression: Documented in about 50 cases; can involve unilateral and bilateral cases and in the latter one or both eyes (2,11,12,58,59); it has been suggested that spontaneous regression and expression may be influenced by immune mechanisms (9,15)

Chromosome aberrations: Multiple nonspecific aberrations (18,37); chromosome 13 deletion (26,29,63,84); trisomy 21 (8,26,69, personal case); trisomy 13 (personal case)

most patients with retinoblastoma have apparently normal chromosomes (26,50,82), we consider those with chromosome aberrations a special class and have generally excluded them from the following considerations.

The literature provides statistical data mainly concerning the offspring of *sporadic* cases. The proportion of affected offspring in different series is for the offspring of sporadic unilaterally (SU) affected parents, 6.8% (79), 6.6% (26), 1.2% (13), 15.4% (27), and 0/9 (32), and for the offspring of sporadic bilaterally (SB) affected parents, 52.1% (26), 55.6% (13), and 25% (27). The reported data do not allow a comparison between the proportions of unilaterally versus bilaterally affected persons among the offspring of SU parents and SB parents.

To obtain information about offspring of familial cases we analyzed the reported familial instances of retinoblastoma which are reproduced in Figs. 2 to 4. Figure 2 shows 40 instances where only sibs are affected (group A). Figure 3 shows 68 pedigrees with occurrence in consecutive generations (group B), and Fig. 4 shows 27

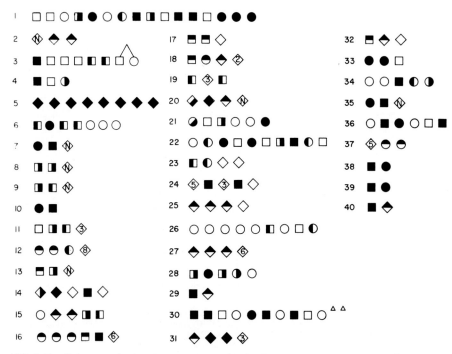

FIG. 2. Familial cases of retinoblastoma reported in the literature: occurrence in sibs. Symbols as in Fig. 1. References: *1* (7, #339); *2* (7, #346); *3* (7, #347); *4* (7, #348); *5* (7, #349); *6* (7, #350); *7* (7, #351); *8* (7, #352); *9* (7, #353); *10* (7, #354); *11* (7, #355); *12* (7, #356); *13* (7, #357); *14* (7, #358); *15* (7, #359); *16* (7, #360); *17* (7, #363); *18* (7, #364); *19* (7, #365); *20* (7, #298); *21* (7, #299); *22* (81); *23* (28, Mazzei); *24* (28, Waardenburg); *25* (28, Ernrooth); *26* (72,KS); *27* (28, Leber); *28* (28, Calderaro); *29* (46, #12); *30* (55, #12); *31* (28, Dabney); *32* (28, Valenti); *33* (55, #77); *34* (55, #115); *35* (28, Adam); *36* (72, BL); *37* (28, Nemoto); *38* (72, Pd); *39* (72, KI); *40* (46, #5).

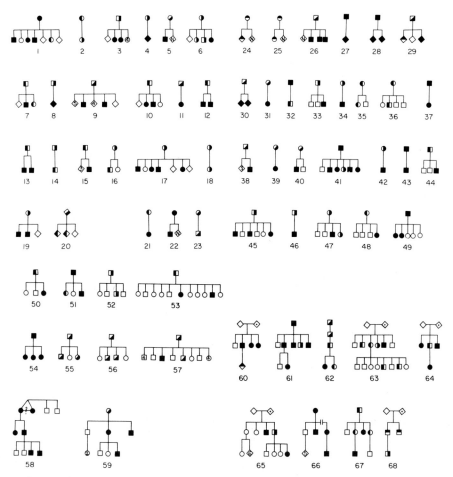

FIG. 3. Familial cases of retinoblastoma reported in the literature: occurrence in consecutive generations. References: *1* (7, #333); *2* (7, #336); *3* (7, #338); *4* (7, #340); *5* (7, #341); *6* (7, #343); *7* (7, #345); *8* (7, #361); *9* (81, Hoeve); *10* (81, Sym); *11* (81, Hemmes); *12* (81, Stallard); *13* (81, Lange); *14* (81, Reimsloh); *15* (81, Lange); *16* (81, Reiser); *17* (81, Griffith); *18* (81, Fietta); *19* (81, v. Hoffmann); *20* (81, Best); *21* (17); *22* (28, Heijl); *23* (28, Kennon); *24* (28, Melanowski); *25* (28, Odinow); *26* (28, Heine); *27* (68, #1); *28* (68, #2); *29* (68, #3); *30* (68, #4); *31* (10, #5); *32* (24, #63); *33* (24, #72); *34* (10, #3); *35* (10, #4); *36* (10, #5); *37* (10, #6); *38* (77, #1); *39* (77, #2); *40* (77, #3); *41* (72, Mp); *42* (72, St); *43* (72, Le); *44* (72, Kr); *45* (72, Mr); *46* (72, Ki); *47* (72, Li); *48* (72, Re); *49* (72, Hg); *50* (72, Hd); *51* (72, Pu); *52* (72, De); *53* (72, vd Ve); *54* (27, #2); *55* (27, #3), *56* (27, #4); *57* (27, #6); *58* (27, #1); *59* (27, #5); *60* (81, Bell 337); *61* (28, Griffith); *62* (81, Sleight); *63* (10, #1); *64* (10, #2); *65* (55, #47); *66* (72, Ko); *67* (72, Da); *68* (46, #23).

families with 2 or more unaffected carriers (group C). The information from these pedigrees is summarized in Table 3. The pedigrees in Fig. 3 include at least 59 and those in Fig. 4 at least 26 instances of male-to-male transmission. The three groups contain a nonsignificant excess of affected males. The proportion of unilateral tumor occurrence in groups A, B, and C is 0.41, 0.43, and 0.48, respectively. In these

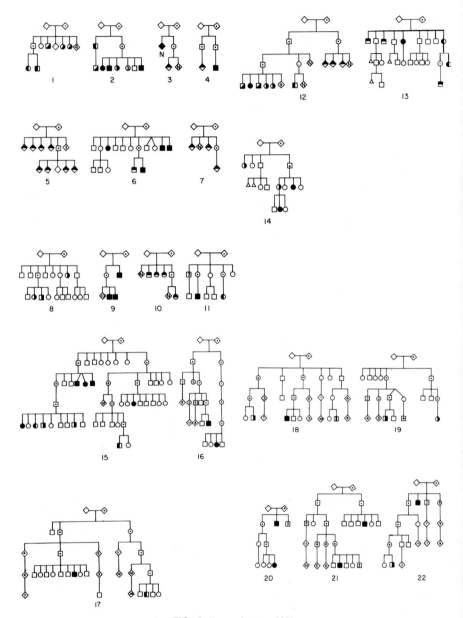

FIG. 4. (legend on p. 425).

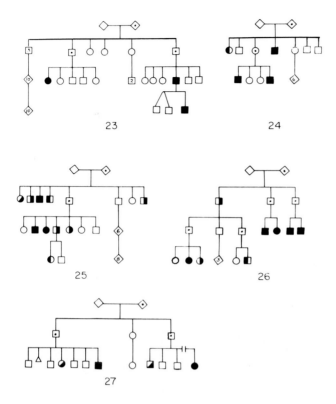

FIG. 4. Familial cases of retinoblastoma reported in the literature: families with at least two unaffected carriers. References: *1* (7, #334); *2* (7, #342); *3* (7, #344); *4* (81, Lukens); *5* (81, Hemmes); *6* (7, #366); *7* (81, v. Graefe); *8* (28, Nemoto); *9* (28, Sabugin); *10* (28, Feinstein); *11* (55, #67); *12* (7, #335); *13* (24, #35); *14* (24, #71); *15* (55, # 60 and #63); *16* (55, #14); *17* (55, #55 and #62); *18* (55, #116); *19* (55, #52); *20* (55, #40); *21* (55, #65); *22* (55, #23); *23* (55, #41); *24* (72, vZw); *25* (72, Hs); *26* (17); *27* (27, #7).

groups we found no statistical difference between bilaterally and unilaterally affected males and females, sex ratios, and unilateral versus bilateral tumor occurrence, and we assume, therefore, that the affected individuals in the three groups form a biologically homogeneous class.

In group B and group C the *offspring of affected parents* shows no significant difference between the sex ratios, the proportions of affected offspring (carrier offspring is here included with the affected offspring), and the proportions of unilaterally versus bilaterally affected persons among the affected offspring. Male

TABLE 3. Retinoblastoma: Summary of familial cases

Number of pedigrees
Group A (affected sibs): 40
Group B (2 generations affected): 68
Group C (with 2 or more carriers): 27
Total: 135

1. Number of affected individuals:	Total	Group A 121	Group B 199	Group C 112	Total 432
Sex: Affected eye[a]					
male					
bilateral		24	62	31	117
right		12	11	9	32
left		12	18	7	37
unilateral		—	16	5	21
unknown		6	2	5	13
female					
bilateral		18	39	14	71
right		2	15	10	27
left		8	12	7	27
unilateral		1	7	4	12
unknown		8	3	3	14
unknown					
bilateral		12	8	1	21
right		1	—	—	1
left		—	2	—	2
unilateral		1	1	—	2
unknown		16	3	16	35

2. Offspring of affected individuals

Parent	Group B						Group C			Total
sex[a]	M	M	M	F	F	UNK	M	M	F	
affected eye [a]	B	A	U	B	U	U	B	U	U	
number	11	1	30	6	22	1	1	3	2	77
Offspring normal										
male	9	—	60+	6	23+	—	2	2	2	104+
female	5	—	18	2	13	—	2	2	1	43
sex unknown	4	—	25	2	6	—	—	—	1	38
	—	—	17+	2+	4+	—	—	—	—	23+
Offspring affected [a]										
male	26	U 1	49	11	31	2	1	2	2	125
female	U 2,B 9		U 9,B 19	B 7	U 5,B 11		B 1	U 1		65
sex unknown	U 2,B 9		U 5,B 11	U 1,B 3	U 6,B 8			U 1	U 1,B 1	48
	B 3,A 1		B 4,A 1		B 1	U 2				12
Offspring carrier										
male	—	—	—	—	—	—	2	2	1	3
female	—	—	—	—	—	—	2	2	1	2
										1
Total	35	1	109+	17	54+	2	3	6	5	232+

3. Offspring of carriers

Parent	Group A	Group B	Group C			Total
			M	F	Unk	
sex [b]	—	—	M	F	Unk	
number	40	5	38	28	27	138
Offspring normal						
male	93	5	117	81+	70+	366+
female	19	3	53	22	35	132
unknown	24	2	35	19	27	107
Offspring affected [a]						
male	50+	—	29+	40+	8+	127+
female	121	14	51	24	34	244
	U 24,B 24,A 6	U 5,B 4	U 12,B 13	U 3,B 10,A 2	U 6,B 7,A 3	
	U 11,B 18,A 8	U 2,B 3	U 9,B 11,A 1	U 3,B 1	U 7,B 2,A 2	
	U 2,B 12,A 16	—	A 5	A 5	B 1,A 6	
Offspring carrier						
male	—	—	12	13	36	61
female	—	—	5	9	21	35
	—	—	7	4	15	26
Total	214+	19	180+	118+	140+	671+

[a] Affected eye: B, bilateral; U, unilateral; A, affected but site unknown.
[b] In Group A and B all carriers were of undetermined sex except for one female in Group A.

and female parents produced similar series of offspring, but unilaterally (FU) affected parents and bilaterally (FB) affected parents produced significantly different series. When compared to the offspring of FU parents, the offspring of FB parents contained a significantly ($p < 0.02$) higher proportion of affected offspring and also a significantly ($p < 0.02$) higher proportion of bilaterally affected persons. The offspring of FU parents included 49% normal, 49% affected, and 2% carrier individuals, and the offspring of FB parents included 31% normal and 69% affected individuals. FU and FB parents had 35% and 14% unilaterally affected offspring, respectively.

The *offspring of carriers* in groups A and B differ from the offspring of carriers in group C apparently because of strong ascertainment bias: sibships in group A were, of course, selected for an increased number of affected persons and against carriers among them. Thus, there is a significant difference in the proportion of affected persons ($p < 0.001$); however, the proportion of males:females and unilaterally:bilaterally affected offspring in the three groups is similar. Male and female carriers in group C have similar offspring. Thus, we assume that carriers in all three groups are biologically homogeneous. Carriers had 54.5% normal, 36.4% affected, and 9.1% carrier offspring. This indicates a rate of telomutation of at least 0.364. Among the offspring of carriers, 47% of cases were unilaterally affected.

In Table 4 the offspring of affected persons (SU,SB,FU,FB) and of carriers (C) are compared for the proportion of affected persons among them. The offspring of carriers and the offspring of SU parents appear to form a distinct class. The significant differences between the offspring of FU parents and the offspring of FB parents have already been pointed out. The table also shows that the proportion of affected persons among the offspring of SB parents is not significantly different from the offspring of FU parents or of FB parents. Here it would be useful to compare the proportion of unilaterally versus bilaterally affected offspring, but for SB parents such data are not available.

Three previous studies included data on the offspring of familial cases. Briard-Guillemot et al. (13) found in their personal series among 165 offspring of unaffected carriers, 58.2% normal, 30.3% affected, and 11.5% carrier individuals. The differences between these and our values are not statistically significant ($p < 0.7$). In 1949

TABLE 4. *Offspring of persons with retinoblastoma*

	C	FB	FU	SB
SU	0.001	0.001	0.001	0.001
SB	0.05	0.1	0.7	
FU	0.01	0.01		
FB	0.001			

Difference between the offspring of sporadic (S), familial (F), unilaterally (U), and bilaterally (B) affected parents and the offspring of carriers (C). Listed are the *p* values. Since normal and carrier offspring cannot be distinguished among the offspring of sporadic parents, those numbers have been combined also among the offspring of carrier and FU parents. The data of Vogel (79) are used for SU parents and the data of François et al. (26) for SB parents. (See text.)

Franceschetti and Bischler reported an excellent statistical analysis on retino-blastoma (25), but their paper was superseded in 1955 by that of Kaelin, a student of Franceschetti, who presented an extensive review of reported familial retinoblastoma cases (42) which included a number of the pedigrees shown in Figs. 2 to 4. Kaelin grouped his material of familial RB cases into four classes: affected sibs with negative family history (class A), consecutive transmission over one (class B) or several (class D) generations; and, transmission by normal individuals (class C). He reviewed the cases reported up to 1952 and noted that these occurred in a single sibship in 37% of cases, in 48% of cases in consecutive generations, and in families with an unaffected carrier parent in 15% of cases. Kaelin's material showed a slight excess of males. Unilateral occurrence was 82% in sporadic cases, 53% in class A, 55% in class C, and 78% in classes B plus D. The proportion of affected offspring was close to 50% for an affected parent (classes B and D) and also for an unaffected parent who had affected relatives (class C), and it was slightly over 30% for an unaffected parent in class A. Kaelin found that FB cases tend to have bilaterally affected children but that FU cases did not have predominantly unilaterally affected offspring.

Pleiotropy

Expression of the RB gene may not be limited to the eye in all cases. We suspect that the RB gene may be a cause of true mosaic pleiotropy which may be evident in two ways: (1) Different members of the same family may be affected by different tumors (including retinoblastoma), presumably all caused by the RB gene; and (2) a patient with retinoblastoma may subsequently (or, possibly, antecedently) develop another malignancy, also caused by the RB gene. Evidence for the first is provided by such reports on retinoblastoma families as the one by Rados (67) who documented the occurrence of a pontine glioma in a female first cousin of a boy with bilateral retinoblastoma. Similar observations were presented by Falls and Neel (24), Macklin (55), and Gordon (27). With improved treatment of retinoblastoma, the occurrence of subsequent malignancies in the same patient has been increasingly recognized. Kitchin and Ellsworth (44) saw 48 subsequent tumors in a series of 1,130 patients with retinoblastoma. At least 13 tumors appeared unrelated to radiation; they included 10 osteogenic sarcomas, two thyroid tumors, and one Wilms' tumor. With one exception they all occurred in patients with bilateral retinoblastoma. The association of retinoblastoma and osteogenic sarcoma was pointed out previously by Jensen and Miller (40). Schimke et al. (73) described two sibs with bilateral retinoblastoma who subsequently both developed osteogenic sarcoma of the femur. Strong and Knudson (76) reported rhabdomyosarcoma, melanoma, and acute lymphoblastic leukemia in one bilaterally and two unilaterally affected patients. Hoefnagel et al. (36) followed a male with surgically removed left retinoblastoma from 1½ years until 9½ years when he developed acute lymphoblastic leukemia. Gordon (27) observed a male in whom bilateral retinoblastoma (Fig. 3, pedigree 54) developed at 2 years and who at 40 years developed fibrosarcoma of the thigh. In his series of 114 index cases, Gordon found a parent to have a malignant neoplasm other than retinoblastoma in 6.7% of unilaterally affected patients and 9.6% of bilaterally affected patients (27).

Interpretation

Interpretation of the genetic data on retinoblastoma centers on the sporadic occurrence of most cases contrasted to familial occurrence in a significant proportion of cases. Since 1930 Franceschetti has suggested an autosomal dominant mutation as the cause of the familial cases and a somatic mutation as the cause of the sporadic cases (25). In 1954 Vogel concluded that 25% of RB cases were due to an autosomal dominant gene with 80% penetrance and that 75% of RB cases were sporadic and of unknown etiology (78). Presently, the Knudson two-mutation model provides a widely accepted explanation for the sporadic occurrence of a genetic disorder in some families and familial occurrence in others (46–48). Knudson proposed that two mutations are necessary for every case of RB and suggested that sporadic occurrence was due to two somatic mutations, while familial cases are due to an inherited germinal and a second somatic mutation. More recently, Briard-Guillemot and her colleagues proposed that a small chromosome deletion could account for sporadic as well as familial cases of RB (13): a heritable small chromosome break might be repaired in subsequent generations to produce normal offspring or might not be repaired to produce affected offspring. A similar hypothesis was suggested by Hashem and Khalifa (29).

We would like to pursue the implications of the Auerbach delayed mutation model with respect to the genetic data on retinoblastoma. Neel (61), Knudson (46), and François et al. (26) have made reference to the Auerbach model for pedigrees of RB with multiple unaffected carriers. And, prior to Auerbach's paper, Jzikowitz (41) and Kaelin (42) recognized the occurrence of RB in sibships, in consecutive generations, and in families with unaffected "connecting" relatives, and they concluded that these instances were caused by a uniform genetic mechanism. Jzikowitz, who published his thesis in 1938, explicitly compared the inheritance of retinoblastoma with phenomena observed in *Drosophila* and *Antirrhinum majus* which we consider to represent delayed mutation (41).

We present the following interpretation to show that the genetic data on retinoblastoma can be explained by a single autosomal dominant mutation which can be either complete or delayed according to the Auerbach model and which can occur in germinal as well as in somatic cells. Exceptions to this general explanation are those cases of retinoblastoma which are associated with constitutional chromosome aberrations. Specific aspects of this interpretation with respect to genetic counseling are presented elsewhere (35).

Numerous instances of male-to-male transmission and a risk of about 0.5 to the offspring of familial cases (i.e., those affected individuals who themselves have affected sibs, parents, or more distant relatives) suggest that retinoblastoma is due to an autosomal mutation with high ($\sim$100%) penetrance. Differences in the pedigree patterns and the laterality of the tumor could depend on whether the mutation occurred during somatic (mitotic) or germinal (meiotic) cell divisions and whether the mutational process is delayed or complete. A relatively high frequency of mutation during *somatic* cell division is suggested by the high number of sporadic cases of unilaterally affected individuals who have a significantly lower risk of producing affected offspring than the familial cases. Mutation during *germinal* cell division is suggested by sporadic bilateral cases who have a risk of 0.5 of producing affected offspring. Apparent examples of such cases are given in Fig. 3 by pedigrees 1, 22, 27, 28, 37, 41, 43, 49, 51, 54, 58, 61, and 66. It is difficult to estimate the true proportion of cases due to germinal mutation, but the number appears to be smaller than the number of cases due to somatic mutation. Indirect evidence for the occurrence of mutation during germ cell development is the increased paternal age (17,64) for sporadic bilateral cases.

The pedigrees in Fig. 4 of distantly related affected family members suggest delayed mutation with transmission of a premutated allele according to the rules of autosomal dominant inheritance. Delayed mutation at the retinoblastoma locus can occur apparently both during germinal and somatic cell division. Pedigree 23 suggests telomutation in the germ cells of a carrier who has a bilaterally affected son who, in turn, is the father of a bilaterally affected male. Pedigrees 13 and 26 suggest somatic telomutation in two unilaterally affected persons who have carrier offspring.

It appears that complete mutation at the RB locus, too, occurs during germinal and somatic cell division. Complete mutation during germinal cell division is suggested by the high proportion of sporadic, bilaterally affected (SB) parents who transmit the condition to their children. Complete mutation during somatic divisions is suggested by the significantly lower proportion of affected individuals among the offspring of SU parents than among the offspring of carriers.

The proportion of cases due to delayed and complete mutation and to mutation during somatic and germinal cell division is different for SU, SB, FU, and FB cases. SU cases usually inherit the normal, but sometimes the premutant allele, and they usually are due to somatic, but perhaps sometimes also to germinal delayed or complete mutation. Vogel (79) found in his series of 135 SU parents who had 21 affected and 290 normal offspring that the 21 affected offspring were born to 15 different parents, whereas 120 parents had only normal children. One might perhaps conclude that the 15 parents, i.e., roughly 10% of SU cases, are carriers of the premutant allele with a risk of 0.36 for producing affected offspring, and that roughly 90% of SU cases have a negligible risk of producing affected offspring. Sporadic, bilaterally affected individuals are presumed to be due to (delayed or complete) germinal mutation. The data do not allow us to determine whether an important minor proportion of SB cases exists which is due to somatic mutation. It is difficult to judge the proportion of delayed versus complete mutation in SB cases other than by analogy to the SU cases. While the magnitude of this proportion may be of interest, it is of no practical importance in genetic counseling.

Familial cases of retinoblastoma with occurrence in consecutive generations can be due to transmission of the premutant allele and successive somatic delayed mutation or they can be due to (delayed or complete) germinal mutation and subsequent transmission of the mutant allele. Occurrence in sibs of unaffected parents can be due to (germinal or somatic) delayed mutation or, perhaps less likely, to germinal mosaicism. A correlation for FU and FB cases between their parents (carrier, unilaterally affected, and bilaterally affected) and their offspring (proportion of normal, affected, and carrier individuals and unilaterally versus bilaterally affected cases) may be helpful in determining the relative frequency of the premutant versus the mutant allele in FU and FB cases. Figures 3 and 4 include FU and FB cases with each type of parent, but the data concerning their offspring are limited. Eight FU cases with a carrier parent (Fig. 3, pedigrees 63-65; Fig. 4, pedigrees 2, 13, 14, 25, 26) had 13 normal, 5 unilaterally affected, 3 bilaterally affected, and 3 carrier offspring. The offspring of these 8 FU parents and the offspring of carriers (Table 3) are very similar with respect to the number of normal, unilaterally affected, bilaterally affected, and carrier individuals. This suggests that most, if not all, FU cases who have a carrier parent are due to somatic mutation of a premutated allele and have the same risk of affected and of carrier offspring as carriers. Presumably essentially all FU and FB cases with a bilaterally affected parent and presumably also most, but not all, cases with a unilaterally affected parent have inherited the mutant allele. The difference between the proportion of unilaterally affected offspring among FB parents (14%), FU parents (35%), and carrier parents (47%) in Table 3 suggests that the FU case population consists of roughly 60% of carriers of the premutated allele and of 40% of individuals with the mutated allele. The proportion of FB cases who inherited the premutated allele is undetermined, but probably very small.

DISCUSSION

The data shown here for carotid body tumors and for retinoblastoma, and the data we presented previously on achondroplasia and the Wiedemann-Beckwith syndrome indicate regularities in the patterns of pedigrees which are consistent for the individual condition but differ from one condition to another. On the clinical level it cannot be determined whether these factors which correlate with the different patterns (namely, the type of cell division and the sex and fitness of affected persons and carriers) influence the consecutive mutational processes at that particular locus, or whether they influence segregation or expression of the premutant and mutant alleles.

It is of interest to consider the phenomenon of delayed mutation from three different angles: genetic instability, cryptic mutation, and nonexpression of a genetic trait.

The process of delayed mutation has some features in common with the phenomenon of spontaneous instabilities described in lower organisms. These instances of genetically controlled high mutability at particular loci are relatively frequent and well-studied in yeast, certain bacteria, and *Drosophila*. In many cases their occurrence can be related to chromosome translocations, small chromosome duplications or deletions, mutator genes, or transposable controlling elements. A recent review of the subject is provided by Auerbach and Kilbey (5). They make the distinction between *replication errors* (when a changed DNA-template continues to cause mutational changes at each successive replication) and *replicating instabilities* (premutational changes that can replicate in the unstable state to produce mutations in *several* lines of descent). Only those instabilities which replicate as instabilities are comparable to the delayed mutation model.

Since the premutated gene is phenotypically not detectable, the process of delayed mutation may be considered to involve a cryptic mutation. The premutated gene requires some genetic qualities to be detectable. Such qualities may be related to gene replication, recombination, conversion, DNA repair, etc. Several aspects of cryptic mutations were recently delineated by Lamb who pointed out that almost one in four base substitution mutations are expected to be cryptic changes (52). Lamb pointed out the effects of cryptic mutations on conversion and recombination. We suspect that these mechanisms may be relevant to the differences in the pedigree patterns which we observed in the various conditions.

Nonexpression of a genetic trait can clinically be observed at the level of cell, tissue, and organ development, and with respect to the whole organism or an entire generation. Variable expressivity refers to nonexpression within parts of an organism, and decreased penetrance describes nonexpression of a genetic trait in an organism as a whole. Delayed mutation is a genetic mechanism for nonexpression of a genetic trait in an entire generation; this necessarily includes nonexpression of the trait in an organism with its organs, tissues, and cells. Introduction of the term *phenotrance* as a measure of phenotypic expression of a genetic trait in generations is helpful for the understanding of these differences. A single recessive gene can be considered to have a phenotrance of 0 and an always-expressed dominant allele, the phenotrance 1; the phenotrance may be said to be decreased when expression of the trait in generations is decreased over what is expected from its penetrance in individuals. The pedigrees in Fig. 4 show decreased phenotrance but essentially complete penetrance. Offspring of mutant parents can show decreased penetrance but not (usually) decreased phenotrance. However, carrier parents may produce sibships with both decreased phenotrance and decreased penetrance. In a sibship with decreased phenotrance one sib may be a carrier (with or without being affected due to somatic telomutation) and others may be affected or nonaffected mutants. The carrier sib is definitely genetically different from his mutant sib by the same mechanism which prevented expression of the trait in previous generations. Thus, there is a vertical and a horizontal measure of phenotrance; these need not be of the same magnitude if, for instance, two or more consecutive mutational changes occur at the particular locus.

Since the term phenotrance makes reference to the phenotype and not to the etiology of genetic nonexpression, it covers not only delayed mutation proper but also other causes of nonexpression in generations which may involve segregation, epistatic genetic factors, genetic inactivation, imprinting, etc. Phenotypic lag can be considered one type of decreased phenotrance. We have indicated above the difficulty of distinguishing between these possibilities on the basis of clinical material, and, strictly speaking, the data presented concern decreased phenotrance with delayed mutation as a likely but not the only possible explanation.

The data on retinoblastoma (RB) may serve to clarify these points. Mutant individuals with early and late onset, unilateral and bilateral involvement, and metastatic and nonmetastatic course illustrate variable expressivity. The mechanisms of variable expressivity in RB are undetermined, but in general, they appear to involve physiologic and developmental processes. The pedigrees of Figs. 2 to 4 do not include any certain examples of decreased penetrance, and none are known to us from the literature with the possible exception of cases of spontaneous regression of RB. The mechanisms of decreased penetrance have not been elucidated in any condition, but they may be quite different from those of variable expressivity and of decreased phenotrance. However, one could assume for a moment that the mechanisms of variable expressivity in RB also could lead to decreased penetrance, and one can then estimate this to occur in 2% of cases on the basis that 14% of mutant individuals are unilaterally affected.

A distinction between variable expressivity, decreased penetrance, and decreased phenotrance is relevant to considerations concerning the Knudson two-mutation and the Auerbach delayed mutation model. Both models involve a two-phase mutational process, but they are concerned with different steps in tumor development. The Auerbach model concerns the events before, and the Knudson model the events after, the fully mutant gene has arisen. Thus, the Auerbach model does not exclude a subsequent mutational process while the Knudson model does not exclude delayed mutation in the process leading to the first mutation; in fact, Knudson has stated in his original paper that in some families with RB, delayed mutation is a likely explanation (46).

The Knudson model implies that oncogenesis is complete only in cells which develop into a tumor and explains why only so very few of the mutants develop into cancer cells. The Auerbach model is an explanation for decreased phenotrance, and, in our interpretation, implies that the (fully) mutant gene, once it has arisen by delayed or complete mutation, is sufficient to cause cancer. High penetrance of the RB gene makes it, in our opinion, unnecessary to postulate a further mutational process. We consider development or nondevelopment of tumor foci, tumor growth, unilateral and bilateral involvement in mutant individuals to represent variable expressivity related to oncoplasia. Although not fully understood, this type of variable expressivity is also observed in many other dominant human neoplasia syndromes such as Gardner's syndrome, neurofibromatosis, and intestinal polyposis as well as in nonneoplastic syndromes.

ACKNOWLEDGMENTS

This work was supported by USPHS/NIH Grant GM 20130: Publication No. 1866 from the University of Wisconsin Genetics Laboratory. I thank Dr. John M. Opitz for continued and stimulating discussion and for his review of the manuscript. I thank Mrs. Priscilla Medler and Mr. James Olson for their meticulous technical assistance.

REFERENCES

1. Aherne, G. E. S., and Roberts, D. F. (1975): Retinoblastoma - a clinical survey and its genetic implications. *Clin. Genet.*, 8:275–290.

2. Andersen, S. R., and Jensen, O. A. (1974): Retinoblastoma with necrosis of central retinal artery and vein and partial spontaneous regression. *Acta Ophthalmol.*, 52:183–193.
3. Arias-Stella, J. (1969): Human carotid body at high altitudes. *Am. J. Pathol.*, 55:82a.
4. Auerbach, C. (1956): A possible case of delayed mutation in man. *Ann. Hum. Genet.*, 20:266–269.
5. Auerbach, C., and Kilbey, B. J. (1971): Mutation in eukaryotes. *Ann. Rev. Genet.*, 5:163–218.
6. Beard, M., and McQuarrie, D. G. (1968): Brotherly lumps. *Minn. Med.*, 51:79–82.
7. Bell, J. (1922): Giloma retinae. In: *The Treasury of Human Inheritance. Vol 2.* Cambridge University Press, London.
8. Bentley, D. (1975): A case of Down's syndrome complicated by retinoblastoma and celiac disease. *Pediatrics*, 56:131–133.
9. Bertrams, J., Schildberg, P., Höpping, W., Böhme, U., and Albert, E. (1973): HL-A antigens in retinoblastoma. *Tissue Antigens*, 3:78–87.
10. Böhringer, H. R. (1956): Statistik, Klinik und Genetik der schweizerischen Retinoblastomfälle (1925–1954). *Arch. Julius Klaus Stift. Vererbungsforsch.*, 31:1–16.
11. Boniuk, M., and Zimmerman, L. E. (1962): Spontaneous regression of retinoblastoma. *Int. Ophthalmol. Clin.*, 2:525–542.
12. Boniuk, M., and Girard, L. J. (1969): Spontaneous regression of bilateral retinoblastoma. *Trans. Am. Acad. Ophthalmol. Otol.*, 73:194–198.
13. Briard-Guillemot, M. L., Bonaiti-Pellié, C., Feingold, J., and Frézal, J. (1974): Étude génétique du rétinoblastome. *Humangenetik*, 24:271–284.
14. Chase, W. H. (1933): Familial and bilateral tumours of the carotid body. *J. Pathol. Bacteriol.*, 36:1–12.
15. Char, D. H., Ellsworth, R., Rabson, A. S., Albert, D. M., and Herberman, R. B. (1974): Cell-mediated immunity to a retinoblastoma tissue culture line in patients with retinoblastoma. *Am. J. Ophthalmol.*, 78:5–11.
16. Chedid, A., and Jao, W. (1974): Hereditary tumours of the carotid bodies and chronic obstructive pulmonary disease. *Cancer*, 33:1635–1641.
17. Czeizel, A., and Gárdonyi, J. (1974): Retinoblastoma in Hungary, 1960-1968. *Humangenetik*, 22:153–158.
18. Czeizel, A., Csósz, L., Gárdonyi, J., Remenár, L., and Ruziscka, P. (1974): Chromosome studies in twelve patients with retinoblastoma. *Humangenetik*, 22:159-166.
19. DelFante, F. M., and Watkins, E. (1967): Chemodectoma of the heart in a patient with multiple chemodectomas and family history. *Lahey Clinic Found. Bull.*, 16:224–229.
20. Desai, M. G., and Patel, C. C. (1961): Heredo-familial carotid body tumors. *Clin. Radiol.*, 12:214–218.
21. Devesa, S. (1975): The incidence of retinoblastoma. *Am. J. Ophthalmol.*, 80:263–265.
22. Dollfus, M. A., and Auvert, B. (cited by Kaelin).
23. Edwards, C., Heath, D., and Harris, P. (1971): The carotid body in emphysema and left ventricular hypertrophy. *J. Pathol.*, 104:1–13.
24. Falls, H. F., and Neel, J. V. (1951): Genetics of retinoblastoma. *Arch. Ophthalmol.*, 46:367–389.
25. Franceschetti, A., and Bischler, V. (1949): Rétinoblastome et hérédite. *Arch. Julius Klaus Stift. Vererbungsforsch.*, 21:322–328.
26. François, J., Matton, M. T., DeBie, S., Tanaka, Y., and Vandenbulcke, D. (1975): Genesis and genetics of retinoblastoma. *Ophthalmologica*, 170:405–425.
27. Gordon, H. (1974): Family studies in retinoblastoma. *Birth Defects*, 10:185–190.
28. Griffith, A. D., and Sorsby, A. (1944): The genetics of retinoblastoma. *Br. J. Ophthalmol.*, 28:279–293.
29. Hashem, N., and Khalifa, S. (1975): Retinoblastoma. A model of hereditary fragile chromosomal regions. *Hum. Hered.*, 25:35–49.
30. Hayes, H. M., and Fraumeni, J. F., Jr. (1974): Chemodectomas in dogs: Epidemiologic comparisons with man. *J. Natl. Cancer Inst.*, 52:1455–1458.
31. Heath, D., Edwards, C., and Harris, P. (1970): Postmortem size and structure of the human carotid body. *Thorax*, 25:129–140.
32. Hemmes, G. D. (1931): Untersuchungen nach dem Vorkommen von Glioma retinae bei Verwandten von mit dieser Krankheit Behafteten. *Klin. Monatsbl. Augenheilkd.*, 86:331–335.
33. Herrmann, J., and Opitz, J. M. (1977): Delayed mutation as a cause of genetic disease in man: Achondroplasia and the Wiedemann-Beckwith syndrome. In: *Proceedings of the Workshop on Regulation of Cell Proliferation and Differentiation*, edited by W. W. Nichols and R. W. Miller. Plenum, New York. *(In press.)*
34. Hermann, J. (1975): Delayed mutation as a cause of human disease. *Am. J. Hum. Genet.*, 27:43a.

35. Herrmann, J. (1976): Delayed mutation as a cause of retinoblastoma: Application to genetic counseling. *Birth Defects,* 12/1:79–90.
36. Hoefnagel, D., McIntyre, O. R., Storrs, R. C., Sullivan, P. B., and Maurer, L. H. (1973): Retinoblastoma followed by acute lymphoblastic leukaemia. *Lancet,* 1:725.
37. Inoue, S., Ravindranath, Y., Ottenbreit, M. J., Thompson, R. I., and Zuelzer, W. W. (1975): Chromosome analysis of metastatic retinoblastoma cells. *Humangenetik*, 25:111–118.
38. James, A. G., and Saleeby, R. (1953): The management of carotid body tumors. *Surgery,* 34:104–110.
39. Jensen, A. D. (1965): Retinoblastoma in Denmark 1943-1958. *Acta Ophthalmol. (Kbh),* 43:821–840.
40. Jensen, R. D., and Miller, R. W. (1971): Retinoblastoma: Epidemiologic characteristics. *N. Engl. J. Med.,* 285:307–311.
41. Jzikowitz, M. (1938): Les tumeurs malignes de la rétine. Thesis, Paris.
42. Kaelin, A. (1955): Statistische Prüf- und Schätzverfahren für die relative Häufigkeit von Merkmalsträgern in Geschwisterreihen bei einem der Auslese unterworfenen Material mit Anwendung auf das Retinagliom. *Arch. Julius Stift. Vererbungsforsch.,* 30:263–485.
43. Katz, A. D. (1964): Carotid body tumors in a large family group. *Am. J. Surg.,* 108:570–573.
44. Kitchin, F. D., and Ellsworth, R. M. (1974): Pleiotropic effects of the gene for retinoblastoma. *J. Med. Genet.,* 11:244–246.
45. Kline, P. S., Thomas, R. A., and McNamara, W. L. (1949): Bilateral carotid body tumor. *Am. J. Surg.,* 77:120–123.
46. Knudson, A. G., Jr. (1971): Mutation and cancer: Statistical study of retinoblastoma. *Proc. Natl. Acad. Sci. U.S.A.,* 68:820–823.
47. Knudson, A. G., Jr., Strong, L. C., and Anderson, B. E. (1973): Heredity and cancer in man. *Progr. Med. Genet.,* 9:113–158.
48. Knudson, A. G., Jr. (1974): Heredity and human cancer. *Am. J. Path.,* 77:77–84.
49. Kroll, A. J., Alexander, B., Cochius, F., and Pechet, L. (1964): Hereditary deficiencies of clotting factors VIII and X associated with carotid body tumors. *N. Engl. J. Med.,* 270:6–13.
50. Ladda, R., Atkins, L., Littlefield, J., and Pruett, R. (1973): Retinoblastoma: Chromosome banding in patients with heritable tumour. *Lancet,* 2:506.
51. Lahey, F. H., and Warren, K. W. (1951): A long term appraisal of carotid body tumors with remarks on their removal. *Surg. Gynecol. Obstet.,* 92:481–491.
52. Lamb, B. C. (1975): Cryptic mutations: Their predicted biochemical basis, frequencies and effects on gene conversion. *Mol. Gen. Genet.,* 137:305–314.
53. LeCompte, P. M. (1951): Tumors of the carotid body and related structures (chemoreceptor system). In: *Atlas of Tumor Pathology (Section IV, Fascicle 16).* AFIP, Washington, D.C.
54. Lewison, E. F., and Weinberg, T. (1950): Carotid body tumors. *Surgery,* 27:437–448.
55. Macklin, M. T. (1960): A study of retinoblastoma in Ohio. *Am. J. Hum. Genet.,* 12:1–43.
56. McGuirt, W. F., and Harker, L. A. (1975): Carotid body tumors. *Arch. Otolaryngol.,* 101:58–62.
57. McNealy, R. W., and Hedin, R. F. (1939): Surgery of carotid body tumors. *J. Int. Col. Surg.,* 2:285–294.
58. Mehra, K. S., and Gupta, I.M. (1974): Unilaterally regressing retinoblastoma with massive optic nerve involvement in a bilateral lesion. *Ann. Ophthalmol.,* 6:919–922.
59. Morris, W. E., and LaPiana, F. G. (1974): Spontaneous regression of bilateral multifocal retinoblastoma with preservation of normal visual acuity. *Ann. Ophthalmol.,* 6:1192–1194.
60. Mouren, P., Poinso, Y., Pellet, W., Lavieille, J., Soubeyrand, J., Mouren, M. C., and Gouron, P. (1975): Les tumeurs du glomus jugulaire. *Sem. Hôp. Paris,* 51:1917–1926.
61. Neel, J. V. (1962): Mutations in the human population. In: *Methodology in Human Genetics,* edited by W. J. Burdette, p. 208. Holden-Day, San Francisco.
62. Olson, J. R., and Abell, M. R. (1969): Nonfunctional, nonchromaffin paragangliomas of the retroperitoneum. *Cancer,* 23:1358–1367.
63. Orye, E., Delbeke, M. J., and Vandenbeele, B. (1974): Retinoblastoma and long arm deletion of chromosome 13. Attempts to define the deleted segment. *Clin. Genet.,* 5:457–464.
64. Pellié, C., Briard, M. L., Feingold, J., and Frézal, J. (1973): Parental age in retinoblastoma. *Humangenetik,* 20:59–62.
65. Phelps, F. W., Case, S. W., and Snyder, G. A. C. (1937): Primary tumors of the carotid body. *West. J. Surg.,* 45:42–46.
66. Pratt, L. W. (1973): Familial carotid body tumors. *Arch. Otolaryngol.,* 97:334–336.
67. Rados, A. (1946): Occurrence of glioma of retina and brain in collateral lines in same family. *Arch. Ophthalmol.,* 35:1–12.
68. Reese, A. B. (1949): Heredity and retinoblastoma. *Arch. Ophthalmol.,* 42:119–122.

69. Rethoré, M. O., Saraux, H., Prieur, M., Dutrillaux, B., Meer, J-J., and Lejeune, J. (1972): Syndrome 48, XXY, +21 et rétinoblastoma. *Arch. Fr. Pédiatr.*, 29:533–539.

70. Rush, B. F. (1963): Familial bilateral carotid body tumors. *Ann. Surg.*, 157:633–636.

71. Saldana, M., Salem, L. E., and Travezan, R. (1973): High altitude hypoxia and chemodectomas. *Hum. Pathol.*, 4:251–263.

72. Schappert-Kimmijser, J., Hemmes, G. D., and Nijland, R. (1966): The heredity of retinoblastoma. *Ophthalmologica*, 151:197–213.

73. Schimke, R. N., Lowman, J. T., and Cowan, G. A. B. (1974): Retinoblastoma and osteogenic sarcoma in siblings. *Cancer*, 34:2077–2079.

74. Shamblin, W. R., ReMine, W. H., Sheps, S. G., and Harrison, E. G. Jr. (1971): Carotid body tumor (chemodectoma)—clinicopathologic analysis of ninety cases. *Am. J. Surg.*, 122:732–739.

75. Sprong, D. H., and Kirby, F. G. (1949): Familial carotid body tumors: Report of nine cases in eleven siblings. *Ann. West. Med. Surg.*, 3:241–242.

76. Strong, L. C., and Knudson, A. G., Jr. (1973): Second cancers in retinoblastoma. *Lancet*, 2:1086.

77. Tucker, D. P., Steinberg, A. G., and Cogan, D. G. (1957): Frequency of genetic transmission of sporadic retinoblastoma. *Arch. Ophthalmol.*, 57:532–535.

78. Vogel, F. (1954): Über Genetik and Mutationsrate des Retinoblastoms. *Z. Menschl. Vererb. Konstitutionslehre*, 32:308–336.

79. Vogel, F. (1967): Genetic prognosis in retinoblastoma. In: *Modern Trends in Ophthalmology*, edited by A. Sorsby, pp. 34–42. Butterworth, London.

80. Warburg, M. (1974): Retinoblastoma. In: *Genetic and Metabolic Eye Disease*, edited by Morton F. Goldberg. Little, Brown, Boston.

81. Weller, C. V. (1941): The inheritance of retinoblastoma and its relationship to practical eugenics. *Cancer Res.*, 1:517–535.

82. Wiener, S., Reese, A. B., and Hyman, G. A. (1963): Chromosome studies in retinoblastoma. *Arch. Ophthalmol.*, 69:311–313.

83. Wilson, H. (1970): Carotid body tumors: Familial and bilateral. *Ann. Surg.*, 171:843–846.

84. Wilson, M. G., Towner, J. W., and Fujimoto, A. (1973): Retinoblastoma and D-chromosome deletions. *Am. J. Hum. Genet.*, 25:57–61.

Discussion

Hirschhorn: Could you give a possible molecular explanation for premutation?

Herrmann: I could only speculate that it is some change in DNA that would make subsequent change at the same locus much more likely, perhaps by several orders of magnitude. Ethylation of N-7 in guanine has been suggested as a possible DNA change leading to the initiation of GC to AT transitions.

Yerganian: In an earlier study, Armenian hamsters were treated with ethyl methanesulfonate (100 mg/kg) and bred with normal females [*Science*, 172:171–174 (1971)]. The F_1 male progeny was screened for induced translocations [*Lab. Anim. Sci.*, 24:62–65, (1974)], and cytologically normal males were bred to normal females. The resulting F_2 males were then treated with urethan (100/kg). To our surprise, 50% of the males exhibited specific breaks at the junction of the early and late replicating segments of the X chromosome in 86% of the cells examined at diakinesis 6 days after urethan treatment. Hence, a site-specific, latent anomaly had been retained in the premutated state for two generations after an ancestral exposure to ethyl methanesulfonate, with the mutational process being completed only when the required energy was provided via urethan. In many respects, this parallels Auerbach's findings regarding fractional (mosaic) mutations in *Drosophila* induced by chemical mutagens [*Science*, 158:1141 (1967)].

Herrmann: There are other analogous experiments in different organisms using spontaneous and chemically and radiation-induced mutagens. I believe they show just what we see in man—that mutational events are basically similar in various species, strains, or loci, but different mechanisms may operate for different animals and loci. For instance, the pedigree patterns in familial carotid body tumors are consistent but very different from those of achondroplasia and retinoblastoma families.

Comings: Sister chromatid exchanges tend to occur preferentially between the hetero-chromatin and euchromatin junctions. This may be a secondary phenomenon unrelated to specific sites in the DNA. Dr. Herrmann, the essence of the definition of premutation you just gave is that an initial event predisposes to a subsequent event. The important point is, "What happens in a single cell?" In an organism you can get selection for a rare somatic mutation, and that is exactly what Dr. Knudson postulates. You must be able to reduce your hypothesis to a single cell level or it will disappear.

Herrmann: In phage, yeast, and *Drosophila,* consecutive mutations have been shown to occur in single cells and at specific sites.

Comings: But, I meant directly in reference to retinoblastoma.

Herrmann: That is hard to do, but might be approached with Dr. Fialkow's techniques.

Genetics of Human Cancer, edited by J. J.
Mulvihill, R. W. Miller, and J. F. Fraumeni, Jr.
Raven Press, New York, 1977.

41

Clonal Origin and Stem Cell Evolution of Human Tumors

Philip J. Fialkow

Medical Service, Veterans Administration Hospital, Seattle, Washington 98108, and the Departments of Medicine and Genetics, University of Washington, Seattle, Washington 98195

Studies of tumorigenesis are limited by the necessary proscription against direct investigation in human subjects, and, therefore, generally provide only indirect evidence concerning causative factors. One such indirect approach takes advantage of naturally occurring cell labels to ask such questions as, ''Does the neoplasm arise from one or from many cells?'' This information is important because it provides clues to the tumor's mode of origin. For example, if a neoplasm is initiated by a rare, random event such as ''spontaneous'' somatic mutation, single cell (clonal) origin would be expected. In contrast, multicellular origin might be seen for a tumor caused by cell-to-cell spread of a virus.

This question can be investigated in subjects with two (or more) genetically distinct cell types, i.e., in subjects with mosaicism. Both cell types will be found in normal tissues, but neoplasms with unicellular origin should contain only one type. Chromosomal and immunoglobulin mosaicism have been employed, but the most generally applicable system is the mosaicism that occurs in females consequent to random inactivation of one X chromosome in each somatic cell. The X-linked glucose-6-phosphate dehydrogenase (G-6-PD) locus is an especially useful marker for this purpose.

Females heterozygous for the usual G-6-PD gene, Gd^B, and a variant allele such as Gd^A, have two cell populations, one producing G-6-PD B and the other, G-6-PD A. These enzymes are easily distinguished by electrophoresis. Tumors with unicellular origin should exhibit only one type of G-6-PD (B *or* A) (single-enzyme phenotypes), whereas those arising from multiple cells might have both B and A enzymes (double-enzyme phenotypes). Selected examples of tumors studied with the G-6-PD system are discussed in this chapter. Extensive reviews appear elsewhere (16,17).

NEOPLASMS WITH STEM CELL ORIGIN

Chronic Myelocytic Leukemia

Clonal Origin

Although the Philadelphia (Ph^1) chromosome rearrangement is present in 90 to 100% of dividing marrow cells in typical cases of chronic myelocytic leukemia (CML), clonal origin of the disease is not necessarily indicated since it is conceivable that the Ph^1 chromosome anomaly arises independently in many cells.

G-6-PD.

Thus far eight G-6-PD heterozygotes with Ph^1-positive CML have been studied (4,18; R. Jacobson and P.J. Fialkow, *unpublished data*). As expected, both B and A enzymes (double-enzyme phenotypes) were found in skin fibroblasts, but in each case only a single G-6-PD type was observed in the CML granulocytes, i.e., they had single-enzyme phenotypes. Four patients typed as B and four as A. These findings in CML granulocytes contrast sharply with those in blood cells from nonleukemic G-6-PD heterozygotes which almost invariably exhibit both B and A enzyme types (15). The fact that single-enzyme phenotypes occur in CML granulocytes, but not in normal white cells, strongly favors a clonal origin of CML. However, this conclusion obviously applies only to the stage at which the disease is clinically apparent. Conceivably, at an earlier phase many cells might be affected but one clone evolves by the time leukemia is manifest.

Other markers.

Numerous other lines of evidence also indicate that at the time the diagnosis is made, the CML stem cells are all derived from a single clone. For example, in patients whose number 22 chromosomes (or number 9) can be distinguished from one another, formation of the Ph^1 anomaly always involves the same number 22 (or 9) (29,33,34). Evidence for unicellular origin is also provided by studies with 6-phosphogluconate dehydrogenase isoenzymes and Rh antigens in one patient (21,22) and in studies of patients with sex chromosome mosaicism (26,43).

Stem Cell Origin

In Gd^B/Gd^A heterozygotes with CML, the single-enzyme phenotypes occur in red cells as well as in granulocytes (4,18), and Ph^1 is found in red cell precursors (12,50). In contrast, both B and A enzymes are found in red cells from nonleukemic Gd^B/Gd^A heterozygotes (15). Thus, the CML clone arises in a stem cell common to granulocytes and erythrocytes but not to skin fibroblasts. Similarly, we have found single-enzyme phenotypes in platelets and cultured monocytes *(unpublished studies)*. Blood lymphocytes stimulated to divide *in vitro* by phytohemagglutinin apparently are Ph^1-negative, but this does not necessarily exclude the possibility that lymphocytes emanate from the CML stem cell. For example, the phytohemagglutinin-responsive cells are presumably long-lived and may have antedated the development of the CML clone. Furthermore, they may reflect only one subtype of lymphocyte, and other lymphocytes are also possibly descendants of the CML stem cell.

Are There Any Normal Stem Cells in CML?

The single-enzyme G-6-PD phenotypes and Ph^1 data do not exclude the presence of a small population of normal stem cells, which would not be detected if they contributed less than 5% of the dividing marrow cells or 5 to 10% of the total enzyme activity. The presence of some normal stem cells in CML is suggested by the observation of a few Ph^1-negative colonies in cultures of stem cells from two CML patients (10). However, other investigations have found such colonies to be uniformly Ph^1-positive (3,44,54). Further evidence is provided by the occasional reports of CML patients with unusual sensitivity to busulfan who, after recovery from profound marrow insufficiency, manifest a Ph^1-negative population (25,30), and by a preliminary report of the appearance of such cells in some patients treated with intensive therapy (11). The question of whether there are normal stem cells could be further investigated by determining G-6-PD phenotypes of stem cell colonies grown from heterozygotes with CML.

Pathogenesis of CML

Genetic marker studies indicate that the alteration responsible for development of CML occurs in marrow stem cells. However, morphologically this disease is not considered a stem cell leukemia. The predominant picture in the marrow is an overabundance of myelocytes and more mature granulocytic cells with little evidence of increased stem cells. To reconcile these morphological observations with the genetic marker data, it is necessary to postulate that the normal stem cell population is totally or largely replaced by CML stem cells. Although normoblasts and megakaryocytes originate from the CML stem cell and are Ph^1-positive, erythrocytes and platelets generally are not greatly increased in number. In contrast, the same Ph^1 anomaly in granulocyte precursors makes them exempt from normal growth-control mechanisms.

In a small proportion of Ph^1-positive patients, a relatively large fraction of dividing marrow cells lacks the chromosome anomaly, even early in the course of the disease. A possible explanation for this unusual situation is that in these cases, Ph^1 occurs in a stem cell that has already undergone differentiation towards the granulocytic line, so that the Ph^1-negative marrow cells are normoblasts. Alternatively, the disease may always involve a multipotential marrow stem cell, but in these few patients the Ph^1-positive clone only partially replaces the normal marrow stem cells.

Ph^1 is detected in 90 to 100% of dividing marrow cells from typical CML patients and is highly specific and characteristic of that disease; it is present throughout the course of CML and in some patients has been observed in marrow cells years before the onset of overt leukemia (9). For these reasons, many investigators believe that

Ph[1] is intimately involved in the pathogenesis of CML and may be its immediate cause. However, the primary causes (that presumably induce Ph[1]) remain largely unknown.

Etiological Implications of Clonal Origin

Among etiologic factors postulated for CML are "spontaneous" or radiation-induced genetic accidents, viruses, and physiologic defects in marrow homeostasis. The "spontaneous" mutation hypothesis requires that the tumor would begin in one cell; the genetic marker data are in accord with this suggestion. Defective homeostasis implies that the basic abnormality is not intrinsic to the marrow cells themselves, but is found in the mechanisms which regulate marrow proliferation and maturation. In so far as this hypothesis predicts multicellular origin, the genetic marker data make it unlikely to be correct. With a viral or radiation cause, the origin could be from one or many cells. For example, if the virus were only one of several factors necessary for tumorigenesis, or if the oncogenic change induced by the virus were rare, clonal origin would be found (e.g., chromosome abnormalities in many cells might be induced, but only the rare cell which happened to have Ph[1] would evolve into CML). Alternatively, the putative oncogenic virus might have specific affinity for the DNA in the involved regions of chromosomes 22 and 9, in which case Ph[1] could be induced in multiple cells. The probable clonal origin of CML makes this latter possibility less likely and also virtually excludes any pathogenetic hypothesis based on continuous cell recruitment (i.e., the ability of a cell that has undergone leukemic transformation to continuously induce other cells to become a part of the neoplasm, possibly by transfer of an infectious agent).

Blastic Transformation

Since CML is often associated with prolonged survival unless myelofibrosis or acute blastic transformation occurs, it can be regarded as a preleukemic condition. What factors determine its progression to acute, malignant leukemia? During blastic transformation Ph[1] and the single-enzyme phenotypes persist, indicating that the acute malignancy occurs in preexisting CML cells. It is difficult to determine by the use of Ph[1] and G-6-PD markers whether blastic transformation involves one or many cells since by the time transformation occurs, all or most of the hematopoietic cells are Ph[1]-positive and have a single-enzyme phenotype. However, sequential chromosome analyses suggest that a single CML subclone evolves to blastic transformation (6,32). Unicellular origin is also suggested by study of a patient with constitutional sex chromosome mosaicism (45).

In most patients, blastic transformation is characterized by overabundance of very immature granulocyte precursors such as myeloblasts and promyelocytes. However, the possibility has been raised that occasionally lymphoblastic conversion of CML may occur (8)—a suggestion based on morphologic characteristics and steroid responsiveness. Evidence in rodents suggests a stem cell pluripotent for myeloid and lymphoid cells (47) and there are suggestive data in man as well (5). If CML involved such a pluripotent stem cell, lymphoblastic conversion might occur. This question can be approached through G-6-PD studies of lymphocyte subpopulations in CML. An alternative explanation for lymphoblastic conversion in CML, if it indeed occurs, is that patients with CML are predisposed by virtue of the disease or its therapy to develop acute lymphoblastic leukemia. Were this the case, the lymphoblastic cells in individuals with mosaicism would sometimes manifest genetic markers (e.g., G-6-PD) different from those detected in the CML clone.

Polycythemia Vera

Stem Cell Origin and Probable Clonal Origin

Single-enzyme phenotypes were found in erythrocytes from two Gd^B/Gd^A patients with this disease suggesting that it has clonal origin (2). As the same single-enzyme phenotypes were found in granulocytes and platelets, it can be concluded that polycythemia vera is a stem cell disorder. Blood lymphocytes displayed a normal double-enzyme phenotype indicating that at least a major lymphocyte population does not emanate from the abnormal polycythemia vera cells.

Are There Any Normal Stem Cells in Polycythemia Vera?

Detailed analyses of single erythroid colonies grown in semisolid medium indicate that there are some residual normal stem cells (48). The number of colonies derived from normal progenitor stem cells was increased by erythropoietin treatment indicating that these residual normal cells retain their sensitivity to that hormone. Preliminary studies suggest that polycythemia vera stem cells as well as normal stem cells respond to erythropoietin, but we do not yet know the relative sensitivity of the two populations to the hormone.

Pathogenesis and Etiology

The implications of stem cell origin and probable clonal origin of polycythemia vera for its etiology and pathogenesis are similar to those discussed above for CML. The G-6-PD data make very unlikely the previously postulated mechanism that polycythemia results from a primary defect in erythropoietin homeostasis.

Acute Transformation

The prevalence of acute leukemia is significantly elevated in polycythemia vera, but it is uncertain if this is related to therapy, if it is part of the disease's natural history and/or if polycythemia vera patients have increased susceptibility to develop acute leukemia in previously uninvolved cells. This latter possibility would be supported by the observation that, for example, preleukemic cells from Gd^B/Gd^A-polycythemia patient typed as A, but the leukemic cells typed as B/A or B.

Idiopathic Myelofibrosis

Myelofibrosis may develop in the course of CML or polycythemia vera, but most cases occur without obvious predisposition. Although many think that the disorder is neoplastic, the identity of the neoplastic cell is much debated. Thus far, only a single G-6-PD heterozygote with this disease is known to have been studied. The same enzyme type was found in blood granulocytes, red cells, and platelets (R. Jacobson and P. J. Fialkow, *in preparation*), indicating that a basic abnormality resides in hematopoietic stem cells. Furthermore, the data suggest that these cells are clonally derived and by inference, that the disease is "neoplastic." Clonal origin argues strongly against one previously postulated pathogenetic mechanism, altered marrow and spleen microenvironment. According to this hypothesis, damage to reticuloendothelial stroma (microenvironment), which directs stem cells into one or another differentiated pathway, results in hematopoietic cell hyperplasia and marrow fibrosis. In contrast to blood cells, cultured marrow fibroblasts displayed the normal double-enzyme phenotype, suggesting that the marrow fibrosis which predominates the clinical picture may be a secondary phenomenon. Similar conclusions are reached using chromosomal markers (57; P. J. Fialkow, R. Jacobson, and A. Salo, *unpublished data*).

Lymphoproliferative Disorders

These disorders have been most extensively studied with immunoglobulin (Ig) markers. A given Ig-synthesizing cell is committed to the production of molecules with only one light chain and one variable region (idiotype). Normal lymphoid tissue consists of a mixture of cells synthesizing many Ig molecules. All the immunocytes in a tumor with clonal origin synthesize the same Ig, whereas several Igs should be synthesized in a neoplasm with multicellular origin.

The progenitors of antibody-secreting cells, B lymphocytes, also synthesize Igs and although the molecules generally are not secreted, they are easily detected on the B lymphocytes' surfaces where they function as antigen receptors. When stimulated by antigen, B lymphocytes become large blast-like cells ("immunoblasts") and ultimately differentiate into antibody-secreting plasma cells. Neoplasia may affect a cell along any step in this pathway.

Multiple Myeloma

The predominant finding in this disease is a clonal proliferation of plasma cells, but recently it has been shown in some patients that circulating B lymphocytes bear the same "monoclonal" Ig on their surfaces as is found in the serum (1,42). Thus, multiple myeloma appears to be fundamentally a clonal disorder of B lymphocytes (or their progenitors) that ultimately differentiate into antibody-secreting plasma cells. Overabundance of the latter cells is the predominant clinical manifestation.

Chronic Lymphocytic Leukemia

The leukemia cell surfaces in almost every patient with this malignant proliferation of B lymphocytes bear monoclonal Ig (51,53). The fact that the monoclonal Ig is rarely found in the serum of leukemia patients suggests that in contrast to other B lymphocyte clonal proliferations, such as multiple myeloma and Waldenström's macroglobulinemia, in chronic lymphocytic leukemia there is a maturation block in the proliferating clone.

Waldenström's Macroglobulinemia

This disease has some features of multiple myeloma and others of chronic lymphocytic leukemia, being characterized by monoclonal IgM in the serum and proliferation in the marrow of pleomorphic B cells (e.g., B lymphocytes, "plasmacytoid-lymphocytes," and plasma cells). The surfaces of these lymphoid cells bear the same monoclonal Ig found in the serum (49,58). Thus, Waldenström's macroglobulinemia reflects proliferation of a clone of immunocytes that continues to differentiate and ultimately forms mature plasma cells. Moreover, although blood lymphocyte counts are not increased in most patients, many circulating lymphocytes have membrane-bound monoclonal IgM. In this sense, the disease may be regarded as a form of leukemia.

Idiopathic Chronic Cold Agglutinin Disease

Cold agglutinins in this disease have specificity for I and i red cell antigens (36,41) and are monoclonal (28). As in Waldenström's macroglobulinemia, the surfaces of blood lymphocytes also bear monoclonal IgM (14). Thus, in one sense this disease may also be considered a B cell neoplasm.

Many other benign and malignant neoplasms have been studied with cell markers and the data suggest single cell origin for most of them (reviewed in refs. 16 and 17). However, at least one carcinoma of the colon (7) and perhaps some carcinomas of the cervix (55) may be exceptions. Some benign hereditary and viral tumors also have multicellular origin.

HEREDITARY TUMORS

Among the tumors that might be expected to have multicellular origins are neoplasms that develop in a subject with innate predisposition to tumorigenesis (e.g., in a patient with a genetic disease strongly associated with tumor development). In this case, there are a large number of target cells predisposed to neoplasia by virtue of the inherited mutation.

Multiple Neurofibromatosis

Tumors and the overlying normal skin were studied from seven separate sites in each of two unrelated G-6-PD heterozygotes with this dominantly inherited syndrome (23). Each neurofibroma had a double-enzyme phenotype very similar to that of the overlying normal skin indicating multicellular origin for the neurofibroma as it occurs in von Recklinghausen's disease. Alternate possibilities to explain the double-enzyme phenotypes, such as that the neurofibromas contain both B and A enzymes because they are "contaminated" with nonneoplastic cells or because both X chromosomes are active in individual neurofibroma cells, have been excluded (23).

It has been estimated that the hereditary neurofibroma originates from hundreds or even thousands of cells (23). The initial tumorigenic step is a germinal mutation, but since the neurofibroma starts from so many cells, the factors which determine its formation are not "spontaneous" mutation-like events. Rather, tumor induction involves many cells initially as might be seen with neoplasms induced by hormonal changes. Increased levels of nerve-growth factor have been described in patients with hereditary neurofibromatosis (52). Another possibility is that the oncogenic mechanism alters only a single cell and adjacent normal cells are recruited to form the tumor.

In contrast to hereditary neurofibromas, single-enzyme phenotypes indicating clonal origin are found in sporadically occurring neurofibromas (P. J. Fialkow and R. Jacobson, *unpublished observations*). These data indicate that although the biological and histological features of the hereditary and sporadic tumors are similar, there is a fundamental difference in the tumorigenic mechanisms.

Patients with neurofibromatosis are at a significantly increased risk to develop sarcomatous transformation of their tumors. Does the malignant change involve only a single, preexisting neurofibroma cell or is an entire field of cells altered? This question could be answered with G-6-PD studies of appropriate sarcomas.

Other Hereditary Tumors

Results of G-6-PD studies in another dominantly inherited disease characterized by tumor formation, multiple trichoepitheliomas, are compatible with multiple cell origin (31). However, since this neoplasm consists of a mixture of epithelial cells and fibroblasts, the data are difficult to interpret.

Although the data indicate multiple cell origin for hereditary neurofibromas, this cannot be expanded into a general interpretation regarding all hereditary tumors. For example, from what is known about the molecular abnormality in xeroderma pigmentosum, one probable oncogenic mechanism, somatic mutation secondary to a defect in DNA repair, predicts that each of the multiple tumors arising in a patient with this disease will have single cell origin. Knudson and his colleagues have recently amassed data suggesting that two sequential mutations are necessary for the development of the embryonal neoplasms (retinoblastoma, neuroblastoma, and Wilms' tumor) (e.g., ref. 39). In autosomal dominant retinoblastoma, the first mutation is inherited through the germ cell and neoplasms are often multiple and bilateral. On the other hand, in nonhereditary retinoblastoma both mutations are somatic; tumors are unilateral and single. If this hypothesis is correct, retinoblastoma of the hereditary as well as the sporadic type, should have clonal origin. In contrast, if the second step is not mutational, hereditary retinoblastomas might have double-enzyme phenotypes whereas the sporadic forms would have clonal origin and, therefore, single-enzyme phenotype.

VIRAL AND PUTATIVE VIRAL TUMORS

In addition to innate susceptibility, the nature of the external oncogenic agent may be a major factor in determining the number of cells initially affected. For example, multicellular origin will occur when tumors are caused by cell-to-cell spread and transformation by oncogenic viruses. The only neoplasms in man with proven viral cause are warts.

Warts

Condylomata Acuminata ("Venereal" Warts)

These rapidly growing benign "neoplasms" occur at mucocutaneous junctions such as the vulva. They are caused by a papovavirus. Each growth consists of cauliflower-like clumps of small individual verrucous subunits. Double-enzyme phenotypes were found in each of four warts from two G-6-PD heterozygotes (27). Epithelial remnants from even the smallest verrucal subunits have multicellular origin. Detailed analysis of one wart suggests that it developed from about 4,000 to 5,000 cells. Since these lesions arise from so many cells, it is likely that the tumorigenic virus is highly infectious on a cellular level. What are the factors which limit the growth of warts and prevent their transformation to malignant neoplasms? One possibility is that the growth of condyloma acuminatum is limited by immunological surveillance, perhaps against viral antigens, and malignant outgrowth occurs only if this control is breeched by an altered clone of cells. Alternatively, a malignant tumor may develop only if a virally infected cell is the site of one or more additional events such as a genetic change. Either of these possibilities would be supported by the findings that malignancies which develop from condylomata acuminata have unicellular origin.

Verruca Vulgaris (Common Warts)

The common wart is also caused by a papovavirus but in contrast to the double-enzyme phenotypes found in "venereal" warts, single-enzyme phenotypes were found in six common warts from as many patients (46). Although these findings are compatible with clonal origin, an alternative explanation is that the common wart arises from several cells but that, in each of the six lesions studied, all the transformed cells happened to have the same G-6-PD phenotype. If this interpretation were correct, further study of common warts should reveal some with double-enzyme phenotypes.

If in fact, common warts have unicellular origin—whereas "venereal" warts have multiple cell origin and the common and "venereal" wart papovaviruses are the same—there may be a significant effect of initial inoculum size and/or of local environmental conditions on the facility of viral spread and the pattern of "tumorigenesis."

Burkitt Lymphoma

This malignant lymphoblastic disease occurs with notable frequency in some regions of Africa and New Guinea. Patients usually have multiple tumors in the jaw, orbit, gonads, kidneys, mesentery, retroperitoneal and paravertebral structures, liver, and spleen (13). There is much circumstantial evidence for a viral cause (38) and the putative agent is Epstein-Barr virus (EBV), a ubiquitous DNA herpesvirus.

Although a viral cause is postulated for Burkitt lymphoma and the clinical presentation suggests multifocal disease, G-6-PD and immunoglobulin marker data indicate clonal origin (19,20, and *unpublished observations*).

Implications of Clonal Origin for Putative Viral Cause of Burkitt Lymphoma

Despite the fact that viruses may infect many cells, clonal origin of a tumor does not necessarily exclude viral cause. For example, single cell origin may occur if the oncogenic change induced by the virus is a relatively rare one such as a specific chromosomal alteration like the recently described rearrangement involving chromosome numbers 14 (35,40,59) and 8 (59). Another possibility is that tumor formation is dependent not only upon the virus, but also upon cofactors, at least one of which is rare. For example, another way to look at the Burkitt lymphoma chromosome rearrangement is that it does not arise as a consequence of the putative oncogenic virus, but rather is a necessary precondition (perhaps arising from a "spontaneous" genetic accident) before the virus can induce malignant transformation in a cell or before a virus-transformed cell can develop into clinical malignancy. Alternatively, EBV may promote tumorigenesis merely by stimulating cell division of lymphocytes and thereby enhancing the likelihood for mutations and chromosomal rearrangements to occur. Finally, clonal origin would also be seen if multiple cells are transformed initially, but only a rare clone escapes surveillance mechanisms. In any event, the contrast between the unicellular origin of the malignant putative viral disease, Burkitt lymphoma, and the multicellular origin of the benign viral "tumor," venereal wart, suggests that virus-infected cells give rise to a malignant clone only if one or more additional events occur.

Burkitt Recurrences

The majority of patients with this disease undergo therapeutically induced "complete" remissions, but tumors reappear in at least 60% of cases. Are these true recurrences of the old disease, in other words, reemergence of the originally detected malignant cell lines, or are they "new" inductions of disease? If they are true recurrences of the old disease, they should have the same genetic markers as were found in the initial tumors. On the other hand, if they are new malignant cell lines, they may have discordant genetic markers. G-6-PD and immunoglobulin phenotypes of 27 early (less than 3 months) recurrent tumors were concordant with the phenotypes in the initial tumors, indicating that early relapses are reemergences of the original malignant clones (20). In contrast, phenotypes in three of nine relapses that occurred after 5 months were discordant with those of the initial tumors, indicating that some "late" recurrences may be the result of newly induced malignant clones (20). Similar suggestions have been made on the basis of clinical observations (60). Early relapses tend to appear at previously involved anatomic sites whereas late regrowths often occur in hitherto uninvolved organs. Furthermore, the prognosis for late recurrences is similar to that for initial presentations, whereas early relapses respond very poorly to therapy (61).

The finding that some late recurrences are due to emergence of a second malignant clone is compatible with the existence of predisposing factors to Burkitt lymphoma. These may be endogenous changes or environmental factors. However, recurrences could be associated with therapy which is generally immunosuppressive and may favor the emergence of a new clone due to escape from immunologic surveillance. It is noteworthy that even discordant late recurrences have clonal origin. Thus, continuous recruitment of hitherto normal cells to the malignancy rarely if ever occurs in Burkitt lymphoma despite its putative viral etiology.

Acute Lymphoblastic Leukemia

Another malignant lymphoblastic disease with putative viral etiology is acute lymphoblastic leukemia. Thus far, no reports of G-6-PD heterozygotes with this disease have appeared, but studies with chromosomal markers have provided evidence for the development of leukemia in more than one cell line in each of two patients under very exceptional circumstances (24,56). Both patients were girls who were treated with 1,000 rad whole-body irradiation followed in one day by a marrow transplant from a histocompatible brother. Leukemia relapses occurred, respectively, on the 62nd and 135th day after transplantation. In each case, leukemia cells containing Y chromosome and, therefore, of *donor* origin were demonstrated. Several possible mechanisms underlying these recurrences in donor cells have been discussed (24,56), but perhaps the most likely one is new induction of disease by an oncogenic virus. Irradiation has been shown to activate leukemogenic virus in rodents (37), and possibly a similar activation occurred in the patients and led to transformation of susceptible donor cells. It is of considerable interest now to know if untreated acute lymphoblastic leukemia has unicellular or multicellular origin.

CONCLUDING REMARKS

Results reviewed in this communication illustrate that study of neoplasms arising in patients with mosaicism can provide important information about tumorigenesis. The type of information gained in this way includes the substantiation of stem cell origin of several hematopoietic disorders including chronic myelocytic leukemia, polycythemia vera, and idiopathic myelofibrosis. The genetic marker data also suggest that these diseases have single cell origin.

The G-6-PD system has confirmed the hypothesis that at least some benign hereditary and viral neoplasms have multicellular origin. However, Burkitt lymphoma, a malignancy in man for which there is much circumstantial evidence for a viral cause, has clonal origin. Of particular note is the observation that early relapses of Burkitt lymphoma represent reemergence of the original malignant cell lines, whereas some late recurrences may be the result of the emergence of "new" tumor lines. However, even for these late recurrences, the individual tumors are clonal. Thus, continuous recruitment of normal cells to the malignancy does not occur in Burkitt lymphoma.   At present, genetic marker approaches are limited essentially to neoplasms that synthesize immunoglobulin or arise in G-6-PD heterozygotes. When other suitable mosaic systems are discovered, many more tumors can be investigated.

ACKNOWLEDGMENT

Studies done in the author's laboratory were supported by Grants GM 15253 and CA 16448 from the National Institutes of Health, DHEW.

REFERENCES

1. Abdou, N. I., and Abdou, N. L. (1975): The monoclonal nature of lymphocytes in multiple myeloma: Effects of therapy. *Ann. Intern. Med.*, 83:42–45.
2. Adamson, J. W., Fialkow, P. J., Murphy, S., Prchal, J. F., and Steinmann, L. (1976): Polycythemia vera: Stem cell and probable clonal origin of the disease. *N. Engl. J. Med.*, 295:913–916.
3. Aye, M. T., Till, J. E., and McCulloch, E. A. (1973): Cytological studies of granulopoietic colonies from two patients with chronic myelogenous leukemia. *Exp. Hematol.*, 1:115–118.
4. Barr, R. D., and Fialkow, P. J. (1973): Clonal origin of chronic myelocytic leukemia. *N. Engl. J. Med.*, 289:307–309.
5. Barr, R. D., Whang-Peng, J., and Perry, S. (1975): Hematopoietic stem cells in human peripheral blood. *Science*, 190:284–285.
6. Berger, R. (1965): Chromosomes et leucémies humaines, la notion d'evolution clonale. *Ann. Genet.*, 8:70–82.
7. Beutler, E., Collins, Z., and Irwin, L. E. (1967): Value of genetic variants of glucose-6-phosphate dehydrogenase in tracing the origin of malignant tumors. *N. Engl. J. Med.*, 276:389–391.
8. Boggs, D. R. (1974): Hematopoietic stem cell theory in relation to possible lymphoblastic conversion of chronic myeloid leukemia. *Blood*, 44:449-453.
9. Canellos, G. P., and Whang-Peng, J. (1972): Philadelphia-chromosome-positive preleukaemic state. *Lancet*, 2:1227–1229
10. Chervenick, P. A., Ellis, L. D., Pan, S. F., and Lawson, A. L. (1971): Human leukemic cells: *In vitro* growth of colonies containing the Philadelphia (Ph¹) chromosome. *Science*, 174:1134–1136.
11. Clarkson, B. D., Dowling, M. D., Gee T. S., Cunningham, I., Hopfan, S., Knapper, W. H., Vaartaja, T., and Haghbin, M. (1974): Radical therapy for chronic granulocytic leukemia (CGL). *Abstr. of 15th Congr. Intl. Soc. Hematol.*, Jerusalem, p. 136.
12. Clein, G. P., and Flemans, R. J. (1966): Involvement of the erythroid series in blastic crisis of chronic myeloid leukaemia: Further evidence for the presence of Philadelphia chromosome in erythroblasts. *Br. J. Haematol.*, 12:754–758.

13. Davies, J. N. P. (1975): Burkitt's tumor: pathology and diagnosis. In: *Lymphoproliferative Diseases,* edited by D. W. Molander, p. 290. Charles C. Thomas, Springfield, Illinois.

14. Feizi, T., Wernet, P., Kunkel, H. G., and Douglas, S. D. (1973). Lymphocytes forming red cell rosettes in the cold in patients with chronic cold agglutinin disease. *Blood,* 42:753–762.

15. Fialkow, P. J. (1973): Primordial cell pool size and lineage relationships of five human cell types. *Ann. Hum. Genet.,* 37:39–48.

16. Fialkow, P. J. (1974): The origin and development of human tumors studied with cell markers. *N. Engl. J. Med.,* 291:26–35.

17. Fialkow, P. J. (1976): Clonal origin of human tumors. *Cancer Reviews,* 458:283–321.

18. Fialkow, P. J., Gartler, S. M., and Yoshida, A. (1967): Clonal origin of chronic myelocytic leukemia in man. *Proc. Natl. Acad. Sci. USA,* 58:1468–1471.

19. Fialkow, P. J., Klein, G., Gartler, S. M., and Clifford, P. (1970): Clonal origin for individual Burkitt tumours. *Lancet,* 1:384–386.

20. Fialkow, P. J., Klein, E., Klein, G., Clifford, P., and Singh, S. (1973): Immunoglobulin and G-6-PD as markers of cellular origin in Burkitt lymphoma. *J. Exp. Med.,* 138:89–102.

21. Fialkow, P. J., Lisker, R., Detter, J., Giblett, E. R., and Zavala, C. (1969): 6-Phosphogluconate dehydrogenase: Hemizygous manifestation in a patient with leukemia. *Science,* 163:194–195.

22. Fialkow, P. J., Lisker, R., Giblett, E. R., Zavala, C., Cobo, A., and Detter, J. (1972): Genetic markers in chronic myelocytic leukaemia: Evidence opposing autosomal inactivation and favouring 6-PGD-Rh linkage. *Ann. Hum. Genet.,* 35:321–326.

23. Fialkow, P. J., Sagebiel, R. W., Gartler, S. M., and Rimoin, D. L. (1971): Multiple cell origin of hereditary neurofibromas. *N. Engl. J. Med.,* 284:298–300.

24. Fialkow, P. J., Thomas, E. D., Bryant, J. I., and Neiman, P. E. (1971): Leukaemic transformation of engrafted human marrow cells in vivo. *Lancet,* 1:251–255.

25. Finney, R., McDonald, G. A., Baikie, A. G., and Douglas, A. S. (1972): Chronic granulocytic leukaemia with Ph[1] negative cells in bone marrow and a ten year remission after busulphan hypoplasia. *Br. J. Haematol.,* 23:283–288.

26. Fitzgerald, P. H., Pickering, A. F., and Eiby, J. R. (1971): Clonal origin of the Philadelphia chromosome and chronic myeloid leukaemia: Evidence from a sex chromosome mosaic. *Br. J. Haematol.,* 21:473–480.

27. Friedman, J. M., and Fialkow, P. J. (1976): Viral "tumorigenesis" in man: Cell markers in condylomata acuminata. *Int. J. Cancer,* 17:57–61.

28. Fudenberg, H. H., and Kunkel, H. G. (1957): Physical properties of the red cell agglutinins in acquired hemolytic anemia. *J. Exp. Med.,* 106:689–702.

29. Gahrton, G., Lindsten, J., and Zech, L. (1974): Clonal origin of the Philadelphia chromosome from either the paternal or the maternal chromosome number 22. *Blood,* 43:837–840.

30. Galton, D. A. G. (1972): Thyroid tumours, lymphomas, granulocytic leukaemia. In: *Proceedings of the 2nd Padua Seminar on Clinical Oncology,* Piccin Medical Books, Padua.

31. Gartler, S. M., Ziprkowski, L., Krakowski, A., Ezra, R., Szeinberg, A., and Adam, A. (1966): Glucose-6-phosphate dehydrogenase as a tracer in the study of hereditary multiple trichoepithelioma. *Am. J. Hum. Genet.,* 18:282–287.

32. Grouchy, J. de, Nava, C. de, Cantu, J. M., Bilski-Pasquier, G., and Bousser, J. (1966): Models for clonal evolution: A study of chronic myelogenous leukemia. *Am. J. Hum. Genet.,* 18:485–503.

33. Hayata, I., Kakati, S., and Sandberg, A. A. (1974): On the monoclonal origin of chronic myelocytic leukemia. *Proc. Japan Acad.,* 50:381–385.

34. Hossfeld, D. K. (1975): Additional chromosomal indication for the unicellular origin of chronic myelocytic leukemia. *Z. Krebsforsch.,* 83:269–273.

35. Jarvis, J. E., Ball, G., Rickinson, A. B., and Epstein, M. A. (1974): Cytogenetic studies on human lymphoblastoid cell lines from Burkitt's lymphomas and other sources. *Int. J. Cancer,* 14:716–721.

36. Jenkins, W. J., Marsh, W. L., Noades, J., Tippet, P., Sanger, R., and Race, R. R. (1960): The I antigen and antibody. *Vox Sang.,* 5:97–121.

37. Kaplan, H. S. (1967): On the natural history of the murine leukemias: Presidential address. *Cancer Res.,* 27:1325–1340.

38. Klein, G. (1975): The Epstein-Barr virus and neoplasia. *N. Engl. J. Med.,* 293:1353–1357.

39. Knudson, A. G., Jr. (1973): Mutation and human cancer. *Adv. Cancer Res.,* 17:317–352.

40. Manolov, G., and Manolova, Y. (1972): Marker band in one chromosome 14 from Burkitt lymphomas. *Nature,* 237:33–34.

41. Marsh, W. L. (1961): Anti-i: A cold antibody defining the Ii relationship in human red cells. *Br. J. Haematol.*, 7:200-209.

42. Mellstedt, H., Hammerström, S., and Holm, G. (1974): Monoclonal lymphocyte population in human plasma cell myeloma. *Clin. Exp. Immunol.*, 17:371–384.

43. Moore, M. A. S., Ekert, H., Fitzgerald, M. G., and Carmichael, A. (1974): Evidence for the clonal origin of chronic myeloid leukemia from a sex chromosome mosaic: Clinical, cytogenetic, and marrow culture studies. *Blood*, 43:15–22.

44. Moore, M. A. S., and Metcalf, D.(1973): Cytogenetic analysis of human acute and chronic myeloid leukemic cells cloned in agar culture. *Int. J. Cancer*, 11:143–152.

45. Motomura, S., Ogi, K., and Horie, M. (1973): Monoclonal origin of acute transformation of chronic myelogenous leukemia. *Acta Haematol.*, 49:300–305.

46. Murray, R. F., Hobbs, J., and Payne, B. (1971): Possible clonal origin of common warts (verruca vulgaris). *Nature*, 232:51–52.

47. Nowell, P. C., and Wilson, D. B. (1971): Lymphocytes and hemic stem cells. *Am. J. Pathol.*, 65:641–651.

48. Prchal, J. F., Adamson, J. W., Steinmann, L., and Fialkow, P. J. (1976): Human erythroid colony formation *in vitro*: Evidence for clonal origin. *J. Cell. Physiol. (in press)*.

49. Preud'homme, J. L., and Seligmann, M. (1972): Surface bound immunoglobulins as a cell marker in human lymphoproliferative diseases. *Blood*, 40:777–794.

50. Rastrick, J. M., Fitzgerald, P. H., and Gunz, F. W. (1968): Direct evidence for presence of Ph[1] chromosome in erythroid cells. *Br. Med. J.*, 1:96–98.

51. Salsano, F., Frøland, S. S., Natvig, J. B., and Michaelsen, T. E. (1974): Same idiotype of B-lymphocyte membrane IgD and IgM. Formal evidence for monoclonality of chronic lymphocytic leukemia cells. *Scand. J. Immunol.*, 3:841–846.

52. Schenkein, I., Bueker, E. D., Helson, L., Axelrod, F., and Dancis, J. (1974): Increased nerve growth stimulating activity in disseminated neurofibromatosis. *N. Engl. J. Med.*, 290:613–614.

53. Schroer, K. R., Briles, D. E., Van Boxel, J. A., and Davie, J. M. (1974): Idiotypic uniformity of cell surface immunoglobulin in chronic lymphocytic leukemia: Evidence for monoclonal proliferation. *J. Exp. Med.*, 140:1416–1420.

54. Shadduck, R. K., and Nankin, H. R. (1971): Cellular origin of granulocytic colonies in chronic myeloid leukaemia. *Lancet*, 2:1097–1098.

55. Smith, J. W., Townsend, D. E., and Sparkes, R. S. (1971): Genetic variants of glucose-6-phosphate dehydrogenase in the study of carcinoma of the cervix. *Cancer*, 28:529–532.

56. Thomas, E. D., Bryant, J. I., Buckner, C. D., Clift, R. A., Fefer, A., Johnson, F. L., Neiman, P. E., Ramberg, R. E., and Storb, R. (1972): Leukaemic transformation of engrafted human marrow cells in vivo. *Lancet*, 1:1310–1313.

57. Van Slyck, E. J., Weiss, L., and Dully, M. (1970): Chromosomal evidence for the secondary role of fibroblastic proliferation in acute myelofibrosis. *Blood*, 36:729–735.

58. Werner, P., Feizi, T., and Kunkel, H. G. (1972): Idiotypic determinants of immunoglobulin M detected on the surface of human lymphocytes by cytotoxicity assays. *J. Exp. Med.*, 136:650–655.

59. Zech, L., Haglund, U., Nilsson, K., and Klein, G. (1976): Characteristic chromosomal abnormalities in biopsies and lymphoid cell lines from patients with Burkitt and non-Burkitt lymphomas. *Int. J. Cancer*, 17:47-56.

60. Ziegler, J. L., Bluming, A. Z., Fass, L., and Morrow, R. H., Jr. (1972): Relapse patterns in Burkitt's lymphoma. *Cancer Res.*, 32:1267–1272.

61. Ziegler, J. L., and Magrath, I. T. (1974): Burkitt's lymphoma. *Pathobiol. Annu.*, 4:129–142.

Discussion

Gallo: Have you looked at acute myelogenous leukemia (AML)?

Fialkow: We have not had the opportunity to use G-6-PD markers, because we have not located any G-6-PD heterozygotes with AML. Chromosomal markers, however, suggest that AML is a stem cell disorder because, when found, the markers are also seen in cells synthesizing hemoglobin, presumably red cell precursors [*Lancet,* 2:1178–1179 (1974)].

Harnden: I worry when you compare the multicellular nature of *benign* neoplasms like neurofibromas with the clonal nature of fully malignant neoplasms. Would it be possible to look first at a benign tumor in a patient with neurofibromatosis, and later at the same patient's malignant neurofibrosarcoma to see whether the tumor becomes clonal?

Fialkow: We would like to do that, but again have not yet encountered a G-6-PD heterozygote with neurofibromatosis that has gone on to develop malignancy. We have looked at sporadically occurring neurofibromas; these are of single cell origin (P.J. Fialkow and R. Jacobson: *unpublished observations*) in contrast to the multicellular origin of genetic neurofibromas.

Harnden: Perhaps you could follow malignant degeneration in another disease, say, multiple polyposis.

Miller: Epidemiologically, the tumor that seems most heavily influenced virally or environmentally is cancer of the uterine cervix. Would it be good to study, especially as it is common?

Fialkow: It has been studied extensively; we have about 50 cases. But, there are problems in studying carcinoma biopsies because they typically are not a homogeneous population of cells; rather, they have remnants of normal epithelium, stroma, and inflammatory cells that confuse analysis. Despite these problems, our data and a report by Park and Jones [*Am. J. Obstet. Gynecol.,* 102:106–109 (1968)] suggest a single cell origin. A third study of seven tumors suggested multicellular origin in two [*Cancer,* 28:529–539 (1971)]. Preinvasive cervical cancers (cervical dysplasia and carcinoma in situ) have single enzyme phenotypes and thus are likely to be clonal. Personally, I think almost all invasive cervical carcinomas are clonal.

Gatti: Do you have evidence as to the origin of leukemia after bone marrow transplantation?

Fialkow: Again, we have no data on G-6-PD heterozygotes. Chromosomal markers strongly suggest multicellular origins in leukemia arising after bone marrow transplantation for acute lymphoblastic leukemia. In collaboration with Thomas' group, we documented by sex chromosome markers that two relapses after transplantation arose in donor cells. Cell kinetics also argue a multicellular origin rather than a clonal proliferation in this unusual circumstance.

Fuscaldo: In patients with polycythemia vera and essential thrombocythemia, we have reported the presence of oncornavirus-like particles in platelets [*J. Natl. Cancer Inst.,* 55:1069–1074 (1975)].

Miller: Are there any opportunities in the USSR or in Japan to make similar studies in relation to some other gene?

Fialkow: Unfortunately, the only known polymorphic X-linked trait demonstrable at the cellular level is G-6-PD. The Xg locus is not inactivated and therefore would not be suitable. G-6-PD variants may be electrophorectic or quantitative: the first are essentially confined to black populations, the second are found worldwide in varying frequencies. But I do not like to work with quantitative variants because neoplastic cells may have many nonspecific quantitative changes. The only other known marker useful for this purpose is immunoglobulin, either secreted or on the cell surface but is applicable only to tumors that synthesize immunoglobulin.

Genetics of Human Cancer, edited by J. J.
Mulvihill, R. W. Miller, and J. F. Fraumeni, Jr.
Raven Press, New York, 1977.

42

RNA Viruses, Genes, and Cancer

Robert C. Gallo

Laboratory of Tumor Cell Biology, National Cancer Institute, Bethesda, Maryland 20014

No human cancer has been shown to be unambiguously caused by a virus. The best evidence for associating a virus with human cancer is the Epstein-Barr virus (EBV) with African Burkitt lymphoma. Among the problems encountered in concluding that EBV is indeed the causative agent are the ubiquity of the virus, the lack of clear-cut *mammalian* animal models which show that the herpes viruses or herpes-like viruses cause malignancies under natural conditions, and the few cases of Burkitt lymphoma in which EBV has not been identified. The ubiquity of the virus does not argue against its involvement, but the latter two points present some difficulties. In a recent excellent editorial, George Klein has suggested that genetic change in the host cell may be a prerequisite for EBV to cause Burkitt lymphoma (26). This view is based on the results of cytogenetic studies, especially the commonly seen chromosome 14 marker in the Burkitt cells. Lymphoid cell lines derived from normal donors but containing EBV usually have normal karyotypes, whereas the Burkitt lymphoma cell lines have chromosomal anomalies.

The situation with the RNA tumor viruses (oncornaviruses) is different from EBV. Considerable evidence supports an etiologic role for these viruses in some naturally occurring mammalian neoplasms, especially leukemias and lymphomas (16,20), and justifies their designation as tumor viruses. Yet, like many other viruses, they encompass a spectrum with widely divergent biological activity and genetic content; some may have no pathological effects. Therefore, simply detecting them or their "footprints" is not proof that they cause disease. Moreover, unlike other viruses, the fact that the genetic information for some oncornaviruses is often a part of the genetic content of the normal cell presents a unique problem. Such RNA "tumor" viruses are called endogenous. Detection of their expression is not surprising and may not have anything to do with disease (see below). Thus, human beings, like many vertebrates, may have genetic information for an endogenous virus. If such a virus is isolated, it will be simple to prove it is a human virus. Since it is in reality a cell gene product, molecular hybridization techniques can readily show extensive homology of the viral genomic RNA to DNA of the normal host cells. However, as noted above, detection

455

of partial expression of a complete endogenous virus or its isolation does not mean the virus was relevant to a disease in question. Again, in contrast to EBV, a second problem with the oncornaviruses is obtaining unambiguous evidence that they can be identified in humans. In this brief report I will focus on the myelogenous leukemias and try to summarize the status of three major issues: (1) Have type C RNA tumor viruses or information derived from these viruses been detected in man? (2) If so, where did the virus or viral information come from? Is it endogenous, exogenous, or both? (3) If present, are such viruses involved in the pathogenesis of the myelogenous leukemias of man?

CELLULAR ABNORMALITY OF MYELOGENOUS LEUKEMIAS

As discussed by Fialkow (Chapter 41), chronic myelogenous leukemia in man appears to be a disease of stem cells, primarily a monoclonal hyperproliferation of these cells. Differentiation may not be affected. In contrast, it is not known whether acute myelogenous leukemia (AML) is mono- or multiclonal and less certain that it involves a stem cell. Whatever its cell origin, the phenotypic abnormality in AML appears to involve a block in the differentiation process so that immature cells capable of DNA replication and cell mitosis accumulate. Data from *in vitro* experiments from some laboratories, especially with mouse cell systems, suggest that this block may at least in part be reversible (35). The results were obtained by studying the effect of factors (contained in media obtained after incubation of some normal cells) on leukemic cells plated onto a solid surface and observing their growth and differentiation. Apparently some myelogenous leukemia cells of mice respond to factor (differentiation positive cells) while others do not (differentiation negative cells). Recently, we found a whole human embryo cell strain which produced a factor (or factors) which promoted exponential growth and differentiation of human myelogenous leukemia cells (10,11). All leukemic cells in the population may not respond to our factor and normal myelogenous cells certainly do not. In contrast, different factors derived from other sources of conditioned media have greater effects on normal myelogenous cells than on leukemic ones. Altogether, it seems that some (but not all) myelogenous leukemia cells can be induced to mature to normal *appearing* granulocytes. By inference, at least some of these cells retain their response to putative physiological growth regulators, with wide variations in responsiveness of different cells, strongly suggesting heterogeneity of the leukemic cell population, at least phenotypically. Despite evidence that the leukemias are monoclonal (although AML has apparently not been studied), one wonders whether the functional heterogeneity reflects the presence of different genotypes. Could subtle changes in genetic information occur in various cells after transformation even if they were all derived from one progenitor cell?

RNA TUMOR VIRUSES (ONCORNAVIRUSES): THEIR ORIGIN AND ACQUISITION OF ONCOGENIC INFORMATION

Figure 1 schematically summarizes my thinking about the origin of RNA tumor viruses and how they may become oncogenic. Many studies have shown that in

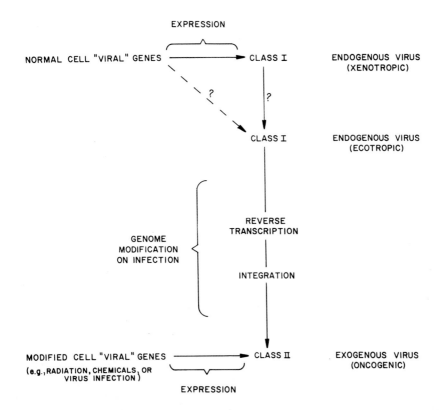

FIG. 1. Scheme for proposed origin of RNA tumor viruses with oncogenic potential. Normal cells of many, and possibly all, vertebrates contain "viral" genes. Their function is unknown. Sometimes they are suppressed or only partially expressed. Therefore, virus particles are not seen. Other times full expression occurs, and virus is released (class 1 virus). Sometimes full expression and release of virus is associated with neoplasia; other times it is not. Therefore, the cause of neoplasia cannot simply be due to "switching on" [activation of an endogenous virogene as originally proposed in the "oncogene" theory (21)]. It may be that some genetic change is required. The released endogenous virus is usually exenotropic (i.e., infects foreign cells but not cells of the host species). By mechanisms not understood, the virus may escape host control and become infectious to other animals of the same species or of other species. This results in genetic change in the virus. We believe this change leads to the acquisition of oncogenic properties (13,16). The virus now contains differences between its RNA genome and DNA from the original host cell, detectable by molecular hybridization. We call this a class 2 virus (16). An alternative mode for origin of a class 2 virus is by direct genetic alteration of the class 1 "viral" genes [i.e., if chemicals, radiation, or an infecting virus interact at or adjacent to the endogenous "viral" genes of the host cell, a putative "hot spot" (13)]. If such alteration occurs, and it is followed by full expression, a class 2 virus is released. In this case, the virus is the *result* and not the cause of the neoplasia. However, once formed, the class 2 virus has the potential to transmit oncogenic information to other cells, and if it escapes from the host and enters other animals of the same or of other species, it could become the primary cause of the disease in the species in question (e.g., cat). I have termed this a virogene "hot-spot model" (13). Leukemia virus may have originated from a species other than cat and now is involved as an etiological agent in cats. Other examples are the gibbon ape and bovine leukemias. Both may be due to infectious virus originating from another species. In any case, with all three (feline, bovine, and gibbon ape), the viruses are infectious for these species and in each case clearly not endogenous to the susceptible animal. It is imperative to know if man ever acquires the disease in a similar manner since this might be preventable.

several vertebrate species the genetic information for oncornaviruses resides in the genome of the normal cell. Thus, the virus can be looked upon as a cell gene product. With others, we assume that this "viral" information has some normal function, perhaps in development; however, there is no proof of this or data which suggest a specific developmental function. But, when these genes are fully expressed, a type C virus is synthesized. Based on the technique of molecular hybridization, we define this endogenous virus as a class 1 virus, namely one in which the RNA genome of the virus can be shown to hybridize completely to DNA from cells of the normal *uninfected* host animal. Most of these viruses are xenotropic, i.e., although released by these cells they cannot infect cells of their host but only infect heterologous cells. Some type C viruses are able to infect cells of their host, when they escape from cell control; they become ecotropic presumably as a consequence of genetic change in the host, the virus, or both. After repeated infections, still greater genetic change may occur, perhaps by infidelity of the reverse transcriptase (1), a catalytic reaction required for each infection (16). More likely, the greatest change occurs upon recombination of the viral genetic information with that of the host. In other words, after infection, it is not only the host which is changed but also the virus, which may lose some of its information and acquire some from the host. The greatest genetic change may occur when the virus infects cells of a new species. In many instances, the new viruses are really laboratory creations, produced by the investigator who may repeatedly infect homologous and heterologous cells *in vitro* and *in vivo* with the virus. Such laboratory creations probably include most murine ecotropic leukemia and sarcoma viruses, like the Rauscher leukemia virus and the various murine sarcoma viruses. It has sometimes been implied that simply because they may have been "created" in the laboratory they are not as interesting as the "natural viruses." However, the various manipulations resulted in an important property, namely, oncogenic potential. To me it seems to be of the utmost interest that this trait may have been induced by laboratory experiments that simply involved repeated infection by virus of different host cells. In any case, what can occur rapidly under laboratory conditions may also occur naturally with time. Thus, feline leukemia virus is an infectious agent of cats, associated with cat leukemia and other feline diseases (7), but probably originating from another species (5). Feline leukemia is particularly interesting in that many cats are infected but only a rare animal acquires the disease. This could be due to chance requirements (e.g., infection of the right cell at the right time or integration into the right chromosome at the right site), variation in host susceptibility, or other required environmental exposures (e.g., certain chemicals and radiation). Recently, evidence suggests that the cause of leukemias in cows and in some primates may also involve a role for an infectious virus which originated from another species.

SUBHUMAN PRIMATE TYPE C RNA TUMOR VIRUSES

These viruses are of special interest because (1) they are the first type C viruses to be obtained from animals closely related to humans; (2) in some cases they appear to have been involved in the cause of spontaneous neoplasia in these lower primates; (3) usually the animals have been in close proximity to humans or, in fact, the animals had been inoculated with human material, raising the possibility of their transmission from man; (4) some molecules (certain proteins and nucleic acids) have been found in some human leukemia cells related or identical to molecules present in some of these viruses which again raises the possibility that man may harbor related or identical viruses to these so-called subhuman primate viruses; and (5) recently, highly related or identical viruses have, in fact, been isolated from humans by five independent laboratories.

Viruses belonging to class 1 and 2 categories have been isolated from primates. The class 1 virus was first identified in the placenta of baboons (22) and subsequently isolated (4). These are typical endogenous viruses. Hence DNA proviruses (virogenes) can be found in DNA from apparently all normal baboons. To date they have not been shown to cause disease. In a very interesting study, viruses of this type were isolated from baboon lymphomas which developed following inoculation with human leukemic blood (19). In view of the fact that these viruses can be isolated from normal baboons, it is difficult to infer that the human blood was the source of virus. Yet, studies from our laboratory (37) and others (33) have indicated that "baboon" type C virus may be isolated from human cells (see section on human studies), and recent experiments from our laboratory have shown that DNA from tissues of some leukemic patients contains a portion of the DNA provirus of the baboon endogenous virus (34,44). These new results provide unequivocal evidence that viruses isolated from human tissues related to or identical to what we call baboon endogenous virus may not be laboratory contaminants. We can say that the DNA from these patients contained the requisite genetic information to give rise to this type of virus.

A second group of primate type C viruses are class 2 viruses which have been isolated from gibbon apes and from a woolly monkey. These viruses are infectious for primates. To date there is one isolate (38,42) of the so-called "woolly monkey" virus or simian sarcoma virus (SSV). It was obtained from a spontaneous fibrosarcoma of a pet animal raised in captivity and exposed to humans and several household pets. Surprisingly, this virus is highly related to the so-called gibbon ape leukemia virus (GaLV). The GaLV has been isolated from several gibbons (25). The first isolates came from a group of gibbons injected with human blood from patients with malaria (6). Several of these animals developed leukemias or lymphomas; whereas, none of the control (untreated) animals developed neoplasia. Clearly, SSV and GaLV are infectious viruses and not endogenous to primates. Sometimes they can (and have) infected animals without provoking disease. Therefore, it is possible sometimes to detect them in normal animals (24,40). GaLV can induce leukemias in gibbons (23), and SSV has been shown to induce sarcomas in marmosets (24). It is clear that these viruses (GALV or SSV) are not endogenous to any primates. They appear to have originated from a rodent, probably a mouse, in the past and entered primates as an infectious agent (27,43).

EVIDENCE FOR "HUMAN" TYPE C VIRUSES OR VIRUS COMPONENTS

Several reports show that fresh uncultured blood cells from some patients with leukemia contain reverse transcriptase (2,12,17,28,30,36,39,41) which in certain cases is related by immunological tests specifically to reverse transcriptase from the SSV-GaLV virus group (12,14,30,39). Other studies have reported detection of high molecular weight RNA with some nucleic acid sequences related (by molecular hybridization tests) to the RNA genome of some type C virus (2,3,14,15,28,29). Our results show that the relationship is closest to the RNA of the above-mentioned primate type C viruses (15,29), a finding confirmed by Mak et al. (28). It appears that these molecules are encapsulated in a structure exhibiting biophysical properties of an RNA tumor virus (2,14,15,28,29,36) but there is no convincing evidence that these particles contain viral structural proteins. Recent studies have indicated that whole infectious type C virus may be isolated from human cells. Thus, we reported isolation of virus from a 61-year-old lady with AML (9). The isolate consists of two components, one related to SSV and one related to BaEV (34,37). It has been transmitted now to many secondary cells (37). Virus isolates were subsequently reported by Panem et al. from human embryo (32). Again the isolates appear to consist of two components, one related to SSV (32) and one to BaEV (14). Additionally, Nooter et al (31) and Gableman et al. (8) reported isolation of virus from leukemic patients related to SSV. Despite the worrisome fact that the viruses we have isolated from the AML patient are highly related and possibly identical to viruses previously obtained from subhuman primates, we are confident that they do not represent laboratory contaminants. Our reasons are several: (1) in over 4 years work with over 100 human cell lines we have not had a known contamination with type C virus; (2) we have reidentified the virus from three independent specimens obtained over a 14-month interval from the same patient (11); (3) as discussed above, similar independent findings have been made by other investigators; (4) Aoki (*personal communication*) has recently found antibodies widespread in the human population to a viral envelope protein that appears to be directed specifically against this virus group; (5) the fresh uncultured blood cells of this patient contained reverse transcriptase related to reverse transcriptase from SSV (30); (6) fresh uncultured blood cells from this patient contained RNA related to the RNA of the virus isolates (34); (7) finally, and most compelling, we have recently identified the DNA provirus of the BaEV component of our isolate in the DNA of this patient's spleen (34). There is no way of explaining this by contamination.

The immunological data taken at face value suggest that these viruses are widespread in the human population. If this does turn out to be the case, the data will be best explained by assuming widespread infection early in life, possibly *in utero*. They do not say that the virus caused the disease. However, by analogy with some animal models, we propose that this viral information is causatively involved but in a complex way which probably depends on other factors. As noted earlier, these factors may include host genetic traits, chance (e.g., infection of the right cell at the right time and integration into the right chromosomal site), and perhaps environmental inducing events.

REFERENCES

1. Battula, N. and Loeb, L. A. (1975): On the fidelity of DNA replication. *J. Biol. Chem.*, 250:4405–4409.
2. Baxt, W., Hehlman, R., and Spiegelman, S. (1972): Human leukemic cells contain reverse transcriptase associated with a high molecular weight virus-related RNA. *Nature [New Biol.]*, 240:72–75.
3. Baxt, W. G., and Spiegelman, S. (1972): Nuclear DNA sequences present in human leukemic cells and absent in normal leukocytes. *Proc. Natl. Acad. Sci. USA*, 69:3737–3741.
4. Benveniste, R. E., Lieber, M. M., Livingston, D. M., Sherr, C. J., Todaro, G. J., and Kalter, S. S. (1974): Infectious C type virus isolated from baboon placenta. *Nature*, 248:17–20.
5. Benveniste, R. E., Sherr, C. J., and Todaro, G. J. (1975): Evolution of type C viral genes. Origin of feline leukemia virus. *Science*, 190:886–888.
6. DePaoli, A., Johnsen, D. O., and Noll, W. W. (1973): Granulocytic leukemia in whitehanded gibbons. *J. Am. Vet. Med. Assoc.*, 163:624–629.
7. Essex, M., Sliski, A., Cotter, S. M., Jakowski, R. M., and Hardy, W. D. (1975): Immunosurveillance of naturally occurring feline leukemia. *Science*, 190:790–792.
8. Gabelman, N., Waxman, S., Smith, W., and Douglas, S. D. (1975): Appearance of C type virus like particles after cocultivation of a human tumor cell line with rat (XC) cells. *Int. J. Cancer*, 16:355–369.
9. Gallagher, R. E., and Gallo, R. C. (1975): Type-C RNA tumor virus isolated from cultured human acute myelogenous leukemia cells. *Science*, 187:350–353.
10. Gallagher, R. E., and Gallo, R. C. (1976): Continuous production of complete type-C virus by exponentially-growing cultured leukocytes from one of sixteen patients with myelogenous leukemia. In: *Proc. 2nd Int. Congress on Pathological Physiology, Prague, Czechoslovakia, 1975*.
11. Gallagher, R. E., Salahuddin, S. Z., Hall, W. T., McCredie, K. B., and Gallo, R. C. (1975): Growth and differentiation in culture of leukemic leukocytes from a patient with acute myelogenous leukemia and re-identification of a type-C virus. *Proc. Natl. Acad. Sci. USA*, 72:4137–4141.
12. Gallagher, R. E., Todaro, G. H., Smith, R. G., Livingston, D. M., and Gallo, R. C. (1974): Relationship between RNA-directed DNA polymerase (reverse transcriptase) from human acute leukemic blood cells and primate type-C viruses. *Proc. Natl. Acad. Sci. USA*, 71:1309–1313.
13. Gallo, R. C. (1974): On the origin of human acute myeloblastic leukemia: Virus "hot spot" hypothesis In: *Modern Trends in Human Leukemia* edited by R. Neth, R. C. Gallo, S. Spiegelman, and F. Stohlman, pp. 227–236. Lehmanns Verlag, Munich.
14. Gallo, R. C., Gallagher, R. E., Miller, N. R., Mondal, H., Saxinger, W. C., Mayer, R. J., Smith, R. G., and Gillespie, D. H. (1975): Relationships between components in primate RNA tumor viruses and in the cytoplasm of human leukemic cells: Implications to leukemogenesis. *Cold Spring Harbor Symp. Quant. Biol.*, 39:933–961.
15. Gallo, R. C., Miller, N. R., Saxinger, W. C., and Gillespie, D. (1973): Primate RNA tumor virus-like DNA synthesized endogenously by RNA-dependent DNA polymerase in virus-like particles from fresh human acute leukemic blood cells. *Proc. Natl. Acad. Sci. USA*, 70:3219–3224.
16. Gallo, R. C., and Ting, R. C. (1972): Cancer viruses. *CRC Crit. Rev. Clin. Lab. Sci.*, 3:403–449.
17. Gallo, R. C., Yang, S. S., and Ting, R. C. (1970): RNA dependent DNA polymerase of human acute leukaemic cells. *Nature*, 228:927–929.
18. Gillespie, D., and Gallo, R. C. (1975): RNA processing and the origin and evolution of RNA tumor viruses. *Science*, 188:802–811.
19. Goldberg, R. J., Scolnick, E. M., Parks, W. P., Yakovleva, L. A., and Lapin, B. A. (1974): Isolation of a primate type-C virus from a lymphomatous baboon. *Int. J. Cancer*, 14:722–730.
20. Gross, L. (1970): *Oncogenic Viruses*. Pergamon Press, New York.
21. Huebner, R., and Todaro, G. J. (1969): Oncogenes of RNA tumor viruses as determinants of cancer. *Proc. Natl. Acad. Sci. USA*, 64:1087–1094.
22. Kalter, S. S., Helmike, R. J., and Panigel, M. (1973): Observations of apparent C-type particles in baboon *(Papio cyanocephalus)* placentas. *Science*, 179:1332–1333.
23. Kawakami, T. G., and Buckley, P. M. (1974): Antigenic studies in gibbon type-C viruses. *Transplant. Proc.*, 6:193–196.

24. Kawakami, T. G., Buckley, P. M., McDowell, T. S., and DePaoli, A. (1973): Antibodies to simian C type virus antigen in sera of gibbons (*Hylobates* sp.). *Nature* [*New Biol.*], 246:105–107.

25. Kawakami, T. G., Huff, S. D., Buckley, P. M., Dungworth, D. L., Snyder, S. P., and Gilden, R. (1972): C-type associated with gibbon lymphosarcoma., *Nature* [*New Biol.*], 235:170–171.

26. Klein, G. (1975): The Epstein-Barr virus and neoplasia. *N. Engl. J. Med.,* 293:1353–1357.

27. Lieber, M. M., Sherr, C. J., Todaro, G. J., Benveniste, R. E., Callahan, R., and Coon, H. G. (1975): Isolation from the Asian mouse *Mus caroli* of an endogenous type C virus related to infectious primate type C viruses. *Proc. Natl. Acad. Sci. USA,* 72:2315–2319.

28. Mak, T., Kurtz, S., Manaster, J., and Housman, D. (1975): Viral-related information in oncornavirus-like particles isolated from cultures of marrow cells from leukemic patients in remission and relapse. *Proc. Natl. Acad. Sci. USA,* 72:623–627.

29. Miller, N.R., Saxinger, W.C., Reitz, M.S., Gallagher, R.E., Wu, A.M., Gallo, R.C., and Gillespie, D. (1974): Systematics of RNA tumor viruses and virus-like particles of human origin. *Proc. Natl. Acad. Sci. USA,* 71:3177–3181.

30. Mondal, H., Gallagher, R. E., and Gallo, R. C. (1975): RNA-directed DNA polymerase from human leukemic blood cells and from primate type-C virus-producing cells: High and low molecular weight forms with variant biochemical and immunological properties. *Proc. Natl. Acad. Sci. USA,* 72:1194–1198.

31. Nooter, K., Aarssen, A. M., Bentvelzen, P., de Groot, F. G., and van Pelt, F. G. (1975): Isolation of infectious C type oncornavirus from human leukaemic bone marrow cells. *Nature,* 256:595–597.

32. Panem, S., Prochownik, E.V., Reale, F.R., and Kirsten, W.H. (1975): Isolation of type C virions from a normal human fibroblast strain. *Science* 189:297–299.

33. Prochownik, E. V., Panem, S., and Kirsten, W. H. (1976): Primate type-C related particles in normal human cells: Isolation of two infectious components from a strain of fetal lung fibroblasts. *Nature. (In press.)*

34. Reitz, M. S., Miller, N. R., Wong-Staal, F., Gallagher, R. E., Gallo, R. C., and Gillespie, D. H. (1976): Primate type-C virus nucleic acid sequences (woolly monkey and baboon type) in tissues from a patient with acute myelogenous leukemia and in viruses isolated from cultured cells of the same patient. *Proc. Natl. Acad. Sci. USA,* 73:2113–2117.

35. Sachs, L. (1974): Regulation of membrane changes, differentiation, and malignancy in carcinogenesis. *Harvey Lect.,* 68:1–35.

36. Sarngadharan, M. G., Sarin, P. S., Reitz, M. S., and Gallo, R. C. (1972): Reverse transcriptase activity of human acute leukemic cells: Purification of the enzyme, response to AMV 70S RNA, and characterization of the DNA product. *Nature* [*New Biol.*], 240:67–72.

37. Teich, N. M., Weiss, R. A., Salahuddin, S. Z., Gallagher, R. E., Gillespie, D., and Gallo, R. C. (1975): Infective transmission and characterisation of a C-type virus released by cultured human myeloid leukaemia cells. *Nature,* 256:551–555.

38. Theilen, G. H., Gould, D., Fowler, M., and Dungworth, D. L. (1971): C-type in tumor tissue of a woolly monkey (Lagothrix spp.) with fibrosarcoma. *J. Natl. Cancer Inst.,* 47:881–889.

39. Todaro, G. J., and Gallo, R. C. (1973): Immunological relationship of DNA polymerase from human acute leukaemia cells and primate and mouse leukaemia virus reverse transcriptase. *Nature,* 244:206–209.

40. Todaro, G. J., Lieber, M. M., Benveniste, R. E., Sherr, C. J., Gibbs, C. J., and Gajdusek, D. C. (1975): Infectious primate type C viruses: Three isolates belonging to a new subgroup from the brains of normal gibbons. *Virology,* 67:335–343.

41. Witkin, S. S., Ohno, T., and Spiegelman, S. (1975): Purification of RNA instructed DNA polymerase from human leukemic spleens. *Proc. Natl. Acad. Sci. USA,* 72:4133–4136.

42. Wolfe, L. G., Deinhardt, F., Theilen, G. H., Rabin, H., Kawakami, T. G., and Bustad, L. K. (1971): Induction of tumors in marmoset monkeys by simian sarcoma virus, type I (Lagothrix): A preliminary report. *J. Natl. Cancer Inst.,* 47:1115–1120.

43. Wong-Staal, F., Gallo, R. C., and Gillespie, D. (1975): Genetic relationship of a primate RNA tumor virus genome to genes in normal mice. *Nature,* 256:670–672.

44. Wong-Staal, F., Gillespie, D. H., and Gallo, R. C. (1976): Proviral sequences of baboon endogenous type C RNA virus in DNA of human leukaemic tissues. *Nature,* 262:190–195.

Discussion

Koprowski: I wonder whether we should not extend now the spectrum of potentially oncogenic viruses beyond just C-type RNA viral particles? The crucial point you made was the integration of the virus into the cell genome. Certainly other viruses not classified as oncogenic today may become integrated into the cellular DNA and prove ultimately to be oncogenic. For example, it is alleged that reverse transcriptase was found in Newcastle disease, a paramyxovirus. Transfection (transmission of infection by DNA extracted from virus infected cells) with nontumorigenic RNA was described for tick-borne encephalitis (an arbovirus B), for respiratory syncytial (a paramyxovirus), and for HA-2 (another paramyxovirus). Does this similarity to oncornaviruses make these viruses to be classified potential, if not real, "tumor viruses?"

Finally, I am not so enthusiastic as you about the role of viruses in human cancer; today, I accept only the wart virus as proven to cause human neoplasia. For other cancers, we still need much more evidence even to postulate their viral etiology.

Gallo: I do not dare to say that we have proved that any viruses cause human cancer. I personally believe viral information is involved in the disease that I limit myself to—acute myelogenous leukemia; I would not be working on it otherwise. I think we are going to be in a position soon to establish conclusively the presence of viral information very clearly in a certain number of people by immunologic and molecular studies that are being pursued.

Warts are almost not worth mentioning. As for other potential oncogenic viruses, I agree that RNA viruses other than the classic oncornaviruses could either carry reverse transcriptase or induce a putative reverse transcriptase in a host cell. This newly synthesized DNA might integrate into DNA of the host. Once integration occurs, you have the potential for genetic damage or change including oncogenesis. Several laboratories have reported such behavior with a few RNA viruses other than the classic oncornaviruses. I hesitate to discuss it because: (a) some are very common viruses of infectious diseases; (b) in fact, we have no data suggesting they are oncogenic; and (c) I am not convinced that these reports are correct.

Moreover, evidence that such viruses are oncogenic will be difficult to collect. For instance, if you find genetic information of herpes I virus in a cancer of the lip I would say that it was from an earlier unrelated cold sore. Further, their ubiquity and the lack of animal models thwart valid evidence. In short, it has to be considered a theoretical possibility, although not at the moment a matter for public concern.

Hirschhorn: I have two comments. First, I suspect that some of the viruses that Dr. Gallo and others mention are related to what others call environmental agents in general. And still, as Dr. Gallo implied, something in the host is necessary before agents, such as mutagens, radiation, or viruses, can induce the cell to become malignant.

Second, as a medical geneticist, I worry about the use of the term, "dominance." We understand little about so-called dominant inheritance in man; it can be vague. For example, for only two or three disorders is there even a rudimentary idea about the molecular basis. Also, the phenomenon of sporadic mutations and their increasing frequency with advanced paternal age raise the question of whether some of these dominant traits may, in fact, represent more than a single gene mutation. They could be double mutant events as postulated by Dr. Herrmann and Dr. Knudson (and their hypotheses are not all that different, I believe). Finally, some families interpreted as dominant patterns of cancer have such an enormous frequency that Mendelian expectations are surpassed.

Genetics of Human Cancer, edited by J. J.
Mulvihill, R. W. Miller, and J. F. Fraumeni, Jr.
Raven Press, New York, 1977.

43

Clinical Genetics and Cancer

John M. Opitz and Jürgen Herrmann

*Clinical Genetics Center, Departments of Medical Genetics and Pediatrics, University of
Wisconsin, Madison, Wisconsin 53706*

Clinical genetics is one of the most intensely interesting and productive branches of
human biology and medicine at the present time.

WHAT IS CLINICAL GENETICS?

The term has as many uses and misuses as the term "genetic counseling," and
depending on the departmental or college tensions underlying its teaching and on
whether the subject of attention is called a *patient, proband* (or *propositus),* or
counselee, clinical genetics is considered to involve mainly one or all of the following
three areas of activity.

Clinical and Diagnostic Activities

These constitute the efficient and expert clinical and laboratory evaluation of the
patient with the goal of making a medical diagnosis. Though medical qualifications
are a professional prerequisite for this activity, it is sadly evident that most medical
schools do not adequately teach the epistemological basis for performing this task
properly, i.e., in learning to tell normal from abnormal structure and function, in
being able to give a complete and qualitatively and quantitatively adequate description of the patient's abnormalities, but, above all, in being able to analyze the
patient's phenotype for pathogenetic and etiologic clues. This leaves many physicians deficient in dealing with birth defects and genetic disorders. We find that even
after two years of good pediatric training, two additional years of clinical training are
required to acquire the rudiments of effective *phenotype analysis.*

Genetic Analysis

This involves analysis of physical, functional, biochemical, cytogenetic, and other
laboratory and genealogic data to determine cause and recurrence risk for single

individuals *(probands, propositi),* families, or defined populations. This activity can be performed by nonmedical persons, is frequently the subject of Ph.D. dissertations in departments of medical or human genetics in the U.S., does *not* qualify the graduate of such a program to perform all three phases of clinical genetics, and is frequently regarded by basic science geneticists as the most important, if not the sole activity deserving the designation "genetic counseling." It includes, to a variable extent, genetic epidemiology and studies leading to the formulation of empiric risk figures. An excellent text dealing with this topic is that by Murphy and Chase (14).

Genetic Counseling

Genetic counseling proper is all of those professional activities which help and sustain the *counselee* from the moment of ascertainment or referral, through the diagnostic work-up to the point when the clinical, prognostic, therapeutic, and genetic conclusions are put before the counselees and/or their relatives in the most effective and supportive way, and attempts are made to enlist the counselee's collaboration in examining consequences and options concerning therapy and reproductive choices, and to support the counselees in their attempt to obtain help in effecting their decisions. This can be a potentially mischievous activity if performed by physicians with inadequate counseling skills and genetic knowledge or by human geneticists without clinical expertise or training in counseling proper. It is *not* true that all physicians are ipso facto good and effective counselors; most of the harm done by genetic counseling is not due to the facts, but the way they were presented.

Medical genetics fortunately has taken a lesson from psychiatry, which, at least in the U.S., has for a long time used social workers to assist in patient care, by encouraging the training of genetic associates or assistants from diverse professional backgrounds and fitting them for the task of counseling proper (and other related activities), usually through a masters degree program in genetics, interviewing, guidance and counseling, and other pertinent courses. Lack of clinical skills and of sophistication in the methods of human genetics limits their activities to major medical centers where they usually work as members of various teams, such as in the genetics clinic, muscular dystrophy clinic, hemophilia center, etc. We envision excellent results from the extensive collaboration of such skilled professionals in cancer centers and registries concerned with the familial occurrence of cancer and outrightly hereditary forms of cancer.

CLINICAL GENETICS IN MEDICAL NOSOLOGY

What is the most important task of clinical genetics besides providing teaching and clinical services? We think it is to do nosology, as well as possible, both in the narrower sense of establishing and differentiating "disease categories" on pathogenetic and/or etiologic grounds, and in the broader sense of grouping these disorders into larger, "biologically meaningful" groups. This activity, under the best of circumstances, is comparable respectively to differentiating white-throated from white-crowned sparrows on the basis of their cladogenetic differences, and to the grouping together of such sauropsidian relatives as birds and reptiles on the basis of the many anatomical, developmental, reproductive, sex-determining mechanisms, and other cytogenetic characteristics they share in common. A "sauropsidian" grouping in cancer is: All of xeroderma pigmentosums (XP); an initial nosologic grouping is the division of XP into the two classes with and without CNS defects (i.e., the DeSanctis-Cacchione and non-DeSanctis-Cacchione forms of XP); and, the white-throated sparrows are sorted from the white-crowned sparrows in XP by the complementation studies of Robbins, Lutzner et al. *(this volume)* which have resulted in the division of XP into five different complementations, hence etiologically discrete and different groups or entities. An analogous story is that of the many mucopolysaccharidoses (or, speaking in old terms, of gargoylism or the many forms of dysostosis multiplex), at first sorted on clinical grounds and urinary acid mucopolysaccharide criteria into types I to VII (i.e., Hurler disease, Hunter disease, etc.) and then sorted into subtypes on the basis of the Neufeld complementation assay, and finally defined by a specific inborn error of metabolism (i.e., the biochemical sorting of the Sanfilippo disease into types A and B, respectively, due to heparan sulfate sulfatase and N-acetyl-α-D-glucosaminidase deficiency).

What are the methods of genetic nosology? Broadly speaking they are, or should be, identical to those of general medical nosology:

1. Analyses of the history of gestation, parturition, growth, development, medical, and social events.

2. Taking inventory of the static, structural findings in the person, a skill of value not only to the clinician but to the pathologist as well, including:

i. the physical examination, supplemented as necessary by anthropometric measurements, dermatoglyphic prints, casts, etc.,

ii. photographic studies,

iii. radiological studies,

iv. methods of anatomy and pathology,

v. methods which lead to inferences on the developmental origins of observed differences and the testing of etiologic and pathogenetic hypotheses,

vi. methods of embryology [e.g., the classical studies of Emil Witschi on the overripeness of the egg as a cause of twinning, malformation, cancer, and chromosomal abnormalities (20,21) and the studies of Lash on the relationship between the development of the limbs and kidneys (10)],

vii. methods of teratology,

viii. methods of developmental genetics.

3. Laboratory studies of functional abnormalities, either primary or secondary to other structural and/or functional changes.

4. Statistical analysis of objective phenotypic manifestations, including all-or-none manifestations, age of onset data, anthropometric data, and other objectively scoreable or measurable phenotypic data, etc., in order to determine, among others:

i. whether relative frequencies of manifestations and combinations of manifestations allow for the postulation of new syndromes in the stochastic manner first introduced into clinical medicine by von Pfaundler (18) and Günther (6), and those recently exemplified by the "epidemiological" definition by Miller and co-workers (11) of such nosological entities and formal genesis syndromes as the hemihypertrophy-Wilms' tumor "syndrome," the aniridia-Wilms' tumor syndrome, etc.;

ii. whether *n* patients with overlapping manifestations fall into one or more different nosologic groups by discriminant functions and other methods. Examples are, first, the recent statistical studies of many patients with the Brachmann-deLange syndrome (12), which led to the conclusion that however the data were analyzed, it was not possible to demonstrate phenotypic or etiologic heterogeneity in that group of patients; and, second, the statistical studies by Herrmann and co-workers (8) on the limbs in the Hanhart syndrome, Möbius syndrome, Poland anomaly, the ankyloglossia superior syndrome, aglossia-adactylia syndrome, and other related entities which led to the conclusion that all of these disorders fall either into a Hanhart-Möbius or a Poland-Möbius syndrome and that all the other entities are synonymous with one or the other of these two disorders;

iii. whether within-group analysis of manifestations can lead to prognostic statements. This is exemplified by the studies by Barr and co-workers on the Brachmann-deLange syndrome which showed that the degree of intrauterine growth retardation, microcephaly, reduction in fingertip total ridge count, and severity of limb defects was directly related to the incidence of seizures and the severity of the patients' mental retardation (2);

iv. whether allelic modifications can be detected as, for example, Renwick did in analyzing patellocondylar ratios in nail-patella syndrome patients to detect normal alleles modifying the expression of the mutant gene (19). (Many other examples could be cited of such statistical studies which are the bread and butter of many human geneticists, but still performed too rarely by clinicians who have a far greater opportunity to make pertinent observations and to collect informative data than have basic science human geneticists.)

5. Causal studies—on individuals, families, and groups of unrelated individuals with a multitude of methods including somatic and germinal, *in vivo* and *in vitro* cytogenetic analyses, *in vivo* and *in vitro* biochemical and immunological studies, somatic cell genetic studies (e.g., the complementation studies in XP), pedigree studies (including linkage and association studies), twin studies (especially with that splendid coidentical twin family study method of Nance, *this volume*), and epidemiological studies of environmental and genetic oncogenic hypotheses in man and his animals (pets and other domesticated animals), either prospective, retrospective or "laterospective."

THE RESULTS OF GENETIC NOSOLOGY

Numerous insights can be expected from applying these nosologic methods to genetic and congenital disorders, including those with neoplastic features:

1. Pathogenesis, i.e., processes of differentiation, dedifferentiation, metaplasia, and neoplasia, which, if they lead to cancer, are collectively called *oncoplasia*. This should also lead to better understanding of the natural history of the disorder and

prognosis in individual cases.

2. The action of different environmental causes; i.e., viruses and other infectious agents; ultraviolet light, roentgen rays and other physical agents; pre- and postnatal exposure to hormones and other oncogenic chemicals.

3. The action of different mutant genes and classes of mutant genes, e.g., the difference between types I, II, and III of the autosomal dominant multiple endocrine neoplasia (MEN) "syndromes" and the five types of XP on one hand, and that of pleiotropic autosomal dominant mutations and pleiotropic autosomal recessive traits predisposing either to chromosome breakage, anemia, leukemia, and other malignancies, or to immunological deficiencies and lymphoreticular malignancies on the other hand. In this connection we are not sure of the correctness of Gerald's surmise *(this volume)* that all of these autosomal recessive traits will be found to be inborn errors of metabolism, especially not with respect to those autosomal recessive traits which are associated with true multiple congenital anomaly (MCA) syndromes (e.g., the Fanconi MCA/anemia syndrome).

4. The delineation of new syndromes and, ultimately, their cause. The aniridia-Wilms' tumor, McCune-Albright and diGeorge syndromes remain stubbornly sporadic and "idiopathic." At least in the latter instance, there is good reason to think that the constellation of anomalies of the thyroid, parathyroid, thymus, and aortic arch represents a single developmental field defect, and that this may some day perhaps be found as a component manifestation of a causal genesis Mendelian or chromosome mutation syndrome; however, the aniridia-Wilms' tumor syndrome is a true MCA/mental retardation (MR) syndrome, and unless a subtle chromosome defect is demonstrated (either cytologically or through deletion mapping), this syndrome will remain as 'idiopathic" as the Hallermann-Streiff syndrome or the Rubinstein-Taybi syndrome, which are all "stuck" on the formal genesis level of syndrome definition.

In this connection caution in interpreting cytogenetic data is indicated. Ataxia telangiectasia is clearly an autosomal recessive trait; therefore, the cytogenetic abnormalities found in these cases cannot be its cause but must be a consequence of the basic genetic trait. A similar argument applies to the Brachmann-deLange syndrome (12), although the evidence for its autosomal recessive inheritance is less (equal sex ratio, possibly excessive parental consanguinity, but only a 1 to 2% segregation ratio). However, in chronic myelogenous leukemia the argument is not quite so firm; rare familial cases suggest genetic "predisposition" or an outright Mendelian trait in some cases. However, the constancy of involvement of 22q, specifically translocations taking material away from 22q, suggests a more direct pathogenetic relationship between the cytogenetic defect and the onset of the disease. This cytogenetic defect, like that of mosaic trisomy 7 leukemia, seems to be postnatally acquired.

THE FOUR GROUPS OF SYNDROMES AND GENETIC DISORDERS

Finally, in the aforementioned "sauropsidian" manner the many congenital and genetic disorders delineated by genetic nosology can be assigned to four major groups for general biological, prognostic, and other purposes (5,7,15,16):

1. Deformities and deformity syndromes, e.g., the Potter syndrome, the arthrogryposes, etc. (In many of these cases the pathogenesis of the deformities is fairly easy to discern. So far as we know, these patients, if they live, do not have an increased risk of cancer.)
2. Malformations and malformation syndromes.
3. Dysplasia and polydysplasia syndromes.
4. Inborn errors of metabolism and metabolic diseases.

A number of conditions share characteristics of more than one group: the symptomatic anomaly syndromes (e.g., congenital Minamata and rubella disease) have manifestations of groups 1 and 2; dysplasia/malformation syndromes [e.g., the nevoid basal cell carcinoma syndrome, Elejalde syndrome (4), etc.] share characteristics of groups 2 and 3; and the metabolic dysplasias (e.g., stilbestrol-induced congenital vaginal adenosis) overlap with groups 3 and 4.

With insights provided by the biological nature of the entities in these groups and the results of phenotypic analysis and causal studies in individual disorders, we would like to offer a few generalizations and illustrative examples.

Malformations are abnormalities of structural development of one or more organs, body regions, or complex anatomical structures. All malformations are developmental field defects or complexes (DFCs), i.e., complex disturbances of development of one or more structures differentiating at about the same time. These structures can be contiguous, in which case the defect is called a monotopic DFC, or noncontiguous, in which case it is termed a polytopic DFC. The alobar holoprosencephaly DFC is a classic example of the former, the acrorenal DFCs of the latter. A simpler, normal developmental and functional polytopic relationship is seen in Petrakis' studies of the relationship between dry and sticky ear wax and nonlactational breast secretion, involving in both cases apocrine glands *(this volume)*. Ipsilateral absence of breast and axillary apocrine glands in the new dominant trait studied by Pallister and coworkers (17) probably should be considered a polytopic DFC, especially if a developmental relationship can be established between these gland defects and the ipsilateral limb defects seen in individuals severely affected with this trait. The studies by Bersu et al. (3) and Herrmann et al. (8) on the Hanhart-Möbius-Poland defects make it likely that at least the limb, oral, and rare anal defects seen in the Hanhart syndrome represent a single, polytopic DFC.

By definition, DFCs are etiologically nonspecific, hence nonpathognomonic, and may occur sporadically, as Mendelian traits, and as components of true MCA syndromes.

Dysplasias are abnormalities of tissue development and include all of the moles, nevi, café-au-lait spots, lentigines, hemangiomata, exostoses, enchondromata, polyps, etc., mentioned throughout this volume, as well as dystopias, dyssynchronies, other hamartomata, teratomata, and probably many neoplasms. Individual dysplasias also are etiologically nonspecific, and like malformations, occur sporadically, as Mendelian (mostly autosomal dominant) traits and as components of MCA and multidysplasia syndromes, such as the Gardner syndrome, the Cowden syndrome, the MEN syndromes, etc.

Some malformations may, in fact, represent the consequences of fetal dysplasia with subsequent maturation of tissue so that the malformed organ is histologically normal. The nevoid basal cell carcinoma syndrome has been cited as a possible example in which the vertebral or rib anomalies, or both, may represent "healed" fetal dysplasia. This line of thinking should perhaps be pursued in all syndromes or cases with cancer *and* apparently true malformations as component manifestations.

We think that all gross chromosome imbalance syndromes are MCA/dysplasia syndromes and that they *all* have an increased risk of neoplasia or outright cancer, either on the basis of the aneuploidy, or the dysplasia, or both. The Down syndrome (DS)-leukemia association is well-documented; a DS-retinoblastoma relationship is emerging, and the occurrences of retinoblastoma or retinoblastoma-like lesions in two 13-trisomy patients and Wilms' tumor in the 18-trisomy syndrome are not surprising in view of their common, gross retinal and renal dysplasia. To date, no inborn error of metabolism has been found in true MCA syndromes of chromosomal or gene mutational origin, and the occurrence of cancer in them should probably be regarded as a direct consequence of maldifferentiation, before or after birth.

Depending on type and basic condition many, but by no means all, dysplasias may be premalignant lesions. It is remarkable that in the polymultidysplasia condition par excellence, tuberous sclerosis, so few outright metastasizing cancers have been described. Different dysplasias in the same individual have different neoplastic or oncoplastic potentials; in the Gardner syndrome there appears to be no danger of cancer in the skin lesions, but a high risk in the intestinal polyps. In osteogenesis imperfecta there is a very small but definite risk of osteogenic sarcoma; whereas, in polyostotic fibrous dysplasia there is a more appreciable risk of osteogenic sarcoma occurring in one of the osseous lesions.

In general, single congenital anomalies (DFCs) and most MCA syndromes are not associated with an increased risk of neoplasia. However, several exceptions are known and challenge the developmental geneticist for explanation:

A. Single congenital anomalies/DFCs

1. the Wilms' tumor-leukemia/aplastic anemia "syndrome"—an autosomal dominant trait (5)

2. the apparently nonspecific renal malformation-Wilms' tumor association

3. the pseudohermaphroditism-Wilms' tumor syndrome

4. the Poland anomaly-leukemia association

5. the autosomal dominant presacral teratoma with sacral, anal, and other local developmental defects, and rare occurrence of teratocarcinoma arising in the teratoma (1)

6. the hypodysplastic gonad/gonadoblastoma association in which endocrine stimulation may promote neoplastic transformation and proliferation of such cells

7. the diGeorge "syndrome" or DFC-lymphoma association.

B. MCA and MCA/dysplasia syndromes

1. chromosome imbalance syndromes mentioned previously

2. the Fanconi MCA/anemia syndrome; the pathogenesis of the leukemia in these patients is presently unknown (it is interesting that the often highly abnormal

kidneys are apparently not associated with an increased risk of Wilms' tumor.)
   3. the aniridia-Wilms' tumor syndrome
   4. the nevoid basal cell carcinoma syndrome
   5. the hemihypertrophy-Wilms' tumor association
   6. the Wiedemann-Beckwith syndrome.

The latter two entities provide important etiologic, nosologic and pathogenetic questions embodied in Miller's diagram of phenotypic-statistical relationships between these and other entities (11), Meadow's case of the mother with hemihypertrophy and child affected with Wilms' tumor *(this volume, p. 60)*, and Dr. Bruce Beckwith's observation *(personal communication)* that children with Wilms' tumor may have a larger-than-normal birthweight. We have a nosologic "hunch" that many cases of the hemihypertrophy-Wilms' tumor syndrome and many Wilms' tumor children, in whom no other congenital anomalies are recorded, in fact have the Wiedemann-Beckwith syndrome, but have not done and know of no pertinent studies addressed to that hypothesis. Etiologically, the Wiedemann-Beckwith syndrome is particularly fascinating, and has been interpreted by Herrmann as an example of premutation (9). Pathogenetically, the following hypothesis has been made about this condition (5). The mutation may interfere with the mitotic process (perhaps to produce polyploidy) and leads, in many tissues, to nucleomegaly (with increased DNA content/cell volume) and cytomegaly. Such cells and tissues may mature and differentiate more slowly than normally and lead to the dyssynchronous dysplasias seen especially in kidneys and skeletal muscle which may show, after birth, respectively, persistence of cortical glomerulogenesis and persistence of myoblasts; they may not be able to divide fast enough for normal growth and differentiation, hence some hypoplasia and even aplasia. Such cells frequently function abnormally and lead to the hyperinsulinism and other functional abnormalities of the Wiedemann-Beckwith syndrome. An apparently increased capacity to transformation may explain the many cancers (pre- and postnatal) that have been seen in affected patients; the abnormal cells in this syndrome also lead to abnormal and incomplete development, i.e., true multiple congenital anomalies associated with a characteristic facies. Finally, extensive nucleocytomegaly leads to histomegaly and organomegaly and its secondary effects, such as exomphalocele, disturbance of facial growth due to macroglossia, etc.

CONCLUSION

In this volume, there are examples of infectious cancers, pre- and postnatally chemically induced cancers, developmental cancers with or without associated malformations, and cancers representing apparent or proven interaction of environment and genetic constitution (such as the autosomal recessive disorders, epidermodysplasia verruciformis and XP, discussed by Lutzner and others). Mulvihill has compiled an inventory of around 160 human Mendelian traits associated with a risk of cancer development (13). In view of this extraordinary etiologic, pathogenetic diversity and complexity of the tumors discussed at this conference, we find it difficult to see how one can maintain the view that the causal/pathogenetic events leading to cancerous transformation are simple, the same or very similar in all cancers, or dependent on only a few genetic changes.

ACKNOWLEDGMENT

This work was supported by DHEW/USPHS Grant 20130-02 from the National Institute of General Medical Sciences: Paper No. 1946 from the University of Wisconsin Genetics Laboratory.

REFERENCES

1. Ashcraft, K. W., Holder, T. M., and Harris, D. J. (1975): Familial presacral teratomas. *Birth Defects,* 11(5):143–146.
2. Barr, A., Grabow, J., Matthews,C. G., Grosse, F. R., Motl, M. L., and Opitz, J. M. (1971): Studies of malformation syndromes XXVB: Neurologic manifestations of the Brachmann-deLange syndrome. *Neuropädiatrie,* 3:46–66.
3. Bersu, E. T., Pettersen, J. C., Charbonneau, W. J., and Opitz, J. M. (1976): Studies of malformation syndromes of man XXXXI A: Anatomical studies in the Hanhart syndrome. *Eur. J. Pediatr.,* 122:1–17)
4. Elejalde, B. R., Gilbert, E. F., Giraldo, C., and Jimenez, R. (1976): Acrocephalopolydactylous dysplasia: A previously undescribed autosomal recessive malformation/dysplasia syndrome *(in preparation).*
5. Gilbert, E. F., Herrmann, J., and Opitz, J. M. (1977): Dysplasia, malformations and neoplasia, especially with respect to the Wiedemann-Beckwith syndrome. In: *Proceedings of the Workshop on Regulation of Cell Proliferation and Differentiation,* edited by W. W. Nichols and R. W. Miller. Plenum, New York *(in press).*
6. Günther, H. (1948): Anomaliekomplex und Zufallssyndromie. *Zentralbl. Allg. Pathol.,* 84:6–16.
7. Hermann, J., and Opitz, J. M. (1974): Naming and nomenclature of syndromes. *Birth Defects,* 10(7):69–86.
8. Herrmann, J., Pallister, P. D., Gilbert, E. F., Viseskul, C., Bersu, E. T., Pettersen, J. C., and Opitz, J. M. (1976): Studies of malformation syndromes of man XXXXI B: Nosologic studies in the Hanhart and the Möbius syndrome *Eur. J. Pediatr.,* 122:19–55.
9. Herrmann, J., and Opitz, J. M. (1977): Delayed mutation as a cause of genetic disease in man: Achondroplasia and the Wiedemann-Beckwith syndrome. In: *Proceedings of the Workshop on Regulation of Cell Proliferation and Differentiation,* edited by W. W. Nichols and R. W. Miller. Plenum, New York *(in press).*
10. Lash, J. W. (1964): Normal embryology and teratogenesis. *Am. J. Obstet. Gynecol.,* 90:1193–1207.
11. Miller, R. W., Fraumeni, J. F., Jr., and Manning, M.D. (1964): Association of Wilms' tumor with aniridia, hemihypertrophy, and other congenital malformations. *N. Engl. J. Med.,* 270:922–927.
12. Motl, M. L., and Opitz, J. M. (1971): Studies of malformation syndromes XXVA: Phenotypic and genetic studies of the Brachmann-deLange syndrome. *Hum. Hered.,* 21:1–16.
13. Mulvihill, J. J. (1975): Congenital and genetic disease. In: *Persons at High Risk of Cancer: An Approach to Cancer Etiology and Control.* edited by J. F. Fraumeni, Jr., pp. 3–35. Academic Press, New York.
14. Murphy, E. A., and Chase, G. A. (1975): *Principles of Genetic Counseling.* Year Book Medical Publishers, Chicago, Ill.
15. Opitz, J. M., and Herrmann, J. (1975): Prolegómenos al estudio de los síndromes humanos. *Bol. Med. Hosp. Infant. Méx.,* 32:881–901.
16. Opitz, J. M., and Herrmann, J. (1976): The study of genetic diseases and congenital malformations in man. *Birth Defects (in press).*
17. Pallister, P. D., Herrmann, J., and Opitz, J. M. (1976): Studies of malformation syndromes in man XXXXII: A pleiotropic dominant mutation affecting skeletal, sexual and apocrine-mammary development. *Birth Defects,* 12(5):247–254.
18. Pfaundler, M. von, and Seht, L. (1921): Über Syntropie von Krankheitszuständen. *Z. Kinderheilkd.,* 30:100–120.
19. Renwick, J. H. (1956): Nail-patella syndrome: evidence for modification by alleles at the main locus. *Ann. Hum. Genet.,* 21:159–169.

20. Witschi, E. (1952): Overripeness of the egg as a cause of twinning and teratogenesis. *Cancer Res.*, 12:763–786.
21. Witschi, E., and Laguens, R. (1963): Chromosomal aberrations in embryos from overripe eggs. *Dev. Biol.*, 7:605–616.

Genetics of Human Cancer, edited by J. J. Mulvihill, R. W. Miller, and J. F. Fraumeni, Jr. Raven Press, New York, 1977.

44

View of a Mammalian Cancer Geneticist

Walter E. Heston

Laboratory of Biology, National Cancer Institute, National Institutes of Health, Bethesda, Maryland 20014

Rapid advances are being made in the area of genetics of cancer. It is good to see the work now being carried from the clinic into the basic laboratory as is well illustrated by the chapters of Dr. Li and Dr. Blattner in this volume. It is in the basic laboratory that the full answers to many of the questions will be found, and exciting new techniques are being introduced. Somatic cell hybridization discussed by Dr. Minna would justify a whole conference. This technique opens up so many opportunities for learning, not only about genes that may be involved in the etiology of cancer in man, but also for the identification of oncogenic viruses.

The geneticist should become an oncologist attacking the problem of human cancer with a genetic perspective rather than a human geneticist conducting some projects on cancer. In so doing he finds himself in a unique position to contribute to the understanding of cancer because he is in the middle of the problem. Genetics is the hub of the biology wheel with reactions either feeding into the gene or radiating out from the gene. Cancer is a problem in biology with genes at the center, and it is where the radiating pathways meet other disciplines that opportunities leading to major discoveries often are found.

The picture is well illustrated by mammary cancer in the mouse that has probably been studied more extensively than any other cancer. Relation of the causative factors are diagrammed in Fig. 1. Mammary cancer can be induced by both physical and chemical carcinogens, and the action of both sets of agents is on the genome of the cell. Thus, it is on this common ground of the geneticist and the carcinogenicist that the opportunities lie for finding what the carcinogens are doing, e.g., altering some enzyme, interrupting some DNA repair mechanism, causing the release of a provirus that has been repressed by a regulator gene, or affecting some other gene action.

At the opposite end of the line of contact between the geneticist and carcinogenicist, there is also an opportunity for the geneticist to make a unique contribution. Our greatest failure in providing good health for the people of this country today is not

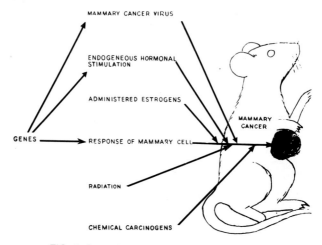

FIG. 1. Causation of mammary cancer in mice.

because of lack of knowledge of disease or how to treat it, and not because of deficiency of hospital care, but because of failing to get members of society to do something for themselves in response to health information available. The excessive cigarette smoking among our high school and even junior high school students well illustrates how miserably we are failing in this area. Human geneticists are especially good at counseling both because of their training and their natural inclination. Here they could make a great contribution, not only in counseling individuals, but also in counseling society. As a mammalian geneticist, I have been called in to help the Environmental Protection Agency in their effort to get some carcinogens taken off the market. During the hearings it has occurred to me that my testimony could have been more effective had I been a human geneticist working on cancer in man.

A second set of factors shown in Fig. 1 which influence the occurrence of mammary tumors are the hormones. For years we have known that the genes are related to the hormones not only in controlling the output of a given hormone but also in controlling mammary cell response to the hormone (4,7). When one attends a conference on hormones today he hears a lot about hormone receptor sites and realizes that in their study of hormone action the endocrinologists are getting close to the gene. Thus, in this area, the geneticist joins with the endocrinologist in taking advantage of opportunities for gaining more information on the action of these factors in the malignant transformation of the cell.

But the opportunities for the human geneticist in cancer that I would like to stress most are in the area where the geneticist meets the virologist. As a biologist it seems to me that, in view of the demonstration of viruses that cause cancer in chickens, mice, cats, and probably subhuman primates, we cannot expect the human animal to have escaped oncogenic viruses. From our work with mice, it would seem that human geneticists have an opportunity to make a significant contribution in the discovery of these viruses in man and in understanding how, in their relation to the genome of the cell, they are affecting the malignant transformation. At this point it is clear that virologists are not going to identify human oncogenic viruses without some input from the genetic perspective.

The chapter on viruses by Dr. Robert C. Gallo has stressed the importance of the cell genome illustrating the need for geneticists in this area of research. I should like to give further emphasis with a brief historical review of the contribution geneticists have made in the discovery and understanding of the nature of some of these oncogenic viruses, particularly the mammary tumor virus of the mouse. After Dr. Peyton Rous had discovered the sarcoma virus in chickens that now bears his name (16), he met opposition to the virus concept of cancer from Dr. James Murphy. Murphy (11) argued that, since the fowl tumor group was composed of many different types, each with a specific agent, one must assume an infinite variety of such agents. For this reason, he proposed that these agents could not be looked upon as extraneous infectious agents as were the viruses, but that they must be of *endogenous origin*. He further compared them in their transformation of cells with the transforming agent of pneumococcus, proposed that they not be considered as viruses, and suggested that they be called "transmissible mutagens." Murphy published these ideas in 1931, probably before Gallo and Croce, who are now talking about endogenous oncogenic viruses, were born. These new concepts could have offered opportunities to cancer virology had Murphy and Rous joined forces. Instead, with this opposition to the classical concept of viruses, the viral approach to cancer went into a decline, and when I entered the cancer field in 1938, Dr. Rous was practically out of the field, working on wound healing.

Who then revived the viral theory of cancer?—largely geneticists under the direction of Dr. C. C. Little at the Jackson Laboratory in Bar Harbor, Maine. After having developed inbred strains of mice, with both high and low incidence of mammary tumors, they proceeded to make reciprocal crosses between these high and low tumor strains and discovered that the causative factor was transmitted through the mother as an extrachromosomal factor (8). A similar observation was published a year later by Korteweg (9) in Amsterdam who had reciprocally crossed a high and a low mammary tumor strain that he had previously obtained from Little. This discovery led through Bittner's (2) demonstration that the agent was transmitted through the milk to the final identification of the agent as the mouse mammary tumor virus (MMTV), an RNA virus seen in its mature form as the B particle—the first virus to be accepted without question in the United States as an oncogenic virus. It should be emphasized that this virus was discovered by geneticists using genetic techniques.

Subsequent research on this virus has been a joint effort between virologists and geneticists with recent significant input from cellular and molecular biologists. Bittner, although naming the virus, never considered the mouse mammary tumor as strictly a viral disease but said there were three sets of factors involved: the virus, the hormonal factors, and the genetic factors (3). By 1945, we (6) had shown that the virus in strain C3H was controlled by genes and recognized that it was much more an integral part of the cell than other viruses such as the smallpox virus. We discussed the possibility of its being endogenous and thought it might represent some form of a gene mutation. Later it was shown that in our strain, C3HfB, mammary tumors could arise in the absence of the milk-transmitted virus and were caused by factors transmitted by the male as well as the female (5). These factors were at first thought to be genes until the Berkeley group (12,15) found B particles which they labeled as nodule-inducing virus (NIV) in contrast with the milk-transmitted MMTV. Subsequently, Mühlbock (10) developed a strain, GR, which had a very high incidence of mammary tumors that were caused by MMTV transmitted by the milk, the egg, and sperm.

Another geneticist who made a signal contribution to research on oncogenic viruses was Dr. P. Bentvelzen of the Netherlands Cancer Institute who had gotten his doctorate in Drosophila genetics, had then spent a year in our laboratory where he became interested in the genetics of mouse mammary tumors, and later spent some time at the Jacob and Monod School where he learned about repressors. In Amsterdam where he was studying crosses between strain GR and low mammary tumor strains, he came up with his hypothesis of the genetic transmission of the mouse mammary tumor virus (1). Using the concept of the provirus as Temin (17) had conceived it in the replication of C type oncogenic viruses, Bentvelzen proposed that the viral information was inherited as a provirus integrated in the genome of the mouse as a structural gene and that the provirus was under the control of a regulator gene acting through a repressor which could be released by a mutation of the regulator gene or some other means and through transcription from RNA which through replication and maturation finally produced the B particle. From the ratios of tumor to nontumor females in the F_2 and backcross generations, Bentvelzen concluded that the virus was transmitted as a single dominant gene. This conclusion later seemed to be confirmed by the observations of van Nie, Hilgers, and Lenselink (14) on the segregation of induced early mammary tumors (EMT) and the closely correlated MMTV antigen. It was not clear, however, whether this segregating gene was the viral information or the regulator gene if indeed there was but a single dominant gene. Nandi and Helmich (13) came up with ratios that would fit a two-gene hypothesis.

Thus, here again were questions about this virus to be answered by genetic techniques. During the past two years, in collaboration with immunologist Dr. Wade Parks of the Laboratory of Tumor Virus Genetics, we have been studying hybrids between strains GR and C57BL with particular emphasis on the second backcross to see if single gene segregation in the first backcross could be confirmed. Final analyses of the data are yet to be made, but it now appears that the segregation is not that of the provirus. Although approximately 50% of the first backcross females had virus present in their milk in early lactations, most of the females that were negative became positive by the fifth or sixth lactations. Thus, it appeared that all the hybrids had the provirus that could be activated by factors, some of which were associated with aging. The segregation observed must, therefore, have been that of regulator genes. Furthermore, results from the second backcross did not confirm a single gene but suggest multiple gene inheritance. Second backcross families from first backcross females negative at early lactation contained positive females, and those from positive first backcross females had an excess of positive females over the 50% expectancy, some with 100% positive. Of the second backcross female progeny of the first backcross males, all families had positive females in percentages varying up to 100% with no evidence of grouping of the families.

This brief review of the work with the mouse emphasizes the opportunities for human geneticists to make a contribution in the area of possible human tumor viruses. Only they can best define the most appropriate families or individuals in which to look for virus. Genetic techniques will be essential in helping to reveal the presence of any virus and once the virus is discovered, genetic perspective will be of assistance in understanding how the virus is genetically transmitted and in determining the nature of its action in bringing about the malignant transformation of the cell.

REFERENCES

1. Bentvelzen, P. (1972): Hereditary infections with mammary tumor viruses in mice. In: *RNA Viruses and Host Genome in Oncogenesis,* edited by P. Emmelot and P. Bentvelzen, pp. 309–337. North-Holland, Amsterdam.
2. Bittner, J. J. (1937): Breast cancer and mother's milk. Relation of nursing to the theory of extra-chromosomal causation of breast cancer in mice—A preliminary report. *J. Hered.,* 28: 363–365.
3. Bittner, J. J. (1942): Observation on the genetic susceptibility for the development of mammary cancer in mice. *Cancer Res.,* 2:540–545.
4. Heston, W. E., and Andervont, H. B. (1944): Importance of genetic influence on the occurrence of mammary tumors in virgin female mice. *J. Natl. Cancer Inst.,* 4:403–407.
5. Heston, W. E., and Deringer, M. K. (1952): Test for a maternal influence in the development of mammary gland tumors in agent-free C3Hb mice. *J. Natl. Cancer Inst.,* 13:167–175.
6. Heston, W. E., Deringer, M. K., and Andervont, H. B. (1945): Gene-milk agent relationship in mammary-tumor development. *J. Natl. Cancer Inst.,* 5:289–307.
7. Huseby, R. A., and Bittner, J. J. (1948): Studies on the inherited hormonal influence. *Acta Unio Int. Contra Concrum,* 6:197–205.
8. Jackson Laboratory Staff (1933): The existence of non-chromosomal influence in the incidence of mammary tumors in mice. *Science,* 78:465–466.
9. Korteweg, R. (1934): Proefondervindelijke onderzoekingen aangaande erfelijkheid van kanker. *Ned. Tijdschr. Geneeskd.* 78:240–245.
10. Mühlbock, O. (1965): A note on a new inbred mouse strain GR/A. *Eur. J. Cancer,* 1:123–124.
11. Murphy, J. B. (1931): Discussion of some properties of the causative agent of a chicken tumor. *Trans. Assoc. Am. Physicians,* 46:182–187.
12. Nandi, S. (1966): Interactions among hormonal, viral, and genetic factors in mouse mammary tumorigenesis. *Can. Cancer Conf.,* 6:69–81.
13. Nandi, S., and Helmich, C. (1974): Transmission of the mammary tumor virus by the GR mouse strain. II. Genetic studies. *J. Natl. Cancer Inst.,* 52:1567–1570.
14. Nie, R. van, Hilgers, J., and Lenselink, M. (1972): Genetical analysis of mammary tumor development and mammary tumor virus expression in the GR mouse strain. In: *Researches Fondamentales sur les Tumeurs Mammaires,* pp. 21–29. Ministere de la Santé Publique, Paris.
15. Pitelka, D. R., Bern, H. A., Nandi, S., and DeOme, K. B. (1964): On the significance of virus-like particles in mammary tissues of C3Hf mice. *J. Natl. Cancer Inst.,* 33:867–885.
16. Rous, P. (1911): A sarcoma of the fowl transmissible by an agent separable from the tumor cells. *J. Exp. Med.,* 13:397–411.
17. Temin, H. M. (1964): Nature of the provirus of Rous sarcoma. *Natl. Cancer Inst. Monogr.,* 17:557–570.

Genetics of Human Cancer, edited by J. J.
Mulvihill, R. W. Miller, and J. F. Fraumeni, Jr.
Raven Press, New York, 1977.

45

Genetics of Human Cancer:
An Epidemiologist's View

Robert W. Miller

Clinical Epidemiology Branch, National Cancer Institute, Bethesda, Maryland 20014

There are no Nobel prizes for epidemiology, but epidemiologists can help point the way. Laboratory scientists who are aware of epidemiologic findings will know better where to place their bets in conducting research. Viruses as a cause of cancer is a case in point.

Epidemiology is a word whose meaning is not widely agreed upon even by epidemiologists. To cover all possibilities, Michael Shimkin has said, "Epidemiology is what an epidemiologist does." I like to think of it as the study of peculiarities in the occurrence of disease as revealed by study of the patient, his family, or the community. Not all of that is epidemiology; some of it is etiology—bedside etiology, if you will. I will come back to this subject later.

It is curious in a way that this volume, which does not include "Epidemiology" in its title and which really does not feature the topic, is nonetheless cosponsored by the Epidemiology Branch of the National Cancer Institute. The reason is to bring together the views of scientists from diverse disciplines, so they can learn what others have to say about an underdeveloped research area, the genetics of human cancer. Through the volume an attempt has been made to give impetus to the coda of our commentaries over the past decade: in determining the causes of human disease, progress is fastest when epidemiology is linked with clinical observations and new laboratory developments.

The book has been panoramic rather than encyclopedic. We should go on from here to have a series of small think-sessions on specific topics that arise from these proceedings. In these think-sessions, one should include some outsiders who have not previously considered the problem at issue.

It is as important to know who gets cancer and why as it is to know what environmental agents induce neoplasia in man. Some of the best leads in this regard come from astute clinical observations. One of the problems in finding such clues to the origins of cancer is that there are not many good, new clue finders. Physicians traditionally think about diagnosis and therapy, rather than about the causes of disease. There is a need to identify young people in medicine, or even before they have decided on a career, who have the capacity to think about cause. They could then be made aware of their talent and advised as to how to make the most of it.

Ultimately each medical school, and perhaps individual departments of medicine or pediatrics, would do well to have a clinical etiologist on its staff. This specialist would not bring in any money, as would a cardiologist or a hematologist, but he would bring in new ideas as he makes ward rounds and sees special circumstances of disease that lend themselves to etiologic exploration through laboratory and epidemiologic research.

Heston has pointed out the need for genetic counseling of society. In a way that is a purpose of this monograph—not genetic counseling of society directly, but genetic counseling of geneticists and clinical oncologists by getting them together to share their information and to know more about what the others are doing.

Genetics of Human Cancer, edited by J. J.
Mulvihill, R. W. Miller, and J. F. Fraumeni, Jr.
Raven Press, New York, 1977.

46

Research Once and Now

Josef Warkany

Cincinnati, Ohio

I am neither a geneticist nor an oncologist and can claim only one outstanding trait, namely, age. Thus, I thought I could describe research methods of my early years and compare them with more recent methods as I see them around me. Before I begin, I would like to state that: Any resemblance to organizations described, living or dead, is purely coincidental.

It may be of interest how we did research some 50 years ago, in a country that just had lost a war and most of its lands; in a country where no money was allotted to young people who were anxious to learn how the statements in their textbooks could be tested and knowledge be expanded. As medical students, we did not have to attend lectures and could work in research institutes that had survived from the golden past. We had to pay for our chemicals and the broken glassware, but the sums were nominal. One could do neurologic research on brain sections and biochemical research with yeast bought at the grocery and red blood cells fetched from the slaughterhouse; micromethods were frowned on and not permitted.

As a resident, I had the good fortune to land in a small babies' hospital that had a sunny laboratory with many shiny bottles. The chief, who was strongly in favor of research, had to approve additional supplies and chemicals. It was the time when vitamin D concentrates became available and spectacular cures of rickets could be achieved. How did these compounds cure rickets? I was able to acquire a rabbit and study the increase of the blood phosphorus level after a single dose of sodium phosphate and could repeat the experiment after the rabbit had been saturated with irradiated ergosterol. There was a marked increase in the rise of these phosphatemic curves, and I was jubilant, thinking I had solved the riddle of vitamin D action. I was ready to publish this work when one of my mentors suggested that I repeat the experiment with another rabbit. So, I approached my chief and said: ''Herr Professor, I need a rabbit.'' Whereupon his amicable attitude changed to indignation, and he said: ''But you already have one.'' And he was right. The following rabbits behaved like the first and the drain on the hospital finances proved unjustified.

In 1932 I came to Cincinnati where I continued my work on vitamin D and phosphorus with rats and rabbits in abundance, but the results seemed to become less important as rickets disappeared. I was left without my favorite disease. I should like to warn you: If you continue your intensive research successfully, the same may happen to you! So I turned to more durable troubles. The Vital Statistics of the United States indicated that congenital malformations had assumed increasing importance in mortality of children, and it seemed that this topic could be an interesting and enduring one. With the help of one capable coworker at a time and with many rats, we made good progress as experimental mammalian teratology proved a worthwhile field of research. After a few years, a foundation expressed an interest in our work and gave us a small grant. About 15 years after we had obtained our first results, three organizations, private and governmental, accepted congenital malformations as spheres of their activity, and I was allowed to work on their granting and planning committees. Let me just state briefly, what a pleasure it was to meet the members of these committees who were from quite different fields, but all interested in promotion of their specialties by recommending funds to sound investigators and by arranging conferences concerned with the subjects to be developed. All the members had done research themselves with a minimum of expense, and the approved grants were usually modest. Politics of any kind was absent, and the peer system worked beautifully. Apparently it was generally appreciated since the funds available were increased with great regularity. Personally, I thought that this system of biomedical research support was one of the great achievements in the United States and recommended to foreign visitors that they study this great achievement of American democracy.

But this paradise did not last. Slowly one hurdle after another was placed in the investigator's path. More reports had to be written, accounting was made complicated, and special project interests made their voices heard. Building and "gadgeteering" replaced ideas. More and more money was requested. Administration had to be expanded, and many other factors and influences reduced the original excellence of the granting systems. It was found out in 1968 that there was not enough money available to continue the systems in their original form. As you know, the paradise is no more.

A few years ago a new faculty member came to Cincinnati. After discussing some of his plans with him, I asked: "Do you do some research?" He answered: "Yes, I am working on a grant application." I thought this was a great joke and told the story many times to entertain my friends.

But alas, now, this is no joke. The research activities of thousands of investigators consist in writing grant applications. How does one go about this now? Let us assume an investigator has a desire to study a biomedical problem and needs some animals, supplies, and equipment. He is located in a hospital or institute with space allotted to research and he goes to his chief or administrator—as I did some 45 years ago—to find out how he could realize his plans. He, too, is encouraged by his chief, but he is told to try for a grant since there are no provisions in the institute's budget for the items needed.

The investigator decides immediately to apply to one of the great sources of funds known for generous support of biomedical research. He writes for a grant application form but is told that since a certain date, investigators have to turn to the Central Application Control Office of the Grantee Institute—if the latter has such an office; or, he is told to describe his future 3- or 5-year program in 300 words, to show that he is worthy of receiving an application form.

And after some time the investigator receives a nice brown package which contains not only the application form but also a generous supply of reading material. There is general information with instructions concerning language and schedule of review. There are three deadlines for submittal, dates of council meetings, and the earliest possible beginning dates which are about 8 months away from the submittal date. This delay is regrettable but understandable because of the careful review policies of the organization. Most of the information proffered is useful, although the inexperienced applicant may be unable to furnish honest answers to some of the questions asked. How can he determine ahead of time the total research period needed and the total amount of direct costs? There is a problem in naming the professional personnel 8 months ahead of the beginning date of the grant, and he sees that there will be difficulties in procuring personnel at the moment of funding.

Concerning description of the research plan the situation is ambiguous. It is certainly justified to ask the applicant to give examples of his approach to a broad research objective. But in sections on methods and procedures, descriptions are requested of the types of experiments, methods, species, numbers of animals per group, techniques to be used, intervals of sampling, means of data evaluation, etc. How can an honest and original investigator put down in writing one or two years ahead of time how many groups of rats or mice and how many individual animals will get which dose of a compound or radiation by this or that method of administration? Should not the investigator have the right to change his mind according to his observations and his reading during the waiting and experimental periods? A severe critic of the 1974 research grant system, the Nobel Prize winner Albert Szent-Györgyi, objected to this request: "If one knows what one will do and find in it, then it is not research any more and is not worth doing. The [Agency] wants detailed projects, wants the applicants to tell exactly what they will do and find during the tenure of their grants, which excludes unexpected discoveries on which progress depends" (2).

In spite of this dilemma our applicant does his best and describes his future experiments with a minimum of deception and bluff, in great detail, hoping that his approach will find favor in the eyes of the reviewers, and that he will, in a year's time, receive funds which will satisfy his burning desire to solve the problem that has aroused his curiosity. His hopes may be dampened when he finds out that his chances of getting support are only one in 20. But he is still of good hope since he is convinced that his project is so superior it cannot be turned down.

So he waits and dreams about his future research, the satisfaction of harvesting the results, and the benefits mankind will derive from them.

After 8 months of waiting, there is a letter from the Director of Granting Services. One out of 20 applicants hears that his grant has been approved, but our friend is not the favored one. He is also not one of the 14 who hear that they were disapproved. He is one of the five lucky ones who are told that the Reviewing Council recommended approval *in time and amount,* but there will be a delay before it can be determined whether or not an award will be made. ''As soon as we are able to develop a definite position, which may take up to 11 months, we will let you know, etc...''

During the following months the applicant's dreams lose some of their rosy tint, but they still deal with the subject of his choice and he can give himself to transcendental meditation. But 20 months after dispatch of his application, a letter arrives which says: ''After review of our current budgetary situation we regret to inform you that we do not have sufficient funds to support your approved research grant application. Please be assured that our not making an award for this application in no way implies prejudice against the submission of other applications.''

It has been said that enthusiasm is the spring of all research, and you can imagine the thrill of our applicant who has learned that his thoughts and methods of approach have been approved—though not funded—and that he is allowed to reenter the cycle and to resubmit. He became also entitled to a pink sheet which specifies the good and bad points of his plans. He is ready for resubmission of the application, mending his ways according to the pink sheet with minor corrections of the title of the grant. Whereas, this was, for instance, ''Etiology of Anencephaly'' before, the new title will be: ''The Role of Anencephaly in Cancer, Heart Disease, and Stroke,'' thus directing his proposal into fields of greater fertility. And now, having done all in his power, he could sit back and look forward to the next 8 months of undiminished enthusiastic waiting. But our applicant is a resourceful and adaptable man. He takes a course in grantsmanship, he studies volumes on grants in general, pores over Guides for the Preparation and Submission of Proposals for Foundation Support, reads a book entitled *Everything You Always Wanted to Know about Grant Applications,* and is cheered by a pamphlet on ''Wooing and Winning Foundation Support''...and many other edifying works of biomedical literature. More important, he has learned to use a clever machine from Savin Business Machines called ''Word Master Unit.'' It tapes his thoughts and plans, making possible multiplication of applications to all foundations that could in any way be related to his project. This ingenious machine permits inserts, deletions, and modifications of his scheme according to the various interests of the foundations. These exercises keep his mind alert and wide awake, preparing it for new ventures of research.

During these fruitful months and years, now being on the roster of American grant applicants, he receives innumerable yellow pages with Requests for Proposals and surely, one of these should be related to his research interests. *There* may be a way to be funded. The RFPs are very democratic procedures but they should be printed on orange paper since they resemble the carrots on sticks held in front of donkeys to make them march. Of course, the donkey never gets the carrot. To an imaginative investigator, contract work is rather dull—unless *he* has designed the plan—but, our applicant hopes that on the way he may make an interesting chance discovery. However, if this should happen, the contractor is in serious trouble and in danger of losing his contract. If his serendipitous findings, i.e., surprising and exciting results, should incite him to research along these unforeseen lines, he has to find new ways of support since a letter may inform him that: "It would appear impracticable and indeed contrary to existing Contract Procedures and Regulations to issue a new contract to a new work scope without the preparation of a contract proposal by the contractor and/or his principal investigator."

Time does not permit to describe the investigator's experience with other organizations, but I can say that some of them also use the carrot system to lure the donkeys.

I ask: What has happened to the splendid granting program of the 1950s? I am too far away from the centers to analyze the decline of these once great American institutions. The answer is not as simple as Dr. Szent-Györgyi thought. He noted that he could not secure a grant since President Nixon took office. It was not a single man who changed the course of the system. Also, I cannot quite agree with Dr. Harold L. Stewart who blamed the abundance of administrators (1). In my experience, most of the administrators are trying to be helpful, but their hands are tied. There were many persons (some well-meaning), governmental and private groups, university officials, lobbyists, and politicians, and—let us be honest—many scientists who contributed to the general decay. Maybe we should never have yielded to the lure of gold. It would take a Thomas Mann or a Cervantes to describe the decline that—in the parlance of modern genetics—has "multifactorial" causation; which means it is the fault of nobody and everybody. That makes counseling and repair most difficult.

I cannot suggest a simple solution to a gigantic problem and cannot imagine that the advice of a small, one-rabbit operator would have any effect. In 1959, Harold L. Stewart, of the National Cancer Institute, gave the Presidential Address at the annual meeting of the American Association for Cancer Research (1). In 13 pages he described the tribulations of the cancer investigator. He, like Szent-Györgyi, pointed out that good research depends on good ideas, enthusiasm, leisure, and freedom from pressures and harassment. And he ended his great address with a utopian, humorous, and frivolous description of an ideal research laboratory. Considering the deterioration of the investigator's lot since his analysis and recommendations of 1959, I shall not follow in his footsteps. Active investigators cannot and should not spend their time repairing the machine which is out of order. We are not trained for this. It has been suggested that the scientific community declare an *application strike*. Have you ever thought of what would happen in such a situation? The vacuums created in some of the buildings dedicated to grant applications could cause implosions with devastating results. I do not want to see that happen and do not recommend extremism.

When I wrote the above description of the present-day hardships of the biomedical investigator, I did not know too many geneticists or oncologists and did not realize that they are a group of people who can do exciting research without the hecatombs of animals and the expensive gadgets which are now considered a necessity of medical research. It seems that they can work with patients, with hospital charts, with pencil and paper, with the contents of good libraries, and with imaginative minds. The sad description I gave of the plight of the average grant-seeking investigator should support that type of research—which in the main consists of *thinking*. I am sure good medical research will go on in spite of the vicissitudes of present-day grantsmanship.

REFERENCES

1. Stewart, H. L. (1959): The cancer investigator. *Cancer Res.*, 19:804–818.
2. Szent-Györgyi, A. (1974): Research grants. *Perspect. Biol. Med.*, 18:41–43.

Genetics of Human Cancer, edited by J. J.
Mulvihill, R. W. Miller, and J. F. Fraumeni, Jr.
Raven Press, New York, 1977.

Appendix

[Ed.: As mentioned by William A. Blattner *(this volume),* the following questionnaire is used by the Epidemiology Branch to elicit medical history from patients of special etiologic interest, because of either their personal medical history or the family occurrence of malignancy. Branch professionals use it as a guide to interviewing, and family members complete it with unclear areas resolved by telephone or letter. Additional questions are added for specific cell types and for detailed gynecologic history. Under continual revision, the present form was developed by Frederick P. Li, Joseph F. Fraumeni, Jr., John J. Mulvihill, Wladimir Wertelecki, Richard B. Everson, Thomas W. Pendergrass, William A. Blattner, and Mark H. Greene.]

Medical History Questionnaire for Cancer Etiology

Date form completed: _____

If you are completing this form for someone else, please answer the questions as if you were that person. Please give your name, address, phone number, and relationship to that person.

Name of the person being studied: _____
Last   First   Middle   Maiden, if any

Street address: _____
City, County, State (Zip): _____
Phone (Area Code); Home: _____ Work: _____
Birthplace (City, County, State): _____
Hospital of birth: _____
Ethnic origins: _____
Birthdate: _____ Present age: _____ Sex: _____ Race: _____
Are you a twin? _____ Identical? _____
Spouse's name (maiden, if any): _____
Physician(s) available for correspondence (use back if necessary):
Name: _____ _____ _____
Street address: _____ _____ _____
City, County: _____ _____ _____
State (Zip): _____ _____ _____
Phone (Area code): _____ _____ _____

1. Authorization to Obtain Medical Information:
   Patient's name: _____ Date: _____
   I hereby give permission to the physicians of the Epidemiology Branch of the National Cancer Institute, Bethesda, Maryland, or their appointed representatives, to review the medical records of myself and my family.

Signature: _____

2. Environmental History:
   A. Have you had any unusual exposures to any poisons, chemicals, or toxic materials? If yes, please give details (use back if necessary). _____
   _____
   _____

489

B. Please list all occupations you have had (use back if necessary).

Type of work or job title, company name	Approximate length of employment

C. Please circle the highest level of education you received.

Grammar and High School   College or Other

1 2 3 4 5 6 7 8 9 10 11 12   13 14 15 16   or greater

3. Personal Medical History:

A. Did you ever have any of the following diseases?   YES   NO   AGE

1) Liver disease (yellow jaundice, hepatitis, other)
2) Lymph node disease (mononucleosis, glandular fever, other)
3) Infections (pneumonia, recurrent skin infections, ear infections, other)
4) Herpes (cold sores, mouth ulcers)
5) Epilepsy or seizures
6) Thyroid disease
7) Diseases of the breast
8) Diseases of the reproductive organs (testis, ovary, uterus, cervix)
9) Allergies (hay fever, drug reactions)
10) Anemia
11) Excessive bleeding, easy bruising, or other blood diseases
12) Disorders of the digestive tract
13) Heart disease
14) Lung disease
15) Disease of the kidneys or bladder
16) Disease of the bones, muscles, or joints
17) Diseases of the skin (eczema, psoriasis, sores, other)
18) Venereal disease
19) Broken bones or other injuries
20) Diseases of the eye (wear glasses, cataracts, other)
21) Tumors or cancer
22) Other, specify _____

Please refer to each "yes" answer above and enter details concerning the nature of the illness, treatment, and physician who you saw. Please list any hospitalizations, include name and address of the hospital and indicate the reason you were hospitalized (use back of sheet if necessary). _____

B. Congenital malformations.

Were you born with any disorders of the following systems?   YES   NO

1) Brain and nervous system (including mental retardation)
2) Heart
3) Kidneys or bladder
4) Bones, muscles, or joints

5) Skin (including birthmarks and moles) _____ _____
6) Others, specify _____ _____ _____
If yes, please describe. Use back if necessary. _____

_____

C. Are there any hereditary conditions or illnesses which run in your family? _____
If yes, please describe. _____

_____

4. Food and Drugs:
    A. Have you ever been placed on special diets, had food restrictions, or craved unusual
foods? Yes _____ No _____
    If yes, please describe. _____

_____

B. Do (Did) you smoke? _____ If yes, what, how much, and how long? _____

C. Do (Did) you drink alcoholic beverages? _____ If yes, please give an estimate of how
much per day (week) you consume(d) and for how long. _____

D. Have you ever taken any of the following? YES NO DATES PHYSICIAN

    1) Thyroid medication ____ ___ _____ _____
    2) Growth hormones ____ ___ _____ _____
    3) Drugs to cause pregnancy ____ ___ _____ _____
    4) Birth control pills ____ ___ _____ _____
    5) Estrogens for menopause ____ ___ _____ _____
    6) Other male or female hormones ____ ___ _____ _____
    7) Cortisone or steroids ____ ___ _____ _____
    8) Dilantin ____ ___ _____ _____
    9) Stimulants or appetite depressants ____ ___ _____ _____
        (diet pills)
    10) Chloromycetin (chloramphenicol) ____ ___ _____ _____
    11) Sulfa drugs ____ ___ _____ _____
    12) Butazolidin (drugs ____ ___ _____ _____
        for arthritis)
    13) Reserpine or other drugs for high ____ ___ _____ _____
        blood pressure
    E. Did your mother take any medications while you were a baby or before your birth? If yes,
please describe. _____

5. Other Considerations:
    Please express any thoughts or observations you might have on the cause of the illness under
study. Add any information you feel is important but not requested (use back if necessary).

_____

_____

_____

6. Family History:
    Please fill in as completely as possible. Include full names (maiden and married for females),
birthdates, dates of death, and places of death (if applicable). Also indicate any miscarriages, if
known. Use the back, if necessary, for additional persons.

	Name, Address, Phone	Date and place of birth	Date and place of death	Illnesses
A. Father's family Your father	_____	_____	_____	_____
	_____	_____	_____	_____
Your father's father	_____	_____	_____	_____
	_____	_____	_____	_____
Your father's mother	_____	_____	_____	_____
	_____	_____	_____	_____
Your father's (1) brothers and sisters (in order of birth)	_____	_____	_____	_____
	_____	_____	_____	_____
(2)	_____	_____	_____	_____
	_____	_____	_____	_____
(3)	_____	_____	_____	_____
	_____	_____	_____	_____
(4)	_____	_____	_____	_____
	_____	_____	_____	_____
B. Mother's family Your mother	_____	_____	_____	_____
	_____	_____	_____	_____
Your mother's father	_____	_____	_____	_____
	_____	_____	_____	_____
Your mother's mother	_____	_____	_____	_____
	_____	_____	_____	_____
Your mother's (1) brothers and sisters (in order of birth)	_____	_____	_____	_____
	_____	_____	_____	_____
(2)	_____	_____	_____	_____
	_____	_____	_____	_____
(3)	_____	_____	_____	_____
	_____	_____	_____	_____
(4)	_____	_____	_____	_____
	_____	_____	_____	_____
C. Your brothers and sisters (in order of birth, oldest to youngest) (1)	_____	_____	_____	_____
	_____	_____	_____	_____
(2)	_____	_____	_____	_____
	_____	_____	_____	_____

(3) _____ _____ _____ _____
      _____ _____ _____ _____

(4) _____ _____ _____ _____
      _____ _____ _____ _____

D. Your children (in order of birth, oldest to youngest)

(1) _____ _____ _____ _____
      _____ _____ _____ _____

(2) _____ _____ _____ _____
      _____ _____ _____ _____

(3) _____ _____ _____ _____
      _____ _____ _____ _____

(4) _____ _____ _____ _____
      _____ _____ _____ _____

E. Any other family members with cancer. Please indicate how they are related to you.

(1) _____ _____ _____ _____
      _____ _____ _____ _____

(2) _____ _____ _____ _____
      _____ _____ _____ _____

(3) _____ _____ _____ _____
      _____ _____ _____ _____

(4) _____ _____ _____ _____
      _____ _____ _____ _____

F. Your spouse (husband or wife) and his or her immediate family

Your spouse _____ _____ _____ _____
              _____ _____ _____ _____

Your spouse's
father   _____ _____ _____ _____
              _____ _____ _____ _____

Your spouse's
mother   _____ _____ _____ _____
              _____ _____ _____ _____

Your spouse's (1) _____ _____ _____ _____
brothers and   _____ _____ _____ _____
sisters (in order of birth)

(2) _____ _____ _____ _____
      _____ _____ _____ _____

(3) _____ _____ _____ _____
      _____ _____ _____ _____

(4) _____ _____ _____ _____
      _____ _____ _____ _____

Subject Index

ABO blood group
  and nail patella syndrome, 321
  and stomach cancer, 20
Achondroplasia, 384, 417
Acoustic neuroma, *see* Neuroma, acoustic
Acrokeratosis verruciformis, 141
ACTH production
  by carcinoid tumors, 189
  by islet cell tumors, 189
  by pheochromocytoma, 187
Actinic keratosis, solar, DNA repair in, 360
Adenocarcinomatosis, familial, 225–226
Adenoma, *see also sites of adenomas*
  sebaceous, in Torre's syndrome, 166
  sebaceum, in tuberous sclerosis, 138, 156–157
Adenosine deaminase levels, in chronic lymphocytic leukemia, 284–285
Adenosis, vaginal
  and adenocarcinoma development, 58, 67
  stilbestrol-induced, 470
Adenovirus
  chromosome damage from, 89, 90
  in fibroblasts from Fanconi's syndrome, 109
Adiposis dolorosa, 177
Adrenal glands
  adenoma of
    in aldosteronism, 138
    in Wermer's syndrome, 138, 188
  cortical neoplasia
    in Beckwith's syndrome, 60, 142
    and congenital hemihypertrophy, 59–60
    and familial cancer, 226, 227, 237
    in Gardner's syndrome, 139
    in Wermer's syndrome, 243
  neuroblastoma origin in medulla, 50
Africa
  Burkitt's lymphoma in, 448, 455
  colonic cancer in, 369
  Ewing's tumor in, 2
  xeroderma pigmentosum in, 214
Agammaglobulinemia
  Bruton type, *see* Bruton's agammaglobulinemia
  Swiss-type, neoplasia with, 152
  X-linked, malignancies with, 339, 340

Age
  and breast cancer incidence, 287
  and cancer association with HLA antigen, 328
  and carcinogenesis, 391–394
  and colorectal cancer onset, 369
  at menarche, factors affecting, 293
Aging
  premature, genodermatoses in, 157–158
  and senescence in hybrid cells, 344
Aglossia-adactylia syndrome, 468
Agranulocytosis, Kostmann's infantile genetic, 141
Ah locus, as marker for cancer, 301–318
Albinism
  and cancer from sunlight, 141, 147–148, 183
Aldosteronism, 138
Alkylnitrosoureas, carcinogenicity of, 66–67
Altitude, and carotid body tumor incidence, 418
Ameloblastoma, in nevoid basal cell carcinoma syndrome, 153
Amenorrhea-galactorrhea syndrome, 138
Amish, malignancies in, 16
Androgens
  affecting female fetus, 31
  levels in breast cancer, 292
Anemia, Fanconi's, *see* Fanconi's anemia
Angiofibroma, in tuberous sclerosis, 156
Angiokeratoma diffusa, 142
Angiolipomas, multiple cutaneous, 172
Angioma
  in blue rubber bleb nevus syndrome, 173
  in Cowden's syndrome, 161, 170
  in Rendu-Osler-Weber disease, 140
  retinal, in Hippel-Lindau syndrome, 138
Angiomatosis
  cutaneous, and macrocephaly, 183
  encephalofacial, *see* Sturge-Weber syndrome
  oculocerebellar, *see* Hippel-Lindau syndrome
Angiomyoma, in Cowden's syndrome, 170
Angiosarcoma, hepatic, from vinyl chloride, 131